Foot and Ankle: Core Knowledge in Orthopaedics

Commissioning Editor: Kim Murphy
Project Development Manager: Pamela Wetherington
Editorial Assistant: Matthew Ray
Project Manager: Rory MacDonald
Design Manager: Steve Stave
Marketing Manager(s) (UK/USA): Richard Jones/Dana Butler

FOOT AND ANKLE: CORE KNOWLEDGE IN ORTHOPAEDICS

Christopher W. DiGiovanni, M.D.

Associate Professor and Chief, Foot and Ankle Service,
Department of Orthopaedic Surgery, Brown Medical School,
Rhode Island Hospital,
Providence, RI

Justin Greisberg, M.D.

Assistant Professor of Orthopaedic Surgery,
Columbia University College of Physicians and Surgeons,
New York, NY

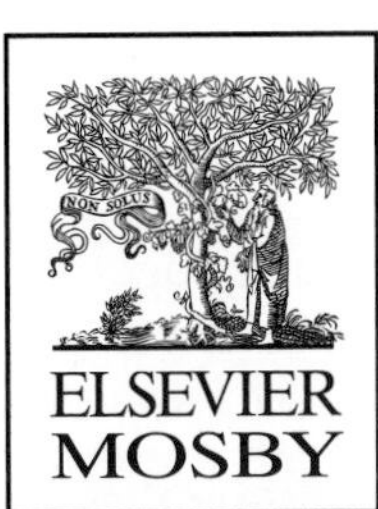

ELSEVIER
MOSBY

ELSEVIER
MOSBY

An affiliate of Elsevier Inc.

First published 2007

ISBN 978-0-323-03735-8

British Library Cataloguing in Publication Data
A catalogue record for this book is available from the British Library

Library of Congress Cataloging in Publication Data
A catalog record for this book is available from the Library of Congress

Notice

Medical knowledge is constantly changing. Standard safety precautions must be followed, but as new research and clinical experience broaden our knowledge, changes in treatment and drug therapy may become necessary or appropriate. Readers are advised to check the most current product information provided by the manufacturer of each drug to be administered to verify the recommended dose, the method and duration of administration, and contraindications. It is the responsibility of the practitioner, relying on experience and knowledge of the patient, to determine dosages and the best treatment for each individual patient. Neither the Publisher nor the author assume any liability for any injury and/or damage to persons or property arising from this publication.

The Publisher

Printed in China

Last digit is the print number: 9 8 7 6 5 4 3 2 1

Contributors

Michael S. Aronow, M.D.
Associate Professor of Orthopaedic Surgery, University of Connecticut School of Medicine, Farmington, CT

Richard J. de Asla, M.D.
Instructor, Orthopaedic Surgery, Harvard Medical School, Massachusetts General Hospital, Boston, MA

Mathieu Assal, M.D.
Médecin Adjoint du Chef de Service, Service de Chirurgie Orthopédique et Traumatologie de l'Appareil Moteur, University Hospital of Geneva, Switzerland

Rahul Banerjee, M.D.
Clinical Instructor, Department of Orthopaedic Surgery, Texas Tech University Health Sciences Center, Interm Chief of Orthopaedic Trauma, William Beaumont Army Medical Center, El Paso, Texas, and Chief of Orthopaedics, 49th Medical Group, Holloman Air Force Base, New Mexico

Stephen K. Benirschke, M.D.
Professor, Department of Orthopaedics and Sports Medicine, University of Washington, Seattle, WA

Eric M. Berkson, M.D.
Orthopaedic Sports Medicine Fellow, Massachusetts General Hospital, Boston, MA

Eric M. Bluman, M.D., Ph.D.
Chief, Orthopaedic Foot and Ankle Surgery, and Chief, Orthopaedic Traumatology, Department of Orthopaedic Surgery, Madigan Army Medical Center, Ft. Lewis, WA

Michael Brage, M.D.
Associate Clinical Professor, Department of Orthopaedics, University of California, Irvine, CA

Lloyd C. Briggs, Jr., M.D., M.S.
Orthopaedic Institute of Ohio, Lima, OH

Margaret Chilvers, M.D.
Michigan International Foot and Ankle Center, Pontiac, MI

Jason Cochran, D.O.
Department of Orthopaedic Surgery, Michigan State University College of Osteopathic Medicine, Ingham Regional Medical Center, Lansing MI

Peter A. Cole, M.D.
Professor and Chief of Orthopedic Traumatology, University of Minnesota Physicians, Regions Hospital, St. Paul, MN

Aaron Colman, M.D.
Sports Medicine Atlantic Orthopaedics, Portsmouth, NH

Gregory J. Della Rocca, M.D., Ph.D.
Acting Instructor, Department of Orthopaedic Surgery, Harborview Medical Center, Seattle, WA

Christopher W. DiGiovanni, M.D.
Associate Professor and Chief, Foot and Ankle Service, Department of Orthopaedic Surgery, Brown Medical School, Rhode Island Hospital, Providence, RI

Craig P. Eberson, M.D.
Assistant Professor, Department of Orthopaedics, Division of Pediatric Orthopaedics and Scoliosis, Brown Medical School, Providence, RI

Eric Gordon, M.D.
Department of Orthopaedic Surgery, New York Orthopaedic Hospital, Columbia-Presbyterian Medical Center, New York, NY

Justin Greisberg, M.D.
Assistant Professor of Orthopaedic Surgery, Columbia University College of Physicians and Surgeons, New York, NY

Jason Heisler, D.O.
Department of Orthopaedic Surgery, Michigan State University College of Osteopathic Medicine, Ingham Regional Medical Center, Lansing MI

Heather E. Hensl, R.P.A.-C.
Physician Assistant, Department of Orthopaedic Surgery, Saint Vincent's Hospital, New York, NY

Anthony Hinz, M.D.
Orthopedic and Neurosurgical Care and Research Center, Bend, OR

Stefan Gerhard Hofstaetter, M.D.
Foot and Ankle Center, Vienna, Austria

Dov Kolker, M.D.
Department of Orthopaedic Surgery, Mount Sinai School of Medicine, New York, NY

Patricia Ann Kramer, Ph.D.
Research Assistant Professor, Department of Anthropology, University of Washington, Seattle, WA

Phillip R. Langer, M.D., M.S.
Department of Orthopedic Surgery, Brown Medical School/Rhode Island Hospital, Providence, RI

Mark Chong Lee, M.D.
Department of Orthopaedics, Brown Medical School, Providence, RI

Kevin J. Logel, M.D.
Department of Orthopaedic Surgery, Union Memorial Hospital, Baltimore, MD

Margaret Lobo, M.D.
Department of Orthopaedic Surgery, Columbia University College of Physicians and Surgeons, New York, NY

Arthur Manoli II, M.D.
Director, Michigan International Foot and Ankle Center, Pontiac, MI

Florian Nickisch, M.D.
OL Miller Foot & Ankle Institute at OrthoCarolina, Charlotte, NC

Martin O'Malley, M.D.
Attending Surgeon, Foot and Ankle Service, The Hospital for Special Surgery, New York, NY

Gregory C. Pomeroy, M.D.
Clinical Associate Professor, University of New England; Director, Portland Orthopaedic Foot and Ankle Center, South Portland, ME

Douglas H. Richie Jr., D.P.M.
Adjunct Associate Professor of Clinical Biomechanics, California School of Podiatric Medicine, Oakland, CA

Matthew M. Roberts, M.D.
Assistant Professor of Orthopaedic Surgery, Hospital for Special Surgery; Instructor in Orthopaedic Surgery, Weill Medical College of Cornell University Hospital, New York, NY

Catherine M. Robertson, M.D.
Department of Orthopaedics, University of California, San Diego, CA

Andrew K. Sands, M.D.
Chief, Foot and Ankle Surgery, and Director, Foot and Ankle Institute, Department of Orthopaedic Surgery, Saint Vincent's Medical Center, New York, NY

Bruce J. Sangeorzan, M.D.
Professor, Department of Orthopaedic Surgery, Harborview Medical Center, Seattle, WA

Jonathan Schiller, M.D.
Department of Orthopaedics, Brown Medical School/Rhode Island Hospital, Providence, RI

Lew C. Schon, M.D.
Director of Foot and Ankle Services, Union Memorial Hospital, Baltimore, MD

Niket Shrivastava, M.D.
Department of Orthopaedic Surgery, Columbia University College of Physicians and Surgeons, New York, NY

Annette M. Smith, M.D., M.S.
Department of Orthopaedic Surgery, Kingsbrook Jewish Medical Center, Brooklyn, NY

Raymond J. Sullivan, M.D.
Assistant Clinical Professor of Orthopaedic Surgery, University of Connecticut School of Medicine, Hartford, CT

Michael P. Swords, D.O.
Assistant Clinical Professor, Michigan State University College of Osteopathic Medicine;
Department of Orthopaedic Surgery, Sparrow Health System, Ingham Regional Medical Center, Lansing, MI; and Mid Michigan Orthopaedic Institute, East Lansing, MI

Ivan S. Tarkin, M.D.
Assistant Professor, Division of Orthopaedic Traumatology, University of Pittsburgh Medical Center, Pittsburgh, PA

Richard M. Terek, M.D., FACS
Associate Professor, Department of Orthopedic Surgery, Brown University, Providence, RI

George H. Theodore, M.D.
Co-director, Foot and Ankle Service, Massachusetts General Hospital; Clinical Instructor, Harvard Medical School, Boston, MA

Hans-Jörg Trnka, M.D., Ph.D.
Foot and Ankle Center, Vienna, Austria

Steven Weinfeld, M.D.
Chief, Foot and Ankle Service, and Assistant Professor of Orthopaedic Surgery, Mount Sinai Medical Center, New York, NY

Preface

Thanks to the dedication of a few pioneering surgeons over the past 50 years, foot and ankle has risen from what was once a forgotten orthopaedic subspecialty to what is today a field at the forefront of modern medicine. Such unprecedented attention has stimulated a remarkable influx of quality research, top notch fellowship trained physicians, and cutting edge innovation. This evolution has enlightened both the public and the medical community at large as to the importance of foot function. We now recognize that many of our more veteran advancements in lower extremity function, such as hip or knee replacement, depend significantly on—and are inseparable from—a well functioning foot and ankle complex. The days of ignoring this part of the anatomy as 'just a foot problem' are gone, and one need only look at the outcomes of polytrauma patients to acknowledge this. After all is said and done, these patients most often complain of their feet. Care of the foot has, partly by necessity, come a long way.

The maturation of foot and ankle into a full-fledged subspecialty of orthopaedic surgery was inevitable. This process, however, has been accelerated by certain individuals who, ahead of their time, displayed a greater appreciation of the unique attributes possessed by the foot. As any comparative anatomist will attest, the foot is what distinguishes us most as human beings. It represents the most evolved structure of our human anatomy, and carries a tremendous responsibility relative to its size. These visionary surgeons were the first to incorporate these principles into clinical practice, laying the foundation for what is now the field of orthopaedic foot and ankle surgery. Nowadays, surgeons who have been inspired by the path of these leaders are fortunately commonplace, resulting in an exponential understanding of foot pathology which has revolutionized the treatment of foot problems. For example, our latest ankle arthroplasty designs are now generating cautious optimism of lasting success, improved surgical techniques have recently demonstrated more favorable and lower risk outcomes in calcaneal fracture management, and arthroscopy of the foot and ankle has now become an effective and routine tool in clinical practice.

Much of the medical research that has brought about these changes was based on retrospective case series and surgeon opinion, now referred to as level IV and V evidence. Although this has been instrumental in helping clinical science flourish, it is no longer sufficient to meet the demands of modern day medicine. Emphasis is now, appropriately, being placed on using evidence-based medicine to drive decisions. Level I and II research (prospective, randomized trials) is emerging as the standard by which to judge all other existing information, because it is less subject to bias.

With these thoughts in mind, we are pleased to compile for you this volume of *Current Knowledge in Orthopaedic Surgery*. Our goal has been to arrange an unbiased, balanced, evidence-based text broaching the most salient topics affecting foot and ankle. With the help of some of the most talented foot and ankle surgeons across the United States, we have been given an opportunity to further the visions of our founding fathers in the field of foot and ankle—for your use. We owe a great debt of gratitude to the many individuals who have devoted substantial time and effort towards this end, without whom this product could never have been completed. We hope you gain as much satisfaction in reading it as we have in putting it together.

Neither of us made this journey alone. We have each been blessed with wonderful colleagues, patients, and hospital staff, all of whom have helped create perspective for editing this text. Most importantly, though, we want to recognize our families, whose endless love and support continue to provide the inspiration, time, and motivation necessary to complete tasks like this one. This text is hence dedicated to our parents for getting us started, to our wives for keeping us going, and to our children for making it all worthwhile.

Acknowledgments

There are a number of devoted orthopaedic surgeons who have been responsible for furthering the field of foot and ankle surgery in recent years. While we would have liked to have spent time with all of these special individuals in our careers, we were at least fortunate to have had the honor of working with a few of these great physicians, who we wish to respectfully mention below.

Michael Ehrlich, MD, continues to drive from his home in Boston to his workplace in Providence every working day as chairman of the Brown University Department of Orthopaedic Surgery, and was the only one never late for our daily 6 AM breakfast meetings. In these didactic conferences, he monitored the program's pulse and educated us in ways that went well beyond being a good technician, test-taker, or thinker. He taught us how to be caring physicians. He convinced us to never settle for 'good enough', and inspired us to be curious and self-critical. Dr. Ehrlich's tireless energy and selflessness remain legendary, and have engendered our academic drive. To this day, his greatest satisfactions have always seemed to be the accomplishments of his students, which he always put before his own remarkable achievements.

Peter Trafton, MD, who just retired from Brown as our chief of orthopaedic trauma, was another icon to whom many of us turned for advice. He was capable of eloquent, introspective discussion on any topic in orthopaedics, and was the one who always made us be sure to equally consider the person connected to the cast. His dedication to teaching and patient care continues to motivate us to maintain and expect the highest standards in our profession.

Sigvard T. Hansen, Jr., MD, our former foot fellowship director, has spent his life challenging dogma and doctrine in orthopaedics. He is one of the true visionaries in the field of foot and ankle surgery. In his sometimes unorthodox but astonishingly competent and successful manner, he has been responsible for major advances in foot care, and has never shied away from the potential controversy created by his occasionally divergent, but frequently correct, opinions. Dr. Hansen continues to inspire countless surgeons in this field with his breakthrough concepts about how the foot works and how it should be managed. We are lucky enough to have experienced his talents and watched him touch the lives of countless patients. Every practitioner in this field owes him a debt of gratitude for being one of the prime motivating forces which has allowed foot and ankle care to transcend the status quo over the past several decades.

Bruce Sangeorzan, MD, remains a great friend and consummate guiding force for us. His ever quiet demeanor is deceiving, because he is the quintessential still water which runs deep, and his voice of reason has always served as a refreshing reminder of what is 'the right thing to do'. He has been a tremendously valuable mentor in a field of ever changing choices, where picking what is most reasonable can often be mired by the temptation to try something new. His commitment to pure and honest research and his reliance on data rather than opinion continues to serve as an example to us all.

Steve Benirschke, MD, our final mentor, has taught us many of the invaluable technical skills we now employ in trauma surgery. His most important contribution has been the realization that 'If you don't have time to do it right the first time, what makes you think you'll have time to do it right the second time?' Dr. Benirschke's compassion for patients is inspiring, as is his extraordinary drive to achieve perfection. Extra time devoted to patient care is rewarded with great outcomes.

These five surgeons have moved us to demand the best from ourselves in medicine. They have led by example, reinforcing the virtues of selflessness, education, and commitment. Never motivated by ego or self-gain when it came to patient care, they have inspired others to follow their path in the pursuit of excellence and quality. They remain teachers, mentors, and friends to whom we owe tremendous gratitude.

Other Volumes in the Core Knowledge in Orthopaedics Series

Spine
Hand and Upper Extremity
Sports Medicine
Trauma
Adult Reconstruction and Arthroplasty
Pediatric Orthopaedics

Contents

1. **Foot and Ankle Anatomy and Biomechanics** 1
Justin Greisberg

2. **Examination of the Foot and Ankle** 10
Matthew M. Roberts and Justin Greisberg

3. **Orthotics** 16
Douglas H. Richie Jr.

4. **Adult Acquired Flatfoot** 38
Margaret Lobo and Justin Greisberg

5. **The Non-neuromuscular Cavus Foot** 58
Margaret Chilvers and Arthur Manoli II

6. **Neuromuscular Foot Deformity** 67
Justin Greisberg, Stefan Gerhard Hofstaetter, and Hans-Jörg Trnka

7. **Diabetic Foot Disorders** 77
Dov Kolker and Steven Weinfeld

8. **Rheumatoid Arthritis and Inflammatory Disorders** 90
Lew C. Schon and Kevin J. Logel

9. **Hallux Valgus** 104
Heather E. Hensl and Andrew K. Sands

10. **First Metatarsophalangeal Disorders** 119
Aaron Colman and Gregory C. Pomeroy

11. **Lesser Toe Disorders** 129
Lloyd C. Briggs Jr.

12. **Common Pediatric Foot and Ankle Conditions** 147
Craig P. Eberson and Jonathan Schiller

13. **Nerve Disorders** 171
Anthony Hinz

14. **Ankle Arthritis** 177
Michael Brage and Catherine M. Robertson

15. **Heel Pain** 195
Eric M. Berkson, Justin Greisberg, and George H. Theodore

16. **Achilles Tendon Problems** 200
Annette M. Smith and Andrew K. Sands

17. **Other Tendon Problems** 209
Eric M. Bluman

18. **Ankle Sprains and Ligament Injuries** 227
Michael S. Aronow and Raymond J. Sullivan

19. **Malleolar Fractures** 240
Stephen K. Benirschke and Patricia Ann Kramer

20. **Tibial Pilon Fractures** 252
Ivan S. Tarkin and Peter A. Cole

21. **Calcaneus Fractures** 267
Rahul Banerjee and Florian Nickisch

22. **Talus Fractures** 283
Michael P. Swords, Jason Cochran, and Jason Heisler

23. **Navicular and Midfoot Injuries** 297
Gregory J. Della Rocca and Bruce J. Sangeorzan

24. **Metatarsal and Phalangeal Fractures** 310
Niket Shrivastava and Justin Greisberg

25. **Tumors of the Foot and Ankle** 321
Phillip R. Langer and Richard M. Terek

26. **Amputations** 339
Mathieu Assal and Eric Gordon

27. **Ankle Arthroscopy** 352
Richard J. de Asla and Martin O'Malley

28. Nail Problems in the Foot 363
Mark Chong Lee and Christopher W. DiGiovanni

29. Enhancement of Bone Healing 376
Rahul Banerjee and Christopher W. DiGiovanni

Index 389

Foot and Ankle Anatomy and Biomechanics

Justin Greisberg[*]

[*]M.D., Assistant Professor of Orthopaedic Surgery, Columbia University College of Physicians and Surgeons, New York, NY

- The foot and ankle comprise a complex "machine" consisting of 26 bones and joints working together. The individual parts do not work in isolation (Fig. 1–1).
- The ankle and hindfoot are one part of this machine, allowing the foot to adapt to uneven terrain while the tibia and the rest of the body remain upright.
- The ankle is the principal joint for plantar flexion and dorsiflexion. The hindfoot joints (the subtalar, the talonavicular, and to a lesser extent the calcaneocuboid) provide a complex motion that can be simply thought of as inversion and eversion. Together, the ankle and hindfoot joints act as a universal joint, so that the foot can be positioned on any irregular surface while the leg remains vertical for bipedal weight bearing.
- Loss of motion from either the ankle or the hindfoot will lead to overload of the other, as the joints attempt to make up for the lost motion. This is why patients with ankle fusions universally develop hindfoot arthritis on x-rays at late follow-up.
- The midfoot bridges the universal joint of the hindfoot to the metatarsal heads. At the joints between the navicular, the cuneiforms, and the medial metatarsals, stability is much more important than flexibility. Arthrodesis of these joints probably does not impair foot function at all.
- Toes, especially the first, provide propulsion during gait. Metatarsophalangeal (MTP) motion is important in this function. Interphalangeal motion is not essential for walking.
- In the normal human foot, contraction of the Achilles pulls on the calcaneal tuberosity at a short distance from the ankle. As the ankle begins to rotate in response to the Achilles contraction, the force is transmitted across a rigid foot to the metatarsal heads, at a distance from the ankle (center of rotation) (Fig. 1–2). The end result is amplification of the Achilles force for propulsion.
- Overall, the human foot has changed from a flexible primate appendage used to grasp tree branches into a rigid lever for bipedal gait.

Hindfoot | Midfoot | Forefoot

Figure 1–1: **Overall schematic of foot. The ankle and hindfoot provide flexibility. The longitudinal arch and the midfoot are more important for stability. The toes remain flexible to facilitate propulsion during gait but are not as important for grasping (as compared with in other primates).**

Evolution of the Modern Foot and Comparative Anatomy

- Human evolution diverged from chimpanzees about 5 million years ago.
- Modern apes do not have a rigid arch. The lever arm for the Achilles tendon is much smaller. The ape foot has less propulsive power than the human foot.
- In fact, the ape foot is better developed for grasping. The first metatarsal is quite mobile at its articulation with the medial cuneiform, so the first ray (hallux) can be used to grasp tree branches (Fig. 1–3).
- The foot of the modern chimpanzee or gorilla is a compromise between a weight-bearing organ and a grasping one. The foot retains the mobile hallux.
- The modern human foot has a tightly packed, immobile first ray. The hallux is no longer able to abduct, because of increased rigidity at the first metatarsocuneiform joint. Adduction of the first metatarsal developed along with stability of the longitudinal arch (Fig. 1–4).

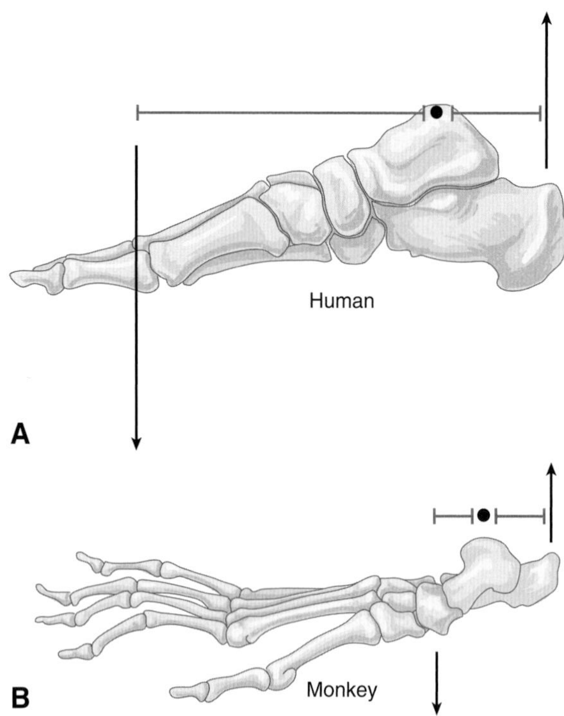

Figure 1–2: **A,** In the normal human, the Achilles tendon acts at a relatively short distance from the center of rotation of the ankle. With a rigid arch, the force of Achilles contraction passes to the metatarsal heads, at a greater distance from the ankle. Thus a small displacement of the Achilles tendon will result in a larger displacement at the forefoot, with strong propulsive forces. **B,** The monkey or primate foot does not have a rigid arch to act as a lever, so that Achilles forces act more on the midfoot than the forefoot. The displacement of Achilles contractions are not amplified, so there is no great propulsion with bipedal gait.

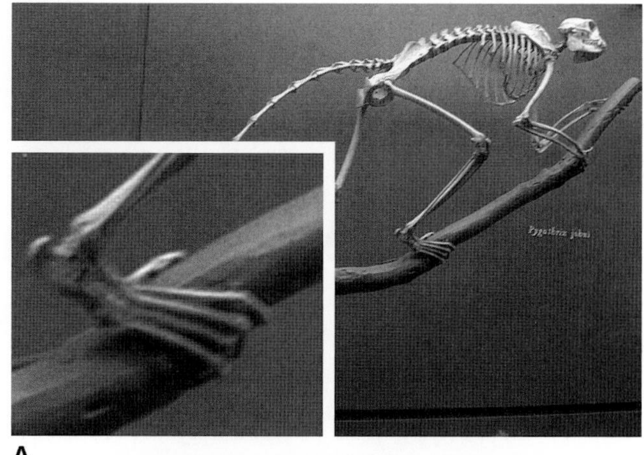

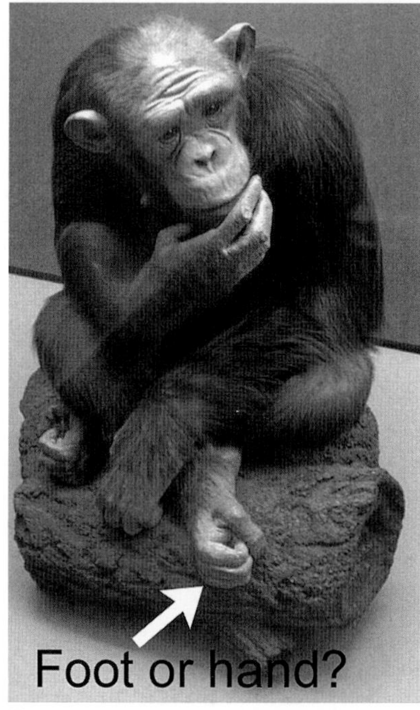

Figure 1–3: **A,** The monkey foot is well adapted for an arboreal lifestyle. The first ray (hallux) is mobile so that it can grasp around a tree branch. **B,** The foot of the chimpanzee is similarly adapted for flexibility, not stability. In this photo, the foot is curled into a fist, more closely resembling the human hand than foot.

- Fossil footprints of a purely bipedal gait are visible from 3.7 million years ago. At that time, human ancestors (*Australopithecines*) had a brain case very much like that of a chimpanzee.
- One theory proposes that development of a modern, bipedal gait was the first step in human evolution. By freeing up the hands from any weight-bearing or tree-climbing obligations, the hands could specifically evolve for fine motor skills and tool use. Such refinement in use of the hands induced rapid expansion of the cerebral cortex.

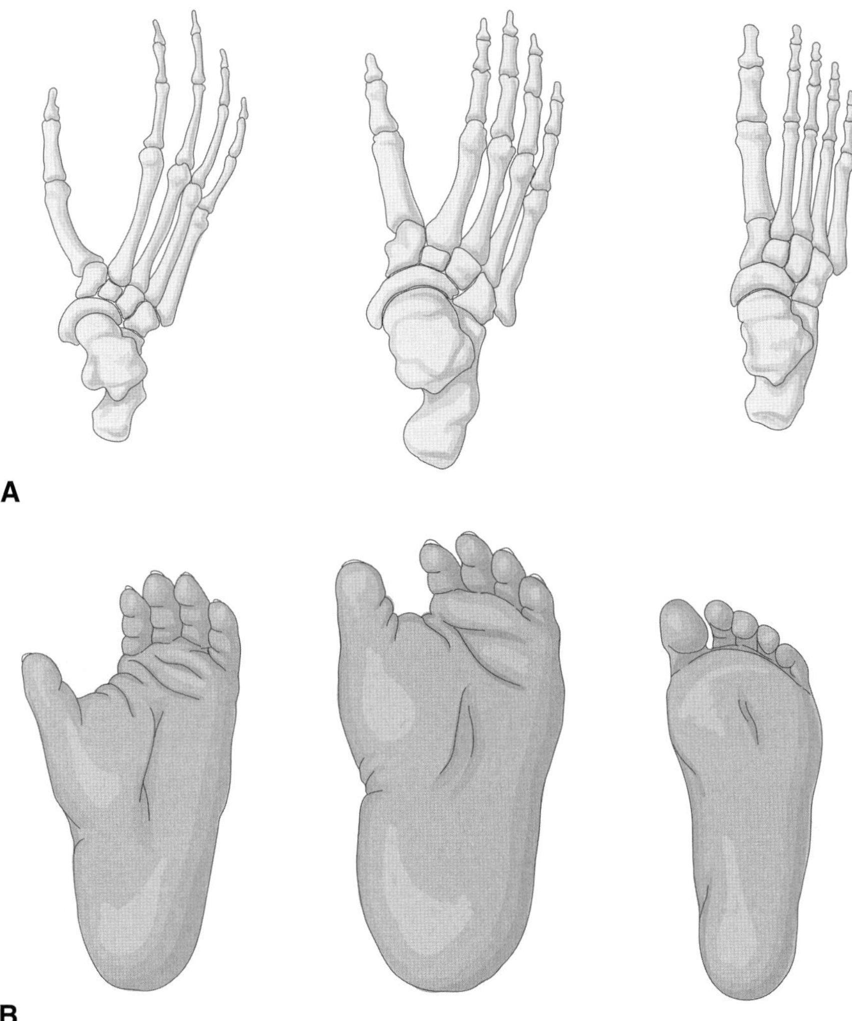

Figure 1–4: **A, From left to right is the chimp foot, the gorilla foot, and the human foot. Both the chimp and human have a medially angulated hallux, with flexibility, not stability. The hallux is packed in tightly with the rest of the forefoot in the human, providing stability and propulsion for gait. B, From left to right, chimp, gorilla, and human feet. The primates have a mobile hallux for grasping, while the human foot is tight for weight bearing.**

- The foot of early hominids (such as *Homo habilis* from 1-2 million years ago) looks very much like a modern human foot.

The Longitudinal Arch

- Compared with other animals, the human foot is well adapted for prolonged walking but perhaps not as good for climbing or running.
- A key anatomical feature of the modern human foot is the longitudinal arch.
- The arch provides some shock absorption while walking and gives room for nerves and vessels to pass to the forefoot without being crushed.
- More importantly, the arch provides a long lever arm for the Achilles tendon to act on the forefoot (see Fig. 1–2). With a stable arch, the joints between the calcaneus and metatarsals are rigid, so that Achilles tendon forces can pass from the calcaneal tuberosity to the metatarsal heads, with rotation at the ankle.
- The rigid lever facilitates propulsion during gait. No other living primate can walk with the sustained bipedal gait of the modern human.

Anatomy of the Foot

- Some articulations are vital for normal function, while others are relatively unimportant for normal walking and running (Table 1–1).

The Ankle

- The tibia and fibula together make a tight socket (mortise) for the talar dome.
- The talar dome is wider anteriorly than posteriorly, so that dorsiflexion tightens up the fit of the talus in

Table 1–1: Importance of Joints of the Foot

JOINT OF THE FOOT	IMPORTANCE
Ankle (tibiotalar)	Essential
Subtalar	Essential
Talonavicular	Essential
Calcaneocuboid	Not essential
Naviculocuneiform	Not essential
Metatarsocuneiform	Not essential
Cuboid-metatarsal	Essential
Metatarsophalangeal	Essential
Interphalangeal	Not essential

the mortise and also causes the fibula to move slightly laterally.

- The joint surfaces are highly conforming, so that weight-bearing forces can be spread out over a broad surface area, minimizing joint pressures.
- Alteration in these conforming surfaces can dramatically decrease contact area and increase pressure, leading to arthritis. This might occur with syndesmotic widening or intraarticular fracture.
- Widening of the mortise by 1 mm increases peak contact pressures almost 50%.
- Several studies have shown that persistent widening of the ankle mortise after injury leads to poorer outcome.
- The cartilage of the joint is relatively thick.
- About one-sixth of weight-bearing forces are borne by the fibula. The remainder passes through the tibia.
- The distal tibial articular surface (plafond) may have as much as 3° of valgus. The mortise is externally rotated 20-30° relative to the knee.

Ankle Ligaments

- Stability for the ankle during standing is primarily through the conforming shape of the joint surfaces. Collateral ligaments play a role while walking and running.
- On the medial side, the superficial deltoid ligament has fibers that pass from the medial malleolus to the talus, navicular, and calcaneus.
- The deep deltoid is most important for stability. It passes from deep inside the medial malleolus to the medial body of the talus.
- A major source of blood supply to the talus enters the body through these medial ligaments.
- The lateral collateral ligaments include the anterior talofibular ligament (ATFL), calcaneofibular ligament (CFL), and posterior talofibular ligament.
- The ATFL provides protection against inversion while the ankle is plantar flexed.
- The CFL is more important when the ankle is dorsiflexed.

The Distal Tibiofibular Syndesmosis

- The distal tibia has a notch posterolaterally for a snug fit with the distal fibula.
- This syndesmosis is held together by the anterior inferior tibiofibular ligament, the posterior inferior tibiofibular ligament, the interosseous ligament and membrane, and the transverse tibiofibular ligaments.

The Talus

- A large part of the talar surface is covered by articular cartilage. The talus is the center of the ankle and hindfoot "universal joint" (Fig. 1–5).
- There are no muscular attachments to the bone.
- The blood supply to the talus is somewhat tenuous. The posterior tibial artery sends an artery to the tarsal canal, which enters the talus through the deltoid medially, and also through the inferior surface in the tarsal canal

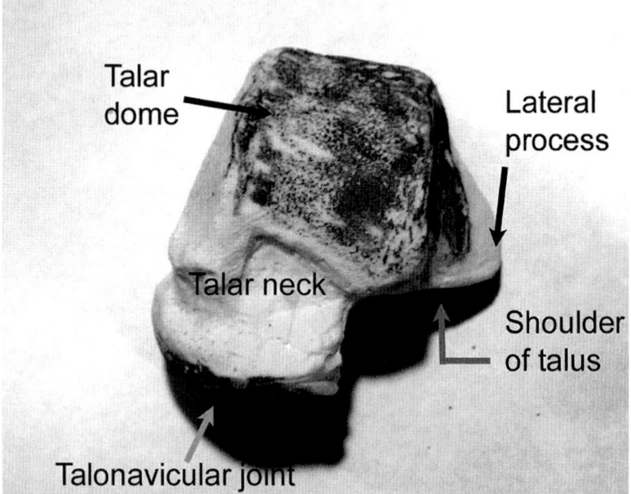

A

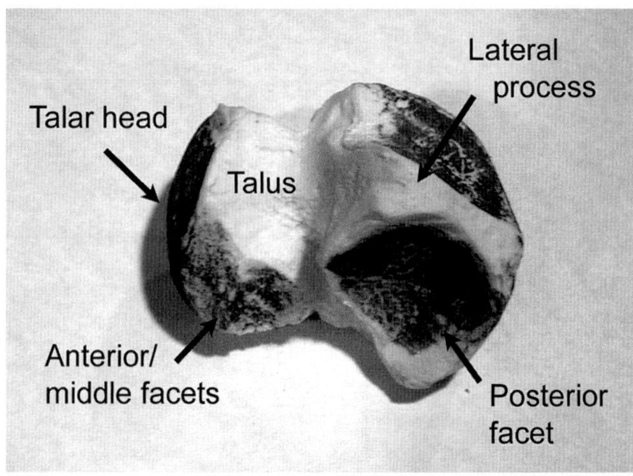

B

Figure 1–5: **A,** View of the talus from above. The articular facets are shaded. Note that the talar neck is relatively medial, and there is a lateral shoulder and process. **B,** A lateral view of the talus shows how the talonavicular joint is contiguous with the anterior facet of the subtalar joint. The function of these joints in providing complex hindfoot motion is closely linked.

(between the posterior and middle facets of the subtalar joint).

- The dorsalis pedis artery provides important blood supply through the dorsal neck.
- The peroneal artery also sends some contributions to the sinus tarsi.
- A fracture or dislocation can easily disrupt some or all of this blood supply, leading to avascular necrosis. Surgical trauma can injure it as well. Although avascular necrosis is rarely seen after surgery, the lack of vascularity may present as surgical non-union. With total ankle arthroplasty, surgical damage to the talus may prevent osseous ingrowth into the implant, with aseptic loosening of the talar component.

The Calcaneus

- In contrast to the talus, the calcaneus has abundant blood supply and soft tissue attachments.
- Fractures of the calcaneus often will have complete disruption of the blood supply to multiple fragments, yet tend to heal well. Old surgeons' joke: That is why it is called the "heal" (heel) bone!
- Occasionally, calcaneus fractures will show avascular necrosis, but less commonly than the talus.
- The calcaneus contains a large, dense, medial projection: the sustentaculum tali. The superior surface of the sustentaculum contains the middle and anterior facets of the subtalar joint. The spring ligament takes its origin here (Fig. 1–6).
- The posterior tibial neurovascular structures pass within a few millimeters of the medial calcaneal wall. When performing a calcaneal osteotomy from the lateral side, it is important to avoid penetrating the medial wall with a saw or osteotome.

Os Trigonum

- The os trigonum is a normal bone found in many patients at the back of the ankle. It may be an ununited posterior process.
- The os may articulate with the posterior facet on the calcaneus.
- It lies just deep to, and lateral to, the flexor hallucis longus tendon.
- It may become irritated, especially in dancers who frequently go into extreme plantar flexion.
- Resection of an os trigonum can be done easily through a posteromedial approach. The commonly used posterolateral approach can lead to injury of the sural nerve.

Hindfoot Joints

- The subtalar joint has three articular facets. The anterior and middle are often contiguous, while the posterior is larger and separate. The posterior facet is saddle-shaped (Fig. 1–7).

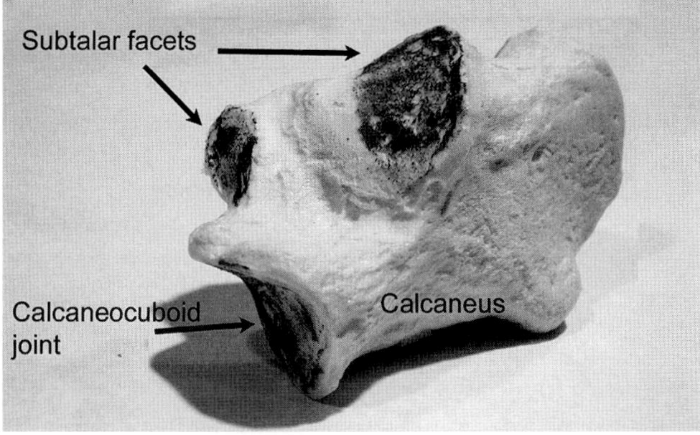

Figure 1–6: A view of the calcaneus from the lateral side.

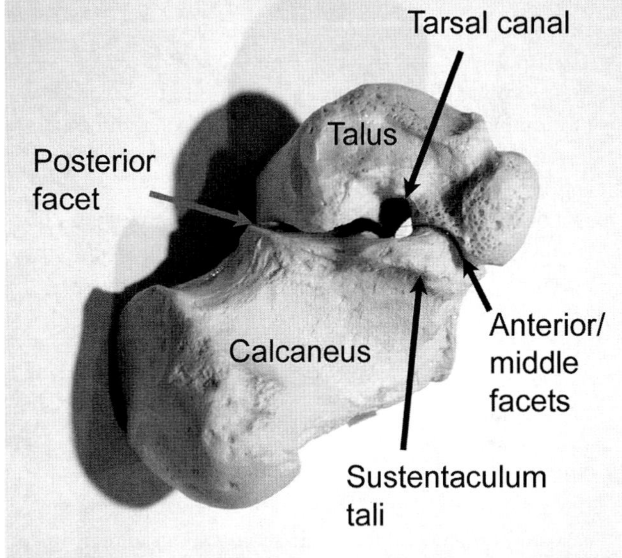

A

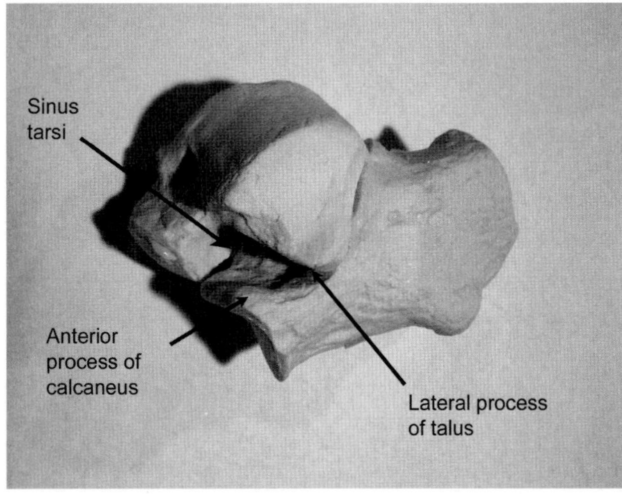

B

Figure 1–7: **A,** Medial view of the subtalar joint. **B,** This lateral view of the subtalar joint shows how the sinus tarsi is formed as the space between the lateral process of the talus and the anterior process of the calcaneus.

- In the past, the subtalar joint was thought to have a single axis of rotation, passing obliquely from posterolateral to anterodorsal. During stance, the axis makes an angle of 41° with the ground.
- More precise biomechanical studies have shown the joint to behave more like a screw, with no one axis of rotation.
- As the calcaneus rotates into eversion, it also passes posteriorly. Inversion is accompanied by forward translation.
- Talonavicular and subtalar motion are tightly coupled. Fusion of the talonavicular joint eliminates all subtalar motion. Fusion of the subtalar joint leaves about 25% of normal talonavicular motion.
- The calcaneocuboid joint is less critical for hindfoot motion. Isolated fusion of the calcaneocuboid does not limit subtalar motion much at all and leaves 67% of talonavicular motion intact.
- The calcaneus and navicular (and the rest of the foot) rotate around the talus (peritalar motion). In general, the motion between other tarsal bones is smaller and much less important than that between the talus, calcaneus, and navicular.
- Although none of these joints have a true single axis of motion, models of hindfoot mechanics often assume they do (Box 1–1).

Hindfoot Ligaments

- There are many interosseous ligaments in and around the subtalar joint. The lateral ligaments provide support against varus stresses.
- The CFL and inferior extensor retinaculum provide some lateral support. Other lateral subtalar supports include the cervical ligament and the interosseous talocalcaneal ligament.
- The spring ligament passes from the sustentaculum tali of the calcaneus to the navicular. It is a key ligament in support of the longitudinal arch.
- The long plantar ligament runs from the calcaneus to the cuboid and is also an arch stabilizer.

Midfoot Joints

- The joints between the navicular and the cuneiforms have little motion.

Box 1–1 Hindfoot Mechanics

- With hindfoot eversion (pronation), the axes of the talonavicular and calcaneocuboid joints are parallel. This alignment effectively unlocks those joints and allows them to flex.
- When the hindfoot is inverted, the axes of these joints are divergent. This "locks" the Chopart joint, making the arch rigid.
- During the heel rise portion of gait, the posterior tibial tendon inverts the hindfoot, making the arch rigid so that forces from the Achilles tendon can be transmitted across the arch to the metatarsal heads. Failure of the posterior tibial tendon leads to arch collapse during heel rise, and ineffective gait.

- The metatarsocuneiform joints are very stable as well.
- There is some motion between the cuboid and fourth and fifth metatarsals. This motion gives some flexibility to the lateral column of the foot, making gait more comfortable. Fusion of these joints should probably be avoided.
- The Lisfranc ligament runs from the medial cuneiform to the second metatarsal base. It is an important stabilizer of the midfoot.
- Strong plantar ligaments bridge from the cuneiforms to the metatarsal bases. The dorsal ligaments are weaker and may be less important for midfoot stability.

The Forefoot

- Motion at the MTP joints is essential during gait, and the metatarsal heads are essential for weight bearing.
- Resection of any metatarsal head should be avoided in general.
- While standing, about 40% of body weight is carried through the first metatarsal; the remainder is divided up among the lesser metatarsal heads.
- The interphalangeal joints are not important for walking. They are important for grasping, although this is not an important task for the human foot.
- Interphalangeal fusion or resection is well tolerated.
- The hallucal sesamoids reside in the tendons of the two flexor hallucis brevis muscles.
- Loss of a sesamoid without repair of the flexor hallucis brevis tendon may lead to varus or valgus at the MTP joint.
- Resection of a single sesamoid is generally well tolerated, but resection of both sesamoids should not be performed.

Plantar Fascia

- The plantar fascia runs from the calcaneal tuberosity to the forefoot. The main (central) band inserts both into the subcutaneous tissue in the ball of the foot and to the septae of the flexor tendons in the toes.
- The plantar fascia supports the longitudinal arch. Complete division of the fascia leads to mild loss of arch height.
- With the "windlass" mechanism, extension at the MTP joints leads to tightening of the fascia and support of the arch (Fig. 1–8).

Plantar Fat Pad

- The plantar subcutaneous layer consists of a specialized collection of adipose tissue within a framework of fibrous lamellae in a complex whorl pattern.
- This fibrous frame gives the plantar fat structural support, allowing it to cushion the foot from the impact of normal walking.
- Damage to the fat pad may occur after high-energy trauma, such as a calcaneus fracture or lawn mower injury.

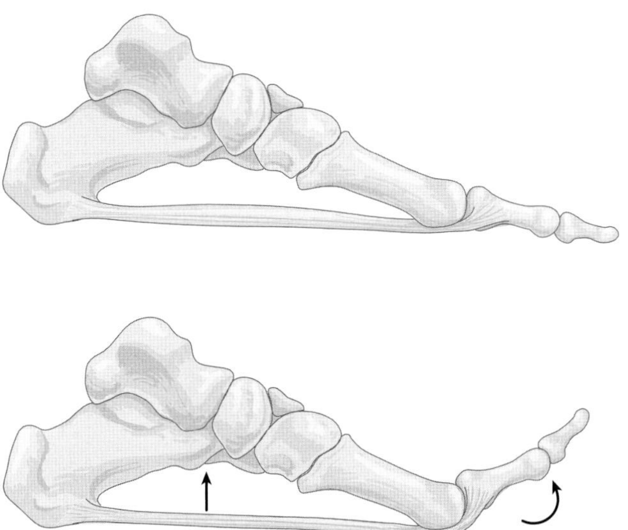

Figure 1–8: Dorsiflexion of the toes tightens the plantar fascia, strengthening the toes.

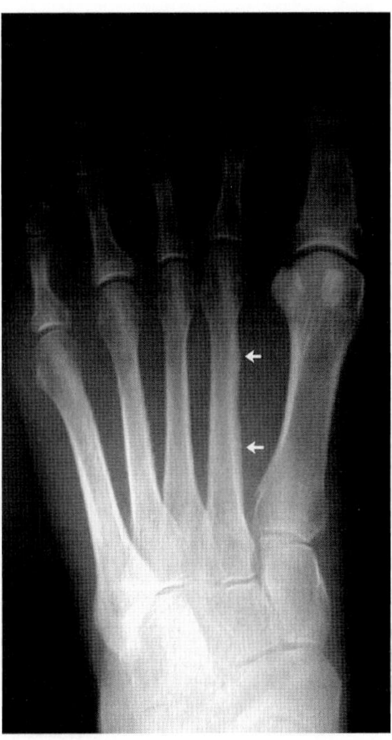

Figure 1–9: This patient complains of pain under the second metatarsal head. She has a mild hallux valgus, with instability of the first metatarsal. The metatarsal instability or hypermobility leads to long-term overload of the second ray, evident as second metatarsal cortical thickening (marked by arrows). Also, note how the second metatarsophalangeal (MTP) joint is slightly deviated medially (compare with the smaller MTP joints). This is a subtle clue to second MTP overload with synovitis.

Instability of the First Ray

- The first ray (medial cuneiform and first metatarsal) is tightly packed with the rest of the foot in the normal human.
- In 1935, Dudley Morton, an anatomist at Columbia University, proposed that instability of the first ray was a source of trouble in the foot. He thought this trait was atavistic, implying a reversion to a more primitive state.
- Possibly because of objections to the concept of evolution in the early twentieth century, his theories were not widely accepted. Controversy continues in modern times.
- Despite continued controversy, it is undeniable that hallux valgus deformity is caused by deformity at the metatarsocuneiform and MTP joints. Because the cuneiform and metatarsal do not change shape with aging, and because hallux valgus is an acquired deformity, there must be instability in the joints to create the deformity.
- Instability of the first ray at the metatarsocuneiform joint leads not only to hallux valgus, but can also lead to elevation of the first metatarsal. Weight-bearing forces will then be transferred to the second metatarsal head. This is often the cause of transfer metatarsalgia (Fig. 1–9).

Arch Height

- The medial longitudinal arch passes through the talonavicular, naviculocuneiform, and metatarsocuneiform joints.
- Instability or sagging at any of these joints can result in a fallen arch or flatfoot.
- Instability at the first metatarsocuneiform joint is seen with hallux valgus deformity. Because this instability is three-dimensional, patients with hallux valgus often have a flatfoot (Fig. 1–10).
- On a weight-bearing lateral radiograph, one indicator of arch integrity is the talometatarsal angle. This angle is determined by the intersection of the axis of the talus with the axis of the first metatarsal. In the normal foot, it is $\pm 4^\circ$.
- Arch height varies. Whether the arch is low or high, the talometatarsal angle should be within the normal range (Fig. 1–11).
- A talometatarsal angle outside the normal range suggests a pathologic process.

The Tripod Model of the Foot

- One model of foot structure depicts the foot as a tripod. The three "legs" of the tripod are the heel, the first metatarsal head, and the fifth metatarsal head. Balance between these three is important for foot support. Elevation or depression of the first metatarsal will tilt the rest of the tripod.
- In some flatfeet, subluxation or sag at the first metatarsocuneiform joint leads to collapse of one leg of the tripod. Without a supporting medial post to balance the foot, the hindfoot can collapse into valgus. The final

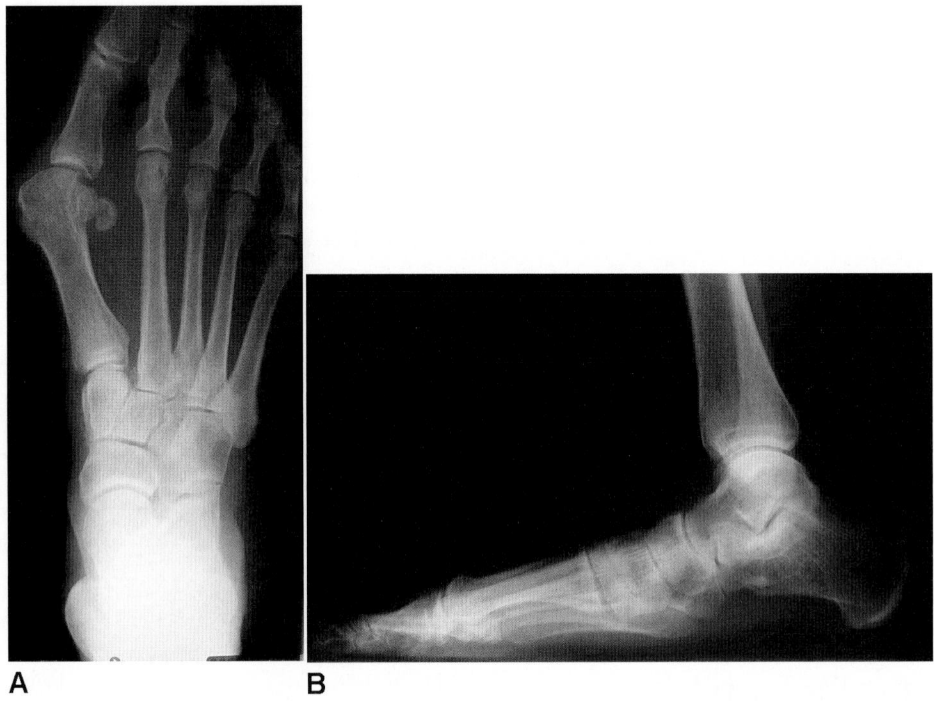

Figure 1–10: **A,** This patient with hallux valgus has medial deviation of the first metatarsal. **B,** A lateral view reveals the flatfoot that is common among patients with hallux valgus. Dorsal angulation of the first metatarsocuneiform joint is clearly visible. This sagging of the medial column of the foot allows the hindfoot to fall into valgus, thus making a flatfoot.

result is a flatfoot. This has been termed forefoot-driven hindfoot valgus. (Collapse at the naviculocuneiform or talonavicular joints can lead to the same end result: hindfoot valgus.)

- By a similar model, plantar flexion of the first metatarsal will drive the hindfoot into varus. This is termed *forefoot-driven hindfoot varus*. The end result is a cavovarus foot.

Structural Diversity in Human Feet

- It is clear that there is a wide spectrum of foot shapes in modern humans. Variations in arch height and first metatarsal alignment lead to abundant diversity.

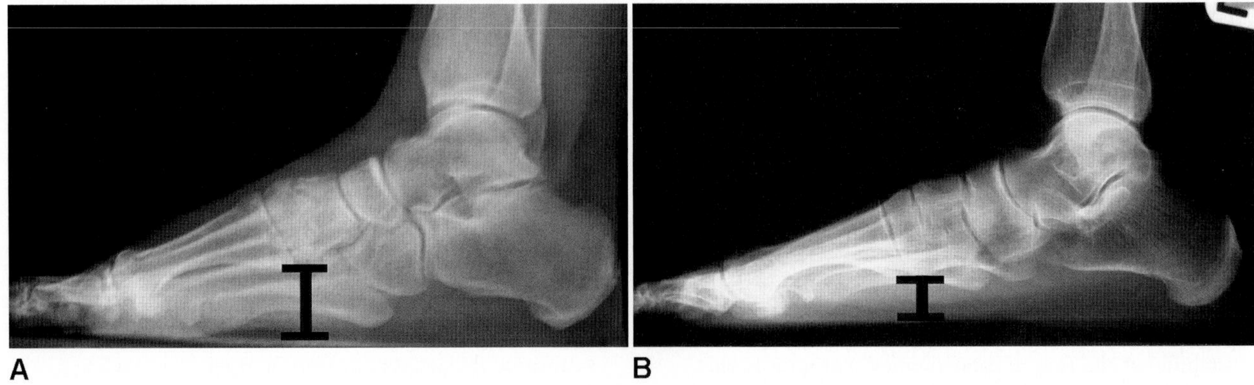

Figure 1–11: **A,** In some feet, the arch will be "high," with a large distance between the medial cuneiform and the floor. **B,** Other feet show a "low" arch. In both A and B, the talometatarsal angle is close to normal. These are variants of normal, not flatfeet. A pathologic flatfoot will show collapse of the arch and increased talometatarsal angle.

- Interestingly, when fossil specimens from prehistoric hominids are evaluated, there is also structural diversity. Rather than implying that early hominids could not walk upright, it suggests that the human foot is a work in progress. It will be interesting to see whether human feet are more uniform 1 million years from now.

The Foot and Ankle in Gait

- As the heel strikes the ground, the ankle moves from dorsiflexion to plantar flexion (foot flat on the ground). Eccentric contraction of the tibialis anterior controls the descent to foot flat.
  - Tibialis anterior rupture or peroneal nerve palsy leads to a gait pattern with uncontrolled "slapping" of the foot on the ground as the limb moves from heel strike to foot flat.
- As the leg moves to midstance, the ankle dorsiflexes about 10°.
- Body weight passes over the foot, and strong gastrocnemius and soleus contractions move the foot to heel rise. The ankle once again plantar flexes.
- The primary functions of the Achilles muscles are to decelerate tibial advance for knee stability, and to stabilize the ankle so the limb can rock on to the forefoot. In routine gait, they are not as important for push-off. As the stride is lengthened, more work is required of the Achilles.
  - Untreated rupture or over-lengthening of the Achilles will prevent effective heel rise. Body weight is kept close to the heel rather than moving to the forefoot. Stride length is shortened, and heel rise is delayed.
- The toe flexors, especially the flexor hallucis longus, are active during late stance, heel rise, and toe-off stages.
- Once the foot leaves the ground, the ankle must dorsiflex to clear the ground. The first toe clears the ground by less than 1 cm during normal gait.
  - Absence of the ankle dorsiflexors (tibialis anterior) leads to a high-steppage gait, where the limb is lifted higher off the ground for clearance.
- Normal cadence for an adult is 101 to 122 steps/min. It is slightly higher in women than in men, and much higher in small children.
- Cadence does not change with aging, but stride length does decrease.

References

Astion DJ, Deland JT et al. (1997) Motion of the hindfoot after simulated arthrodesis. J Bone Joint Surg 79: 241-246.

This well-done experiment reveals the interconnection of the talonavicular, subtalar, and calcaneocuboid joints in complex hindfoot motion. Bottom line: Fusion of the talonavicular joint eliminates virtually all hindfoot motion.

Hansen ST. (2000) Functional Reconstruction of the Foot and Ankle. Philadelphia: Lippincott Williams & Wilkins.

A modern classic, providing logical approaches to foot and ankle function and pathophysiology. A "must read" for any student of the foot.

Morton DJ. (1935) The Human Foot: Its Evolution, Physiology, and Functional Disorders. Morningside Heights: Columbia University Press.

This classic text—written by an anatomist, not a surgeon—is an interesting read emphasizing the importance of first ray stability in some disorders of the human foot.

Olson TR, Seidel MR. (1983) The evolutionary basis of some clinical disorders of the human foot: A comparative survey of the living primates. Foot Ankle Int 3: 322-341.

A thorough review of the foot in humans and primates, again emphasizing the importance of stability of the first ray.

Examination of the Foot and Ankle

Matthew M. Roberts[*] and Justin Greisberg[§]

[*]M.D., Assistant Professor of Orthopaedic Surgery, Hospital for Special Surgery; Instructor in Orthopaedic Surgery, Weill Medical College of Cornell University Hospital, New York, NY
[§]M.D., Assistant Professor of Orthopaedic Surgery, Columbia University College of Physicians and Surgeons, New York, NY

General Points

- Weight matters: Heavy patients who lose weight can eliminate foot pain.
- Are there any other joints involved? The patient's problem could be an inflammatory arthropathy.
- Does the patient smell of smoke? Nicotine inhibits bone and wound healing, leading to higher surgical complication rates.

Inspection

- Examination may begin with the patient sitting on an elevated table, with the leg at eye level for the physician.
- The location and amount of swelling is noted. Swelling may be diffuse, from peripheral edema, or focal, as with inflammation of tendonitis or single-joint arthritis.
- Previous wounds are noted in order to understand the role of previous injury or surgery in current pathology.
- Pigmented lesions should be noted. Subungual hematomas are common, but a pigmented subungual lesion that does not grow out with time raises the possibility of melanoma.
- Is the skin shiny, "wooden," and/or with loss of hair? This could indicate an underlying vasculopathy.
- Does the patient have calluses? Calluses are the clue to where the patient is bearing the most weight. It is normal to have mild callusing under the first metatarsal head or the heel (Fig. 2–1).
- Callusing under the second metatarsal head is an indirect sign of first ray hypermobility/instability.
- Heavy calluses under the first metatarsal head may be present in the cavus foot.
- Thick calluses under the heel will be seen with calcaneus deformity from a weak Achilles.

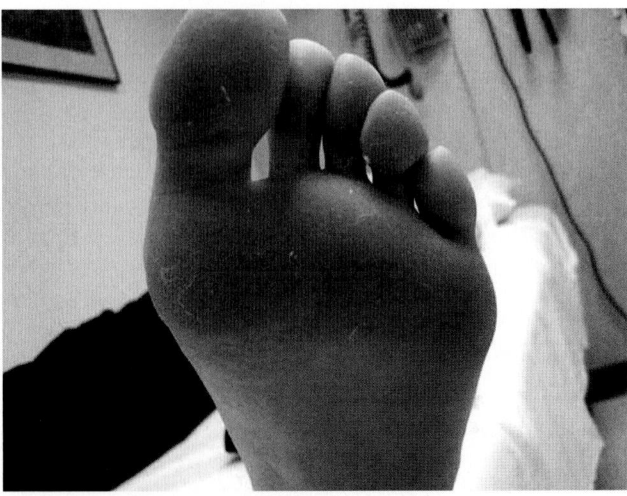

Figure 2–1: **Heavy callusing under the first metatarsal head suggests a cavus foot.**

- Calluses under the navicular may be seen with a collapsed arch (pathologic flatfoot).
- Look at the shoes! Many patients with forefoot deformities will be wearing shoes that are too small for the deformity. A switch to proper-fitting shoes may relieve symptoms.
  - Wear under the lateral shoe suggests cavus or varus alignment, while medial wear is visible with valgus or flatfoot deformity.

Palpation

- Most structures in the foot are superficial and directly palpable. Describe the tenderness anatomically. For example, instead of saying "lateral foot or ankle tenderness," say where it is exactly. Is it the base of the fifth metatarsal, the anterior process of the calcaneus, the peroneal tendons, the distal fibular tip, or the anterior talofibular ligament?

Motion

- Begin with knee motion. Misalignment in the knee can overload the foot, with secondary pain. Stiffness in the knee may be present and may make mild foot deformities or mild ankle stiffness more symptomatic.
- Plantar flexion and dorsiflexion of the foot is mainly through the ankle, although in many cases up to one-third of perceived ankle motion is actually through the subtalar and (especially) the transverse tarsal (talonavicular and calcaneocuboid) joints.
- Subtalar motion is a complex motion with contributions from the three hindfoot joints (talocalcaneal, talonavicular, and calcaneocuboid). The motion is described as inversion and eversion. Hindfoot motion is not purely in the coronal plane. It is a complex motion that is best measured by comparing with the contralateral side. The motion is normal if it is fluid and equal to that of the unaffected side.
- Limitations of hindfoot motion are important to note. A patient with a flatfoot deformity and a "fixed" hindfoot has moderate to severe restriction of subtalar motion, which implies arthrosis or peroneal spasticity. This finding may determine whether a joint-sparing or fusion surgery is indicated for flatfoot reconstruction. An arthritic ankle with decreased subtalar motion may not be a great candidate for an isolated ankle fusion, as this may place more stress on an arthritic joint.
- All the metatarsophalangeal (MTP) joints normally have good motion, especially in extension.

Gastrocnemius Contracture

- When checking ankle dorsiflexion, gastrocnemius contracture may limit passive ankle dorsiflexion. Because the gastrocnemius origin is above the knee on the femoral condyles, a contracted gastrocnemius will limit ankle dorsiflexion with the knee extended but not flexed.
- Normally, passive ankle dorsiflexion should be at least 5 or 10° past neutral. When examining the patient's right foot, the examiner's right hand cups the heel, with the thumb on the navicular tuberosity. The left hand is wrapped around the metatarsal heads to keep them level (Fig. 2–2).
  - It is essential to keep the hindfoot neutral or just slightly inverted. Because of the oblique axis of the subtalar joint, hindfoot eversion will also dorsiflex the forefoot, masking any gastrocnemius equinus.
- Passive ankle dorsiflexion is checked first with the knee extended. The normal ankle dorsiflexes 5 or 10° past neutral. Then the knee is flexed, and dorsiflexion is checked again.

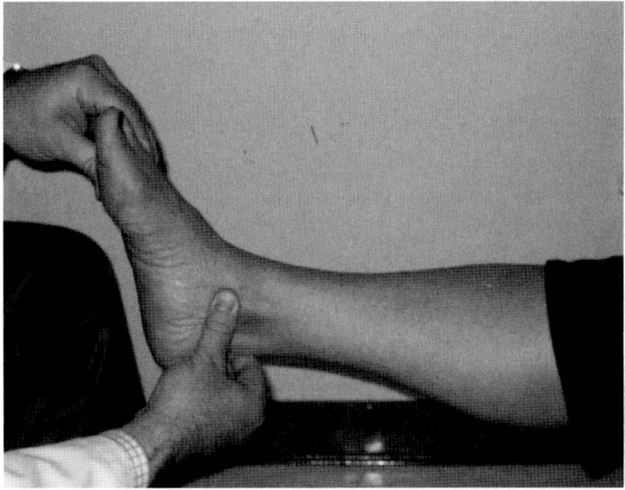

A

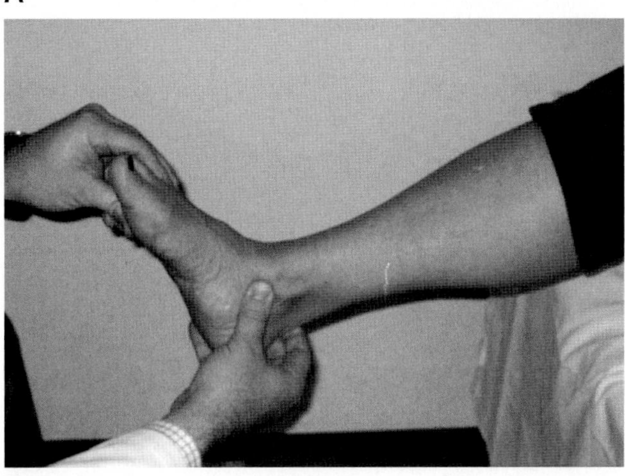

B

Figure 2–2: **A, Equinus measured with hindfoot in neutral and knee extended. The examiner's thumb is over the medial navicular to maintain neutrality of the hindfoot. B, Improved dorsiflexion with knee bent implies gastrocnemius equinus.**

- Limitation of ankle dorsiflexion with the knee extended that corrects with knee flexion indicates gastrocnemius contracture. Limitation of dorsiflexion in all knee positions means that both the soleus and the gastrocnemius are contracted.

Stability

- Anterior drawer and talar tilting tests check for lateral ankle ligament stability.
- The anterior drawer test is done by stabilizing the tibia with one hand and applying an anterior force to the hindfoot with the other hand (Fig. 2–3). The normal ankle will have little translation, with a solid end point. The anterior drawer tests the anterior talofibular ligament.
- The talar tilt test assesses the calcaneofibular ligament. The talus is tilted into inversion, but it is important not to confuse hindfoot inversion with talar tilting relative to the tibia.
- For each of these tests, the result should be compared with that for the other side.
- Both these ankle tests are best done with radiographic imaging to precisely quantify the degree of instability. It also may be helpful to perform these tests with the patient under anesthesia to prevent muscle contraction.
- For ankle injuries, external rotation stress testing is important. Pain with external rotation of the foot relative to the leg suggests an injury, but external rotation stress x-rays are the best test for mortise integrity when evaluating malleolar or syndesmotic injuries.
- There can be instability of the MTP joints, especially the second. This is checked by noting the inferior-superior motion of the phalanx on the metatarsal head with stressing.

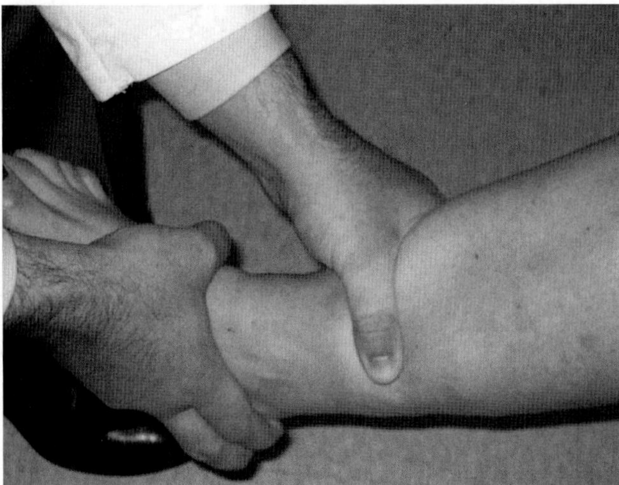

Figure 2–3: Anterior drawer test of the ankle. Stabilize the tibia and translate slightly plantar flexed foot anteriorly.

First Ray Mobility

- As mentioned in Chapter 1, the ideal human foot has evolved to have stability in the first ray, especially at the first metatarsocuneiform joint. This stability gives strength to the medial column, supporting the arch of the foot.
- Instability at the first metatarsocuneiform joint can be three-dimensional, giving rise to a flatfoot, transfer metatarsalgia, and/or hallux valgus.
- Assessing first ray stability is difficult. Several devices have been designed to measure first ray stability. These are outlined further in Chapter 9. However, these devices are not available for regular clinical use.
- Stability of the first ray can be checked on routine physical examination. When examining a right foot, the examiner's left thumb is placed under the lesser metatarsal heads. The examiner's right thumb is placed under the first metatarsal head. Both thumbs apply an equal upward force to the forefoot. Normally, the first metatarsal head should remain even with the second. With hypermobility of the first ray, the first metatarsal head will elevate well above the second.
- Some physicians recommend checking the overall plantar-dorsal translation of the heads, but the important finding clinically is elevation of the first metatarsal above the second.
- A callus beneath the second metatarsal head is indirect evidence of first ray instability.

Strength

- Strength of all the muscle groups is assessed and rated on a 1-5 scale. One is a flicker, 2 is strength unable to overcome gravity, 3 is strength able to overcome gravity, 4 is mildly weak, and 5 is normal.
- It is important to note strength when evaluating neuromuscular patients. If a muscle is to be transferred, it will generally lose one grade of strength, so if a muscle that is graded as 4/5 is transferred for another function, the final strength may be too low to be useful.
- When patients are asked to plantar flex the foot, some patients will push the first ray down more than the others (Fig. 2–4). This is due to *overdrive of the peroneus longus* and is commonly seen with cavus feet. The dynamic plantar flexion of the first ray tends to drive the hindfoot into varus. This process is termed *forefoot-driven hindfoot varus*.
- Some patients will show toe extension when asked to dorsiflex the ankle. This phenomenon, termed *extensor recruitment*, results when the long toe extensors are recruited to assist the tibialis anterior. It may appear in patients with a tight gastrocnemius. In theory, the chronic overactivity of the long toe extensors may lead to clawing of the toes (Fig. 2–5).

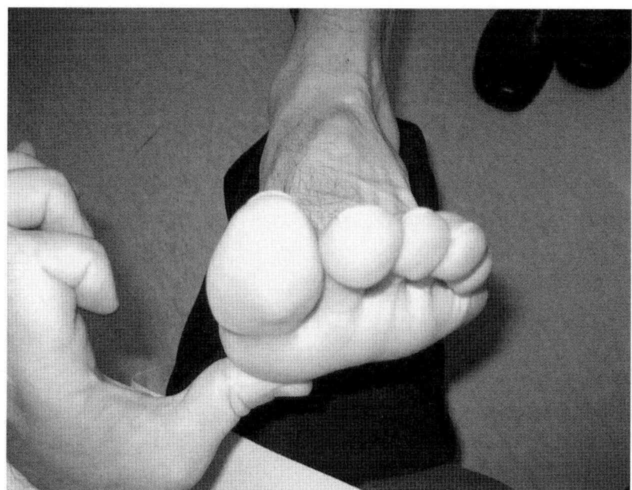

Figure 2–4: An overactive peroneus longus plantar flexes the first metatarsal more than the others.

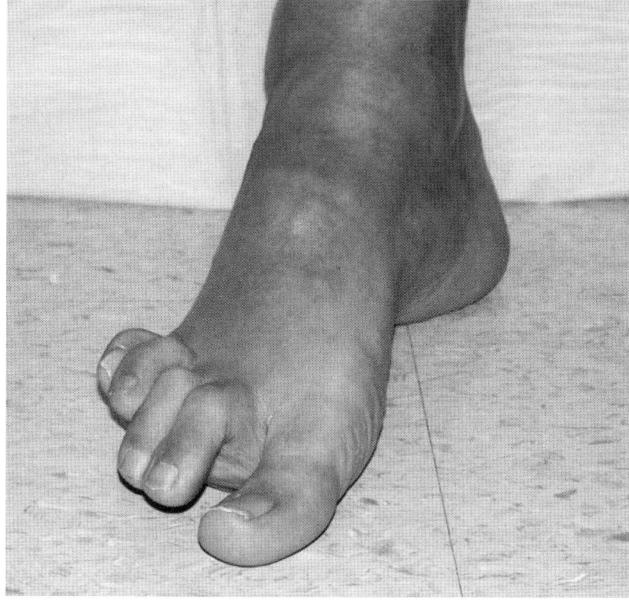

Figure 2–5: This patient has developed claw toes from increased activity of the long toe extensors over time. The foot uses extensor recruitment to "help" ankle dorsiflexion.

Vascular Examination

- Check dorsalis pedis and posterior tibial pulses. The ankle-brachial index can be calculated.
- Look for indirect signs of vascular trouble: loss of hair, ischemic ulcers, or "wooden" skin.

Sensation

- Checking for light touch sensation is obvious and can help when defining previous traumatic nerve injuries.
- However, most diabetic patients with neuropathy will have intact light touch sensation. It is the loss of protective sensation that is important. The Semmes-Weinstein monofilaments are used to check protective sensation. The traditional test is to use the 5.07 (10 g) monofilament on five sites on each foot.
- A recent study found good sensitivity with the use of a smaller force (4.5 g) under the first metatarsal head (Saltzman et al. 2004).
- The dorsal columns can be checked in patients with neurologic disease by testing proprioception at the first MTP.

Alignment

- The patient should stand with both shoes off and both legs visible to a point above the knees. Knee alignment is assessed.
- While looking at the patient from the front, a preliminary judgment about foot alignment can be made. The foot should appear under the leg, not out to the side (as in a valgus flatfoot).
- If the heel is seen medial to the ankle, a varus heel is present. Manoli has termed this the *peek-a-boo heel,* because it "peeks" out from behind the ankle (Fig. 2–6).
- The patient is then viewed from behind. The heel should be in neutral to slight valgus alignment (Fig. 2–7).
- With a planovalgus (flatfoot) deformity, the forefoot will be abducted. The examiner will see the lesser toes lateral to the leg. This has been called the "too many toes" sign (Fig. 2–8).
- The heel rise test is then performed to test for posterior tibial tendon function. While standing on one leg, the patient rises up on to the forefoot. A normal posterior

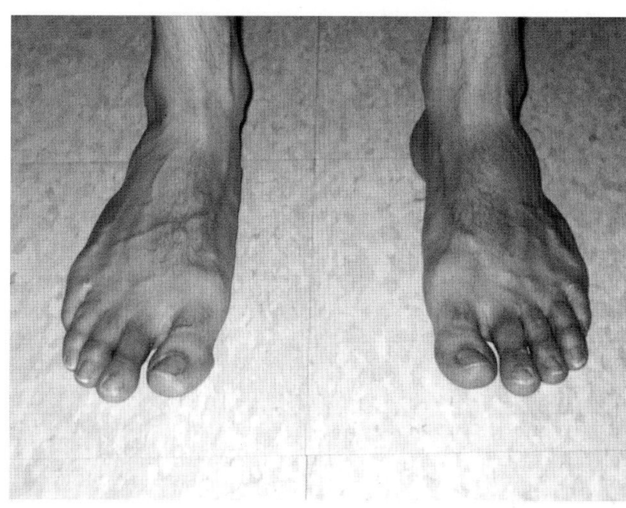

Figure 2–6: The patient's left foot shows a peek-a-boo heel. The heel on the normal right foot is not visible from the front.

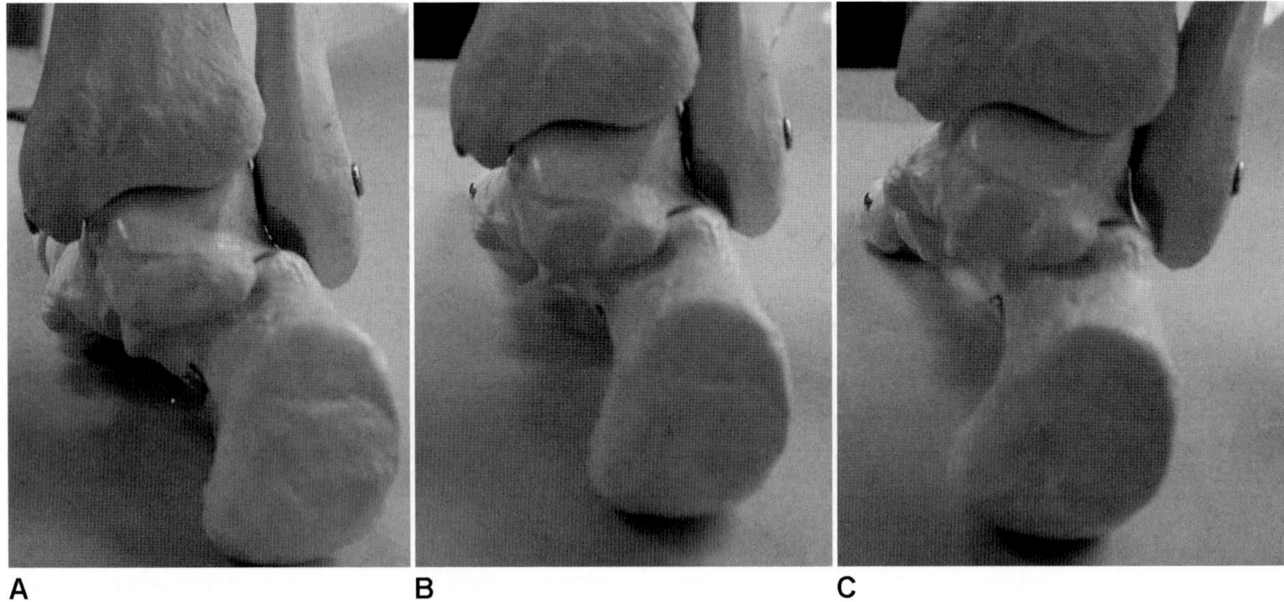

Figure 2–7: **A, The valgus heel is lateral to the leg. B, The neutral heel appears under the leg. C, The varus heel will be medial to the leg.**

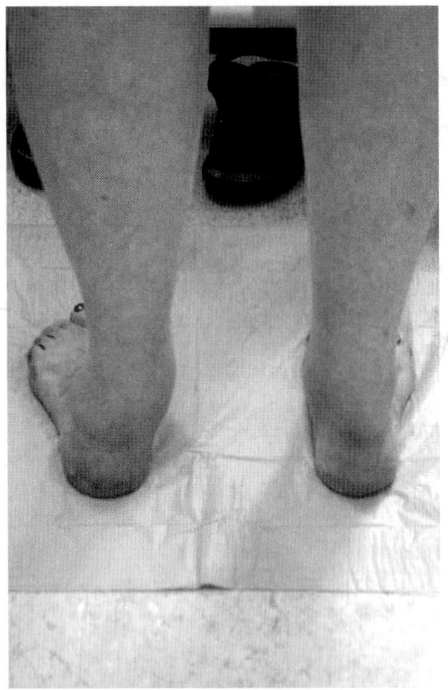

Figure 2–8: **"Too many toes" on the patient's left foot is associated with increased forefoot abduction due to posterior tibial tendon insufficiency.**

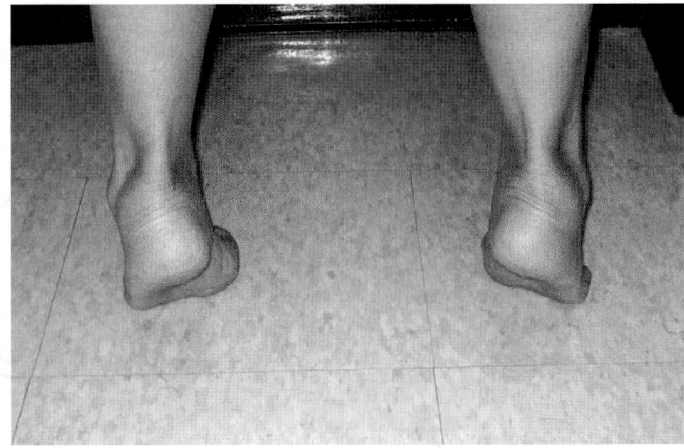

Figure 2–9: **Double-limb heel rise test. Both heels are inverting properly.**

tibial tendon will bring the heel into varus, with no pain. If the heel remains in valgus alignment, or the patient feels pain along the medial hindfoot, then it is likely there is dysfunction of the posterior tibial tendon (Fig. 2–9).

- For the patient with a varus hindfoot (cavus deformity), the Coleman block test is performed. The foot is placed with a block (or a phone book) under the heel and the lateral forefoot. The medial forefoot is allowed to hang over the side. As weight is applied by the patient, the first metatarsal will be able to drop below the level of the block. With a flexible hindfoot, the heel will fall into valgus as the first metatarsal falls below the level of the rest of the foot (termed *forefoot-driven hindfoot varus*). If the hindfoot is stiff in varus, the heel will remain in varus, and no correction will be attained (Fig. 2–10).
- The Coleman block test is based on the tripod model of foot structure, as described in Chapter 1. The first ray supports the hindfoot. Plantar flexion of the first ray drives the heel into varus, and dorsiflexion of the first ray allows the heel to fall into valgus (Fig. 2–11).

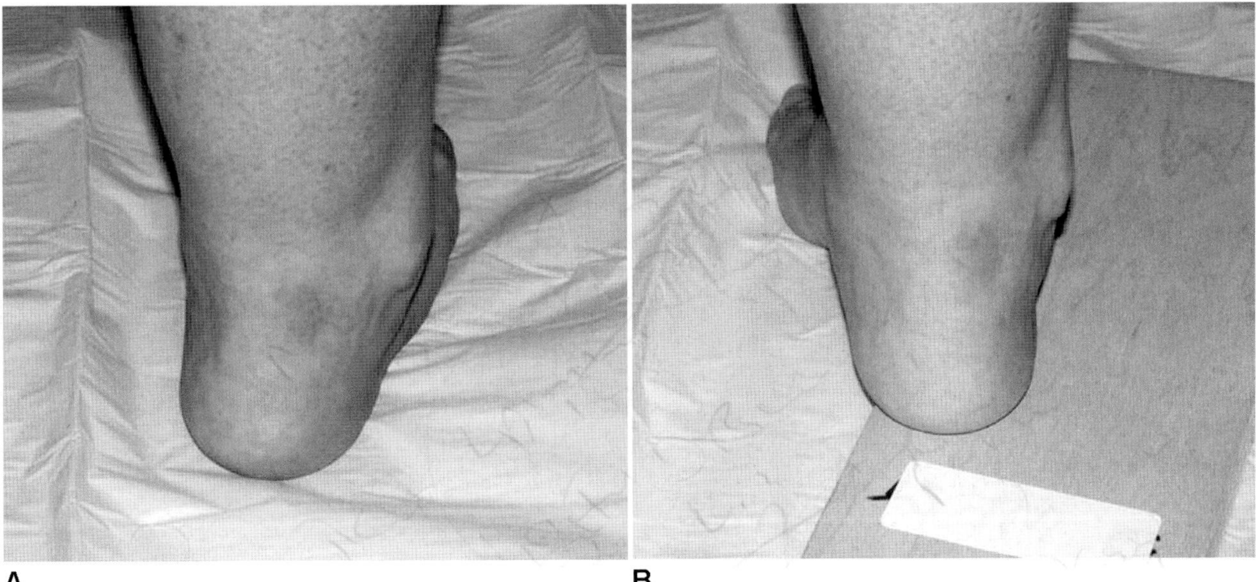

Figure 2–10: **A,** The patient has a cavus foot with heel varus. **B,** With a block under the heel and lateral forefoot, the first metatarsal can "drop down," so the heel shifts to more neutral alignment. This is consistent with forefoot-driven hindfoot varus in this patient.

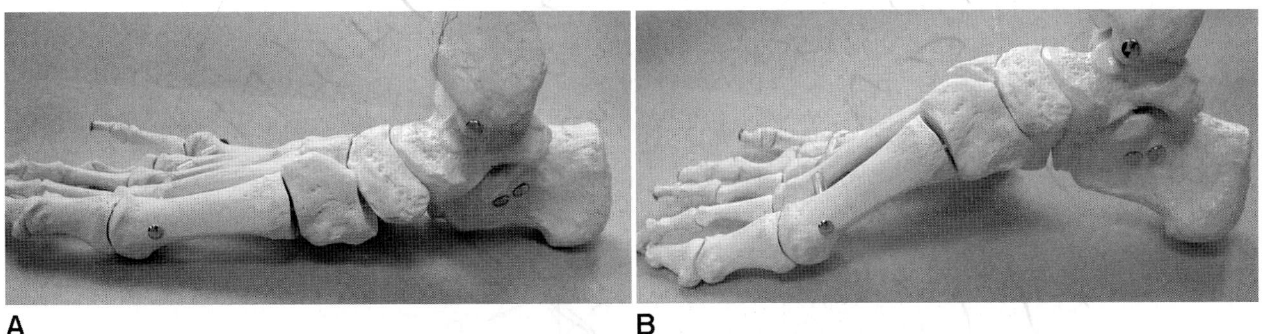

Figure 2–11: **A,** With an unstable first ray (effectively dorsiflexed), the medial column collapses and the hindfoot can fall into valgus. **B,** This foot with a plantar flexed first ray drives the hindfoot into varus. This is commonly seen with many cavus feet.

References

DiGiovanni CW, Kuo R, Tejwani N et al. (2002) Isolated gastrocnemius tightness. J Bone Joint Surg Am 84: 962-970.

A series of patients with foot pathology are compared with a series of patients with normal feet. An increased rate of gastrocnemius contracture was found in those with foot pain. Interestingly, the authors have constructed a device to precisely measure gastrocnemius tightness, although subsequent researchers have questioned the precision of the device.

Manoli A, Graham B. (2005) The subtle cavus foot, "the underpronator." Foot Ankle Int 22(2): 247-264.

Dr. Manoli has presented his observations on a subject that has been ignored too long—the neurologically normal cavus foot.

Morton DJ. (1935) Dorsal hypermobility of the first metatarsal segment: Part III. In: The Human Foot: Its Evolution, Physiology, and Functional Disorders (Morton DJ, ed.). Morningside Heights: Columbia University. pp. 187-195

Morton introduced the concept of first metatarsal instability in human foot disease, but his perspective was more as an anatomist than a clinician. The modern writings of S.T. Hansen, Jr., M.D., and others, have fully developed the concept.

Saltzman CL, Rashid R, Hayes A et al. (2004) 4.5-gram monofilament sensation beneath both first metatarsal heads indicates protective foot sensation in diabetic patients. J Bone Joint Surg 86: 717-723.

In this paper, the authors describe a simple test using one monofilament and one area on the foot to screen for neuropathy. Specifically, the 4.5-g monofilament is applied beneath the first metatarsal head.

Orthotics

Douglas H. Richie Jr.*

*D.P.M., Adjunct Associate Professor of Clinical Biomechanics, California School of Podiatric Medicine, Oakland, CA

Introduction

- Orthosis: An externally applied device used to modify the structural or functional characteristics of the neuromusculoskeletal system. Alternate definition: An apparatus used to support, align, prevent, or correct deformities or to improve the function of movable parts of the body.
- During static stance and during ambulation, the lower extremities are subjected to external forces and moments. During normal function, these forces and moments are resisted or controlled by internal structures of the body. These structures include skeletal segments, ligamentous connections, and muscle-tendon units.
- When internal structures fail, orthoses can modify external forces and moments to allow the body to function in a "normal" manner.
- An external device used to support or improve function of the foot and ankle can take many physical forms. This orthotic can be as simple as a felt pad placed under the metatarsals, or as sophisticated as a composite brace controlling foot and ankle motions.
  - Orthotics prescribed for lower extremity pathologies include foot orthoses (FOs), ankle-foot orthoses (AFOs), knee orthoses, and knee-ankle-foot orthoses.

Types of Orthoses

- Various types of orthoses are commonly prescribed for foot and ankle pathologies. An overview of these orthoses is provided in Table 3–1.
- The basic subcategories of FOs are prefabricated and custom. There are clear differences between the manufacture and design of orthoses in each category, yet advantages or benefit of one type of device over another has yet to be proven.
- Prefabricated devices have the distinct benefit of lower cost compared with custom-fabricated foot orthotics. In addition, prefabricated orthoses can be stocked in the clinic, pedorthic facility, or retail setting for immediate dispensing to the patient.
- The disadvantage of prefabricated orthotic devices is their difficulty in application to limb and foot shapes that fall outside the "average" range.
- Custom molding and contouring of an orthotic device to a body segment may be the critical feature necessary for a successful treatment outcome. Yet the mechanism by which foot orthotics actually achieve their treatment effects remains poorly understood, and thus claims of superiority of custom versus prefabricated devices remain somewhat speculative.
- Prefabricated FOs are available for a wide variety of clinical application. In general, these devices are used to off-load specific areas of the foot, cushion the foot from impact, support the medial longitudinal arch, and provide mild biomechanical control of hindfoot movements.
- Custom FOs fall under two basic categories: accommodative and functional. Functional orthoses are most often used with flexible feet, and work to alter how the foot meets the floor. Accommodative orthoses generally are used with more rigid deformities. Rather

Table 3–1: Types of Orthoses Used for Foot and Ankle Pathologies

	TYPE	EXAMPLES AND DETAILS
Prefabricated	In-shoe pads	Metatarsal pads, callus cushions, medial arch pads, heel pads and cushions
	Flat insoles	Spenco, Sorbothane, Implus
	Contoured insoles	Spenco Polysorb, Apex Lynco, Implus Sof-Sole
	Biomechanical insoles	Superfeet, Ten Seconds Rigid Arch, KLM CP-3000
Custom	Accommodative	Cast technique: direct mold, weight bearing or semi-weight bearing Materials: ethylene vinyl acetate foam, neoprene, polyurethane, cork, polyethylene Uses: total contact orthoses for neuropathic conditions, severe deformity, pressure relief
	Functional	Cast technique: "neutral suspension," vacuum, semi-weight bearing, foam box Materials: polypropylene, polyethylene, TL-2100 Uses: control of forces and joint moments in the lower extremity, sport orthoses, subcalcaneal pain syndrome, chronic ankle instability, adult acquired flatfoot
	Ankle-foot orthoses	Casting: neutral suspension (for functional hinged ankle-foot orthosis), semi-weight bearing, Synthetic Tubular Sock casting sock Materials: polypropylene, polyethylene liner, leather gauntlet closure Uses: adult acquired flatfoot, Charcot arthropathy, drop foot

than attempting to alter foot alignment, accommodative orthoses work to relieve pressure under bony prominences (make the floor fit the foot better).

Prefabricated Foot Orthoses

- The simplest types of prefabricated FOs are in-shoe pads.
- Felt forefoot pads are available to relieve metatarsalgia, sesamoiditis, traumatic neuroma, and intractable plantar keratoma (Fig. 3–1A). These adjust pressure by off-loading adjacent areas and increasing pressure under the pad itself. Thus they are often placed near, but not directly under, the area of pain.
- Heel pads are designed to relieve pressure and symptoms associated with plantar heel spur syndrome and plantar heel fat pad atrophy (Figs 3–1C,D). They distribute forces over a larger area, thus decreasing pressure under the heel.

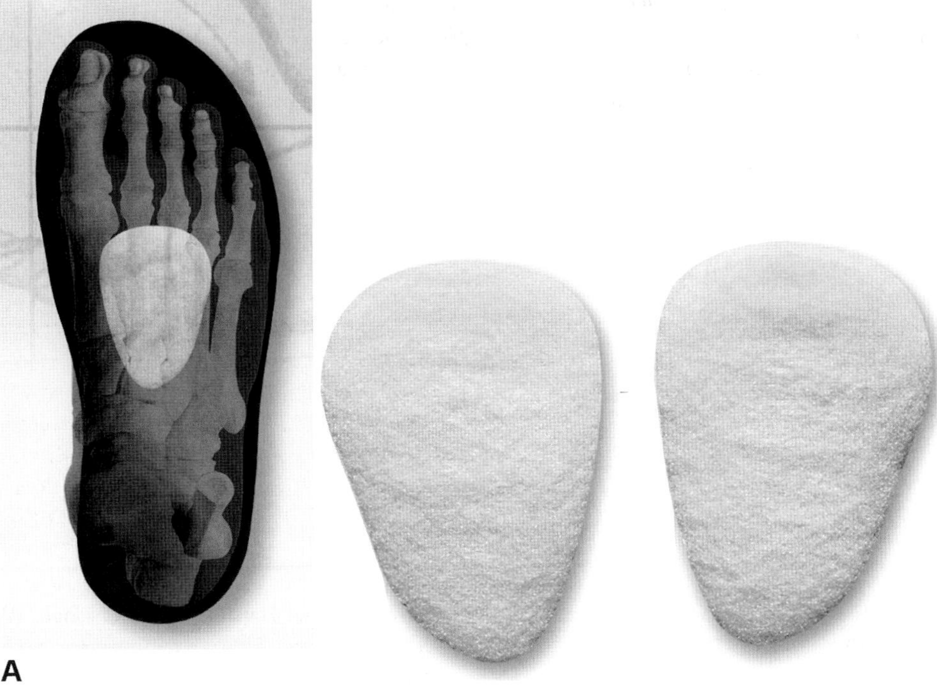

A

Figure 3–1: **A, In-shoe forefoot pads.**

Continued

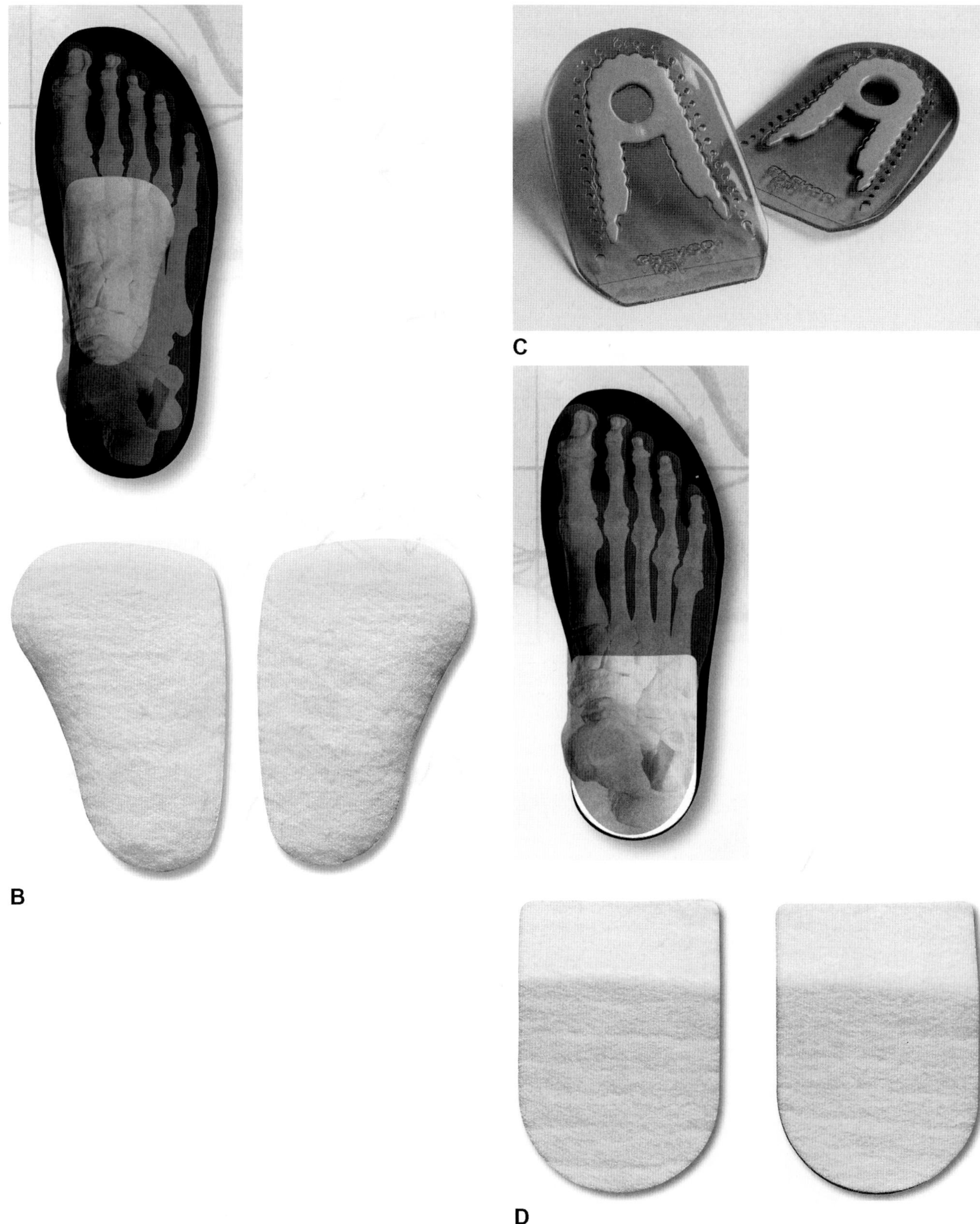

Figure 3–1: Cont'd **B**, Arch pads. **C**, Gel heel pad. **D**, Heel pads. (A, B, and D, courtesy of Hapad, Inc., Bethel Park, PA; C, courtesy of Spenco Medical Corp., Waco, TX.)

- Flat insoles are used primarily for cushioning impact during walking and running. These flat, cushioned insoles can also off-load bony prominences and are used to prevent pressure-induced pathologies of the foot (Fig. 3–2).
- Contoured cushioned prefabricated insoles are also prevalent, and have a wide variety of clinical application for relief of plantar foot pressures, dissipation of impact shock, and enhancement of overall foot comfort. These contoured insoles also function as a softer version of a prefabricated arch support (Fig. 3–3).
- Prefabricated, "biomechanical" semirigid foot orthotics have gained popularity over recent years. These devices are made from materials commonly used in the fabrication of more expensive custom functional FOs. Prefabricated biomechanical devices are contoured to an average shape of a medial and lateral longitudinal arch. In general, these devices lack any heel cup. Sometimes, posting is provided in the rearfoot to enhance pronation control.
- The goal of treatment of these devices is to provide more rigid support and motion control than with softer arch supports (Fig. 3–4).

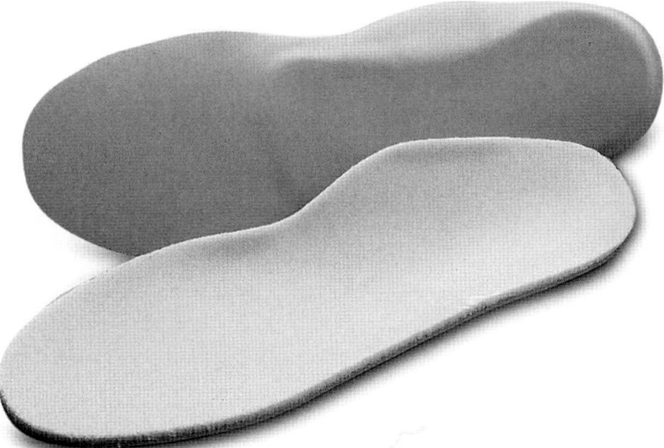

Figure 3–3: Contoured cushioned insoles. (Courtesy of Aetrex Worldwide, Inc., Teaneck, NJ.)

Custom Foot Orthoses

- Custom foot orthotic devices require fabrication to some type of model of the patient's foot. The model on which the orthosis is contoured can be a positive plaster cast, a computer-generated model, or the actual foot of the patient (Fig 3–5).

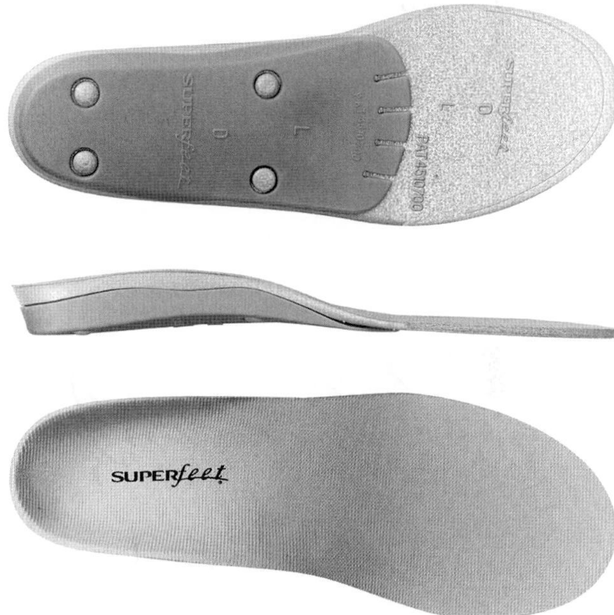

Figure 3–4: Prefabricated biomechanical insoles. (Courtesy of Superfeet Worldwide, LP, Ferndale, WA.)

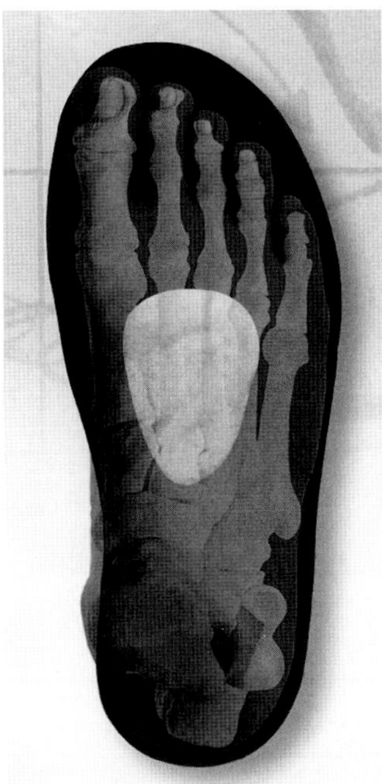

Figure 3–2: Flat cushioned insoles. (Courtesy of Spenco, Inc., Waco, TX.)

- Equally important to the value of any custom foot orthotic is the selection of material composition, which will be unique to the patient's clinical condition or biomechanical needs.
- For simplicity, there are basically two types of custom FOs: accommodative and functional.
- Accommodative FOs are designed to relieve pressure on certain areas of the foot, and to provide support of the foot in its compensated position (Fig. 3–6). The most common use for accommodative foot orthotics is in the management of diabetic foot complications. These devices

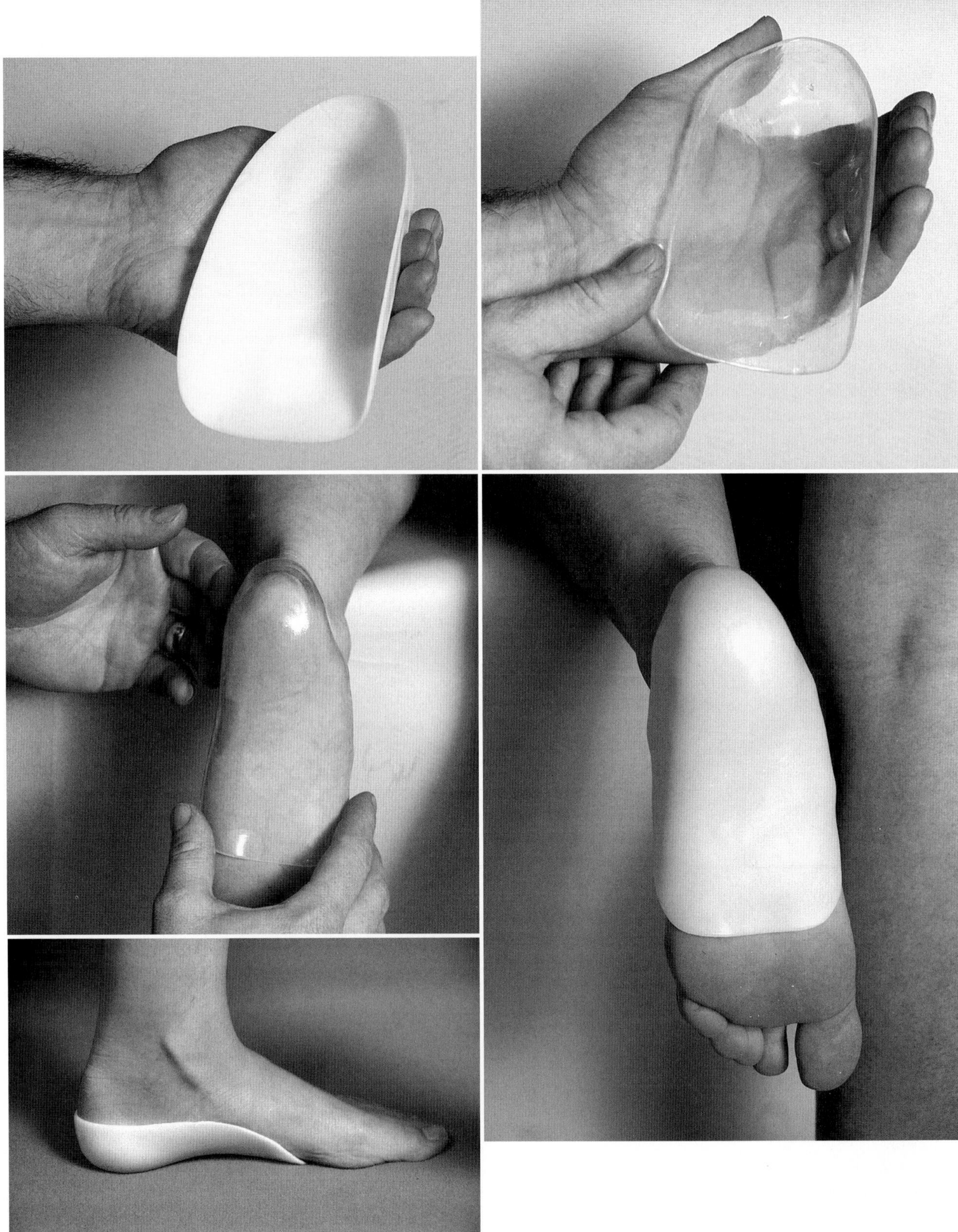

Figure 3–5: Direct molding of foot orthoses to the foot of the patient. (Courtesy of Alimed, Inc. Dedhan, MA.)

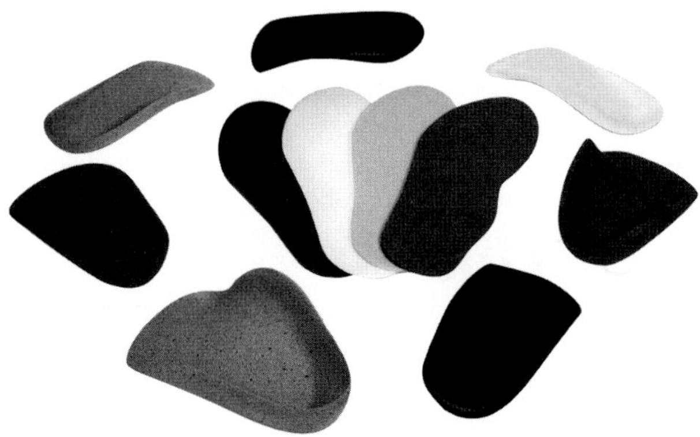

Figure 3–6: **Accommodative orthosis. (Courtesy of KLM Laboratories, Inc., Valencia, CA.)**

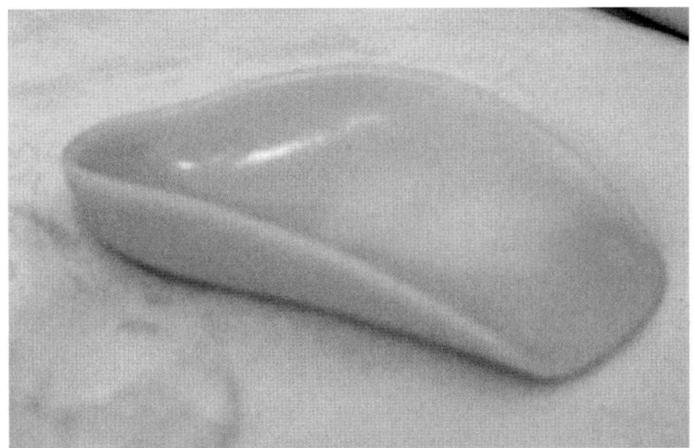

Figure 3–7: **University of California Biomechanics Laboratory orthosis.**

are also known as total contact orthoses, and can disperse plantar pressures to the maximal foot surface area. Most accommodative FOs are fabricated from negative casts taken of the patient in a weight-bearing or semi-weight-bearing position.

- Functional FOs are designed to control forces that act on the foot during the stance phase of gait. These forces are generally pronatory or supinatory forces acting on the subtalar and midtarsal joints.
- While not part of the definition, functional FOs are often expected to correct alignment of the foot. Yet improvements of alignment with functional FOs are relatively modest, as revealed by numerous kinematic studies of these devices (see *Treatment Effects of Orthotics*). Kinetic studies of FOs have confirmed the original definition: These devices can alter forces or moments acting on the joints of the lower extremity.
- A predecessor to the functional FO was the University of California Biomechanics Laboratory orthosis (UCBL). This device is still popular today in the treatment of collapsing flatfoot conditions. The UCBL is a plastic FO with a deep heel cup and very steep medial and lateral flanges (Fig. 3–7). The device is fabricated from a plaster model produced from a semi-weight-bearing cast of the foot.
- The UCBL is best suited to control transverse plane subluxation of the foot by applying force against the lateral wall of the calcaneus, the sustentaculum tali, and the lateral aspect of the fifth metatarsal shaft. These devices have fallen out of favor due to difficulty with shoe fit and the need for multiple adjustments for comfort.
- Functional FOs were developed in the early 1960s by Merton Root, D.P.M., who had developed a classification system of foot morphologies. Several principles apply to functional orthotic development.
- Semirigid to rigid materials are utilized to control significant forces that occur in most foot pathologies (Fig. 3–8).
- Non-weight-bearing, "neutral suspension" casting technique is used. The cast is molded to the foot with no weight across the foot. (As an example, in the case of a flexible flatfoot, the foot is molded when the arch is straight, not when it is collapsed from weight bearing.)

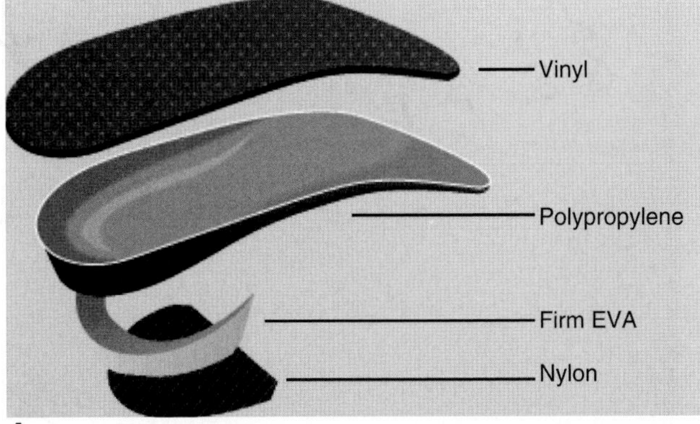

A

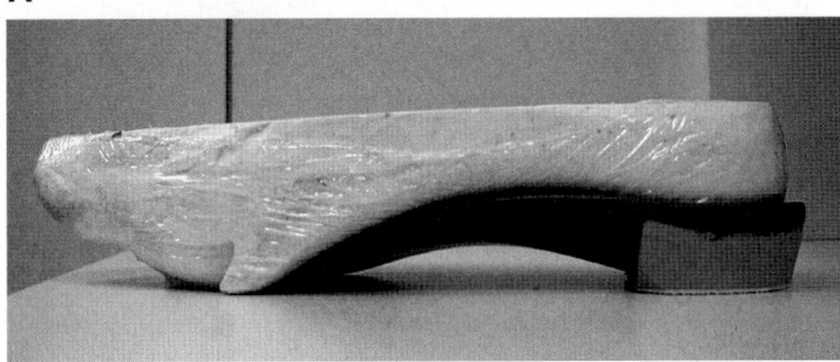

B

Figure 3–8: **A and B, Functional foot orthosis. EVA, ethylene vinyl acetate. (A, courtesy of Paris Orthotics, Ltd., Vancouver, BC, Canada.)**

- Posting is then added to the molded orthosis. In other words, medial or lateral heel wedges are used to tilt the foot in the desired direction.

Casting and Models for Custom Foot Orthoses

- Custom functional FOs can be fabricated from a model of the patient's foot, which can be created from a plaster cast, a digital scan, a pressure scan during dynamic gait, and a direct molded technique to the patient's foot. There are potential shortcomings of each technique.
- Until 10 years ago, the most popular technique for fabrication of custom FOs involved making a "positive" plaster model produced from a negative plaster cast taken of the patient's foot.
- Methods of producing a negative cast of the foot can vary. The most common accepted technique involves an off-weight-bearing, neutral suspension cast taken of the patient's foot. Negative plaster impression casting of a foot is highly dependent on the skill of the practitioner in terms of producing a comfortable, effective foot orthotic device.
- The neutral suspension plaster cast technique attempts to capture a model of the foot in a neutral position at the subtalar joint while the midtarsal joint is pronated and "locked" to end range of motion (Fig. 3–9). This cast will theoretically capture the following characteristics and shape of the foot:
  - intrinsic frontal (coronal) plane deformity of the foot, which can be balanced or adjusted in positive cast correction (Fig. 3–10)
  - the shape of the foot in its presumed "neutral" or "optimal" position of function, void of the influence of ground reaction forces, which would otherwise move the foot to a compensated position
  - the plantar soft tissue contour of the fat pad of the heel and metatarsal weight-bearing surfaces
- The orthosis produced from such a cast technique will have a rounded contoured heel cup, and will contour to the topography of the plantar foot surface.
- A variation of the neutral suspension cast technique utilizes a vacuum cast (Fig. 3–11). This technique requires

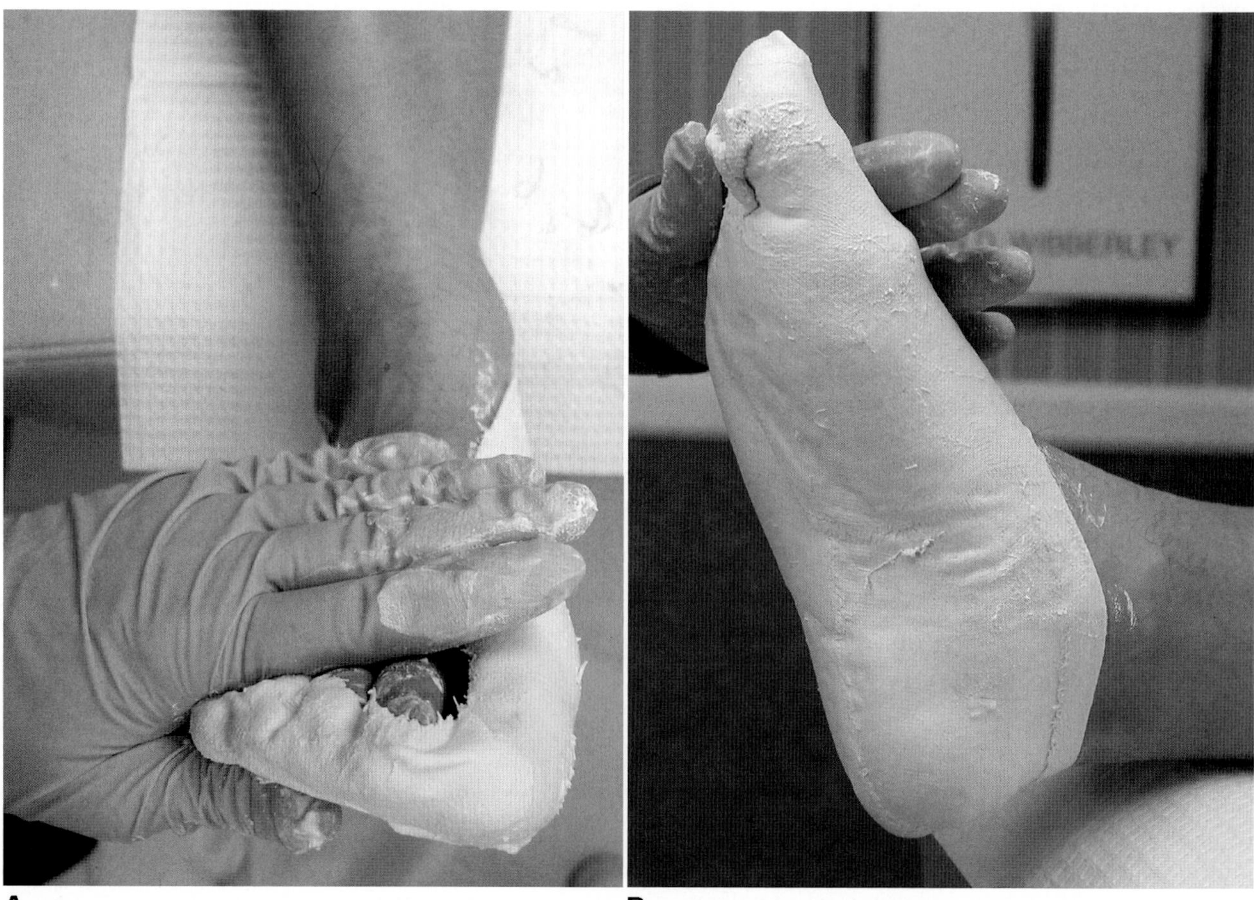

Figure 3–9: Neutral impression cast for functional foot orthosis. A, Foot is positioned in subtalar neutral. B, Forefoot is lifted and pronated.

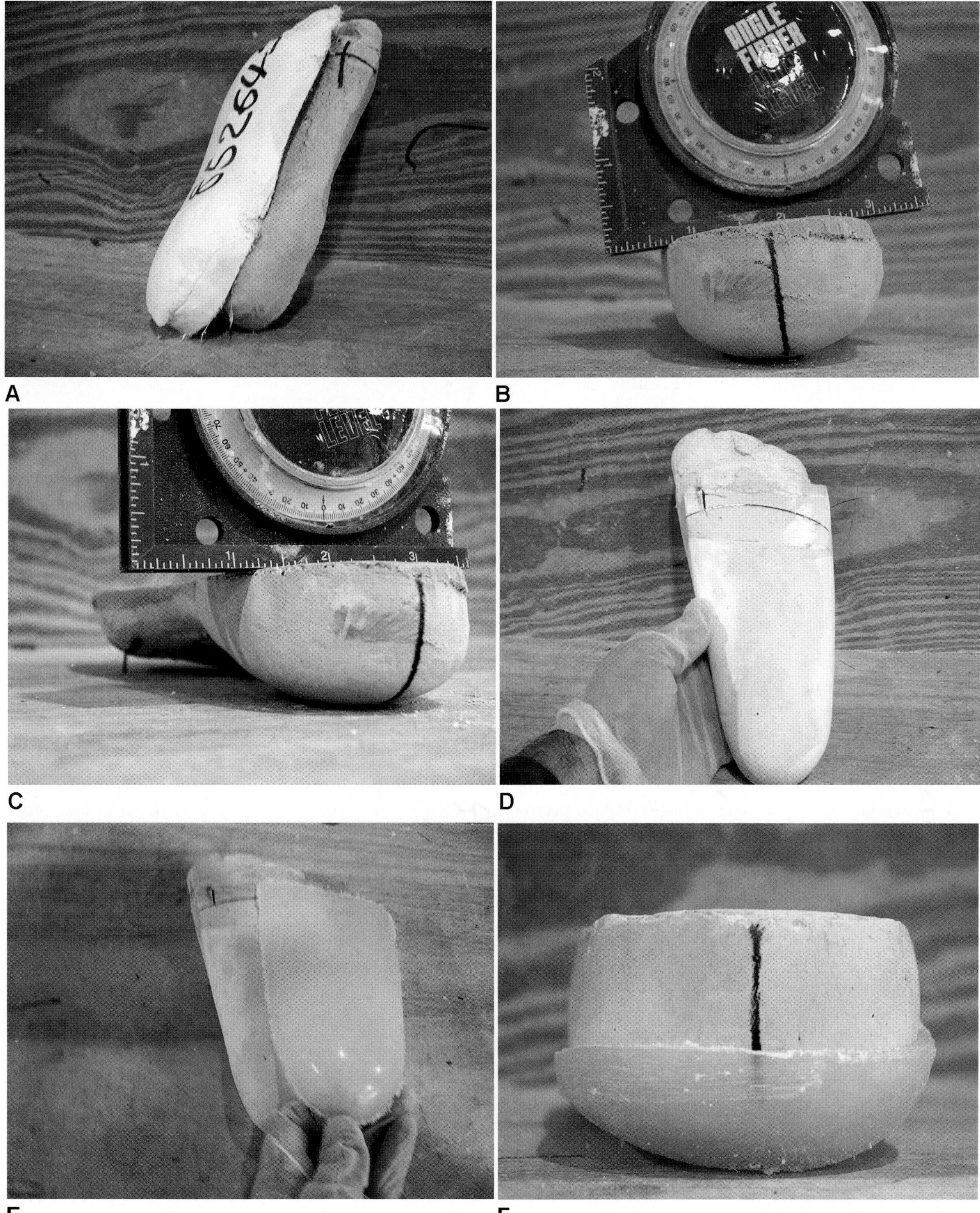

Figure 3–10: **A-F**, Positive cast-balancing functional foot orthosis. A, Positive cast poured from negative cast. **B**, Forefoot to rear foot deformities captured in positive cast. **C**, Positive cast is balanced with heel perpendicular. **D**, Plaster additions to maintain balanced cast and allow soft tissue expansion. **E**, Plastic shell heated and pressed on corrected cast. **F**, Orthosis is balanced identical to positive cast. (A, courtesy Allied OSI Lab, Indianapolis, IN.)

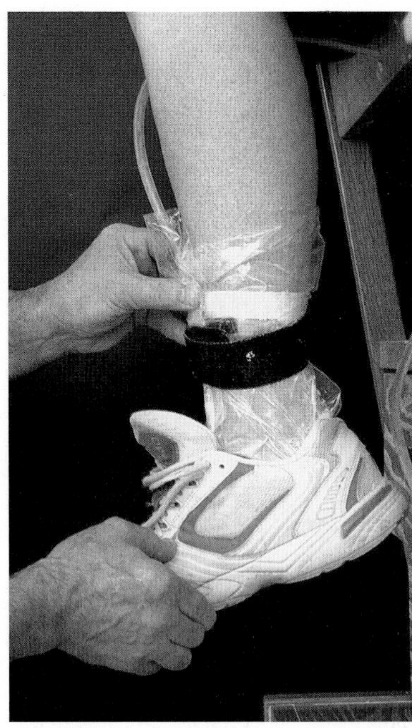

Figure 3–11: Vacuum cast technique. In-shoe negative cast taken with plaster and plastic bag. (Courtesy of Northwest Podiatric Laboratory, Inc., Blaine, WA.)

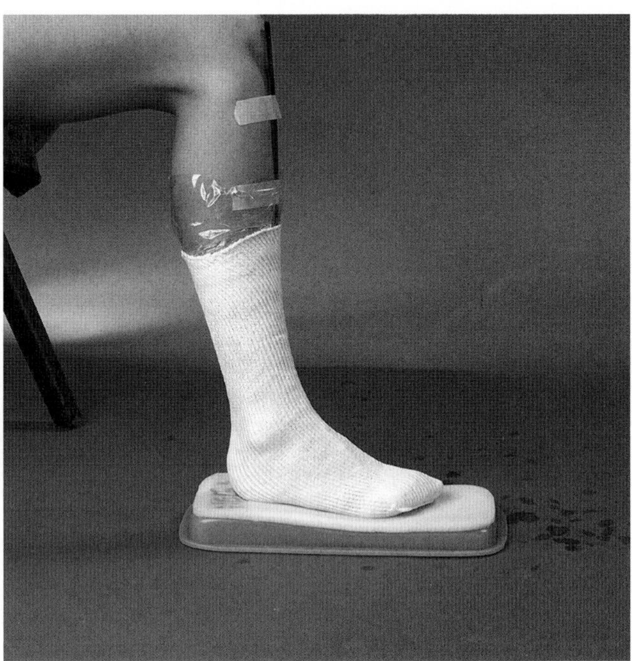

Figure 3–12: Semi-weight-bearing cast technique. Foot is placed on foam block and can be held in alignment or let to rest "as is." (Courtesy of Synthetic Tubular Sock Impression Products, Mill Valley, CA.)

specialized equipment, including a vacuum pump. The cast technique is non-weight bearing and can be used to capture the shape of a foot in a shoe.

- When fit of an orthosis inside a shoe is critical, i.e. with a ski boot or dress shoe, the vacuum cast technique offers a distinct advantage over other methods.
- A semi-weight-bearing negative casting technique places the foot on a foam pad while the practitioner positions the foot in a corrected or "neutral" position at the subtalar joint (Fig. 3–12). The foot will be captured in its somewhat compensated position, but not as fully compensated as it would with full weight bearing.
- A semi-weight-bearing negative cast of the foot will not capture true forefoot varus and valgus deformities, and will not capture the soft tissue topography of the plantar surface of the foot. This technique is best suited for the fabrication of accommodative FOs for patients with significant deformity, such as Charcot arthropathy.
- Foam boxes are a popular technology for producing a negative cast of the foot (BioFoam, Smithers Biomedical Systems, Kent, OH). This technique also utilizes a semi-weight-bearing positioning of the foot (Fig. 3–13). However, the foam is less accurate than plaster in capturing foot topography.
- Foam casting boxes should not be used when a tight conforming FO is desired. As with any semi-weight-bearing cast technique, the positive cast produced from foam boxes will not accurately depict structural forefoot to rearfoot deformities that could be intrinsically balanced. Thus foam boxes are best utilized for the fabrication of accommodative FOs.

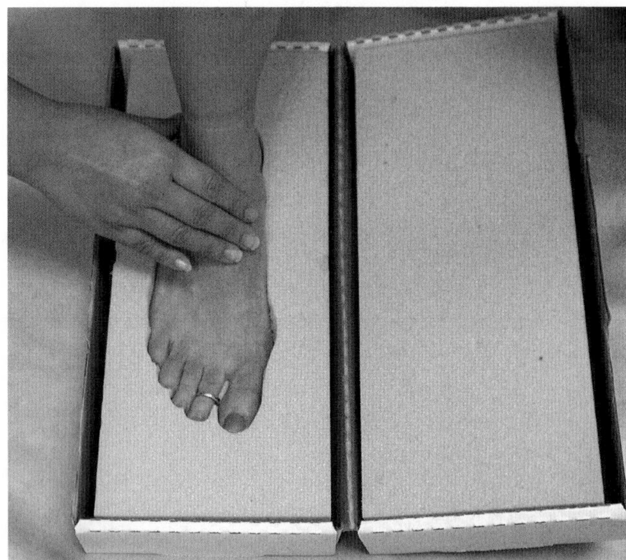

Figure 3–13: Foam box casting technique. Semi-weight bearing with practitioner holding subtalar joint corrected to neutral. (Courtesy of Performance Laboratories Inc., Paterson, NJ.)

- AFOs can be casted using non-weight-bearing or semi-weight-bearing technique. A full foot and leg cast is required, which involves applying plaster or fiberglass casting tape, much the same as applying a short leg walking cast. The cast is bivalved or split for removal.

- Pressure measurements of the foot have been utilized to produce custom foot orthotics. Scientific studies of pressure mapping have disputed whether this technique can accurately depict three-dimensional arch contour and forefoot to rear foot frontal plane deformities, which are captured with traditional negative casting techniques.
- Custom foot orthotics can be produced by directly molding the orthotic material to the foot of the patient. Usually, this is done with a semi-weight-bearing technique. Orthotics made with this technique are shaped to the foot in a compensated position. Therefore orthoses fabricated from a direct mold to the foot of the patient may not fulfill the true definition of a functional FO and are usually utilized as accommodative devices.

Treatment Effects of Orthotics

- The majority of studies of treatment effects of FOs have significant deficiencies that must be noted before any conclusions or recommendations can be made. Many studies are simple retrospective "patient satisfaction" surveys, and few utilize a randomized, controlled, prospective study design. In most cases, the type of orthosis is not described in detail, and description of the foot types of the subjects is often lacking. Still, enough reports have been published that certain consistent findings should be noticed.

Patient Satisfaction Surveys

- Over the past 40 years, numerous patient satisfaction surveys have been published, with 70-80% overall patient satisfaction when foot orthotic devices were used to treat lower extremity injuries.
- Three different studies using semirigid polypropylene custom orthotics to treat patellofemoral pain syndrome have shown that at least 75% of patients report relief of pain attributed to this treatment.
- Another report of 180 people treated with custom rigid orthoses for a variety of athletic injuries revealed that 70% of the patients stated that the orthotics had "definitely helped" their condition, and no adverse effects were reported from use of the rigid orthotics in athletic activity.
- Two rigid types of orthosis materials (Rohadur and TL-61) were studied in the treatment of heel spur syndrome. Thirty-four of 41 patients improved with orthotic therapy and physical therapy combined. Without good controlled studies, it is difficult to know if it was the therapy, orthosis, or just time that helped cure.
- A prospective study compared the treatment effects of two types of FO materials prescribed for 40 professional and recreational athletes. A composite material (TL-2100 SF) was preferred over the standard polypropylene material by the subjects. Overall, 70% of the subjects reported good to excellent relief of symptoms with semirigid, custom orthotic treatment.
- A large retrospective survey of 453 patients, 14 weeks after receiving functional FOs for numerous lower extremity overuse injuries, showed general satisfaction with the orthotic therapy reported by 83% of the subjects.

Effects of Foot Orthotics on Plantar Pressures

- Numerous studies have shown that FOs can significantly reduce vertical force and pressures on various areas of the plantar surface of the foot.
- Peak pressures can be reduced, at the most, by about 20% with an FO. In terms of injury, the significance of this pressure reduction remains speculative.
- FOs have been shown to decrease plantar callus size in patients with diabetes. Patients with leprosy were noted to have improved healing of plantar ulcers with custom FOs.
- A semirigid custom foot orthotic was shown to significantly reduce the incidence of femoral and metatarsal stress fractures in military recruits.
- A prospective 9-week study of military recruits showed that a neoprene insole reduced overuse injuries and tibial stress syndrome from 32 to 23%.

Changes in Foot and Leg Alignment

- Kinematic studies have primarily focused on the effects of foot orthotics on hindfoot alignment. Most of these studies have been performed on running athletes. These studies have demonstrated relatively modest improvements. One study found a mean reduction in hindfoot pronation of 2-3°.
- Rather than causing noticeable change in foot and leg alignment, FOs may have other effects on kinematics. Range of motion of skeletal segments, and velocity of motion, may translate into soft tissue and joint injury.
- Semirigid and soft orthotics have shown a significant effect in reducing the velocity of pronation in both running and walking subjects.
- More recent studies have shown that medially posted custom FOs can reduce the overall range of pronation, the maximum angle of calcaneal eversion, and the range of internal tibial rotation associated with pronation.
- The results of kinematic studies have led most researchers to conclude that these devices do not function to realign the skeleton. These devices can, however, significantly alter kinetics of lower extremity segmental function, as documented by many studies on changes in joint moments with orthotic intervention.

Effect of Foot Orthotics on Joint Moments

- A key area of understanding of orthotic effects on the lower extremity has focused on joint moments. The term *moment* describes a force couple that acts at a distance from an axis of rotation of a specific joint in the body. This force is measured in Newton-meters.
- Much of the recent insight into the treatment effects of FOs has been obtained by studies of joint kinetics. Reduced strain of specific anatomical structures (internal joint moments) has been measured with certain orthotic conditions, and this information can be helpful in designing treatment strategies.
- Wedging of shoe inserts can affect knee joint moments. External varus knee joint moments were reduced by lateral wedged shoe inserts. Also, medial compartment knee joint load was estimated to be reduced with the lateral wedged inserts.
- Medial arch support shoe inserts were shown to reduce lateral patellofemoral joint load during running gait.
- However, some studies have shown that the responses of human subjects to various types of wedging of shoe inserts are subject-specific and unsystematic.
- Mundermann et al (2003) studied various foot orthotic conditions used on 21 runners. Adding a varus post to a flat insert significantly reduced inversion moment at the ankle, as well as maximal external rotation moment at the knee joint.
- Williams et al. (2003) studied the effect of the inverted ("Blake modification") custom FO on various parameters on 11 subjects during running gait. Peak inversion moment of the rear foot was significantly reduced by 54% with the inverted orthosis compared with the no orthosis condition. This indicates that an inverted orthosis can reduce strain on the medial ankle structures, such as the posterior tibial tendon. Peak knee abduction moment increased from no orthosis, to standard orthosis, to inverted orthosis. This indicated that as the foot was inverted, tibial adduction increased, causing increased strain in the knee abduction structures such as the iliotibial band.
- In summary, nearly any type of shoe insert modification that applies medial wedging to the rear foot or molding of the device to the medial arch will significantly reduce rear foot inversion moment during the early phase of running gait. This would indicate a reduced strain of the ankle "invertors," such as the tibialis posterior muscle, and passive structures of the medial ankle, such as the deltoid ligament.

Treatment Effects of Foot Orthoses for Specific Injuries

Heel Pain Syndrome

- Subcalcaneal pain syndrome has been extensively studied in terms of response to treatment with various forms of FOs. Retrospective studies of large groups of patients receiving semirigid and rigid custom FOs report significant improvement of symptoms and high patient satisfaction.
- A well-designed prospective study showed that early-onset subcalcaneal pain responded best to a program of stretching combined with a prefabricated heel pad or arch support, compared with stretching combined with use of a custom semirigid functional FO (Pfeffer et al. 1999).
- However, several retrospective studies of large groups of patients with plantar heel pain have shown disappointing results with the same viscoelastic heel pad used in the aforementioned prospective study.
- A prospective, randomized study compared the results of three types of treatment for long-term, chronic plantar heel pain: corticosteroid injection and non-steroidal antiinflammatory drug, viscoelastic heel cup, and functional FOs. A larger number of patients obtained good to excellent results in the custom foot orthotic group compared with the other groups (Lynch et al. 1998).
- In a static cadaver model, a custom FO has the ability to significantly decrease strain in the central band of the plantar aponeurosis. Devices that contour tightly to the apex of the medial longitudinal arch (talonavicular area) appear to be most effective (Kogler et al. 1996).

Patellofemoral Pain Syndrome

- Foot orthotics have been reported to be very successful in the treatment of patellofemoral pain syndrome, with a success rate of between 70 and 80%. However, most of these studies were not randomized controlled trials, and other adjunctive treatments were utilized.
- Two randomized, controlled studies have shown that an exercise program combined with "soft" orthotics can significantly decrease patellofemoral pain syndrome.

Balance and Postural Control

- The most consistent objective measure of foot orthotic treatment effects have been found in studies of balance and postural control.
- At least four different studies have shown significant improvement in balance control in patients with chronic ankle instability when FOs are utilized.
- Custom-molded foot orthotics have been shown to reduce postural sway in patients after acute ankle sprain, and have been shown to reduce pain while running in these patients.
- Custom-molded FOs appear to reduce postural sway better than flat orthoses. Posting of orthoses appears to also enhance postural control, particularly when medial posting is applied or when pronation of the subtalar joint is controlled.

Material Selection

- Despite the vast array of different types of FOs available, there is not a wide range of materials commonly used in the manufacture of these devices.
- Material selection will usually determine the general classification of the type of orthosis: soft, semirigid, or hard. However, there is little agreement about the true definition and criteria for these categories.
- In terms of stiffness, there is no agreement as to what is standard or acceptable for construction of FOs. Thus it is common to see one orthotic material described as "semirigid" by one author and "rigid" by another.

Materials for Soft Orthoses

- Soft orthoses are primarily used to dissipate plantar pressures and accommodate deformity. For sport application, soft orthoses are used to reduce impact shock.
- Whether custom fabricated from a model of the patient's foot or prefabricated, most soft FOs utilized for the treatment of orthopaedic conditions have a multilayer construction (see Fig. 3–6).
- The choice of materials for these layers usually follows the following principles:
  - a top layer of soft compressible foam or neoprene
  - a middle layer of durable cushioning material such as polyurethane
  - a bottom layer of firmer, non-compressible material such as cork, dense foam, or thin plastic.
- Foam materials and cellular rubbers can have a closed cell or an open cell configuration. Closed cell foams have air pockets that are individually contained and do not connect to each other. Open cell foams have air chambers that connect to each other.
  - Open cell foams dissipate heat and evaporate moisture better than closed cell foams. Open cell foams are generally more durable and resistant to compression deformation than closed cell foams.
  - Closed cell foam materials are susceptible to compression set, and thus are preferred as a top layer for accommodative FOs. High-pressure areas of the foot will collapse the closed air chambers of this material, allowing conformity around bone prominences.
- The most common closed cell foam used in the fabrication of FOs is polyethylene. Polyethylene foams are available under different trade names, and different densities or firmnesses are available.
- Plastazote (BXL Plastics Ltd., ERP Division, Croydon, UK) is the most common closed cell, polyethylene foam used in the foot orthotics industry. It is heat-moldable at 140° and can self-adhere to plastic material at temperatures over 285°. Plastazote is extremely light and is available in three densities or durometers: medium (pink), firm (white) and rigid (black).
- Pelite (Durr-Fillauer Medical Inc., Chattanooga, TN) is another polyethylene foam with similar properties to those of Plastazote. Pelite is available in four durometers and is commonly used as a liner for prosthetics.
- Aliplast is a polyethylene foam also available in four durometers. Manufactured by Allimed Corp., Aliplast is commonly used in direct-molded orthotic fabrication.
- Ethylene vinyl acetate (EVA) is another closed cell foam that has gained popularity in the orthotics industry as a top cover and cushioning material. In the footwear industry, EVA is extensively utilized as a cushioning material in the midsole of athletic shoes.
- Polyurethane is an open cell, thermosetting foam that is not heat moldable.
- Polyurethanes have excellent memory and do not accommodate to pressure or bone prominences.
- The most common polyurethane foam used in the orthotics industry is Poron (Rogers Co., CT). An identical foam is also marketed under the name PPT (Professional Protective Technology). Poron is a good shock attenuator and is very durable. It is commonly used as the middle or bottom layer of laminated soft orthoses. It is not a good top cover due to its poor abrasion resistance.
- Viscoelastic polyurethane such as Sorbothane (Sorbothane, Inc., Kent, OH) and Viscolas (Chattanooga Corp., Chattanooga, TN) is a non-cellular material with unique cushioning properties. Viscoelastic shoe inserts have been demonstrated to have the capacity to attenuate up to 50% of impact shock. However, with high-frequency loading this material may behave in a more rigid fashion, because recovery of shape is very slow. Also, the weight of viscoelastic materials has made them less popular for use in FOs than other foams. Viscoelastic material cannot be ground or heat molded, so its use is limited to prefabricated insoles rather than custom devices.
- Neoprene foam can be used as an inlay for soft orthoses, or can be used as a top cover for any type of orthosis.
- Spenco (Spenco Medical Corp., Waco, TX) is a closed cell neoprene foam with nitrogen bubbles and has a nylon top cover. Developed in 1966, Spenco was originally sold as an athletic shoe insert designed to prevent friction blisters. Now, an entire line of prefabricated Spenco inserts and orthotic arch supports are sold in sporting good stores and pharmacies.
- Spenco material is an excellent top cover for plastic orthotics, as it adds significant cushion and protects the skin from shear stress. Spenco is also very durable and compatible with moisture exposure.
- Lynco (distributed by Apex, NJ) is another form of neoprene but differs from Spenco in being an open cell

foam. Thus Lynco may dissipate heat better than a closed cell foam but may not cushion as well.

- Cork is commonly used as a bottom shell for the construction of custom, soft orthotics. Heat-moldable forms of cork include Thermocork, Birkocork, and Ucocork.
- Non-heat-moldable forms of cork used in orthotic construction include Korex, Orthocork, and Cushion Cork. These types of cork are used in posts and extensions of foot orthotics.
- Brodsky et al. (1988) performed objective testing of five common orthotic insole materials: Plastazote (soft density), Pelite (medium density), PPT, Sorbothane, and Spenco. With cyclic compression testing, Plastazote lost thickness the most, while Sorbothane and PPT did not lose thickness at all. Spenco and PPT performed the best in resistance to shear and compression.
- A final test in this study simulated the ability of a material to reduce force transmitted over a simulated plantar bony prominence. All five materials initially were effective in reducing force. With repetitive load, Plastazote became significantly less effective in this capacity. Sorbothane was the most rigid of the materials and was the least effective in reducing force over a simulated bony prominence.

Materials for Semirigid Orthoses

- Many practitioners interpret the term *semirigid orthosis* to imply that there is a plastic shell of core material comprising the substantial portion of the footplate. It is also known that firmer foams, such as No. 3 Plastazote, can provide the same stiffness as plastic and can be used to fabricate semirigid FOs.
- Others consider any FO that has plastic material in the footplate to be a "rigid" device. Yet rigidity of an FO can vary significantly depending on the type and thickness of the plastic.
- The polyolefin plastics are the material of choice for the fabrication of most custom foot orthotics and ankle-foot orthotics in the USA. Two types of polyolefins are used extensively: polypropylene and polyethylene.
- Polypropylene is more popular than polyethylene for fabrication of FOs, because it is stiffer and more durable. Both materials are thermoplastic, heat moldable, and heat adjustable at temperatures between 360 and 390°F.
- Polyethylene material used for FOs is available in two forms: Ortholene and Sub-Ortholene (Tuefel, Stuttgart, Germany). Ortholene is the stiffer of the two, while Sub-Ortholene is easier to form under heat. Sub-Ortholene is commonly used as a material for the fabrication of "sport orthotics," because it is more flexible than polypropylene. However, Sub-Ortholene is also much more prone to plastic deformation and loss of shape than equivalent thickness of polypropylene.
- Composites have been used for the manufacture of FOs, AFOs, and custom knee braces. Composites consist of a matrix reinforced with a fiber.
- Carbon graphite fiber can be molded to a patient model using thin sheets laminated with liquid resin. This technique, known as "laying up" a composite device, produces an orthosis that is extremely strong and rigid with minimal thickness. The drawback to laminated composite materials is the fact they cannot be heat formed or heat adjusted.
- A proprietary thermoplastic composite known as TL-2100 (Performance Materials, Camarillo, CA) is used extensively in the foot orthotics industry. TL-2100 is thermoformable and heat adjustable. In comparison with polypropylene, TL-2100 can offer equivalent rigidity with less than half the material thickness.

Materials for Rigid Orthoses

- Rigid FOs utilize the same materials as semirigid FOs—the only significant difference is the thickness of the core material of the footplate. Rigid FOs usually do not have a cushioned top cover, which is often found in semirigid orthoses.
- Polypropylene material that is ¼-inch thick will produce a very rigid FO, as will 2.8-mm TL-2100 "rigid" material.
- Rigid FOs usually incorporate polymethyl methacrylate acrylic posts, while semirigid orthoses utilize softer crepe or cork posting materials.

Indications for Soft, Semirigid, and Rigid Orthoses

- Table 3–2 outlines general indications for soft, semirigid, and rigid FOs. These suggestions are based on empiric evidence in the literature. No scientific evidence exists for the superiority of one rigidity over another in the treatment of any lower extremity pathology.
- Rigid orthoses continue to be popular for the treatment of the collapsing flatfoot. Hypermobile foot types appear to tolerate and respond best to rigid orthotic intervention, while rigid cavus feet are best suited to semirigid or soft orthotic designs.
- Soft orthoses tend to be well tolerated by all foot types initially. However, abnormal pronatory or supinatory forces will quickly break down the forgiving materials of these devices, and the intended clinical benefits will be lost.
- Semirigid FOs may be the best devices for most foot and ankle pathologies. When proper impression casting

Table 3–2: Indications for Three Different Categories of Foot Orthoses		
CATEGORY	MATERIAL COMPOSITION	INDICATIONS
Soft	Plastazote Aliplast Pelite Ethylene vinyl acetate Poron (PPT)	Diabetic foot Rheumatoid foot Cavus foot
Semirigid	⅜-inch polypropylene Sub-Ortholene (3 and 4 mm) TL-2100 SF (composite)	Sport injuries Patellofemoral pain syndrome Subcalcaneal pain syndrome Mild to moderate pronation
Rigid	¼-inch polypropylene 5-mm Sub-Ortholene TL-2100 "rigid"	Severe pronation (i.e. flexible, collapsing flatfoot) Tarsal coalition Chronic ankle instability

and positive cast correction are followed, semirigid functional FOs are very well tolerated by most foot types. Positive effects of these devices as reported in patient satisfaction surveys are well documented in the literature.

Specific Indications and Prescription Guidelines for Foot Orthoses

Forefoot Conditions

First Metatarsophalangeal Pathologies

- Conditions that cause painful range of motion of the first metatarsophalangeal (MTP) joint include degenerative joint disease (hallux rigidus), tear of the plantar capsule ("turf toe"), and injuries to the sesamoid apparatus.
- Three basic strategies are available to the clinician when designing an orthotic to alleviate pain in the first MTP joint:
  - block all motion of the joint
  - increase range of motion of the joint
  - off-load plantar pressure and loading of the joint.
- In both turf toe and hallux rigidus, stopping or blocking motion of the first MTP joint is desirable. This can be accomplished by inserting a full-length carbon graphite plate inside the shoe. Plates are available from various manufacturers in various stiffness and toe spring design. The plate makes the shoe into a "hard-soled shoe."
- Another blocking strategy utilizes a footplate extension in a custom functional FO. Here, the plastic footplate is extended across the great toe joint and ends at the tip of the hallux (Fig. 3–14A). Usually, a padded extension is necessary to prevent edge irritation of the plate extension.
- Finally, a rocker sole can be applied to existing footwear to block motion across the first MTP joint, but this may not be as effective or as acceptable to the patient as other strategies.
- Improving range of motion across the first MTP joint is accomplished by facilitating plantar flexion of the first metatarsal head on the fixed hallux during the terminal stance phase of gait. The Kinetic Wedge is a proprietary

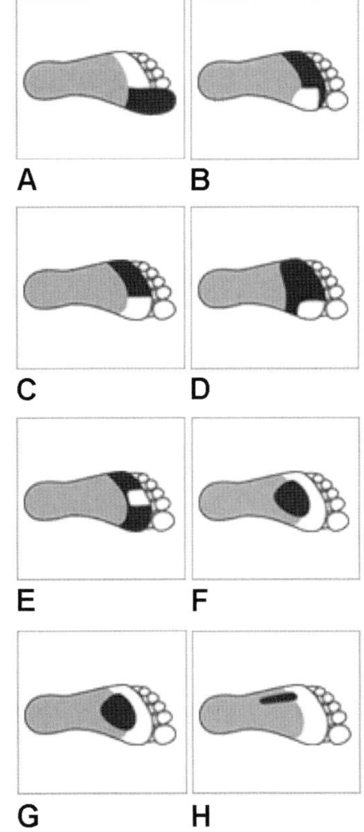

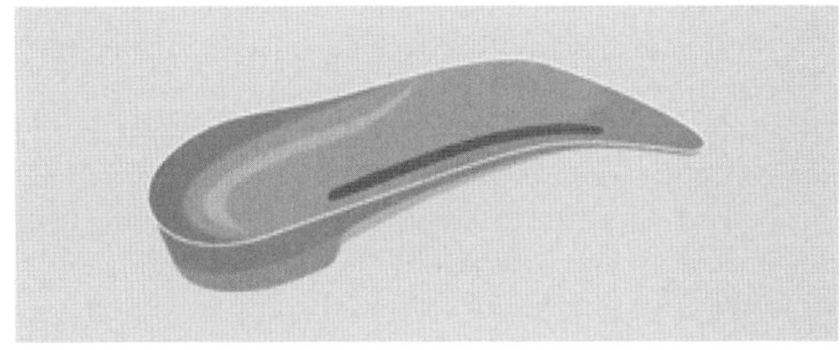

Figure 3–14: Various foot orthotic modifications or additions. **A**, Rigid first extension. **B**, Functional hallux limitus accommodation; **C**, Reverse Morton extension. **D**, Dancer's pad. **E**, Forefoot/metaphalangeal joint lesion accommodation. **F**, Metatarsal pad. **G**, Metatarsal bar. **H**, Neuroma pad. **I**, Fascial accommodation. (Courtesy of Paris Orthotics, Ltd., Vancouver, BC, Canada.)

foot orthotic design with a cutout under the first metatarsal head to facilitate plantar flexion. Another technique is a first ray cutout of the medial aspect of the orthosis footplate, allowing freedom of the first ray to plantar flex off the device during propulsion (Fig. 3–14B).
- A reverse Morton extension on a custom functional FO is also used to plantar flex the first metatarsal below the plane of metatarsals 2–5, and is designed to improve range of motion of the first MTP joint (Fig. 3–14C).
- Off-loading the first MTP joint is used to treat pathologies of the sesamoid bones. A dancer's pad is similar to a reverse Morton extension, but off-loads the plantar aspect of the first metatarsal head and sesamoid apparatus by extending proximal to this area (Fig. 3–14D). A wider custom orthotic footplate with a varus post will elevate the first metatarsal and sesamoids, but may run the risk of creating a hallux limitus condition.

Central Metatarsalgia

- This category includes many diagnoses, including second MTP synovitis, loss of plantar fat pad, and interdigital neuroma.
- Foot orthotic strategies for these conditions involve either:
  - blocking motion of the lesser MTP joints or
  - off-loading the affected metatarsal head.
- Blocking motion across the lesser MTP joints is most useful for arthritis, and can be accomplished with either a rocker sole modification to the footwear, or the application of a carbon graphite plate to the shoe.
- Off-loading the central metatarsal phalangeal joints can be accomplished both indirectly and directly.
- Many cases of bursitis, capsulitis, or callusing around a central metatarsal head are due to failure of the first metatarsal head to accept load during late midstance and terminal stance.
  - Modifications can be added to the functional FO to further enhance stability of the first ray and therefore decrease load under the central metatarsals. A reverse Morton extension is one technique to elevate the lateral metatarsals while allowing the first metatarsal to plantar flex via dynamic mechanisms (Fig. 3–14C).
  - A first ray cutout is an effective way to improve weight bearing under the first metatarsal while decreasing load under the central metatarsals (Fig. 3–14B). A Kinetic Wedge is a proprietary version of a first ray cutout.
- Direct off-loading of the central metatarsals can be accomplished with forefoot extensions added to an FO, with accommodations placed under the area of pathology. Accommodations can be in the form of a cutout or a linear channel created in the padded extension (Fig. 3–14E).
- A metatarsal pad or metatarsal "dome" will off-load the metatarsal head that is located immediately distal (Fig. 3–14F). This may not be due to actual "elevation" of the affected metatarsal. Rather, increased surface area of contact of the orthosis to the plantar surface of the foot occurs (proximal to the metatarsal head) when a metatarsal raise is applied to an FO. In this case, close contouring of the entire orthotic footplate to the plantar surface of the foot may accomplish more than any localized metatarsal pad. (In other words, by increasing the area of contact of the foot with the "floor," the pressure under the foot is decreased.)
- A metatarsal bar applied to an orthosis will theoretically elevate all the metatarsals from the weight-bearing surface, although available movement of these metatarsals in the sagittal plane may be minimal (Fig. 3–14G). A metatarsal bar, whether applied to an orthosis or to a shoe, will also direct ground reaction forces to a more proximal location of the metatarsal, theoretically away from the area of pathology.
- In some mild cases, a cushioned prefabricated orthotic will simply better distribute forces and cushion the area of pain. This is especially helpful in feet with moderate symptoms and minimal deformity.
- When treating interdigital neuroma of the forefoot with any type of shoe insert, a potential aggravation of the condition can occur if there is any compromise of shoe fit. Cushioned, properly fitted footwear is essential in the treatment of forefoot neuromas. Any orthotic designed to treat a neuroma will fail if shoe fit is made tighter.
- Prefabricated "dress orthotics" can be very effective in treating metatarsalgia or neuroma in women wearing pumps and elevated heels (Fig. 3–15).
- For standard footwear, the insertion of a metatarsal pad proximal to the neuroma is a standard practice that has been reported to give relief for patients with mild symptoms of a neuroma.
- For more symptomatic neuromas, the use of a custom functional FO may relieve symptoms due to two mechanisms:
  - off-loading of the metatarsals by directing ground reaction forces to the midfoot
  - decreasing pronation of the foot.
- Foot pronation causes a distal-lateral migration of the forefoot and metatarsals during midstance and terminal stance. This motion is thought to be one mechanism by which the intermetatarsal nerves may be traumatized. Controlling pronation may decrease shear of the third and fourth metatarsals against the plantar digital nerve in the third intermetatarsal space.
- Enhancement of an FO for relief of a neuroma can be accomplished with application of a metatarsal pad or a more oblong "neuroma pad" proximal to the neuroma site (Fig. 3–14H), or the orthotic footplate can be modified by reshaping the positive model to create an elevation between metatarsals 3 and 4 to

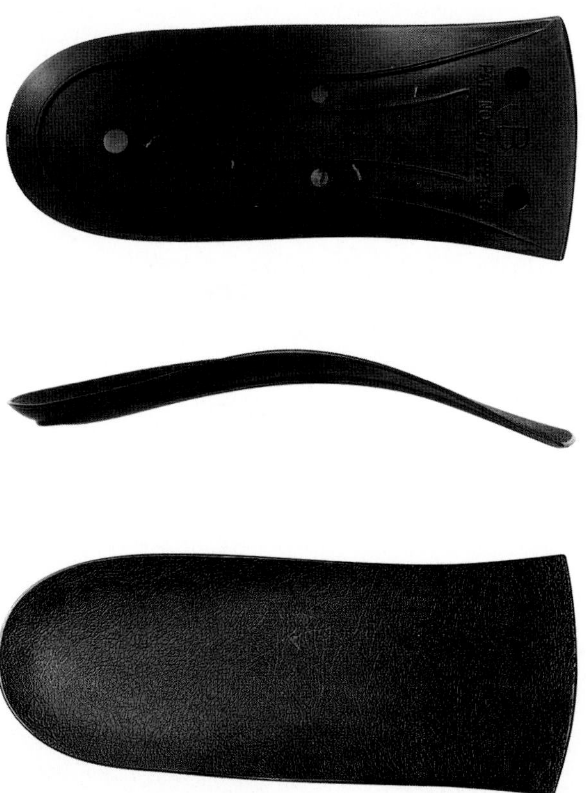

Figure 3–15: Superfeet "dress" prefabricated orthotic. This thin polypropylene shell is designed to off-load pressure in the forefoot in women's pumps and heels. (Courtesy of Superfeet Worldwide, LP, Ferndale, WA.)

theoretically lift and "spread" the metatarsals off the injured nerve.

Heel Pain Syndrome

- Perhaps no other foot condition is most often treated with FOs than subcalcaneal pain syndrome. Probably the majority of people using FOs for heel pain are self-treating with devices purchased in pharmacies or sporting goods stores.
- Most healthcare professionals recommend several types of treatment before prescribing custom foot orthotic devices for subcalcaneal pain syndrome. The cornerstone of this treatment is stretching of the heel cord and use of footwear with heel elevation and stable shank construction.
- When FOs are prescribed by healthcare providers to treat subcalcaneal pain, prefabricated devices are usually preferred as the initial treatment.
- While some practitioners view subcalcaneal pain to be the result of impact shock, the recommendation of a simple heel cushion has resulted in various levels of improvement according to several studies. Viscoelastic heel cups may appear soft on initial examination, but actually behave as a rigid material when repetitive load is applied over a bone prominence. However, any heel pad that elevates the rear foot will conceivably decrease load on the heel cord, which is thought to be a primary contributor to subcalcaneal pain syndrome.
- Most authorities attribute the primary cause of plantar heel pain to an overload of the central band of the plantar aponeurosis. This overload is thought to be due to a combination of tension in the heel cord and elongation of the medial longitudinal arch of the foot.
- Hence most foot orthotic strategies designed to relieve symptoms of plantar heel pain are directed toward providing stability to the medial longitudinal arch of the foot.
- A vast array of prefabricated "arch supports" are available in the commercial marketplace and from professional foot appliance vendors. A broad range of materials, thicknesses, and shapes of these devices allow the prescribing practitioner the ability to select a support best suited for the patient's footwear, lifestyle, and foot type (Fig. 3–16).
- Custom FOs are commonly prescribed for subcalcaneal pain syndrome. The preferred design, material composition, and posting of custom orthoses for subcalcaneal pain vary significantly among various disciplines and among practitioners within any discipline. This reflects poor understanding and agreement of how an FO can off-load strain in the plantar fascia.
- Kogler et al. (1999) studied the effects of various wedges and orthotic designs to decrease strain in the central band of the plantar aponeurosis. A lateral wedge applied under the forefoot reduced strain in the plantar fascia better than a medial wedge or a hindfoot wedge.
- FOs that have close contouring to the talonavicular area also appear to decrease strain in the plantar fascia.
- A heel lift, by itself, could decrease the pitch of the proximal strut of the truss. However, by decreasing load or tension in the heel cord, a heel lift could increase calcaneal pitch and decrease strain on the plantar aponeurosis.
- Semirigid polypropylene material is recommended for the construction of FOs in the treatment of subcalcaneal pain syndrome. Support of the medial arch and resistance to flattening are essential requirements for orthoses designed to decrease strain in the plantar aponeurosis.

Cavus Foot

- The cavus foot predisposes to a number of conditions that may respond to FO therapy. However, the cavus foot type can present a challenge to the practitioner, as these feet are less forgiving and less tolerant of orthotic correction than other foot types.
- Cavus feet are often described as "cavoadductovarus" in terms of alignment, i.e. high arch, forefoot adductus, and hindfoot varus. The varus alignment of the hindfoot in stance may be the result of compensation for a forefoot

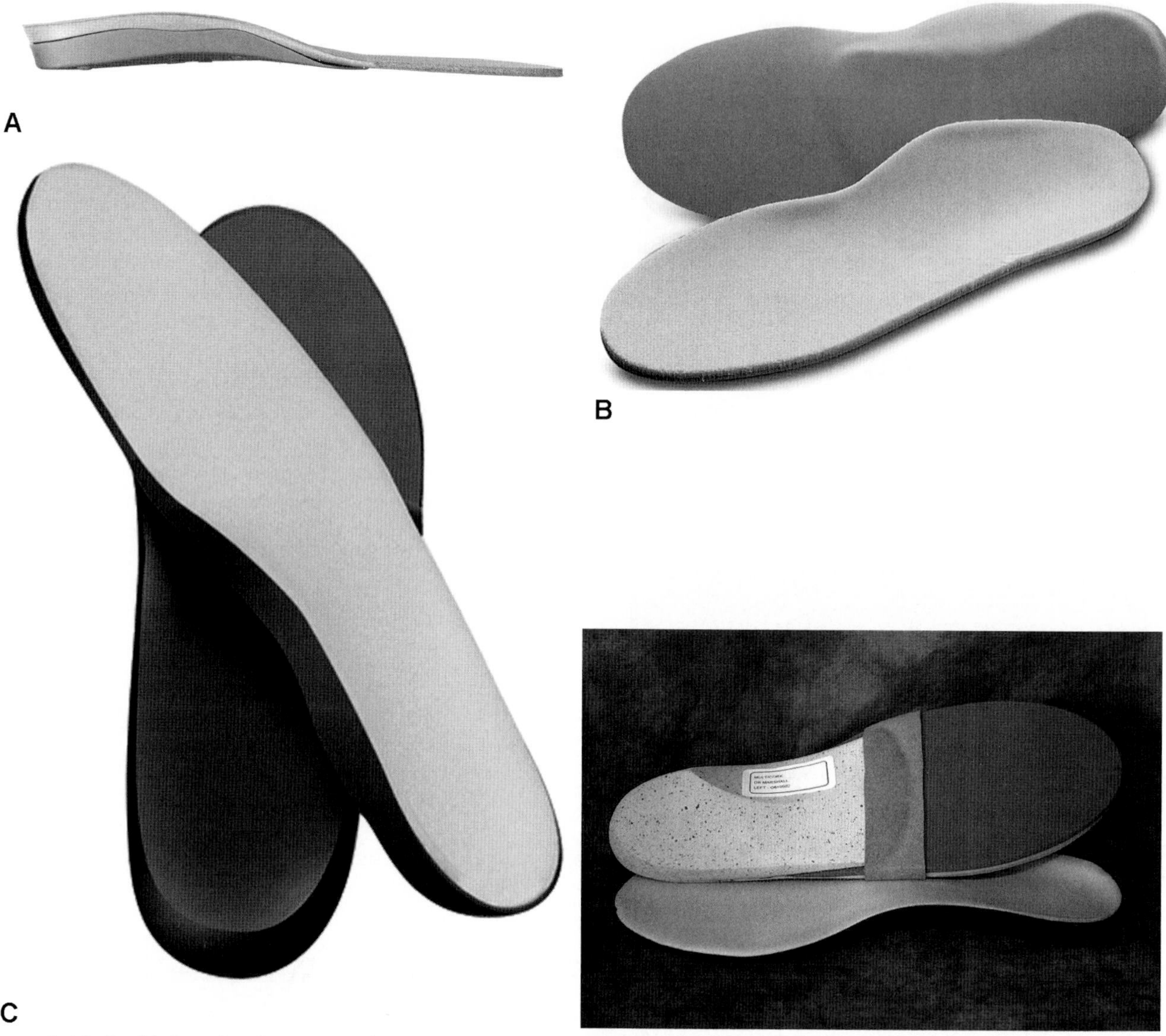

Figure 3–16: **Prefabricated arch supports. (A, courtesy of Superfeet Worldwide, LP, Ferndale, WA; B, courtesy of Aetrex Worldwide, Inc., Teaneck, NJ; C, courtesy of KLM Laboratories, Inc., Valencia, CA.)**

valgus or plantar flexed first ray deformity, or the varus position of the hindfoot may indicate a true positional deformity where subtalar joint range of motion in the direction of eversion is limited.

- When hindfoot varus is secondary to a plantar flexed first ray, a functional FO can be of value to reduce deformity and improve stability in gait. In this case, application of a forefoot valgus post, or a depression under the first metatarsal head, will allow the hindfoot to fall into eversion.
- The ability of an FO to move a hind foot out of varus alignment is dependent on available range of motion of the subtalar joint in the direction of eversion, or pronation. With fixed hindfoot varus, such an orthosis will not correct foot alignment. Thus visible correction of varus alignment may not occur with FO intervention. However, symptoms can improve because FOs can influence joint moments and resultant strain on soft tissue structures.
- Another condition commonly found in cavus feet is the formation of plantar calluses across the forefoot. This may be the result of forefoot equinus, hindfoot equinus, or both.
- Pressure-induced plantar foot pain is associated with the cavus foot because of the rigidity of the foot type and poor shock-absorbing capacity. Also, the cavus foot has less surface area for weight-bearing contact, so forces are focused on the heel and metatarsal heads.
- FOs can reduce high plantar pressures seen in cavus feet by distributing ground reaction forces to the midfoot, and also by providing cushion along the entire plantar surface of the foot.

- The requirements of an FO in treating the cavus foot therefore are geared toward cushioning and reduction of plantar pressures. While soft, accommodative orthotic devices may seem a logical choice, these devices are not ideally suited to reduce varus joint moments and relieve strain on soft tissue structures. Cavus feet, due to less joint mobility, reduce impact shock more poorly than rectus feet, and are likely to crush or bottom out the foam materials used in soft, accommodative orthotics.
- Rigid cavus feet generally are not well suited for rigid FOs. Even semirigid orthotics will not always be tolerated by the cavus foot.
  - A good compromise of cushion and support is best suited for the cavus foot. A thin polypropylene shell (⅛ inch) that is reinforced with Poron on the plantar and dorsal surface (sandwich design) can produce a giving but supportive orthotic device for the cavus foot.
- A top cover of soft polyethylene (pink Plastazote) will protect the Poron layer from abrasion.
- One modification of the orthotic footplate recommended for cavus feet is the incorporation of a plantar fascia "groove" or accommodation (Fig. 3–14I). Most cavus feet have a prominent, tight medial slip of the plantar fascia that bowstrings considerably during terminal stance and tensioning of the windlass mechanism. Any tightly conforming orthotic footplate has the potential to irritate the plantar aponeurosis in the cavus foot.

Lateral Ankle Instability

- Objective measures of positive effects of FOs have been most consistent in studies of subjects with ankle instability.
- FOs, both prefabricated and custom, have been shown to reduce medial-lateral postural sway during single-leg and bipedal stance (Hertel et al. 2001). Improvements in balance and postural control with FOs are more likely in patients after lateral ankle sprain, compared with in healthy subjects. However, similar positive effects of FOs improving balance control have been shown in healthy subjects with excessively pronated feet.
- Possible mechanisms by which FOs can improve balance and postural control include:
  - reducing range of motion of the ankle joint and/or subtalar joint
  - maintaining alignment of the foot in a "neutral" position at the subtalar joint, which may enhance ligament mechanoreceptor function
  - improving tactile sensation on the plantar surface of the foot
  - reducing muscular strain about the ankle.
- FOs fabricated from firm or rigid materials appear to enhance neuromuscular control of the ankle.

Flatfoot

- Perhaps the mildest manifestation of the acquired flatfoot is with tenosynovitis of the posterior tibial tendon (stage 1 of posterior tibial tendon dysfunction). The arch is not collapsed, and the posterior tibial tendon and the key ligaments of the medial arch and hindfoot are intact.
- In stage 1, stabilization of the foot with proper footwear and in-shoe orthoses may protect against progression of deformity, although no validation of the long-term protective effects of this strategy has been reported. The orthosis should provide some arch support with a medial heel post, to encourage hindfoot varus and facilitate the action of the posterior tibial tendon.
- For a foot with visible arch collapse, a slightly different strategy must be followed.
- FOs prescribed for adult acquired flatfoot should be made of semirigid or rigid materials to resist the severe compressive forces that occur in this deformity. One approach is similar to a UCBL—extremely deep heel cup, medial and lateral flanges, and an inverted heel seat using a medial skive technique (Fig. 3–17).
- With a collapsed arch, the talar head or navicular may be prominent medially. A depression or "sweet spot" is often needed in the talonavicular section of the orthotic footplate to avoid irritation.
- For a flexible, mild flatfoot with posterior tibial tendon pain, a low arch support with medial heel post can be used. With intact hindfoot ligaments, inversion of

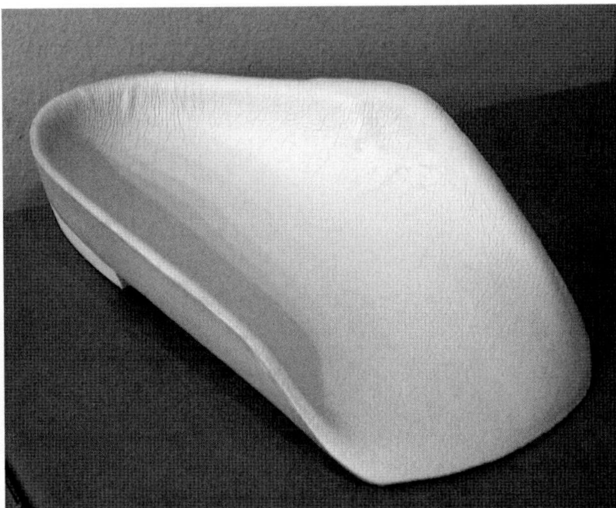

Figure 3–17: Posterior tibial tendon dysfunction orthotic. A custom, functional orthotic with the following additions to enhance control of the adult acquired flatfoot: deep heel cup, high medial and lateral flanges, inverted medial heel post, and "sweet spot" at talonavicular joint prominence. (Courtesy of Allied OSI Orthotics, Indianapolis, IN.)

the subtalar joint will protect the posterior tibial tendon.

- FOs contact only the plantar surface of the foot, and therefore rely on ligament integrity to redirect ground reaction forces and control rotation of the joints that lie above. When medial arch and hindfoot ligaments are attenuated, minimal change will occur in hindfoot alignment when wedges or orthoses are placed under the foot.
- In cases where the supporting ligaments are dramatically attenuated, better control of the foot may be obtained by extending across the ankle with an AFO (Table 3–3).
- AFOs have been shown to be successful in the treatment of various stages of adult acquired flatfoot. In a study of 49 patients with posterior tibial tendon dysfunction, Chao et al. (1996) reported that 67% obtained good to excellent results with either a custom AFO or a UCBL FO. The criteria for prescribing an AFO were fixed deformity, forefoot varus greater than 10°, and excessive body weight (more than 35 lbs over ideal weight).
- Another study used the Arizona AFO (Ernesto Castro, Mesa, AZ) to treat 20 patients in various stages of adult acquired flatfoot deformity (Fig. 3–18). Ninety percent of these patients demonstrated statistically significant improvement of symptoms over a period of 1 year of use of the AFO (Imhauser et al. 2002).
- A recent trend in the non-operative treatment of the adult acquired flatfoot has utilized functional ankle bracing with custom-contoured footplates (Richie braces) (Fig. 3–19). This type of AFO utilizes semirigid leg uprights to control internal rotation of the tibia, as well as a balanced functional orthotic footplate to control subtalar and midtarsal joint movement. Functional ankle bracing is indicated when the adult acquired flatfoot deformity is flexible, and when full ankle motion is desired.
- Hinged AFOs can be used for stage 1 and stage 2 disease, while rigid ankle FOs are recommended for stage 3 and stage 4 disease.

Table 3–3: Comparison of Effects of Foot Orthoses Versus Ankle-Foot Orthoses

FOOT ORTHOSIS	ANKLE-FOOT ORTHOSIS
Controls foot in stance phase only	Controls foot in stance and swing phases
Indirect control on ankle	Direct control on ankle
Indirect control on tibia	Direct control on tibia
Forces applied below axis of rear foot complex	Force applied above and below axis of rear foot complex

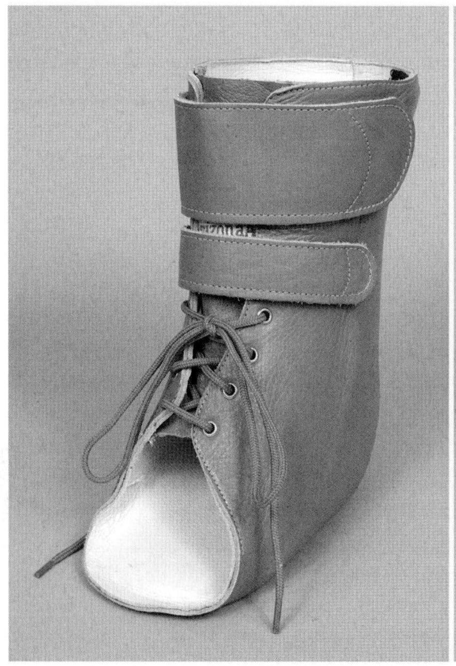

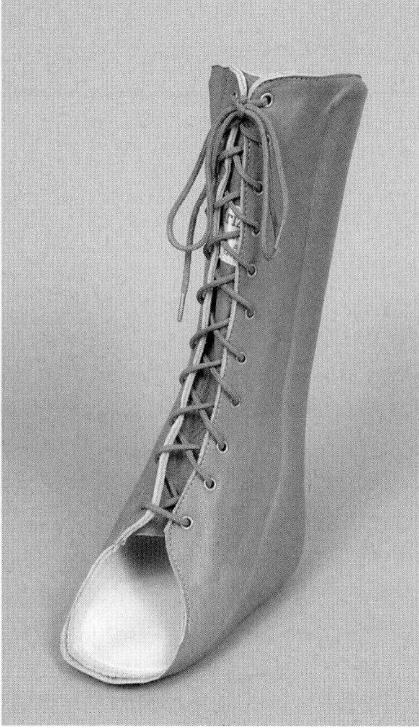

Figure 3–18: Arizona ankle-foot orthosis (AFO). A rigid, solid shell AFO with a leather "gauntlet" closure. (Courtesy of Arizona AFO, Mesa, AZ.)

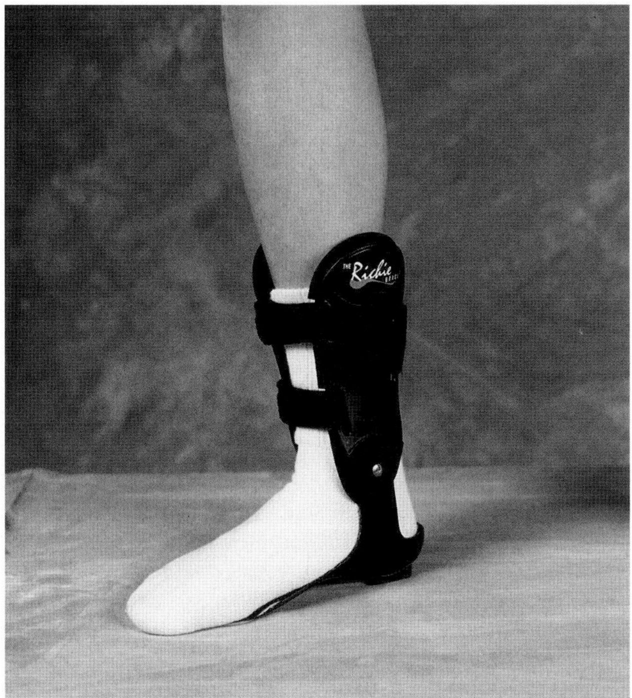

Figure 3–19: Richie-type braces. A custom functional orthotic footplate articulated with semirigid limb supports to control transverse and frontal plane deformities.

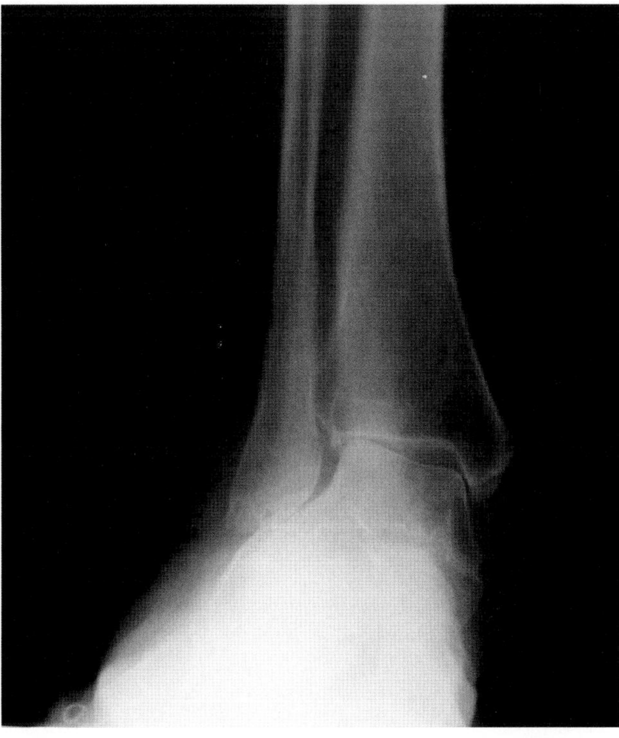

Figure 3–20: Radiograph of stage 4 adult acquired flatfoot.

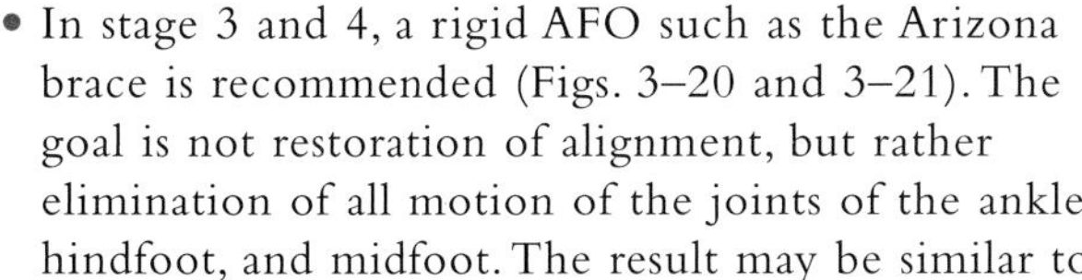

- In stage 3 and 4, a rigid AFO such as the Arizona brace is recommended (Figs. 3–20 and 3–21). The goal is not restoration of alignment, but rather elimination of all motion of the joints of the ankle, hindfoot, and midfoot. The result may be similar to what occurs after a pantalar arthrodesis in terms of translation of increased force proximal to the knee.
- A proposed orthotic treatment protocol for the adult acquired flatfoot is presented in Table 3–4.

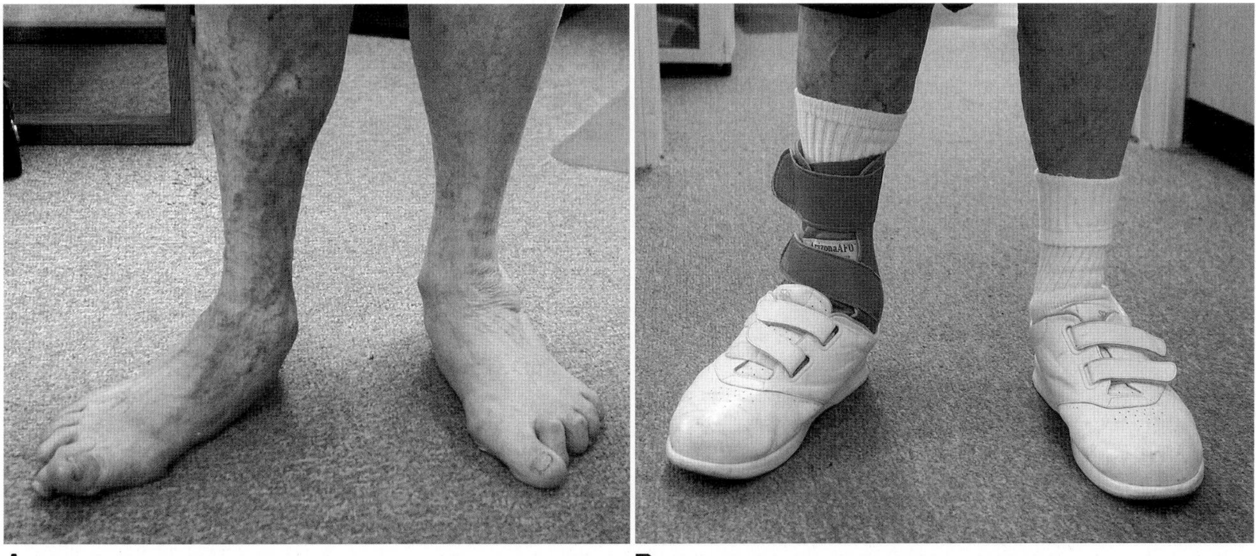

Figure 3–21: Stage 4 adult acquired flatfoot. Same patient in Figure 3–20, before (A) and after (B) fitting with Arizona AFO.

Table 3–4: Comparison of Effects of Foot Orthoses Versus Ankle-Foot Orthose

STAGE(S)	TREATMENT	GOALS
1	Custom rigid or semirigid functional foot orthosis or UCBL	Stabilize preexisting flatfoot Decrease eccentric load on posterior tibial tendon
2	Custom hinged AFO with load on molded footplate (Richie-type AFO)	Preserve ankle motion Decrease hindfoot ligament structures
3 and 4	Solid AFO with "gauntlet" restraint (Arizona-type AFO)	Neutralize sagittal plane deforming force of triceps Eliminate motion in ankle and hindfoot

AFO, ankle-foot orthosis; UCBL, University of California Biomechanics Laboratory orthosis.

References

Augustin JF, Lin SS, Berberian WS et al. (2003) Nonoperative treatment of adult acquired flatfoot with the Arizona brace. Foot Ankle Clin 8(3): 491-502.

Non-operative treatment protocols are presented for various stages of adult acquired flatfoot, along with updated information about the biomechanics of bracing this deformity. Results of treating all three stages of deformity with the Arizona brace show that 90% of patients receive statistically significant improvement of symptoms.

Brodsky JW, Kourosh S, Stills M et al. (1988) Objective evaluation of insert material for diabetic and athletic footwear. Foot Ankle Int 9: 111-116.

This study measures relevant performance characteristics of common insole materials used to treat various foot and ankle pathologies. Loss of thickness due to compression, shear compression, and ability to distribute force were measured. Results provide important guidelines for prescription of off-loading materials used in construction of FOs.

Chao W, Wapner KL, Lee TH et al. (1996) Nonoperative management of posterior tibial tendon dysfunction. Foot Ankle Int 17: 736-741.

The first study to report significant success with either UCBL or custom AFOs in the treatment of stage 2 and 3 posterior tibial tendon dysfunction. Contrary to previous reports, this investigation validates that custom orthotic intervention can delay or obviate surgical reconstruction in older patients with symptomatic flatfoot deformity.

Hertel J, Denegar CR, Buckley WE et al. (2001) Effect of rear-foot orthotics on postural control in healthy subjects. J Sport Rehabil 10: 36.

A comparison of various types of FOs and their effect on balance in healthy subjects. Discussion includes review and comparison with previous studies of FOs in injured subjects.

Imhauser CW, Abidi NA, Frankel DZ et al. (2002) Biomechanical evaluation of the efficacy of external stabilizers in the conservative treatment of acquired flatfoot deformity. Foot Ankle Int 22: 727-737.

A comprehensive laboratory examination of how foot and ankle orthoses may affect the adult acquired flatfoot. Both kinetic (plantar pressures) and kinematic (medial arch and hindfoot alignment) parameters were studied. Both shortcomings and positive influence of orthotic devices are demonstrated, and insight is provided for future design of effective braces for adult acquired flatfoot.

Kogler GF, Solomonidis SE, Paul JP. (1996) Biomechanics of longitudinal arch support mechanisms in foot orthoses and their effect on plantar aponeurosis strain. Clin Biomech 11: 243-252.

A cadaveric study comparing five different orthotic designs and their effect on strain on the central band of the plantar aponeurosis. Devices that best relieved strain in the plantar aponeurosis supported the apical bony structures of the medial longitudinal arch.

Kogler GF, Veer FB, Solomonidis SE. (1999) The influence of medial and lateral placement of orthotic wedges on loading of the plantar aponeurosis. J Bone Joint Surg 81-A: 1403-1413.

A study of static stance cadaver specimens reveals that lateral forefoot wedges can off-load the central band of the plantar aponeurosis more than medial or lateral wedges in any other location under the foot. An in-depth discussion is provided regarding foot mechanics and load on the plantar aponeurosis.

Landorf KB, Keenan AK. (2000) Efficacy of foot orthoses: What does the literature tell us? J Am Podiatr Med Assoc 90: 149-157.

A comprehensive review of the literature relating to FOs, studying six research outcome areas. The results show positive, inconclusive, and negative results in each subject area. Shortcomings of research on FOs to date are discussed.

Lunsford TR. (1997) Strength and materials. In: Atlas of Orthoses and Assistive Devices, 3rd edn (Goldberg B, Hsu JD, eds.). St. Louis: Mosby. pp. 15-66.

A comprehensive review of all aspects of physical behavior and requirements of materials used in orthoses. This entire textbook contains numerous chapters relevant to the foot and ankle surgeon.

Lynch DM, Goforth WP, Martin JE et al. (1998) Conservative treatment of plantar fasciitis: A prospective study. J Am Podiatr Med Assoc 88: 375-380.

A comparison of outcomes with treatment of 103 patients using three common treatments for plantar heel pain: corticosteroid injection (antiinflammatory group), viscoelastic heel cup (accommodative group), and functional FOs with plantar arch taping (mechanical group). Significant improvement was found in the mechanical intervention group compared with in the other interventions.

Mundermann A, Nigg BM, Humble RN et al. (2003) Orthotic comfort is related to kinematics, kinetics and EMG in recreational runners. Med Sci Sports Exerc 35: 1710-1719.

Fifteen kinematic, kinetic, and EMG variables are studied when functional foot orthotics are worn by 21 recreational runners. The concept of comfort of the device correlated with improved biomechanical variables.

Nigg BM, Nurse MA, Stefanyshyn DJ. (1999) Shoe inserts and orthotics for sport and physical activities. Med Sci Sports Exerc 31: S421-S428.

A critical review of published research relevant to FOs and proposed mechanisms of benefit. A new theory of FO treatment effect is proposed involving improved sensory feedback, optimizing muscle function, and supporting a "preferred movement path."

Pfeffer G, Bacchetti P, Deland J et al. (1999) Comparison of custom and prefabricated orthoses in the initial treatment of proximal plantar fasciitis. Foot Ankle Int 20: 214-221.

A multicenter study of 236 patients treated for plantar heel pain of 6 months' duration or less with five different treatment conditions. A prefabricated insert, combined with stretching, produced better results than a custom functional orthotic device.

Rome K, Brown CL. (2004) Randomized clinical trial into the impact of rigid foot orthoses on balance parameters in excessively pronated feet. Clin Rehabil 18: 624-630.

A unique study of postural control using rigid orthoses and monitoring response over a 4-week period of use. Discussion suggests how orthoses can affect neuromuscular control of ankle stability.

Root ML. (1994) Development of the functional foot orthosis. In: Clinics in Podiatric Medicine and Surgery (Jones LJ, eds.). Philadelphia: Saunders. pp. 183-210.

A comprehensive review of the history and development of functional foot orthotic therapy, written by the originator of the technology. A detailed description of the cast corrections and technical designs of the orthotic footplate, as well as clinical guidelines for prescription, are provided.

Williams DS, McClay-Davis I, Baitch SP. (2003) Effect of inverted orthoses on lower-extremity mechanics in runners. Med Sci Sports Exerc 35: 2060-2068.

This study showed that both standard functional FOs and more aggressive inverted orthoses reduced rear foot eversion moment, and increased knee abduction moment, in running subjects. Orthoses that invert the rear foot may decrease soft tissue strain on the ankle invertors and medial knee structures, while increasing strain on the lateral knee structures.

CHAPTER 4

Adult Acquired Flatfoot

Margaret Lobo* and Justin Greisberg§

*M.D., Department of Orthopaedic Surgery, Columbia University College of Physicians and Surgeons, New York, NY
§M.D., Assistant Professor of Orthopaedic Surgery, Columbia University College of Physicians and Surgeons, New York, NY

- Arch height is variable in the population. A "low arched foot" is not pathologic; there is wide individual variation.
- Flatfoot should refer to an abnormal loss of the arch with pain.
- Acquired flatfoot is a common end point of many etiologies (Box 4–1).
  - Posterior tibial tendon (PTT) dysfunction is the most common cause of the adult acquired flatfoot.
  - Other causes include neuropathic (Charcot) degeneration, neuromuscular disease, inflammatory disease, and trauma (fracture malunion or PTT laceration/rupture). Other factors, such as obesity, may play a role.
- Flatfoot describes the end point of a collapsed medial arch with associated deformities of the hindfoot and forefoot.

Box 4–1 Some Causes of an Acquired Flatfoot

- Posterior tibial tendon (PTT) dysfunction—most common cause
- Achilles tendon or gastrocnemius contracture—may cause secondary PTT dysfunction
- Inflammatory arthritis—can cause subluxation of hindfoot joints and/or PTT tendonitis
- Primary midfoot arthritis or midfoot fracture malunion
- Calcaneus or cuboid fracture malunion
- Peroneal muscle spasm—in neuromuscular disease
- Neuropathic deformity—can cause severe deformity
- Coronal plane angulation in the knee, tibia, or ankle—drives the foot into valgus, but foot deformity is secondary

  - The hindfoot progresses into valgus; the forefoot supinates; and the peak pressures and contact forces of the associated joints, such as the subtalar joint, increase.
  - In the sagittal plane, the longitudinal arch collapses, with subluxation of the talonavicular (TN), naviculocuneiform (NC), or first tarsometatarsal (TMT) joints (or a combination of them).
  - In the axial plane, the forefoot abducts, usually through the TN joint.
  - In the coronal plane, heel valgus is seen.
- In three dimensions, the deformity is perhaps best described as dorsolateral peritalar subluxation, because the foot is subluxing dorsally and laterally around the talus. Although the deformity is primarily through the peritalar joints in many flatfeet, it is important to remember that in some feet other joints (such as NC or TMT) may be involved.
- The disease tends to be progressive. Once arch integrity is lost and collapse begins, gravity and weight-bearing forces encourage further destabilization.

The Arches of the Foot

- The medial longitudinal arch comprises the first metatarsal, the medial cuneiform, the navicular, and the talus.
- The lesser longitudinal arch consists of the fourth and fifth metatarsals, cuboid, and lateral calcaneus.
- A transverse arch spans the midfoot, across the midtarsal joints. The second and third metatarsal bases are keystones and help prevent collapse.

Arch Support: Ligaments are the Key Static Supporters of the Arch

- The spring ligament is an important stabilizer of the medial arch. It consists of two parts:
  - the superomedial calcaneonavicular (SMCN) ligament arises from the sustentaculum tali and fans out to insert on the edge of the medial navicular facet
  - the inferior calcaneonavicular ligament runs from the anterior sustentaculum tali and inserts on the plantar aspect of the midnavicular cortex.
- The superficial deltoid originates on the medial malleolus and inserts on the dorsal edge of the SMCN ligament. Its function is to serve as a check rein for the entire complex.
- The plantar fascia also contributes to arch integrity.
  - In biomechanical testing, it fails under load at 1.7-3.4 times body weight (Hintermann 1995).
  - Division of the plantar fascia results in depression of the longitudinal arch and elongation of the medial length of the foot (Sharkey et al. 1998).
  - Its division in the cadaveric feet decreases arch stiffness by 25% (Huang et al. 1993).
  - The long plantar ligament runs from the anterior tuberosity of the inferior surface of the calcaneus. The majority of fibers insert on the cuboid, and the more superficial fibers insert on the second through fifth metatarsals. It is thought to be of secondary importance in arch support.

Dynamic Arch Stabilizers

- The PTT is a powerful inverter and plantar flexor of the foot. It locks the transverse tarsal joints (TN and calcaneocuboid joints).
  - Biomechanical and electromyographic studies suggest that the tendon acts as an arch supporter during gait and loading situations.
  - An imbalance between the PTT and its antagonists (tibialis anterior, peroneal longus and brevis, and triceps surae) may lead to arch collapse. This occurs in muscle imbalance disorders such as cerebral palsy.
- Extrinsic and intrinsic toe flexors also contribute to arch support but have a secondary role. The flexor tendons fail under repetitive stress without a functional PTT.
- Hindfoot motion locks and unlocks the transverse tarsal joints (Fig. 4–1).
  - With subtalar eversion, the transverse tarsal joints are flexible, which keeps the forefoot supple to accommodate uneven surfaces.
  - When the PTT fires just prior to the heel rise portion of gait, the axes of the TN joint and calcaneocuboid joint are divergent, locking the transverse tarsal joints. This creates a rigid medial column and long lever arm for forceful push-off during gait.
- In the normal gait cycle, firing of the PTT just prior to heel rise inverts the heel, bringing the Achilles vector medial to the subtalar joint. Achilles contraction then supports the arch and encourages locking of the transverse tarsal joints. This stabilizes the arch for push-off (Box 4–2).

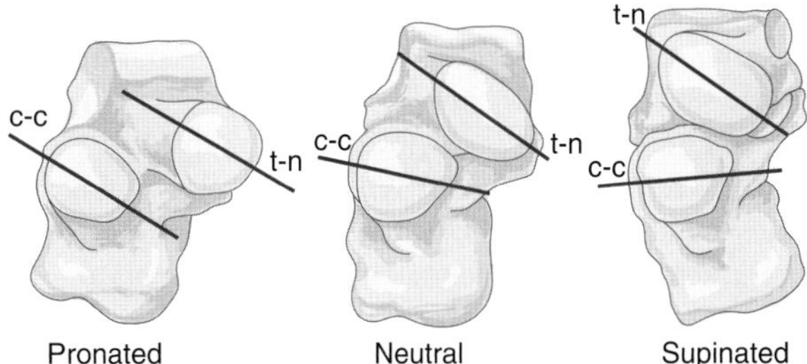

Figure 4–1: The transverse tarsal joint includes the calcaneocuboid and talonavicular joints. In a simplified model, the axes of the joints are divergent in inversion, locking the midfoot. When the foot is everted, the axes are parallel, allowing motion at these joints and unlocking the midfoot.

Box 4–2 The Posterior Tibial Tendon in the Gait Cycle

- After heel contact, the posterior tibial tendon (PTT) serves as a shock absorber that limits hindfoot eversion by eccentric contraction.
- In midstance, the PTT initiates inversion of the hindfoot. This hindfoot inversion forces the axes of the calcaneocuboid and talonavicular joint to become non-parallel, thus locking these joints and rendering the foot rigid for push-off.
- In the propulsive phase, the PTT initiates hindfoot inversion. The Achilles tendon vector shifts medial to the subtalar axis of rotation, which secures hindfoot inversion and transverse tarsal joint position. This optimizes lift and forward propulsion, and the PTT accelerates and assists heel lift.

More About the Three-Dimensional Deformity

- Although arch collapse is traditionally noted in the TN joint, deformity can occur with any combination of TN, NC, and/or first TMT subluxation/collapse.
- Using the "tripod" model of foot structure (Ch. 1), loss of the medial post of the tripod through collapse of any of these joints allows the hindfoot to collapse into valgus.
- Acquired flatfoot is a three-dimensional deformity of hindfoot valgus, longitudinal arch collapse, and forefoot abduction (see Figs 4–5 and 4–6).
  - The talus becomes plantar flexed. The calcaneus everts, and the navicular and cuboid move to a more everted location.
  - With increasing hindfoot valgus, the forefoot assumes a compensatory forefoot supination.
- The lateral column is effectively shortened as the deformity progresses.

- The talus slides anteriorly relative to the calcaneus. hindfoot valgus occurs as a result of rotation through the subtalar and TN joints.
- Achilles contracture is a deforming force that can cause and exacerbate arch failure. When the heel is in valgus, the Achilles insertion lies lateral to the axis of the subtalar joint, so that Achilles contraction promotes subtalar eversion and thus arch collapse.
  - When the PTT fails to invert the hindfoot prior to heel rise, the calcaneal insertion of the Achilles remains lateral to the axis of the subtalar joint. Achilles contraction then leads to hindfoot eversion. The transverse tarsal joints are unlocked, and the arch can sag.
  - Recurrent cycles of this dysfunctional gait can break down the static support of the arch.
  - In some situations, Achilles contracture may precede any other pathology. With Achilles contracture, the talus and calcaneus are plantar flexed. Weight bearing places a dorsiflexion force on the forefoot. Because of the oblique axis of the subtalar joint, subtalar eversion also produces some dorsiflexion. So, in a foot with a tight Achilles tendon, subtalar eversion is necessary to produce a plantigrade foot. With subtalar eversion, the PTT can become secondarily strained and eventually injured.
- Many patients with active PTT tendonitis will have a tight gastrocnemius and a low arch on the "normal" foot.
  - A flatfoot deformity exacerbates Achilles contracture by maintaining the foot in hindfoot valgus and equinus. The Achilles may become more contracted, which further antagonizes PTT function and arch integrity, with a progressive deformity.
- So, an acquired flatfoot can be caused by tightness of the Achilles (especially the gastrocnemius component) and also can result in a contracted Achilles tendon.
- In the deformity, hindfoot and midfoot joint degeneration may develop secondary to increases in joint reactive pressures. With a flatfoot deformity, the subtalar joint facets sublux, so that only half of the articular surface is in contact. The decrease in contact area leads to increased contact pressures (Ananthakrisnan et al. 1999).

Pain from Flatfoot

- The pes planovalgus deformity alters joint mechanics as well as foot and ankle alignment. Pain can occur in the foot, ankle, or even more proximal locations.
- The lower back and hip may be sore from limping or from altered gait mechanics.
- Continued valgus stress on the knee from a valgus foot can lead to medial compartment disease.
- Valgus foot alignment can also lead to valgus ankle deformity, with painful joint degeneration.
- In the foot, pain may be felt medially or laterally, and may arise from inflammation, tendinitis, arthritis, and/or impingement.
- In cases of PTT tendinitis, patients may feel pain only in the medial hindfoot from tenosynovitis, or from a complete or longitudinal tear within the tendon.
- In an advanced flatfoot of any etiology, pain may occur over the medial malleolus and deltoid ligament as the deltoid fibers are tensioned to oppose the worsening hindfoot valgus.

Talocalcaneal Impingement and Calcaneofibular Impingement

- With hindfoot valgus, lateral hindfoot pain can occur as a result of the calcaneus impinging on the distal tip of the fibula or lateral process of the talus.
- Cyst formation and/or sclerosis in this region, either on plain film or computed tomography (CT), should create suspicion of impingement.
- A CT imaging study compared control subjects with patients with severe deformity under 75 N of axial loading. It determined that the prevalence of sinus tarsi impingement was 92% and the prevalence of calcaneofibular impingement was 66% in the flatfoot group versus 0 and 5%, respectively, in the control group. The study patients who had calcaneofibular impingement also had sinus tarsi impingement (Malicky et al. 2002).

Arthritis

- Arthritis may be the causative agent or the end result of a chronic severe deformity.
- Alteration of joint reaction forces causes abnormal loading of the subtalar, tibiotalar, transverse tarsal, and Lisfranc joints, and may result in painful arthritic conditions.

Summary of Etiology of Adult Acquired Flatfoot

- If the normal balance of arch support is disturbed (such as with fracture malunion, PTT injury, or Achilles tightness), persistent abnormally directed weight-bearing forces will tax the remaining support of the arch (such as the PTT or spring ligament), leading to progressive arch collapse.
- Once the deformity is established, it may be difficult to determine which came first—the Achilles contracture, the PTT dysfunction, or the spring ligament rupture.
- Perhaps the most important treatment for an acquired flatfoot is prevention. If the "at risk" foot could be identified, early intervention might prevent the deformity. Once the deformity is established, it is often self-perpetuating and progressive.
- An "at risk" foot would be one with a very tight Achilles and normal PTT function, or one with severe flatfoot deformity but still normal PTT function.

Posterior Tibial Tendon Dysfunction

Tibialis Posterior Anatomy

- The muscle arises from the posterior tibia as a large muscle in the deep posterior compartment of the calf.
- The tendon travels in the medial malleolar groove and inserts broadly into the medial foot.
  - It primarily inserts on to the navicular tuberosity, but multiple slips fan out to insert into the second through fourth metatarsals, into the plantar surface of the cuneiforms, and on the cuboid on the lateral foot.
  - On the plantar surface, it attaches to the deep fascia, the peroneal longus tendon, and the long and short toe flexors.
- A zone of hypovascularity exists 40 mm proximal to the navicular tuberosity and extends proximally over 14 mm of tendon. There is no mesotendon in this region, and surrounding synovial tissue is also hypovascular. This area is subject to mechanical wear.
- It is possible that a transient ischemia creates tendon insufficiency and sets up the cascade of dynamic instability. A diseased PTT has high relative concentrations of type 3 collagen (it is the main collagen in early tendon healing). It has decreased tensile strength, which can cause tendon insufficiency and dysfunction with recurrent use.
- In an evaluation of spontaneously ruptured tendons and controls in an over-35 population, degenerative pathologic changes such as hypoxic degeneration, mucoid degeneration, and tendolipomatosis and calcifying tendinopathy were identified. Of note, these changes were observed in 34% of control tendon specimens. Normal tendon structure was not identified in any of the ruptured tendon specimens. These findings suggest that degenerative tendonopathy is common after age 35 (Kannus and Jozsa 1991).

Posterior Tibial Tendon Disease Progression

- PTT disease progression is a continuum.
- Epidemiology
  - It is more often seen in women in the 45- to 65-year-old age range.
  - It occurs with increased frequency in obese and diabetic patients.
  - About half of patients will relate a traumatic event to the initiation of symptoms.
- As mentioned above, with PTT dysfunction the transverse tarsal joint will not lock during heel rise. Weight-bearing forces across these unlocked joints lead to fatigue failure of the ligaments.
- Additionally, arch-flattening forces, such as the triceps surae and obesity, may contribute to a flatfoot as the repetitive forces of weight bearing cause the deformity to progress.
- Static deformities can cause PTT dysfunction (the arch fails first).
  - The position of forefoot pronation and valgus (arch collapse) will lead to PTT failure and worsening deformity.
  - If the talocalcaneonavicular complex loses stiffness, the PTT insertion sites are in a valgus position. Lengthening of the tendon even 1 cm reduces its efficiency as the primary dynamic stabilizer of the arch.
- A staging system was introduced in 1989 by Johnson and Strom (1989) that included four stages. The system is devised to describe the clinical entity, and offers guidelines for non-operative and operative treatment (Table 4–1).
- Unfortunately, there is no evidence that a foot progresses from one stage to the next over time. It is possible that feet at stage 1 represent a different pathophysiology, with a different natural history, than that of a stage 3 flatfoot.
- Not all feet at any one stage are the same. Although treatment guidelines are often listed by stage, it is important to assess each foot individually. Treatment, especially surgical, cannot be generalized.

Stage 1

- Pain and swelling occur along the course of the tendon and are defined as tenosynovitis or tendinosis.
- Tendon length is unchanged.
- The subtalar joint is flexible.
- The heel inverts on single toe rise, and there is no loss of strength.
- There is no deformity; arch height remains unchanged.
- Radiographs are normal.
- Magnetic resonance imaging (MRI) will demonstrate edema around the tendon and occasional intrasubstance degeneration. Exuberant tenosynovitis may be a hallmark of an inflammatory or rheumatic etiology.

Stage 2

- The tendon is elongated and enlarged, and is functionally incompetent.
- On tendon inspection, there are partial tears and there is evidence of degeneration.
- The patient may be able to perform a single-limb heel rise, but the heel does not invert.
- The foot assumes a pes planovalgus appearance. The arch is collapsed, the hindfoot is in valgus, the forefoot is abducted, and the subtalar joint is everted.
- The subtalar joint remains flexible, and the deformity is passively correctable.
- The Achilles tendon will be contracted.
- There will be a "too many toes" sign.
- Radiographs demonstrate an increased lateral talocalcaneal angle, decreased calcaneal pitch, and lateral peritalar subluxation.

Table 4–1: Stages of Flatfoot and Clinical Findigs

	STAGE 1	STAGE 2	STAGE 3	STAGE 4
PTT disease	Tendinosis	Elongated, functionally incompetent	Elongated, functionally incompetent	Elongated, functionally incompetent
Deformity	Normal	Flexible pes planovalgus deformity Arch is "flatter" than normal	Severe and rigid The subtalar joint is rigid The forefoot is abducted and may be supinated The navicular is rigidly fixed in a laterally subluxed position	Similar to stage 3 but includes valgus tilt of the talus in the ankle
Pain location	Along PTT	Medial ± lateral	Medial ± lateral	Medial ± lateral
"Too many toes"	Absent	Positive	Positive	Positive
Heel rise testing	Normal	Heel will not invert	Unable to complete	Unable to complete
Radiographs	Normal MRI is positive for PTT tenosynovitis	Increased lateral talocalcaneal angle, decreased calcaneal pitch and lateral peritalar subluxation	Peritalar subluxation, plantar flexed talus, and degenerative changes in the subtalar and transverse tarsal joints Lateral impingement may cause a fibular stress fracture	Stage 3 findings and a plantar flexed valgus talus as well as tibiotalar degenerative arthritis

MRI, magnetic resonance imaging; PTT, posterior tibial tendon.

- MRI demonstrates tendon degeneration, possible discontinuity, and changes in the spring ligament.

Stage 3

- Tendon degeneration is pronounced, and it is attenuated or ruptured.
- Single-limb heel rise is often impossible, and the heel cannot be inverted with heel rise.
- The deformity is severe and may be fixed.
  - The subtalar joint is rigid. The forefoot is abducted and may be supinated.
  - The navicular is rigidly fixed in a laterally subluxed position.
- Pain may occur both medially and laterally.
- The "too many toes" sign is grossly positive.
- Radiographs demonstrate peritalar subluxation, plantar flexion of the talus, and often degenerative changes in the subtalar and transverse tarsal joints. Lateral impingement may cause a fibular stress fracture.
- MRI is of little to no benefit in this stage.
- CT may be helpful in assessing degeneration of the midfoot and hindfoot joints. Weight-bearing CT, if available, can give more information about the three-dimensional deformity.

Stage 4

- It includes all findings in stage 3, along with valgus angulation of the talus at the tibiotalar joint secondary to deltoid failure and lateral ankle erosion.
- Radiographs will demonstrate a plantarflexed valgus talus as well as tibiotalar degenerative arthritis.

Other Etiologies of Adult Acquired Flatfoot Deformity

- Rheumatoid or other inflammatory arthropathies can cause PTT dysfunction.
  - Arthrosis can occur at any of the hindfoot or midfoot joints primarily. Subluxation of these arthritic joints will lead to a flatfoot.
  - Inflammatory arthritides can also affect tendons, with all the symptoms of PTT dysfunction.
- Posttraumatic deformity
  - Soft tissue trauma as an etiology of flatfoot is often a subtle diagnosis, as the end-stage deformity, forefoot abduction and hindfoot valgus, is the same.
  - Malunion from navicular, Lisfranc, first metatarsal, and calcaneus fracture can cause settling of the medial longitudinal arch, creating a flatfoot deformity.
  - Flatfoot secondary to midfoot (Lisfranc) malunion is secondary to loss of medial column stability, often at the TMT joint. At the level of the midfoot, the longitudinal arch will break, and the forefoot will drift into abduction. Hindfoot valgus is a secondary compensatory change.
  - A PTT laceration or traumatic rupture will also lead to arch collapse as dynamic support of the arch fails, causing muscle imbalance and eventual arthrosis.
- Neuropathic deformity
  - The characteristic flatfoot deformity has been described in the diabetic neuropathic population, spinal cord

patients, and those with Hansen disease and other neuropathic conditions.
- Charcot neuroarthropathy in the midfoot causes collapse of the medial arch, often with marked deformity. In these cases, it is not PTT dysfunction but rather loss of the normal bony architecture.

Tarsal Coalition

Peroneal Spasm

- Peroneal spasm can be a sign of disease in the peritalar region.
- Protective contraction of any or all of the muscles bridging the peritalar joints may be induced in response to a peritalar insult.
- Patients with a hindfoot coalition have been traditionally thought of as having spastic peroneal tendons. However, the majority of these patients do not have spasm, and peroneal spasm has been identified in patients without tarsal coalitions. These patients should be examined for other peritalar lesions.
- A patient with a tarsal coalition classically will have a unilateral flatfoot, decreased motion, vague foot pain, and peroneal spasm. However, the foot may be normally shaped, with no peroneal spasm. The typical patient presents only with hindfoot pain. The astute clinician will detect a lack of hindfoot motion.
- The coalition may be osseous, cartilaginous, or fibrous, and it may be complete or incomplete.
- Plain x-rays may show dorsal talar beaking. CT examination of the foot can diagnose a coalition (Fig. 4–2). Fibrous coalitions require a high index of suspicion when analyzing the CT.
- The most common coalition is between the calcaneus and the navicular. A middle facet subtalar coalition is the next most common tarsal coalition.
- Once diagnosed, involved joints should be investigated for arthritic changes.
- Coalition resection is appropriate treatment in a non-degenerated calcaneal-navicular coalition. Subtalar arthrodesis may be necessary for subtalar coalitions, as decreased motion, deformity, and peroneal spasm probably exist at the time of diagnosis.

Physical Examination of the Flatfoot

- The physical examination comprises inspection, palpation, range of motion examination, and dynamic strength testing (Box 4–3).
- Inspection
  - Arch height in comparison with the contralateral side should also be noted.
  - The "too many toes" sign confirms forefoot abduction deformity. When viewed from behind, the abducted forefoot will show more toes visible lateral to the leg than normal.
- Heel rise testing (Fig. 4–3)

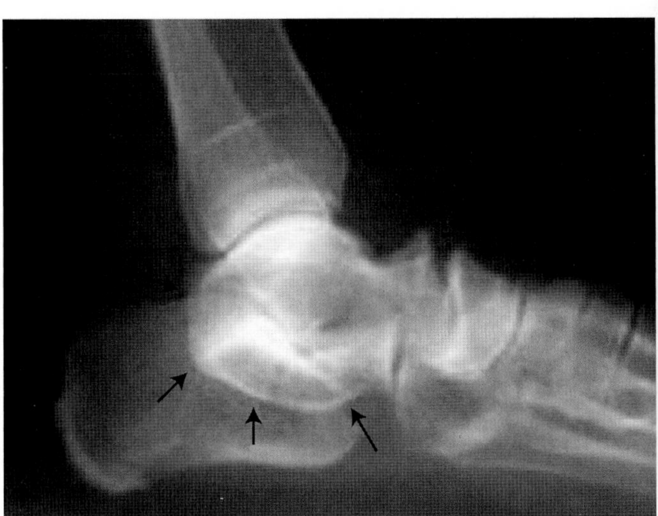

A

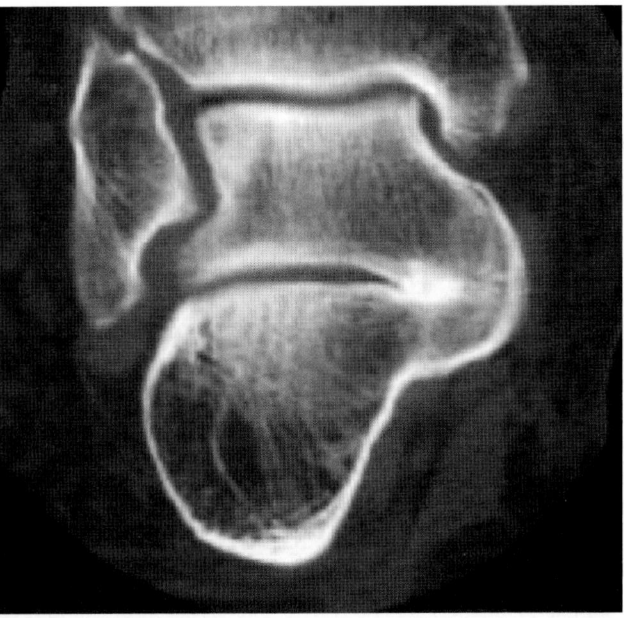

B

Figure 4–2: Tarsal coalition may cause a deformity that resembles the adult acquired flatfoot. It can be diagnosed with computed tomography and may be suspected after noticing dorsal bossing of the talus on lateral radiographs.

Box 4–3 Physical Examination

1. Visualize both legs from the knee down.
2. Observe heel alignment with the patient standing with the feet parallel, shoulder-width apart. Look for heel valgus and forefoot abduction compared with the contralateral foot.
3. Inspect and palpate the course of the posterior tibial tendon (PTT) for tenosynovitis.
4. Look for an inability to perform a single heel rise or the lack of heel inversion in the symptomatic foot. The inability to perform less than 10 heel rises is a stress test and may indicate PTT weakness.
5. Test inversion and eversion muscle power of both feet.
6. Examine the gastroc-soleus complex for contracture with the subtalar joint in the reduced position.
7. Evaluate subtalar motion. In early stages, the hindfoot will be supple and easily reduce. In stages 3 and 4, this maneuver may be painful if secondary subtalar arthrosis exists, or impossible in a rigid deformity.

- In the normal foot, elevation of foot to a tiptoe stance requires a functional PTT to invert the subtalar joint. If normal, this will bring the heel into varus.
- Comparison of the affected and unaffected foot can confirm if the PTT is insufficient by an asymmetric heel position on double heel rise testing.
- An inability to rise up on the affected foot indicates PTT insufficiency or dysfunction.
- It can also serve as a stress test if the patient is unable to perform more than one or two single heel rises.
- Motion examination
  - The flatfoot is diagnosed as either flexible or rigid based on subtalar motion. A rigid deformity implies muscle spasm, advanced arthritis, or a coalition.
  - To examine for an Achilles contracture, the subtalar joint must first be reduced to a neutral starting position. This also allows the examiner to appreciate the degree of forefoot varus and the rigidity of the deformity.
- Palpation
  - Tenderness can occur over the course of the PTT (Fig. 4–4), the plantar fascia, or the spring and deltoid ligaments. Tenderness may also occur on the lateral hindfoot as a result of calcaneofibular or talocalcaneal impingement.
  - Peroneal or tibialis anterior spasm may coexist in patients with a tarsal coalition.

Imaging Studies

- Weight-bearing anteroposterior and lateral views of the foot and an anteroposterior view of the ankle are essential aids in diagnosis.
- Anteroposterior foot (Fig. 4–5)
  - The degree of abnormality in talar alignment can be assessed. The talus becomes increasingly uncovered as the navicular subluxes laterally.
  - The TN coverage angle can determine the degree of uncovering that has occurred.
- Lateral foot (Fig. 4–6)
  - It confirms the loss of alignment between the first metatarsal and talus.

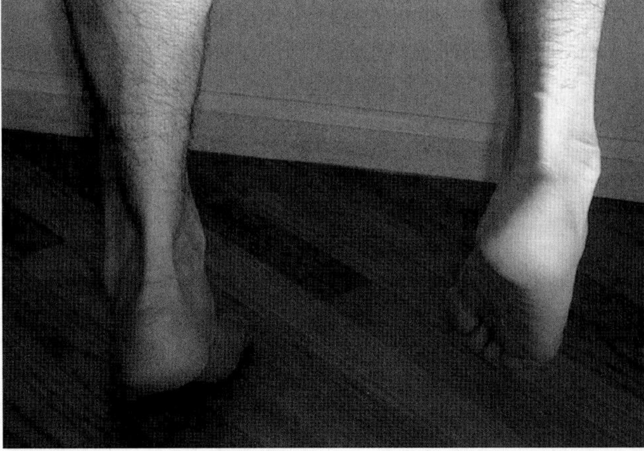
A

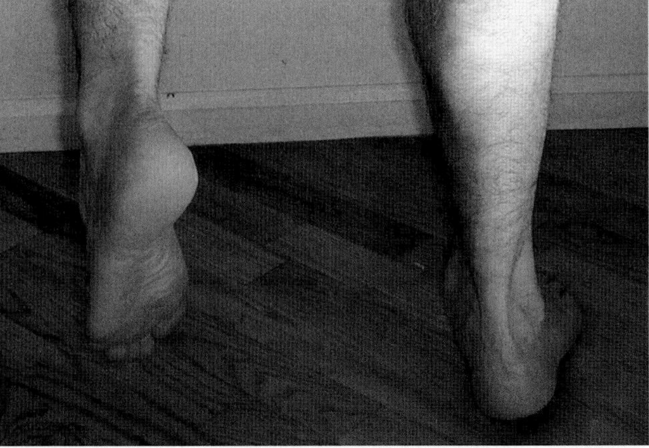
B

Figure 4–3: Single heel rise testing. The elevation of the foot to the toes requires a functional posterior tibial tendon (PTT). A, When competent, the heel will invert and assume a varus orientation. B, PTT dysfunction is confirmed by the inability to complete a single heel rise test or the inability for the heel to shift into a varus position. In this patient, attempted heel rise gets the heel only slightly off the ground, but the heel remains in valgus.

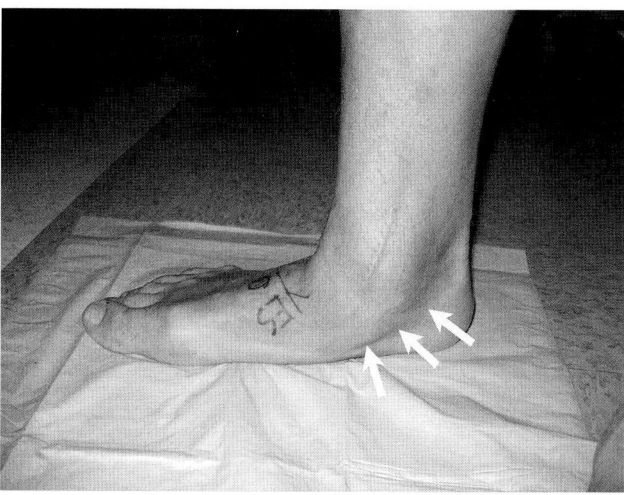

Figure 4–4: **Inspection and palpation along the course of the posterior tibial tendon may demonstrate pain, swelling, and bogginess.**

- Subluxation or sagging is identified at the TN and the naviculocuneiform joints.
- The talus assumes a plantar flexed configuration and the calcaneal pitch decreases as the deformity progresses.
- Anteroposterior ankle (Fig. 4–7)
  - Stage 4 disease is characterized by tibiotalar subluxation secondary to deltoid insufficiency. Talar tilt is determined in this view.
- Degeneration at the midfoot and hindfoot joints can be determined by observing subluxation and loss of joint space, osteophyte formation, and sclerosis.
- Dorsal talar beaking or bossing (see Fig. 4–2), if observed, may be suggestive of a coexisting tarsal coalition.
- MRI is a sensitive and specific test in the determination of PTT pathology (Fig. 4–8). It provides insight into the morphology and internal structure of the tendon.
- Another use of MRI is to evaluate the mid- and hindfoot for underlying disease when determining surgical treatment.

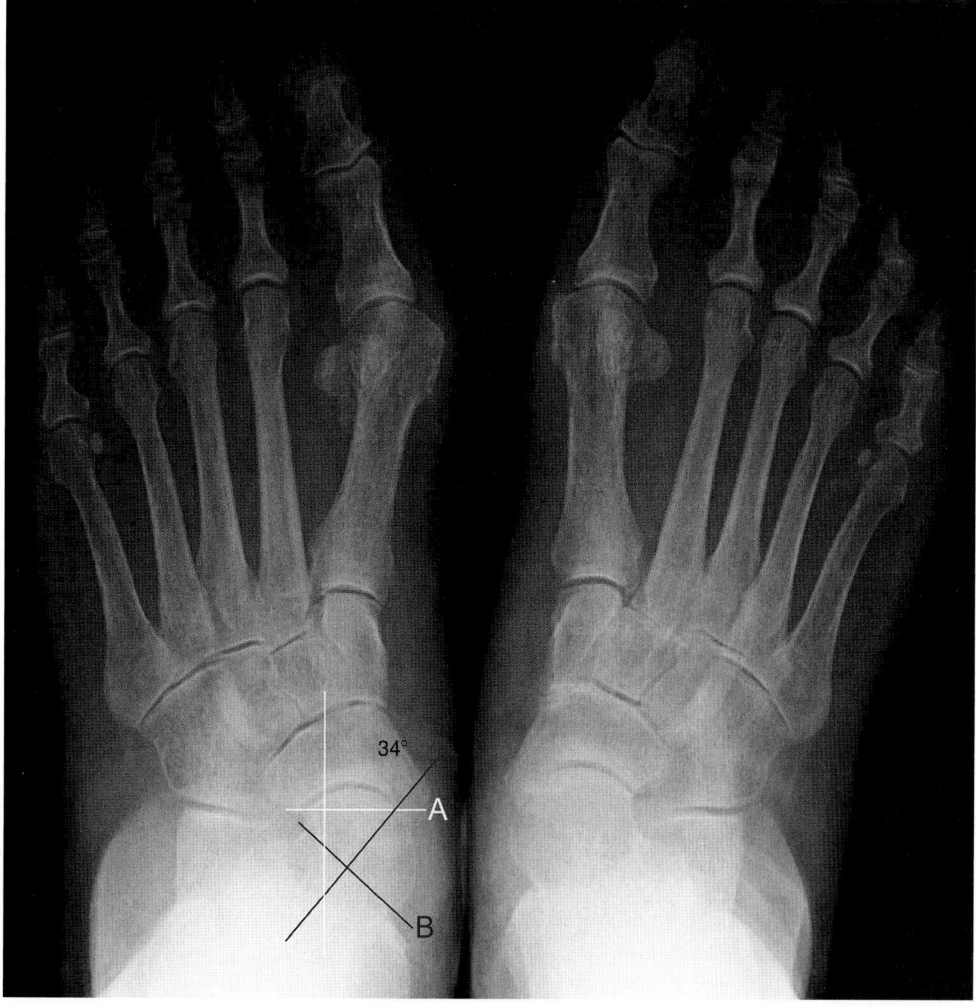

Figure 4–5: **The talonavicular coverage angle can be calculated as a measure of forefoot abduction as the talus becomes increasingly uncovered as the navicular subluxes laterally. Line A connects the articular surfaces of the navicular, and line B connects the articular surfaces of the talus, as described by Sangeorzan (1993). Perpendicular lines are drawn to A and B through the center of the articular surface. It measures 34° in this example.**

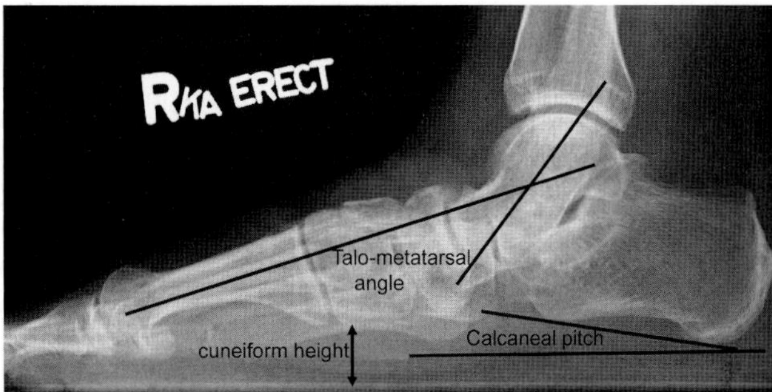

Figure 4–6: The lateral foot radiograph images the loss of alignment between the first metatarsal and midfoot. A talo-first metatarsal angle greater than 4° signifies pes planus; as shown, 32°. The calcaneal pitch angle is also determined on the lateral radiograph; a normal angle is between 17 and 32° (12° in this patient). Arch height loss is documented by a decrease in this angle. A loss of medial cuneiform-floor height is also indicative of loss of arch height. This is shown by the black line.

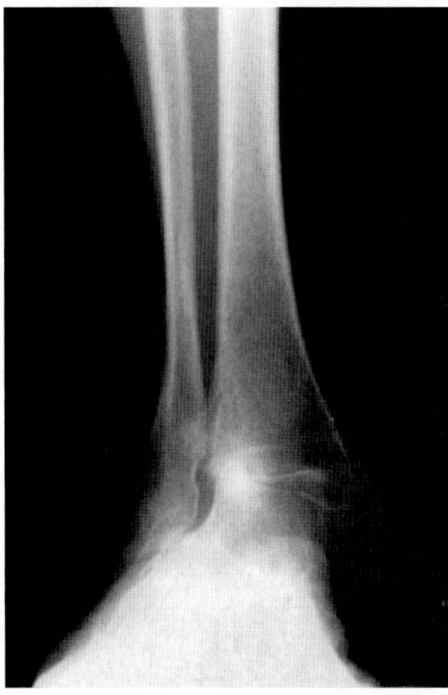

Figure 4–7: Anteroposterior ankle. An anteroposterior view of the ankle is needed to assess overall talar alignment and to evaluate for talar tilt and tibiotalar degeneration in advanced cases.

- Its expense must be considered, as most tendinosis can be determined by history and physical examination.
- Ultrasound is a non-invasive, less expensive modality by which the PTT can be examined.
- Ultrasound can diagnose increased tendon diameter and increased peritendonous space and compare it with the contralateral side.

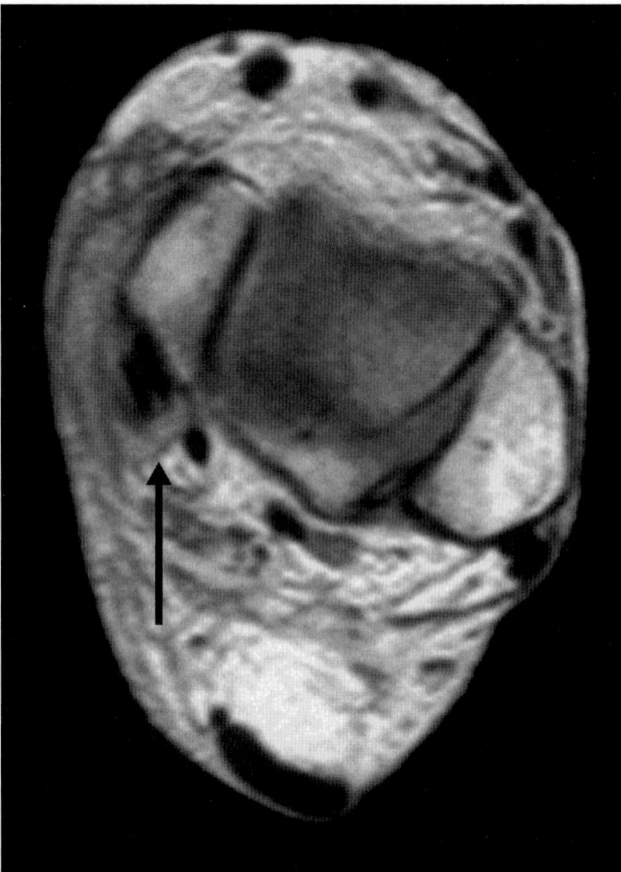

Figure 4–8: Magnetic resonance imaging may demonstrate intrasubstance tears within the tendon, and fluid within the sheath. Increased diameter may also be suggestive of tendinosis.

- Ultrasound diagnosis of stage 1 PTT dysfunction correlates with surgical findings.
- Simulated weight-bearing CT may be useful to better understand the three-dimensional deformity, but hard to obtain in many medical centers.
- Non-weight-bearing CT will more accurately show presence of radiographic arthritis than plain films.

Treatment

- A treatment protocol is devised based on the etiology of the disease; Table 4–2 demonstrates treatment modalities acceptable for the various stages of disease.
- The treatment plan for a rigid flatfoot secondary to tarsal coalition will differ greatly from that of a patient with disease secondary to rheumatoid arthritis. Understanding the etiology of the deformity will dictate the treatment protocol.
- The goal of all treatment modalities is the elimination of pain, both long and short term, and restoration of normal foot biomechanics and orientation.
- Most clinicians argue for a trial of non-operative treatment prior to surgical intervention. In some cases,

Table 4–2: Treatment of Adult Acquired Flatfoot by Stage of Disease

STAGE	FINDING(S)	TREATMENT
1	Pain, swelling No deformity	Casting, arch support Posterior tibial tendon debridement
2	Flexible deformity "Too many toes" sign	Arch support, AFO, UCBL Posterior tibial tendon augmentation Medial/lateral column fusions and osteotomies
3	Rigid deformity	AFO, UCBL Fusions (selective or triple)
4	Rigid deformity Ankle arthritis	Solid AFO bracing Salvage fusion (pantalar or tibiotalocalcaneal)

AFO, ankle-foot orthosis; UCBL, University of California Biomechanics Laboratory orthosis.

such as in a young patient with early deformity and a high likelihood of progression, earlier surgery may halt the disease and avoid the need for more complex surgery later.

Non-operative Treatments

- In flexible flatfoot deformities, the goal of non-operative treatment is to restore normal foot orientation and alleviate pain.
- Anti-inflammatory medications may be helpful.
  - The goal of this treatment is to decrease the inflammation and synovitis surrounding the PTT.
  - Cortisone injections may further jeopardize the PTT and should be avoided.
- With PTT tendonitis, rest with short leg casting often breaks the cycle leading to deformity, and provides pain relief by controlling the symptoms of tendinitis or tenosynovitis.
  - Weight bearing is allowed only if it does not cause pain.
  - After cast removal, a full-length medial arch support is required to maintain PTT support and foot alignment.
- Bracing and orthotics are designed to control progressive heel valgus.
  - By reducing the calcaneus to neutral, the transverse tarsal joint is stiffened and forefoot abduction is decreased.
  - A full-length medial arch support with a medial heel wedge and medial column post will reduce the subtalar joint. This may allow the tendonitis to recede, thus relieving early flatfoot pain.
  - In a more severe but flexible flatfoot deformity, a molded ankle-foot orthosis (AFO) with or without an articulation may be necessary.
  - A University of California Biomechanics Laboratory (UCBL) orthotic is more rigid and provides lateral buttressing of the forefoot to help control severe but flexible abduction deformities of the forefoot.
- In rigid flatfoot, the goal of bracing is to support the foot in situ for pain control and correction of any remaining flexibility of the foot.
  - Bracing requires use of an accommodative device custom molded to the foot deformity.
  - Both articulated and non-articulated custom-molded AFO braces are used. Often, a rocker bottom sole is required in a non-articulated AFO.
  - Skin compromise may occur in a brace that provides too much correction in a patient with a rigid deformity.
- In severe rigid deformities that involve the tibiotalar joint, solid AFOs such as an Arizona brace are the only orthotic option.
- Once arch collapse has occurred, non-protected weight bearing will exacerbate the deformity and lead to secondary degenerative arthritis in the affected joints.
- Bracing and orthotics should probably be tried for several weeks before proceeding to operative intervention. Surgical management is indicated for failure of a well-fitting orthotic to control symptoms.
  - A study by Chao et al. (1996) assessed the results of bracing. They found that 67% of patients (33/49) were treated successfully with UCBL orthosis or AFOs, 24% of patients had fair to poor results but did not seek surgical intervention, and 9% went on to require surgical management. The average time of orthotic wear was between 3 and 6 months for the groups that were not successfully treated with orthotics.

Surgical Principles

- The sources of pain must be addressed.
  - If there is PTT pain, then that should be addressed with tendon repair and augmentation.
  - If there is pain from osseous impingement, arch alignment must be improved to decompress the painful areas.
  - If there is pain from arthritis, the affected joints should probably be fused.
- Surgery should stop the progress of the disease so that no future surgery is needed. In most cases, Achilles tendon (or gastrocnemius) lengthening is an important step to minimize the chance for disease recurrence.
- Any deformity should be realigned, even if not necessary for short-term pain relief. Persistent deformity will place abnormal stresses on the subtalar joint, the ankle, and to a lesser extent the knee, with late joint degeneration.

Surgical Options for Stage 1 Posterior Tibial Tendon Dysfunction

- Active PTT disease with a preserved arch is treated by repairing and augmenting the tendon.
- Achilles tendon contracture can lead to deformity. Surgical lengthening will aid in balancing the deforming force.

- At this early stage, bone work may be avoided. However, in the patient with obesity, or with degenerative or inflammatory disease, consideration should be given to a medial sliding calcaneal osteotomy. This osteotomy moves the insertion of the Achilles tendon to a point medial to the subtalar joint axis, so that the Achilles can further support PTT function.
- For the tendon repair, a medial approach is utilized to inspect the retinaculum, tendon sheath, and tendon (Fig. 4–9).
- Tendon debridement is performed if intratendinous tears or nodularity is encountered. Diseased tendon is excised, and a side to side repair is performed with non-absorbable suture and buried knots.
- The flexor hallucis longus (FHL) and flexor digitorum longus (FDL) are most commonly used to augment the diseased PTT.
  - Advantages of using the FDL include in-phase functioning of the FDL, excursion of the tendon, and proximity of the FDL to the PTT tendon sheath. There is probably no morbidity to transferring the FDL, even in the active patient.
  - The advantages of using the FHL include greater tendon strength and girth in comparison with the FDL.
- After tendon debridement and augmentation, the foot is protected for 6 weeks in a weight-bearing cast. The patient is gradually advanced to regular activities and kept in a medial arch support.
- There have been many studies evaluating the results of surgical debridement and augmentation of stage 1 disease. Most patients get better, but a small minority require augmentation and/or bony realignment (Teasdall and Johnson 1994, Mann 2001).

Surgical Options After Arch Collapse and Prior to Degenerative Changes

- Bony realignments are used in conjunction with PTT debridement and augmentation to protect the soft tissue repair and to correct the underlying deformity.
- The goal is to realign the foot without sacrificing essential hindfoot joints (subtalar, TN). This is done with osteotomies and/or fusions of non-essential joints.
- These hindfoot-sparing procedures cannot overcome advanced collapse of the hindfoot joints, especially when degenerative changes are present.
- While most surgeons agree that bony realignment and medial soft tissue augmentation is the appropriate surgical intervention in a flexible flatfoot, there is wide variation in the method chosen to achieve correction. Bony procedures include medializing calcaneal osteotomy, lateral column lengthening, and/or medial column stabilization.
- These procedures are always combined with soft tissue balancing, including gastrocnemius or Achilles lengthening, and PTT reconstruction.

Medial Sliding Calcaneal Tuberosity Osteotomy

- The combination of medial displacement calcaneal osteotomy and a medial soft tissue reconstruction is currently a popular treatment for patients with milder, flexible deformity and PTT dysfunction.
- Medial displacement calcaneal tuberosity osteotomy corrects hindfoot valgus directly. More importantly, the osteotomy translates the insertion of the Achilles' tendon, so that the tendon runs medial to the axis of the subtalar joint.

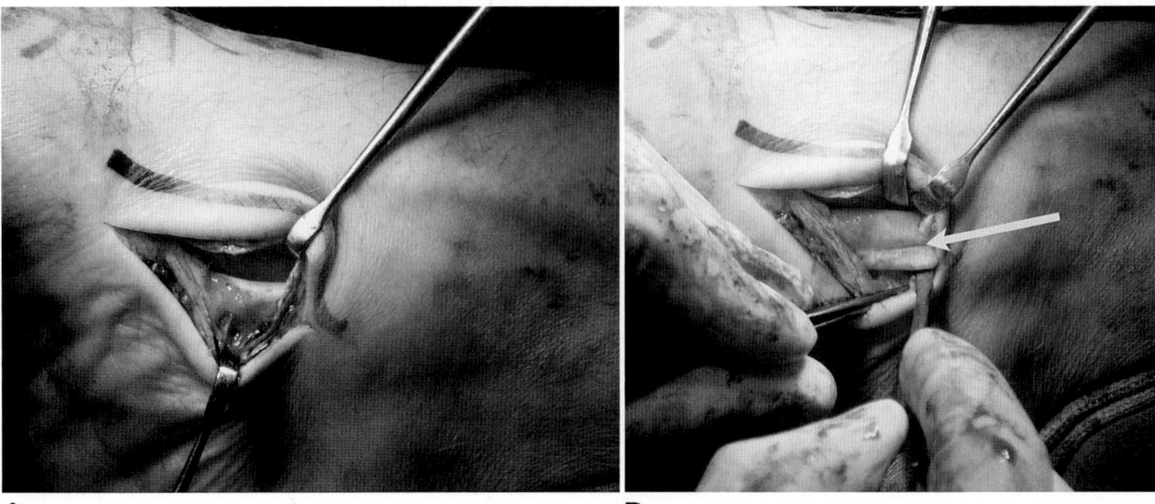

Figure 4–9: **A, At surgery, the posterior tibial tendon is seen to be covered with inflammatory tissue (synovitis). B, With resection of the synovium, a longitudinal tear is seen.**

    - The Achilles tendon then becomes an inverter of the hindfoot, locking the arch and assisting the posterior tibialis.
    - The shift to a more anatomical orientation also decreases the valgus vector from the peroneal brevis and enhances function of the peroneal longus as a plantar flexor of the first metatarsal. This should decrease the abduction moment on the forefoot.
- The flatfoot deformity is only partially corrected with medial calcaneal osteotomy. The procedure inconsistently improves arch height and partially improves TN coverage.
- A recent clinical outcome study by Myerson et al. (2004) demonstrated excellent pain relief (97%) and improvement in function (94%). Subtalar motion was normal in 56 patients, decreased in 66 patients, and moderately decreased in 7 patients. Traditionally, radiographic correction with medial displacement osteotomy and PTT reconstruction yields inconsistent and incomplete correction of alignment. However, in this study, radiographic correction was significant in all four radiographic parameters.

Medial Column Stabilization

- In some flatfeet, medial column collapse occurs at the first metatarsocuneiform or medial NC joint. In these feet, loss of medial column support (loss of the medial post of the tripod) leads to secondary hindfoot valgus.
- In these feet, selective realignment of the metatarsocuneiform and/or NC joints may be performed.
- These feet can be identified by observing collapse of these joints on the lateral weight-bearing radiograph (see Fig. 4–6).
- In some cases, realignment of the medial column joints will result in excellent correction of the arch (Fig. 4–10). In others, addition of a calcaneal osteotomy may be necessary.

Lateral Column Lengthening or Arthrodesis

- Because the subtalar joint acts like a screw, the hindfoot eversion (valgus) of the flatfoot causes the calcaneus to move posteriorly. Although the calcaneus is not truly short, the anterior edge of the bone appears shorter than the talus on weight-bearing anteroposterior radiographs.
- Lengthening of the calcaneus (in the lateral column of the foot) drives the rest of the foot around the talus, through the TN joint.
- The end effect of such lateral column lengthening is to rotate the flexible flatfoot back around the talus, leading to impressive arch correction (Fig. 4–11).
- Such lengthening can be done by inserting a structural graft of bone into an osteotomy of the anterior process of the calcaneus, or into the calcaneocuboid joint.
- When the lateral column is lengthened through the anterior process of the calcaneus, the osteotomy may pass through the middle facet of the subtalar joint. Such an intra-articular osteotomy is undesirable, at least in theory.
- When the lengthening is done through the calcaneocuboid joint (lengthening arthrodesis), the non-union rate is higher.
- In either case, non-unions can occur, so rigid internal fixation is necessary.
- Malunion/malpositioning of the lengthening can lead to fixed forefoot varus, with the first ray not touching the ground.
- Lateral column lengthening dramatically increases calcaneal pitch. It should probably not be used for feet in which the pitch is normal prior to surgery.
- The procedure was first described by Evans in 1975 for treatment of deformity secondary to multiple causes (poliomyelitis, idiopathic calcaneal valgus, rigid flatfoot, talipes equinovalgus, and traumatic division of the PTT in childhood). He reported that the operation was a success in all cases.
- Mosca in 1995 reported his results of the Evans osteotomy. Twenty-nine of 31 patients had a satisfactory clinical result, with creation of a medial arch, decreased talar head prominence, decreased medial pain, and decreased hindfoot valgus.
- Radiographic studies have demonstrated that lateral column lengthening improves talar head coverage by the navicular, reduces forefoot abduction, diminishes hindfoot valgus, and improves sagittal alignment of the arch (Sangeorzan et al. 1993).
- Realignment of the lateral column effects foot alignment in several ways.
    - The peroneal longus lever arm is lengthened. This makes the muscle a more powerful first metatarsal plantar flexor and restores forefoot alignment.
    - The plantar fascia is lengthened. This increases the static support of the arch.
    - The Achilles tendon insertion shifts medially, thereby decreasing its antagonizing effect on the PTT.
- A recent outcome study by Toolan et al. (1999) reviews the results of lateral column lengthening and PTT augmentation in 36 patients (41 feet).
    - Five out of six radiographic parameters were improved significantly.
    - Complications included non-union of the calcaneocuboid joint (20%); sural nerve paresthesias (32%); and additional surgical procedures (71%), such as removal of hardware, revision of fixation, and revision procedures including triple arthrodesis and medial osteotomies.

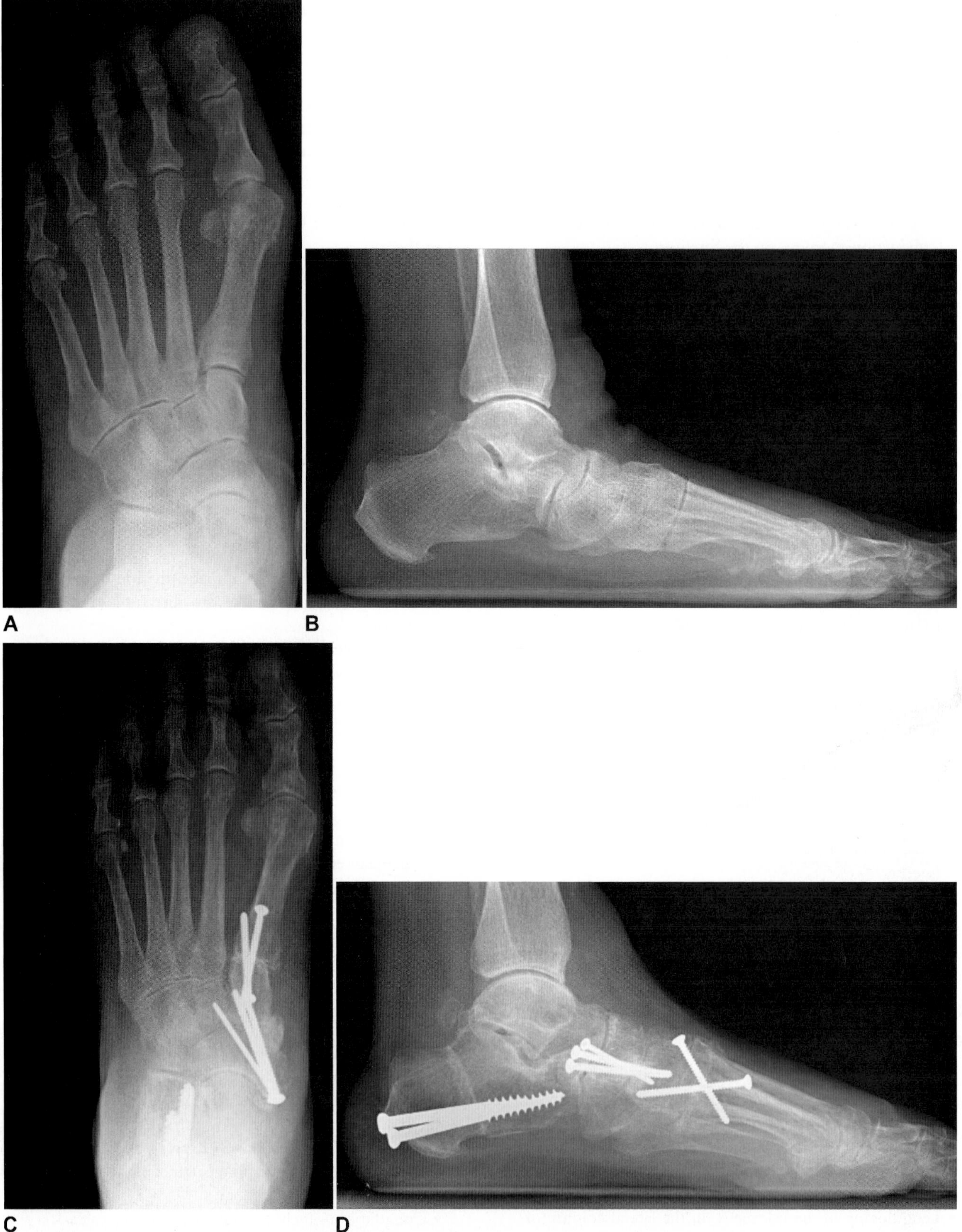

Figure 4–10: **A** and **B**, A 62-year-old woman with a symptomatic flatfoot deformity failed non-operative management. **C** and **D**, She was treated with Achilles lengthening, flexor digitorum longus to posterior tibial tendon transfer, medial column realignment and fusions (naviculocuneiform and tarsometatarsal), and medial sliding calcaneal osteotomy. On the anteroposterior view, note improvement in talonavicular coverage. On the lateral, arch height and talometatarsal angle are improved.

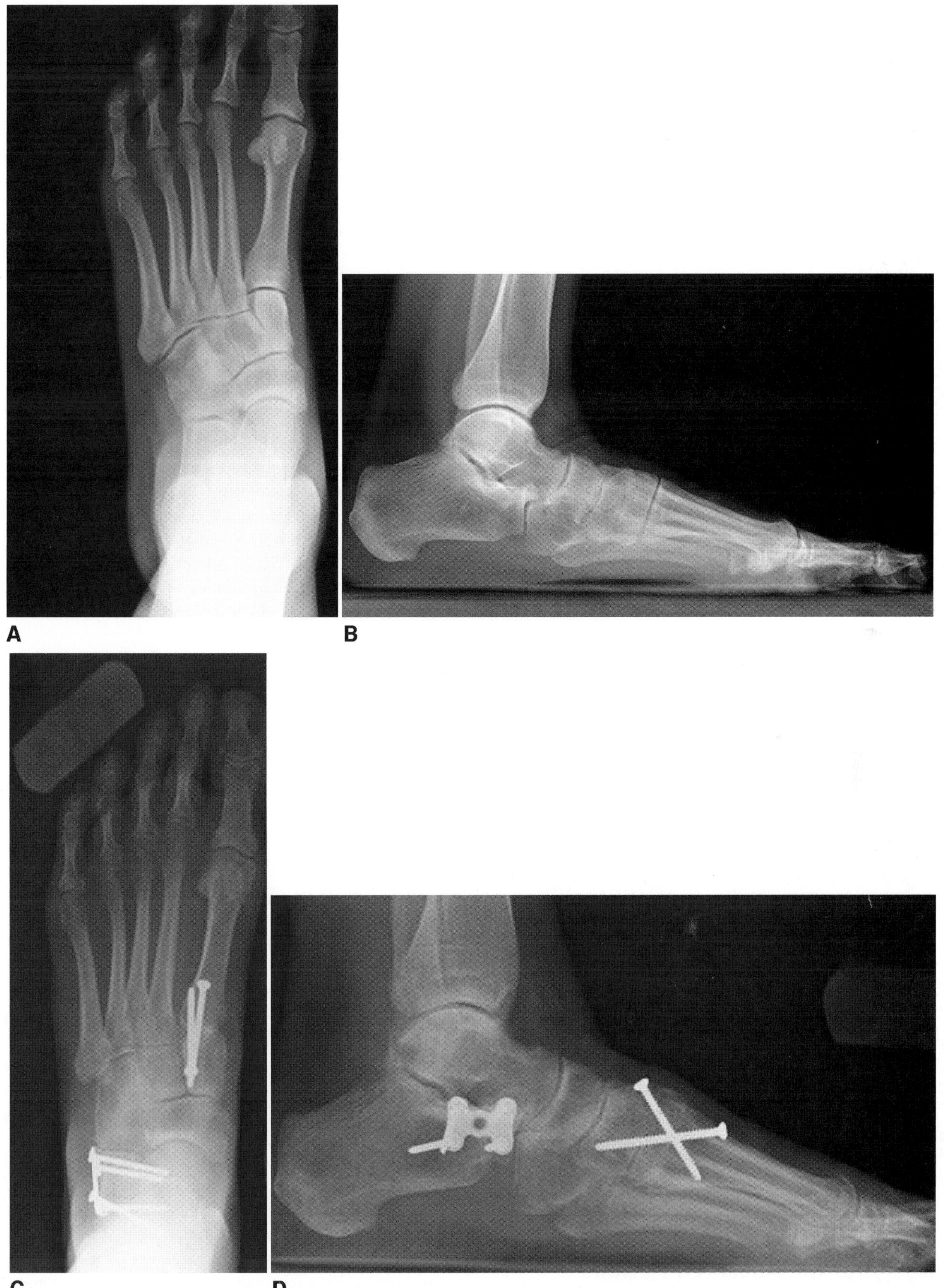

Figure 4–11: **A** and **B**, A 55-year-old woman with a painful deformity over her lateral foot and posterior tibial tendon (PTT), severe hindfoot valgus, forefoot abduction, and arch collapse. **C** and **D**, She was treated with gastrocnemius lengthening, PTT augmentation with flexor digitorum longus, first tarsometatarsal realignment and arthrodesis, and lateral column lengthening (through the anterior process of the calcaneus). She has substantial correction at 1 year post reconstruction.

- Eighty-eight percent were less painful or pain-free, and 85% of patients rated their result as satisfactory; 93% stated that they would have the procedure again if the circumstances were similar.

Combining Medial and Lateral Procedures

- In many feet, a combination of procedures may be needed. The presumption is that the best long-term results will come from more accurate restoration of normal foot structure. Lateral column lengthening or medial displacement osteotomy may be combined with metatarsocuneiform and/or NC realignment and fusion.
- A combination of both medial and lateral column procedures is indicated for a patient with hindfoot valgus, low calcaneal pitch angle, and transverse tarsal joint sag. It is able to correct all aspects of the forefoot and hindfoot deformities in a flexible flatfoot (Chi et al. 1999).

Compensatory Forefoot Supination

- In many flatfeet, collapse of the hindfoot will lead to supination of the forefoot (relative elevation of the first ray). As the hindfoot everts, the first ray must supinate or elevate to stay even with the floor. If this did not occur, the first ray would be driven into the floor.
- After successful hindfoot realignment, many flatfeet will have an elevated first ray (compensatory forefoot supination). In these cases, first metatarsocuneiform plantar flexion arthrodeses can be added to the reconstruction.

Selective Fusions

- Over the years, some surgeons have used isolated TN or subtalar fusions to correct the less severe, flexible flatfoot. Double fusion (TN and calcaneocuboid) has also been advocated.
- Short-term clinical series have shown favorable results.
- Because any of these procedures eliminate the majority of hindfoot motion, there may not be any benefit over triple arthrodesis.
- More importantly, for the less severe flatfoot with more flexible deformity (stage 2 posterior tibial tendonitis), the hindfoot-sparing procedures listed above may lead to better function.
- Of course, for the rare foot with isolated arthritis of one hindfoot joint, isolated fusion of that joint should result in a good outcome. A good example is a patient with posttraumatic arthritis of the TN joint after a navicular fracture.

Surgery for the Advanced Flatfoot

- Triple arthrodesis is historically the "gold standard" procedure for a rigid flatfoot. Arthrodesis of the subtalar, calcaneocuboid, and TN joints is performed with realignment of those joints.
- "In situ" fusion, without realignment, is never appropriate, because persistent deformity can adversely affect adjacent joints (ankle).
- Long-term outcome studies have shown high incidence of degenerative disease in neighboring joints, such as the ankle and midfoot.
- Because of the stiffness that results from triple arthrodesis, it is generally reserved for patients with hindfoot stiffness or arthritis that could not be managed with hindfoot-sparing procedures.
- In one large outcome study, 67 procedures were done on 57 feet, with an average follow-up of 44 years (Saltzman et al. 1999). Many of the study subjects had neuromuscular disease, not flatfoot.
  - Fifty-four patients (95%) were satisfied with the result of the operation, although 78% had some residual deformity, 13 patients had a pseudoarthrosis, and 37 patients had ankle pain.
  - All ankles had degenerative changes on radiographs, and arthritic findings were noted at the NC and TMT joints in the majority of patients.
- Because the most important joints are directly realigned, triple arthrodesis usually leads to good realignment of the hindfoot.
- As mentioned above, it is important to remember that many cases of advanced, rigid flatfoot will have secondary forefoot supination. Realignment of the hindfoot without attention to the forefoot will result in an elevated first metatarsal.
- Residual forefoot supination can be corrected by plantar flexing and fusing the first metatarsocuneiform joint (Fig. 4–12).

Ankle Valgus

- Realignment and pantalar fusion can be performed for the most severe valgus deformities. It results in a stiff straight foot, which is an improvement from a stiff, deformed foot but certainly not ideal.
- Papa and Myerson (1992) presented the results of 21 patients who underwent a pantalar fusion. Eighty-one percent reported improvement, but 95% of patients had lasting pain following the procedure. Those patients who underwent a tibiotalocalcaneal fusion (TN joint left free) instead of a traditional pantalar fusion were more mobile following the procedure.
- An alternative solution is a two-stage reconstruction. hindfoot realignment and fusion (generally triple arthrodesis) is performed initially. At the second stage, 3-6 months later, total ankle arthroplasty is performed.
- Total ankle arthroplasty offers the potential for some motion but has a relatively high complication rate, especially in the foot with severe preexisting deformity (Fig. 4–13).
- The foot deformity must be completely restored to minimize the valgus force across the ankle. Even so, complete incompetence of the deltoid may be a problem to

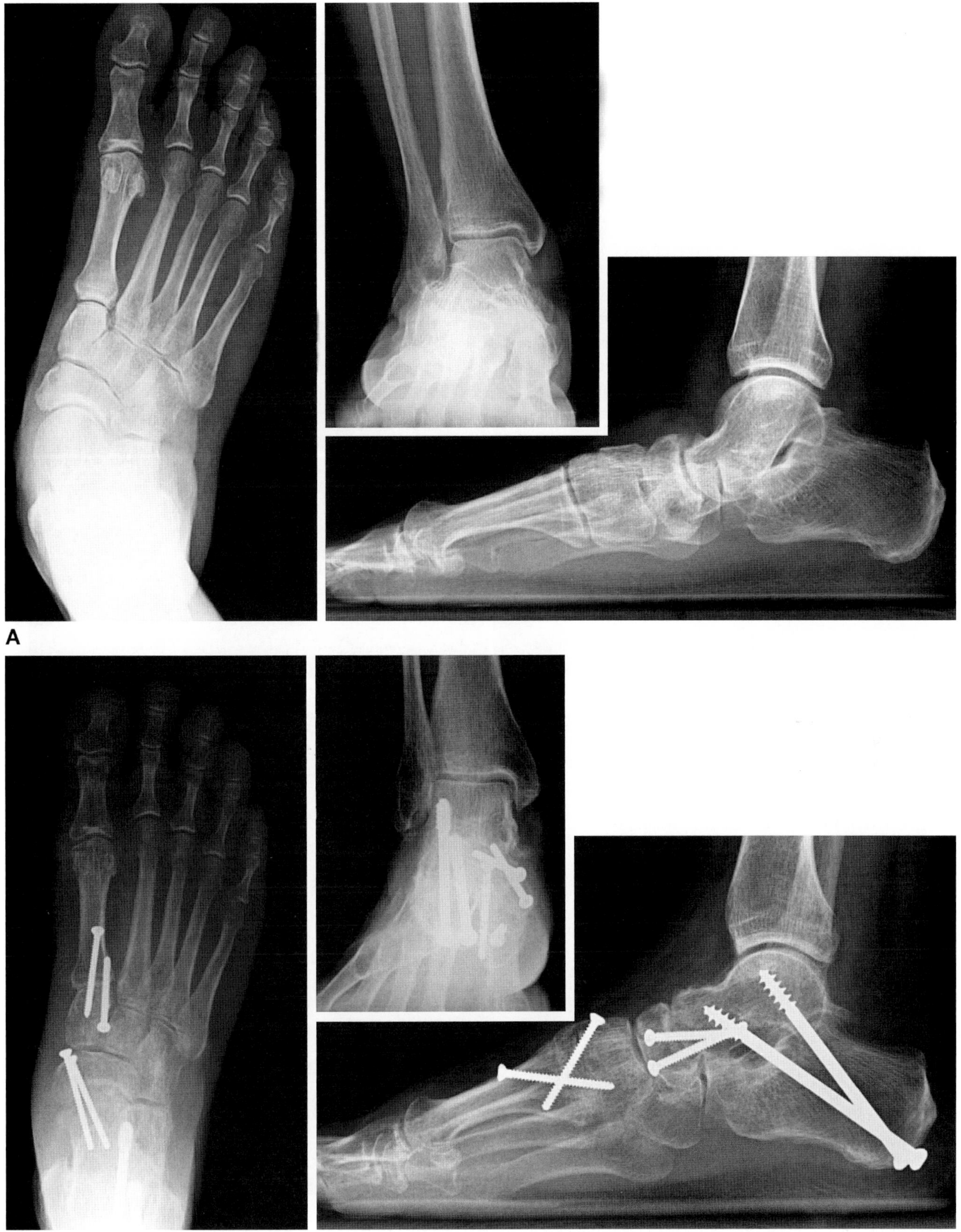

Figure 4–12: **A,** A 57-year-old man with a severe deformity and medial and lateral pain, who has failed orthotic management. **B,** The patient underwent fusion of the talonavicular and subtalar joints to restore hindfoot alignment. Although a triple arthrodesis usually includes the calcaneocuboid joint, that joint was not included in this fusion because it was not necessary. Residual forefoot supination required realignment and fusion of the first tarsometatarsal joint. He achieved excellent alignment with this "triple" arthrodesis.

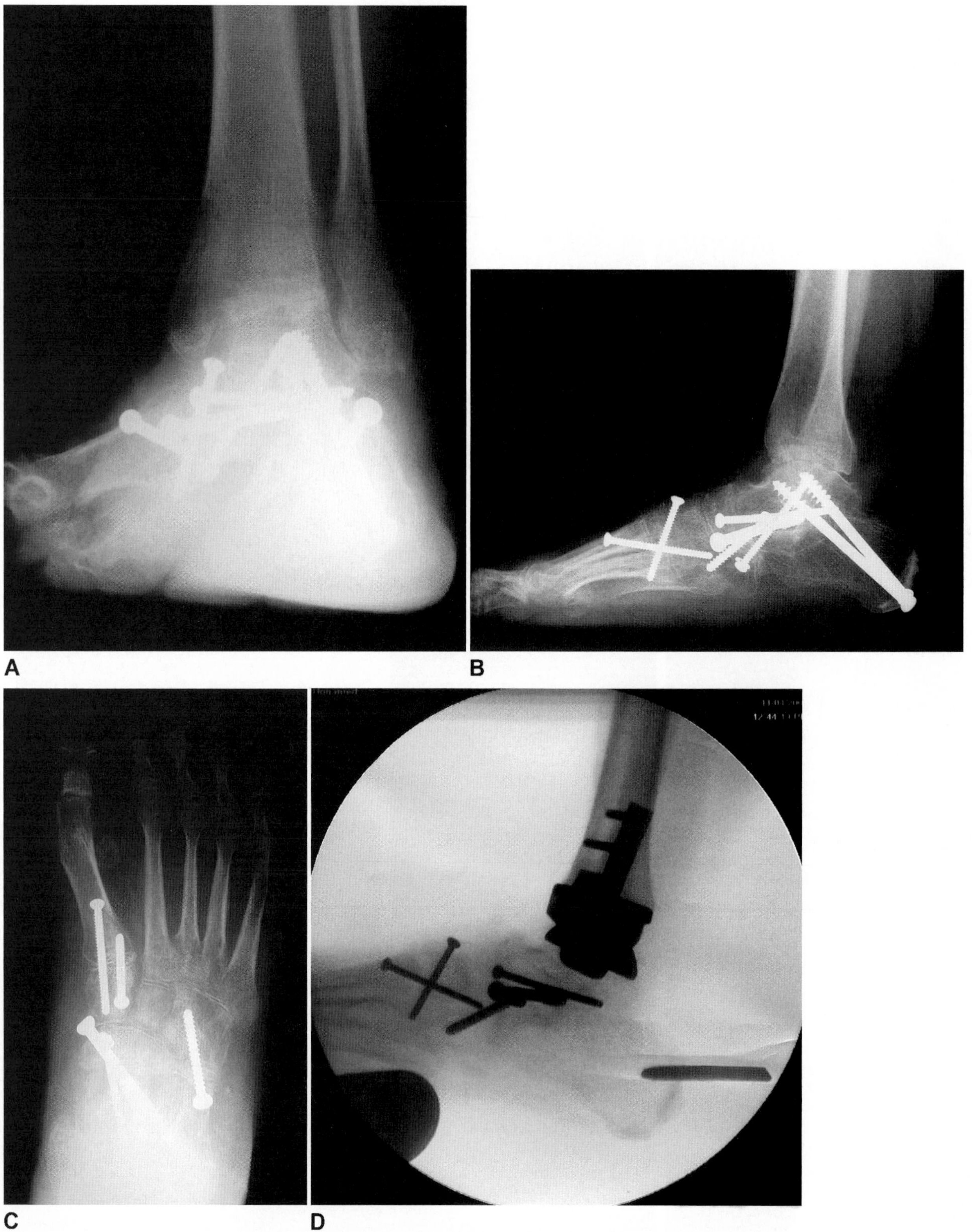

Figure 4–13: This patient suffered from pantalar arthritis from advanced valgus deformity of the hindfoot and ankle, secondary to rheumatoid arthritis. She initially underwent hindfoot realignment and arthrodesis of the subtalar, talonavicular, calcaneocuboid, and metatarsocuneiform joints (quadruple arthrodesis). **A**, The mortise view shows loss of ankle joint space. **B**, restoration of hindfoot alignment after the initial surgery. **C**, restoration of hindfoot alignment after the initial surgery. **D**, Three months later, she underwent total ankle arthroplasty. In the operating room, good alignment was achieved, and a wide-based talar component was used to minimize late subsidence.

Continued

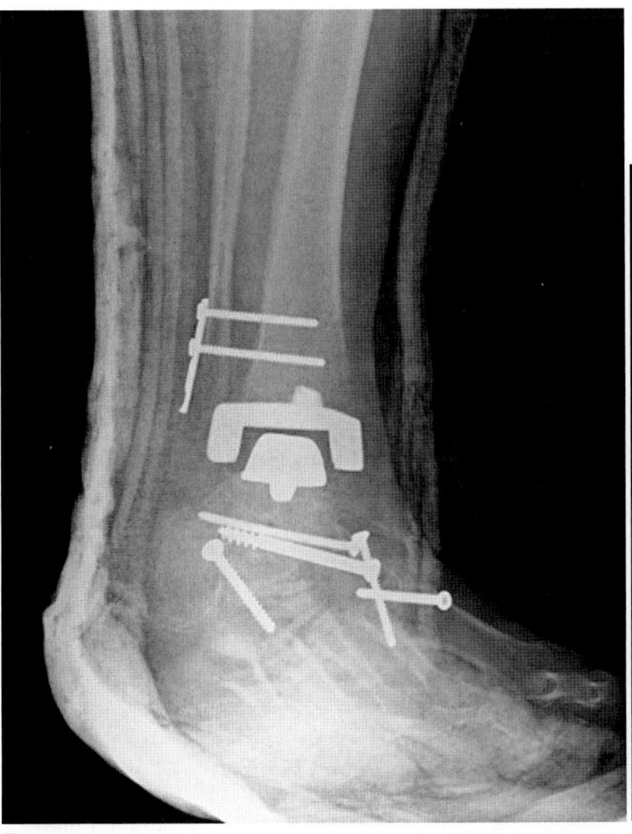

E

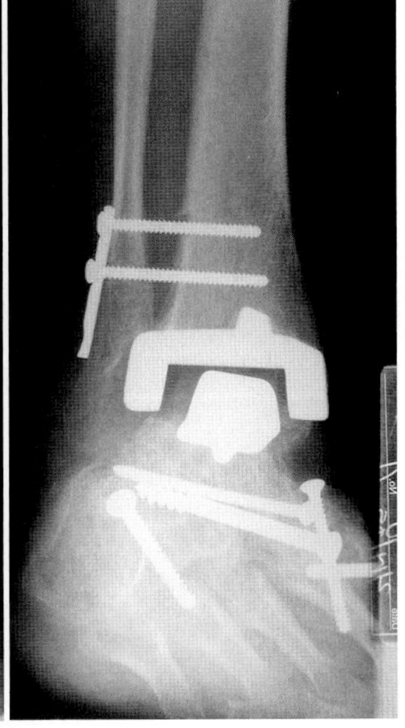

F

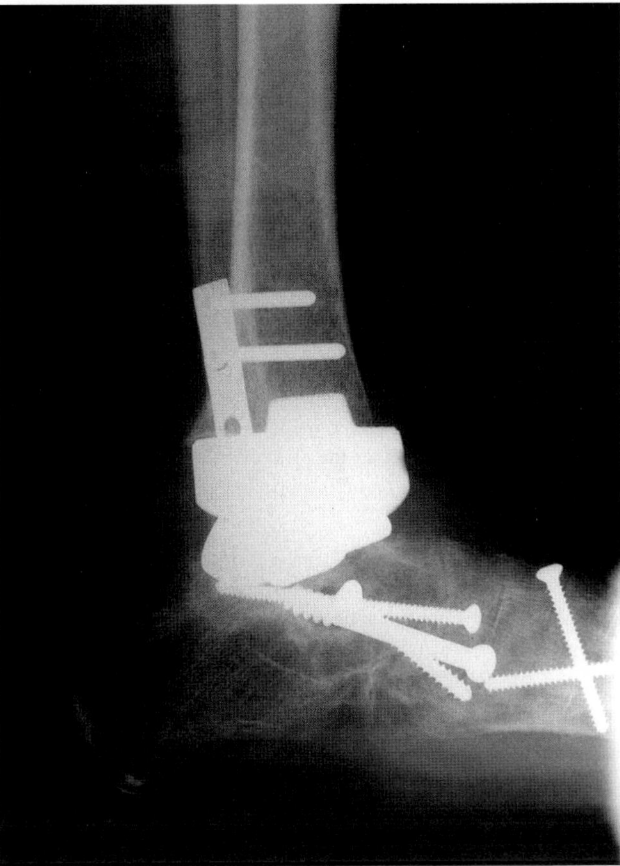

G

Figure 4–13: Cont'd **E**, The mortise view shows good early alignment. **F**, At 5 months postoperatively, the talar component is tilting into valgus and has subsided into the talus. She developed severe lateral ankle impingement pain and requested revision surgery and **G**, At 5 months postoperatively, the talar component is tilting into valgus and has subsided into the talus. She developed severe lateral ankle impingement pain and requested revision surgery.

total ankle arthroplasty, which normally relies on a tensioned deltoid ligament to prevent tilting of the talar component.
- Although the longevity of modern total ankle implants is still unproven, this procedure offers a chance for better function.

Other Procedures

- The patient with deformity from a Lisfranc joint malunion is best treated with multiple joint midfoot realignment. The first, second, and third TMT joints are fused, while the fourth and fifth are generally left mobile, even in the presence of arthritis. Achilles (or gastrocnemius) lengthening is usually required.
- A calcaneal malunion is addressed by tuberosity osteotomy with subtalar fusion and lateral wall decompression. The exact procedure depends on the individual anatomy and will vary.
- For the patient with advanced Charcot deformity, open reduction and internal fixation with arthrodesis is necessary (see Ch. 7).
- Long-term outcome studies for most of the modern flatfoot surgeries are not available.

References

Ananthakrisnan D, Ching R, Tencer A et al. (1999) Subluxation of the talocalcaneal joint in adults who have symptomatic flatfoot. J Bone Joint Surg 81-A: 1147-1154.

Using weight-bearing CT scans, the authors demonstrated subluxation of the subtalar facets with flatfoot, so that only about half of the joint was actually in contact.

Chao W et al. (1996) Nonoperative management of posterior tibial tendon dysfunction. Foot Ankle Int 17(12): 736-741.

Forty-nine patients with PTT dysfunction were treated with orthoses. Forty feet were treated with molded AFOs, and 13 feet were treated with UCBL shoe inserts with medial posting. The authors concluded that patients with PTT dysfunction can be treated by aggressive non-operative management, as 67% of patients had good to excellent results according to a functional scoring system based on pain, function, use of assistive device, distance of ambulation, and patient satisfaction.

Chi TD et al. (1999) The lateral column lengthening and medial column stabilization procedures. Clin Orthop Relat Res 365: 81-90.

The results of medial column stabilization, lateral column lengthening, and combined medial and lateral procedures were reviewed. The study concluded that these procedures effectively correct deformity without disrupting the essential joints of the hindfoot and midfoot, by evaluating pain, function, and radiographic parameters.

Hintermann B. (1995) [Dysfunction of the posterior tibial muscle due to tendon insufficiency]. Orthopade 24(3): 193-199.

This is a review of the dynamic and static supports of the arch in which the focus is on posterior tibialis tendon dysfunction. It recommends early diagnosis and repair or supplementation of the tendon to prevent flatfoot deformity.

Huang CK et al. (1993) Biomechanical evaluation of longitudinal arch stability. Foot Ankle 14(6): 353-357.

This is a study of 12 cadaveric specimens that were loaded after sectioning of the plantar fascia, plantar ligaments, and spring ligament. The study found that the highest relative contribution to arch stability was provided by the plantar fascia, followed by plantar ligaments and spring ligament. The division of the plantar fascia decreased arch stiffness by 25%.

Johnson KA, Strom DE. (1989) Tibialis posterior tendon dysfunction. Clin Orthop Relat Res 239: 196-206.

This paper introduces the staging system of PTT dysfunction. The pain symptoms, clinical signs, and roentgenographic changes for each of these stages are characteristic and reviewed.

Kannus P, Jozsa L. (1991) Histopathological changes preceding spontaneous rupture of a tendon. A controlled study of 891 patients. J Bone Joint Surg Am 73(10): 1507-1525.

A histopathological study of 897 spontaneously ruptured tendons was performed and compared with 445 non-ruptured cadaveric tendons. The findings indicated that degenerative changes are common in the tendons of people who are older than 35 years, and that these changes are associated with spontaneous rupture.

Malicky ES et al. (2002) Talocalcaneal and subfibular impingement in symptomatic flatfoot in adults. J Bone Joint Surg Am 84-A(11): 2005-2009.

Nineteen patients with symptomatic flatfeet and lateral-sided pain were analyzed using CT and weight-bearing x-rays. The study concluded that impingement occurs first within the sinus tarsi and then may involve the calcaneofibular region.

Mann RA. (2001) Posterior tibial tendon dysfunction. Treatment by flexor digitorum longus transfer. Foot Ankle Clin 6(1): vi, 77-87.

A review of the various methods to treat PTT dysfunction. The review focuses on FDL transfer in the attenuated PTT.

Myerson MS, Badekas A, Schon LC. (2004) Treatment of stage II posterior tibial tendon deficiency with flexor digitorum longus tendon transfer and calcaneal osteotomy. Foot Ankle Int 25(7): 445-450.

A retrospective review of 129 patients treated with FDL transfer and medial calcaneal osteotomy for PTT dysfunction. The study concluded—based on radiographic, subjective measurements and function scores—that the procedure yielded excellent results, with minimal complications and a high patient satisfaction rate.

Papa JA, Myerson MS. (1992) Pantalar and tibiotalocalcaneal arthrodesis for post-traumatic osteoarthrosis of the ankle and hindfoot. J Bone Joint Surg Am 74(7): 1042-1049.

Twenty-one patients (13 had a tibiotalocalcaneal fusion and 8 had a pantalar fusion) were evaluated for pain, satisfaction, and return to work. The study found that patients who had had a tibiotalocalcaneal arthrodesis were more mobile and functioned at a higher level than those who had had a pantalar arthrodesis. It concluded that extended arthrodesis of the ankle and hindfoot should be regarded as a salvage operation capable of producing a satisfactory result and usually providing a reasonable alternative to amputation.

Saltzman CL et al. (1999) Triple arthrodesis: twenty-five and forty-four-year average follow-up of the same patients. J Bone Joint Surg Am 81(10): 1391-1402.

A long-term outcome study evaluating patient satisfaction and function following triple arthrodesis for numerous neuromuscular underlying conditions.

Sangeorzan BJ, Mosca V, Hansen ST Jr. (1993) Effect of calcaneal lengthening on relationships among the hindfoot, midfoot, and forefoot. Foot Ankle 14(3): 136-141.

Radiographic parameters of the flatfoot deformity were defined. These parameters were then used to evaluate the corrective power of a lateral column lengthening.

Sharkey NA, Ferris L, Donahue SW. (1998) Biomechanical consequences of plantar fascial release or rupture during gait: Part I—Disruptions in longitudinal arch conformation. Foot Ankle Int 19(12): 812-820.

This is a cadaveric study in which the effect of complete plantar fascia sectioning on arch height was analyzed. Radiographic measurements of height of the arch, base length of the arch, and talo-first metatarsal angle were used to assess contributions to arch support made by the plantar fascia, tibialis posterior, peroneus longus and brevis, and digital flexor muscles. Complete fasciotomy caused significant collapse of the arch in the sagittal plane.

Teasdall RD, Johnson KA. (1994) Surgical treatment of stage I posterior tibial tendon dysfunction. Foot Ankle Int 15(12): 646-648.

A review of 19 patients who underwent synovectomy and debridement for stage 1 PTT dysfunction. Seventy-four percent of patients had complete pain relief, and 84% of patients subjectively reported being "much better" and had a return of function. Two patients underwent subtalar arthrodesis for progressive foot deformity and continued pain.

Toolan BC, Sangeorzan BJ, Hansen ST Jr. (1999) Complex reconstruction for the treatment of dorsolateral peritalar subluxation of the foot. Early results after distraction arthrodesis of the calcaneocuboid joint in conjunction with stabilization of, and transfer of the flexor digitorum longus tendon to, the midfoot to treat acquired pes planovalgus in adults. J Bone Joint Surg Am 81(11): 1545-1560.

The functional and radiographic results of a painful, flexible flatfoot associated with attrition or rupture of the PTT were evaluated in 36 patients (41 feet) treated with calcaneocuboid distraction arthrodesis and medial soft tissue supplementation. The study concluded that relief of pain and the restoration of function achieved through effective correction of the severe pes planovalgus deformity accounted for the satisfactory outcomes in these patients.

The Non-neuromuscular Cavus Foot

Margaret Chilvers[*] and Arthur Manoli II[§]

[*]M.D., Michigan International Foot and Ankle Center, Pontiac, MI
[§]M.D., Director, Michigan International Foot and Ankle Center, Pontiac, MI

- There are a wide variety of foot shapes. The high-arched foot may be referred to as a cavus or cavovarus foot. The cavus foot is traditionally thought of as a manifestation of a neuromuscular condition, but it is commonly found in a less severe form in the normal population.
- There is a normal, bell-shaped distribution of arch height with varying degrees of flat as well as high-arched foot types. The subtle cavus foot has a higher arch than normal but is not associated with any neuromuscular condition.
- The subtle cavus foot is associated with various problems, though, including ankle instability, varus ankle arthrosis, peroneal tendon disorders, lateral foot overload with stress fractures, metatarsalgia and claw toe deformity, ankle impingement syndromes, plantar fasciitis, lateral knee strain, iliotibial band syndrome, and medial knee arthrosis.

Pathomechanics

- During the stance phase of gait, the normal foot position is of hindfoot eversion. This unlocks the transverse tarsal joints and allows the foot to absorb shock. This occurs through the subtalar, talonavicular, and calcaneocuboid joints. If the foot position does not reach this everted position (the cavus hindfoot remains inverted), the shock absorption is decreased.
- There are two main types of cavus foot. The first type is the *forefoot*-driven cavus foot. The cause of the cavus is plantar flexion of the first ray. When the first ray is plantar flexed, as the foot reaches midstance the first metatarsal head hits the ground and stops the progression of the hindfoot into eversion. This keeps the entire foot in varus and eliminates the shock absorption capability of the hindfoot.
  - Another way to think of this is with the "tripod" model of the foot, as described in Chapter 1. A plantar flexed first ray drives the hindfoot into varus.
- The forefoot-driven cavus foot in the non-neuromuscular population is most likely inherited. It is usually associated with peroneus longus hyperactivity (the overactive long peroneal plantar flexes the first metatarsal) and a tight gastrocnemius complex.
- The second type of cavus is the *hindfoot*-driven cavus. The abnormality is a primary varus alignment of the hindfoot.
- Causes of a hindfoot cavus include congenital, untreated or late sequelae of clubfoot, calcaneus fracture malunion, tarsal coalition, and deep posterior compartment scarring as a late consequence of compartment syndrome.
- Whether the primary cause of the cavus is the forefoot or the hindfoot, with time the opposite structure will become a secondary contributor to cavus. For example, if the hindfoot is the primary cause of the cavus, the first metatarsal will plantar flex to meet the ground. At first, the secondary forefoot plantar flexion will be supple, but it will eventually become a stiff, secondary deformity (Manoli and Graham 2005).

Associated Conditions

- With any abnormal posture or alignment, there will eventually be sequelae that develop from the abnormality. With cavus foot alignment, whether forefoot- or hindfoot-driven, there are many associated conditions (Box 5–1).
- A common presenting complaint of a person with cavus is frequent ankle sprains. With hindfoot inversion, the smallest grade can tilt the hindfoot "past the point of no return," causing a lateral ligament sprain. This may be seen with or without ligamentous laxity. The instability may occur within the ankle or less commonly at the subtalar joint.
- Recurrent sprains may lead to anterolateral ankle impingement.
- Peroneal tendons are constantly on stretch with the cavus foot. In addition, they are working to evert the stiff cavus foot and are frequently the site of complaints. The end result can be partial or complete tears of the peroneus brevis.
  - The peroneus longus may be hyperactive and contribute to the cavus by plantar flexing the first ray (Brandes and Smith 2000).
- Lateral foot overload is common with cavus alignment. The majority of the walking stance phase is spent on the lateral aspect of the foot and can lead to fourth or fifth metatarsal stress fractures.
- The cavus foot is a poor shock absorber due to the inability to evert the hindfoot to neutral. This may lead to stress fractures in the tibial shaft, medial plafond, or even tibial plateau.
- A cavus foot is commonly seen with runners who develop iliotibial band symptoms.
- Metatarsalgia under the first ray and sesamoid complaints may develop with a plantar flexed first metatarsal.
- The gastrocnemius is often contracted. This contracture will increase plantar fascia strain and can cause plantar fasciitis. Forefoot equinus from the plantar flexion of the first ray makes the gastrocnemius contracture even worse and plantar fascial strains higher.

Box 5–1 Associated Conditions With Non-neuromuscular Cavus Foot Alignment

- The hindfoot is inverted.
- Predisposes to lateral ligament ankle sprains.
- Recurrent sprains lead to ankle arthritis with varus alignment.
- Persistent varus alignment overloads the peroneals, especially peroneus brevis, with secondary tears.
- Hindfoot varus overloads the lateral column of the foot, with fifth metatarsal stress fractures.
- First metatarsal is plantar flexed.
- Increased pressure under first metatarsal head leads to metatarsalgia.
- Also predisposes to sesamoid stress injuries.
- Arch is high.
- Focuses pressure on forefoot and heel, with pain.
- Clawing of the toes possible from long toe extensors "working" to dorsiflex the midfoot?
- Focuses more pressure on metatarsal heads, with metatarsalgia.
- Shoe-fitting problems with claw toes.
- Varus alignment of foot forces knee into varus.
- Medial knee pain/arthritis.
- Iliotibial band syndrome.

Evaluation of the Patient with a Cavus Foot

- As in all other orthopaedic problems, the first step is careful history. Patients with subtle cavus foot alignment will complain of frequent ankle sprains, ankle pain, lateral foot and ankle pain, arch pain, forefoot pain, or even knee pain. Many times, they have seen other physicians for the same complaints.
- The most important aspect of physical examination is the standing evaluation. With the patient facing forward, line his or her feet parallel and at least six inches apart. In a person with cavus alignment, the medial aspect of the heel will be visible when facing forward. There may also be a bulge or wrinkle under the first metatarsal head (Fig. 5–1A). In contrast, the normal foot or flatfoot will show no medial heel when viewed from the front. This visible medial heel pad has been called the "peek-a-boo" heel sign (Beals and Manoli 1996).
- With the patient still standing, view the patient from behind. Normal hindfoot alignment is about 5° of valgus. In the cavus foot alignment, the calcaneus will be in varus as compared with the midline of the calf. In contrast, the flatfoot will reveal toes lateral to the foot and the classic "too many toes" sign (Fig. 5–1B).
- Once identifying the cavus foot alignment, the most important tool is the 1-inch Coleman block (Coleman and Chesnut 1977). This will differentiate the forefoot-driven cavus from the hindfoot-driven cavus.
  - While observing the patient from behind, place the block under the heel and lateral forefoot. Allow the first two toes to fall off the medial edge of the block. If the hindfoot corrects to a normal valgus alignment, the cavus is forefoot-driven and the hindfoot is flexible (Fig. 5–1C). If there is little or no correction with the block, the hindfoot is stiff in varus (Fig. 5–2).
- Seated examination includes assessment of motion, specifically subtalar motion. A rigid or stiff subtalar joint that is not correctable on the Coleman block may be indicative of a tarsal coalition or arthrosis within the hindfoot. A supple subtalar joint will point to the forefoot as the cause of the cavus.

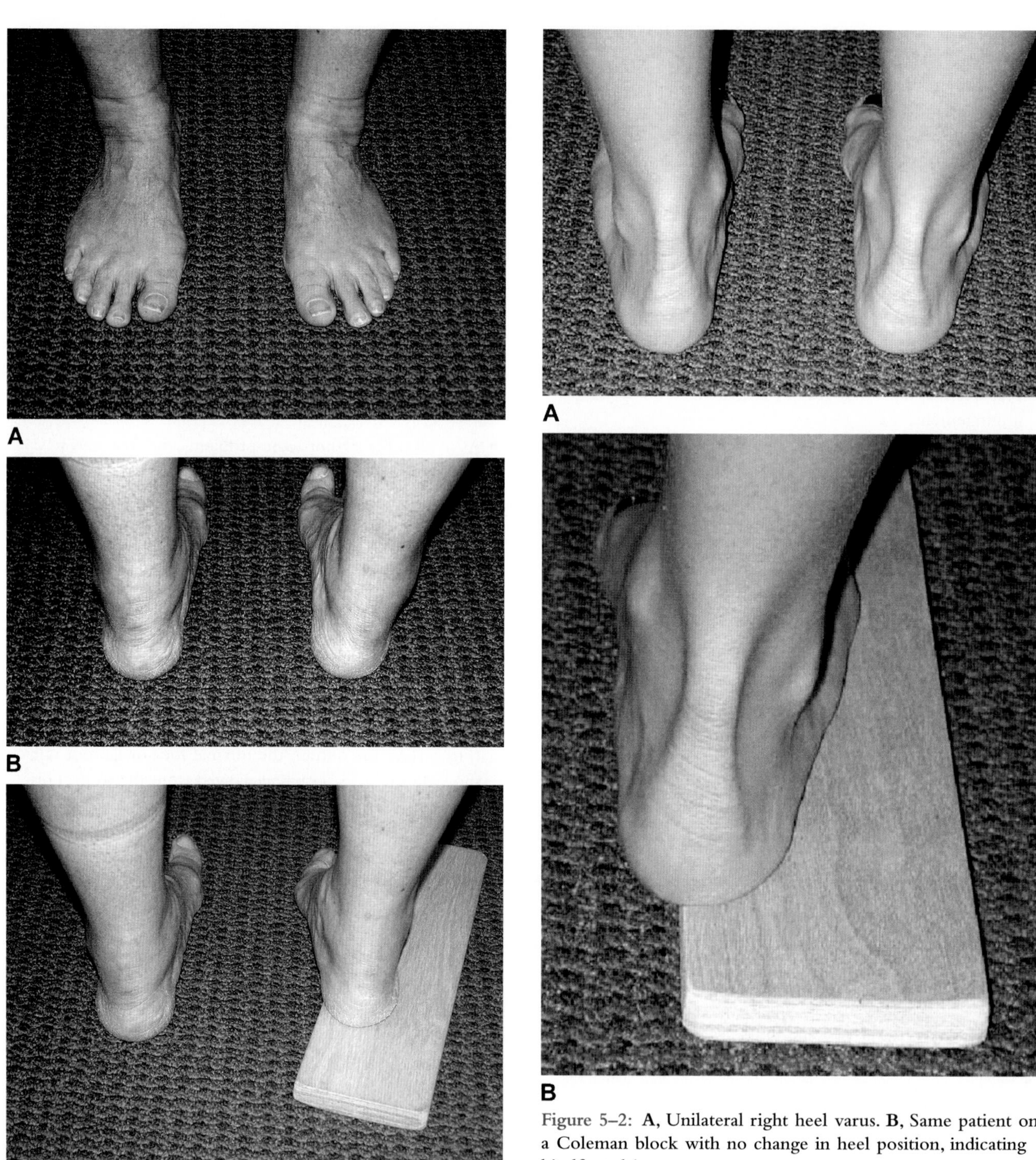

Figure 5–1: **A, Unilateral cavus foot on left (patient's right foot). Note the appearance of the medial heel on the left, while on the opposite side the medial heel is not visible. B, Right varus heel alignment on the same patient, viewed from behind. Note the normal heel alignment of the left foot. C, Correction of heel alignment on Coleman block testing on the same patient. Note the same alignment of both feet while right foot is on the block, implying forefoot-driven cavus.**

Figure 5–2: **A, Unilateral right heel varus. B, Same patient on a Coleman block with no change in heel position, indicating hindfoot-driven cavus.**

- A gastrocnemius contracture should be detected. This is assessed by keeping the hindfoot in a neutral position and dorsiflexing the ankle with the knee extended. An associated gastrocnemius contracture will potentiate the forefoot-driven cavus foot by increasing the relative strength of the peroneus longus as compared with the anterior tibialis (Manoli and Graham 2005) (Fig. 5–3).
- The remainder of the examination is performed in the same manner as for any other orthopaedic examination and

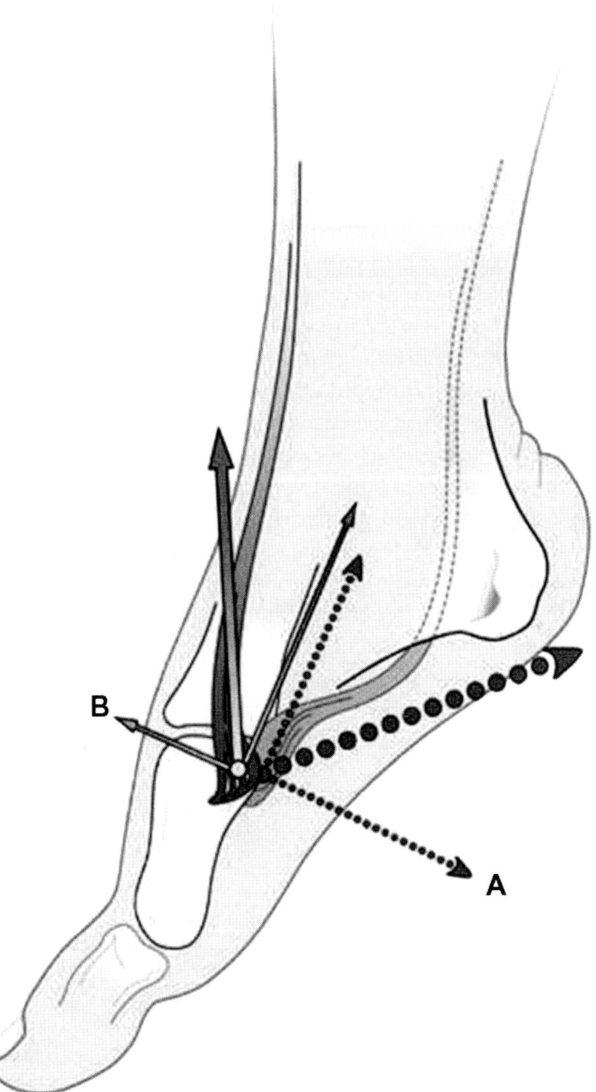

Figure 5–3: **Peroneus longus contribution to cavus foot alignment is potentiated by equinus ankle position. With the foot in equinus, the relative strength of the peroneus longus is greater than the tibialis anterior, leading to first ray plantar flexion.**

is directed to the presenting complaints. Ankle instability is evaluated by testing for ligamentous stability. Ankle impingement signs are directed in the accessory band of the anterior tibiofibular ligament and the anterior ankle capsule. A bone spur may occur at the anterior talofibular ligament. A stress fracture may occur within the fourth or fifth metatarsal. Peroneal tendinopathy may occur, and many times it occurs distally, near the peroneal tubercle.

Imaging

- Radiographic examination should include weight-bearing radiographs of feet and ankles. The anteroposterior ankles and feet should be taken together on the same plate. The lateral radiograph should include the lower one-third of the leg and the foot on one plate.
- On lateral radiographs, the fifth metatarsal base and the inferior aspect of the medial cuneiform should be near the same level. If the fifth metatarsal base is much closer to the floor, the foot is in cavus. If the medial cuneiform is closer to the floor, the foot is in planus (Fig. 5–4).
- Also on the lateral radiograph of the foot-ankle, the Meary lateral talometatarsal angle is measured along the

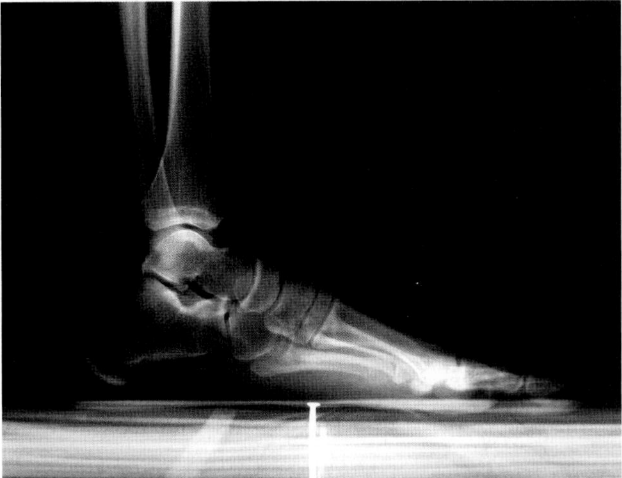

A

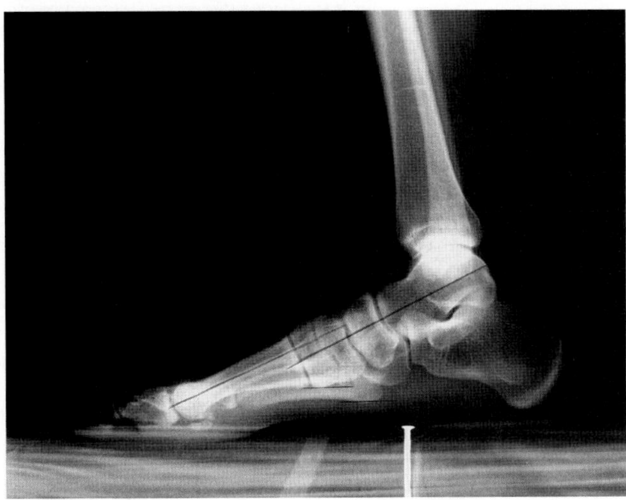

B

Figure 5–4: **A, Standing lateral foot-ankle radiograph of a cavus foot. Note the relative height of the medial cuneiform compared with the fifth metatarsal, and the flexion of the long axis of the first metatarsal compared with the long axis of the talus (Meary angle). B, Standing lateral foot-ankle radiograph of a normal foot. Note that the level of the medial cuneiform is closer to the level of the fifth metatarsal. The long axis of the talus is parallel with the long axis of the first metatarsal.**

Continued

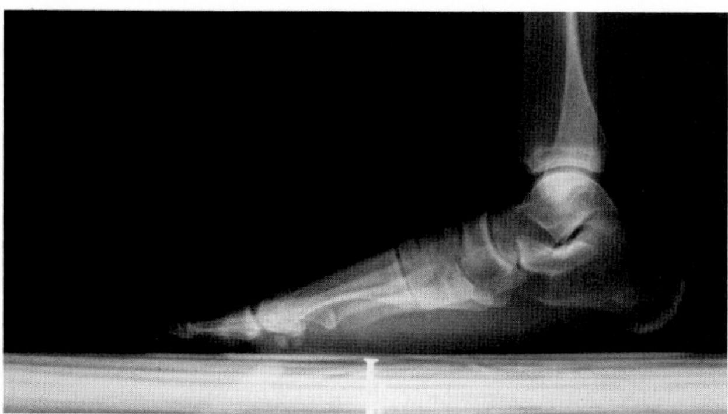

C

Figure 5–4: Cont'd **C, Standing lateral foot-ankle radiograph of a flatfoot. Note that the medial cuneiform is slightly inferior to the fifth metatarsal, and that the long axis of the first metatarsal is dorsiflexed in comparison with the long axis of the talus.**

long axis of the talus and first metatarsal. A normal angle is near 0, while a plantar flexed angle of 20° or more is indicative of a severe neuromuscular cavus foot (Paulos et al. 1980). For the subtle cavus foot, the angle will be 5-10°.

- The last measurement on the lateral radiograph is the calcaneal pitch. A high calcaneal pitch is an angle greater than 30°, and is associated with a hindfoot cavus.
- Normally on anteroposterior radiographs, the talus and calcaneus are divergent, with a talocalcaneal angle of 20-40°. If the angle is less and the talocalcaneal angle is more parallel, the foot is in cavus. Also, the talar head will be completely covered by the navicular in the cavus foot but will be relatively uncovered in the flatfoot. The width of the midfoot is greater in planus feet and progressively gets narrower as the foot is in more cavus (Fig. 5–5).
- On the anteroposterior ankle radiograph, with more severe or longstanding cavus the entire talus may be tipped into varus within the mortise (Fig. 5–6).
- Further tests may be necessary, depending on the associated pathology. For suspicion of stress fractures on the lateral foot, a bone scan is helpful (Fig. 5–7).
- If the foot is rigid with no correction of the foot on the Coleman block test, a computed tomography scan should be obtained in the semicoronal plane perpendicular to the posterior facet of the calcaneus, and axial cuts in the plane of the foot, to determine the presence of a tarsal coalition.
- Magnetic resonance imaging may be utilized to determine pathology within the peroneal tendons.

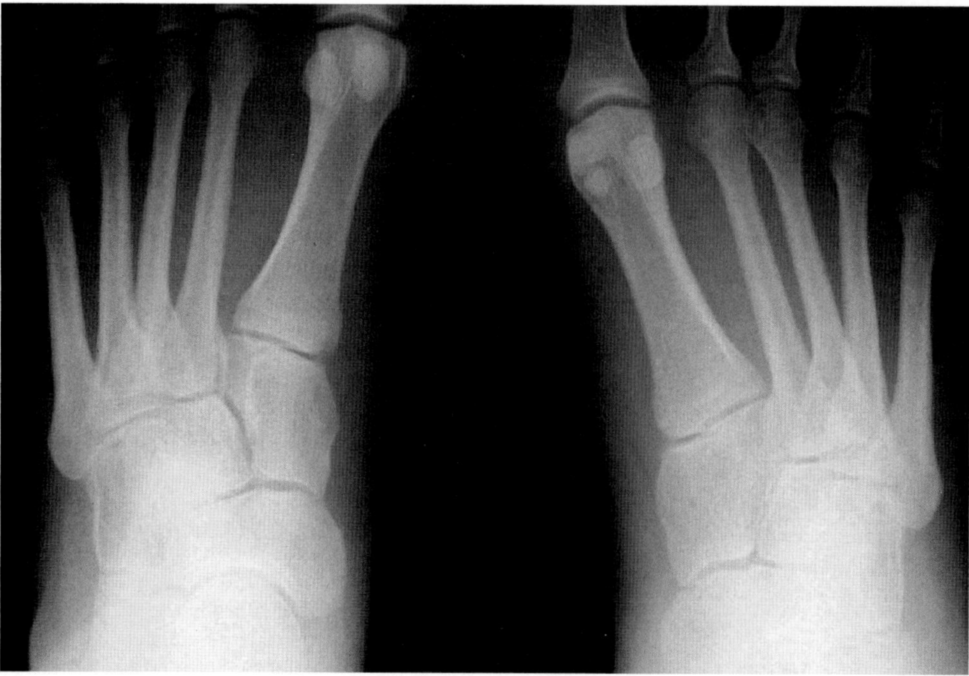

A

Figure 5–5: **A, Standing anteroposterior radiograph of a cavus foot. Note the parallelism of the talus and calcaneus, and the narrow midfoot.**

Continued

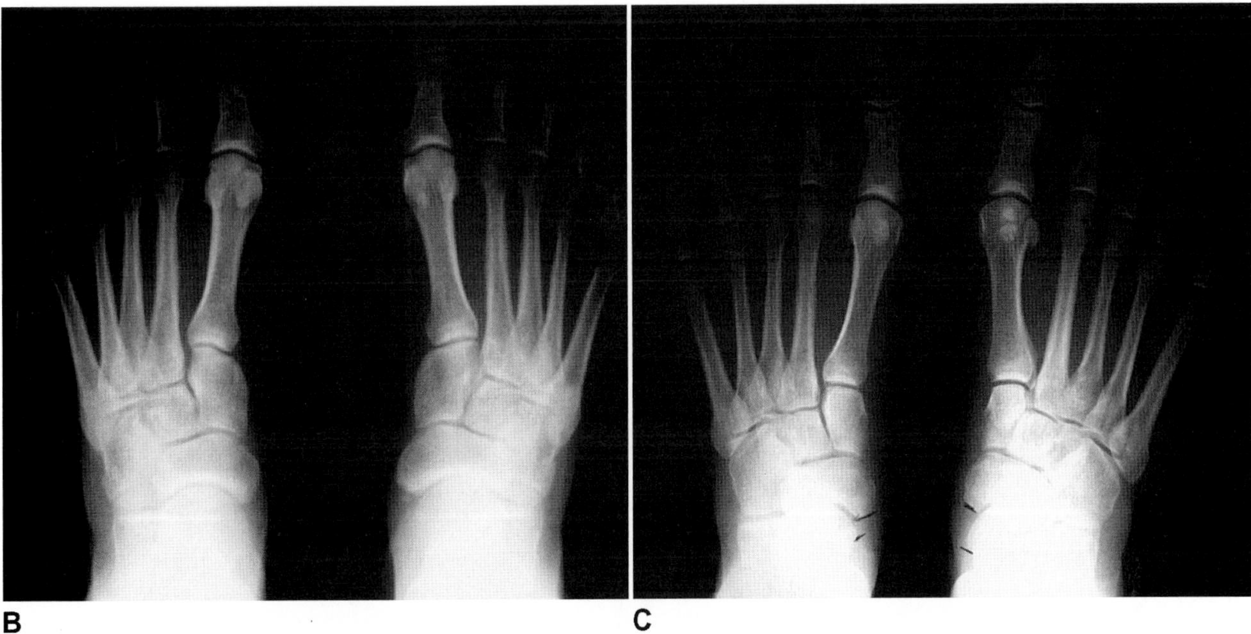

Figure 5–5: Cont'd **B**, Standing anteroposterior radiograph of a normal foot. Note the divergence of the talus and calcaneus. Compare width of midfoot to the cavus midfoot. C, Standing anteroposterior radiograph of a flatfoot. As compared with the normal left foot, there is a greater width of midfoot and uncovering of the right talar head.

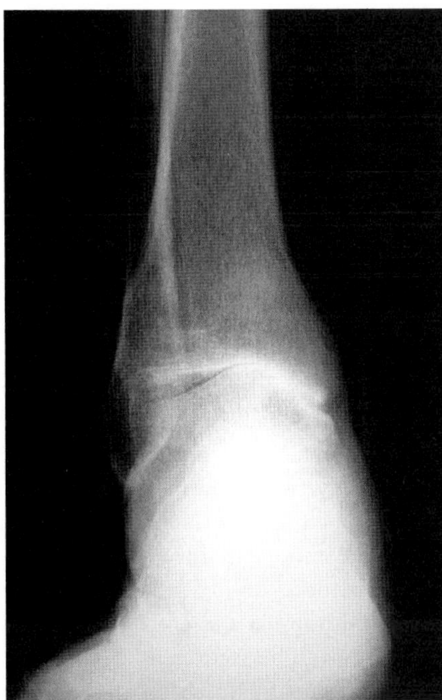

Figure 5–6: Standing anteroposterior ankle radiograph. Note the tipping of the talus under the plafond in the longstanding cavus patient.

Treatment

- Management of the cavus foot should begin non-operatively. A forefoot-driven cavus will have a supple hindfoot, and so a cavus foot orthosis can be utilized.
  - The principles of a cavus foot orthosis are a laterally based forefoot wedge with a recessed area for the first metatarsal head. This recess allows the first metatarsal to plantar flex further, and allows the hindfoot to evert to a neutral/shock-absorbing position (Fig. 5–8).
- Because a tight gastrocnemius complex will potentiate the forefoot-driven cavus, a gastrocnemius stretching program is initiated. Failure of the stretching program after 2 months is an indication for gastrocnemius recession, which generally improves range of motion and complaints associated with the cavus deformity.
- Surgery is indicated for failure of non-operative treatment. Treatment is first directed to the immediate problem, such as a stress fracture, incompetent ankle ligaments, or peroneal tendon tear. Then, the foot is realigned to minimize the chance of recurrence.

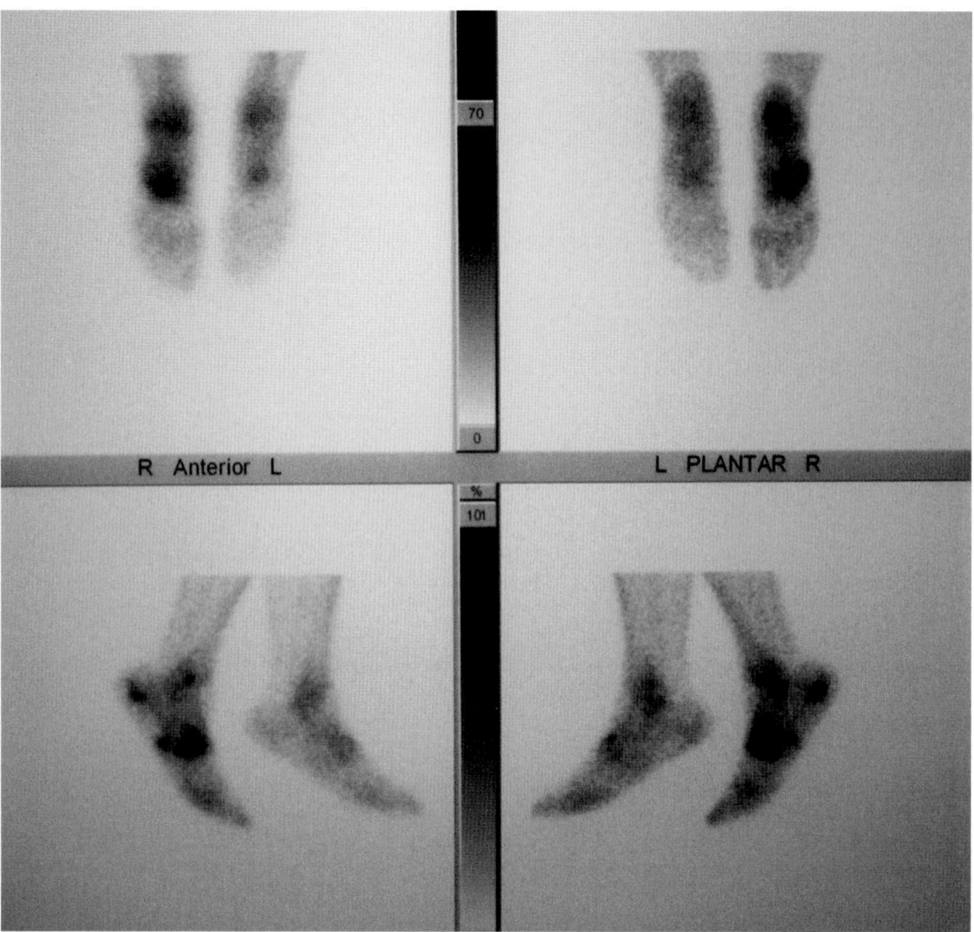

Figure 5–7: **Bone scan indicating stress fracture of right fourth metatarsal base in a patient with subtle cavus foot alignment.**

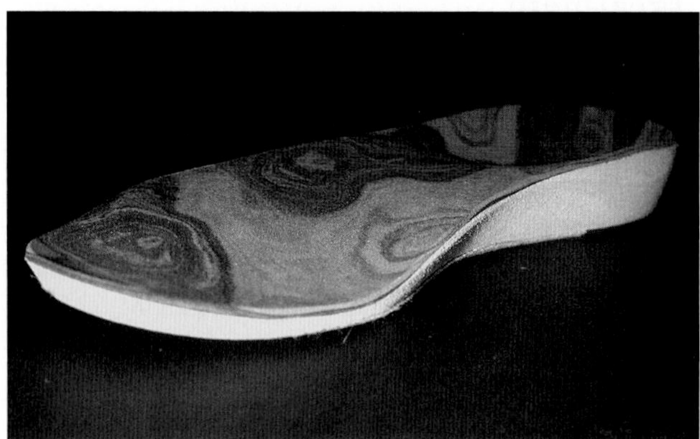

Figure 5–8: **Cavus foot orthotic. Note the hollowed-out recess under the first metatarsal head and the laterally based forefoot wedge and lowered medial arch.**

- Realignment surgery varies, depending on where the deformity resides.
- With a forefoot-driven cavus (plantar flexed first metatarsal), a dorsiflexing osteotomy of the first metatarsal is made (Fig. 5–9). Alternately, a dorsiflexing fusion of the first metatarsocuneiform joint can be easily performed.
- The forefoot-driven cavus foot will usually have an overactive long peroneal. The peroneus longus is then tenodesed to the peroneus brevis. This transfer takes away the deforming force and strengthens the hindfoot evertor (brevis).
- If, after the first metatarsal dorsiflexion osteotomy, there is still plantar flexion of the other rays, multiple dorsiflexion osteotomies may be needed. This is not common in the neurologically normal cavus foot.
- With time, a forefoot-driven cavus foot can develop secondary to hindfoot stiffness in varus. In these cases, a lateral sliding calcaneal tuberosity osteotomy brings the heel out of varus and normalizes forces in the foot and ankle (Fig. 5–10).
- In a very stiff cavovarus foot, a medial partial plantar fasciectomy may be required to allow the posterior tuber to slide laterally. A more extensive medial release of tight structures may be necessary for realignment. The medial talonavicular joint capsule and even some of the spring ligament may need to be sectioned.
- The gastrocnemius contracture should also be addressed with a gastrocnemius recession if the contracture is isolated to the gastrocnemius, or an Achilles tendon lengthening if the entire posterior complex is contracted.

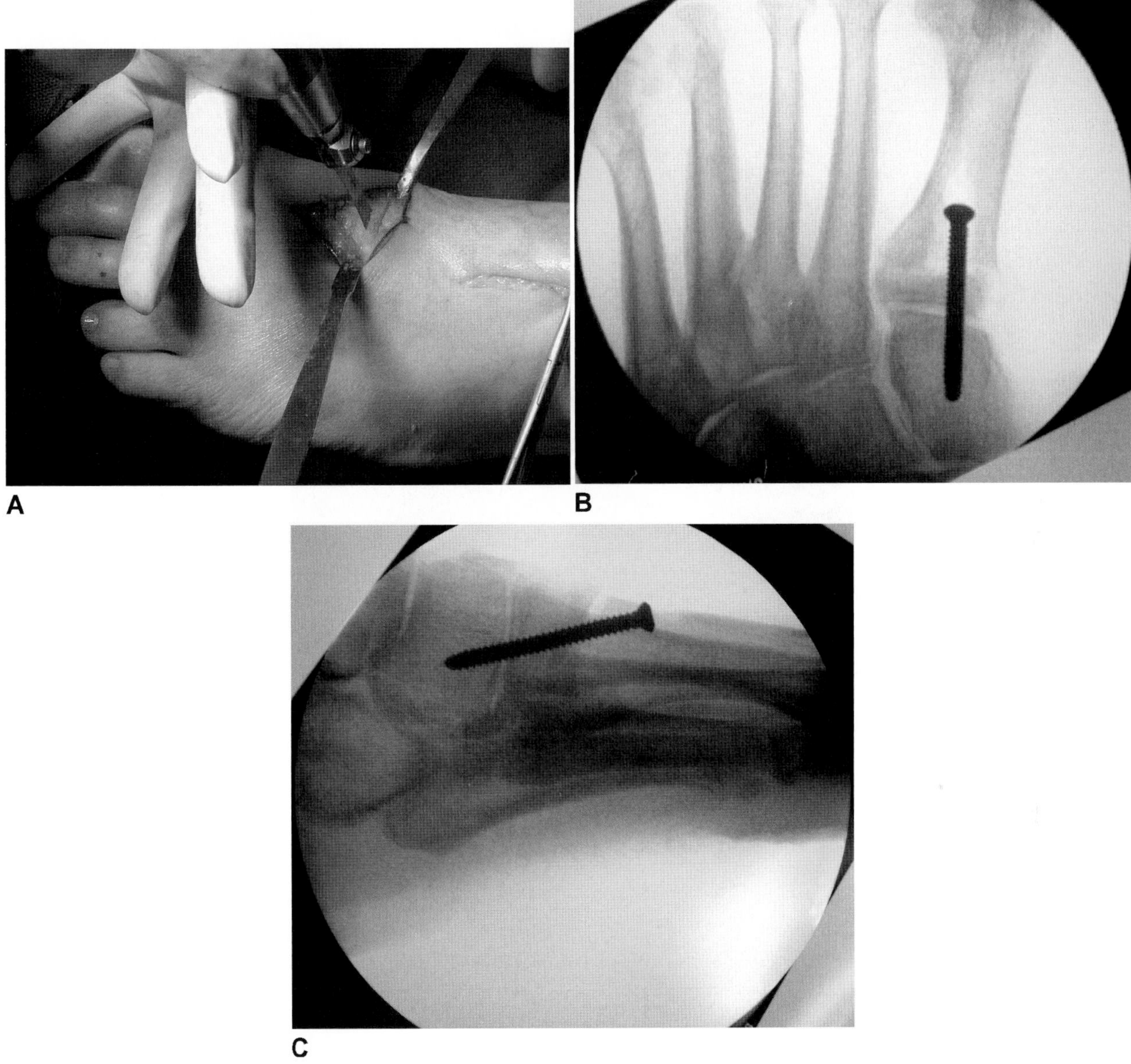

Figure 5–9: **A, Intraoperative first metatarsal dorsiflexion osteotomy is a closing wedge, dorsally based osteotomy. Postoperative B, anteroposterior and C, lateral radiograph showing position and internal fixation for the first metatarsal osteotomy.**

- In a severe cavus foot deformity associated with neuromuscular disease, a triple hindfoot arthrodesis is needed both to achieve the realignment and to maintain the correction. Extensive hindfoot fusion is usually not needed in the neurologically normal cavus foot.

Claw Toe Deformity

- These subtle cavus feet can develop severe claw toes, which contribute to metatarsalgia and can rub on shoes.
- When a shoe with a tall toe box is no longer able to relieve symptoms, surgery is indicated.
- Muscle balance is achieved by transferring the long toe flexor to the extensor over the proximal phalanx. This encourages extension at the interphalangeal joints and flexion at the metatarsophalangeal joint.
- Metatarsophalangeal or interphalangeal capsulotomies are performed as needed. Fixed proximal interphalangeal joint contractures will need formal joint arthroplasty or fusion, with temporary pin fixation.

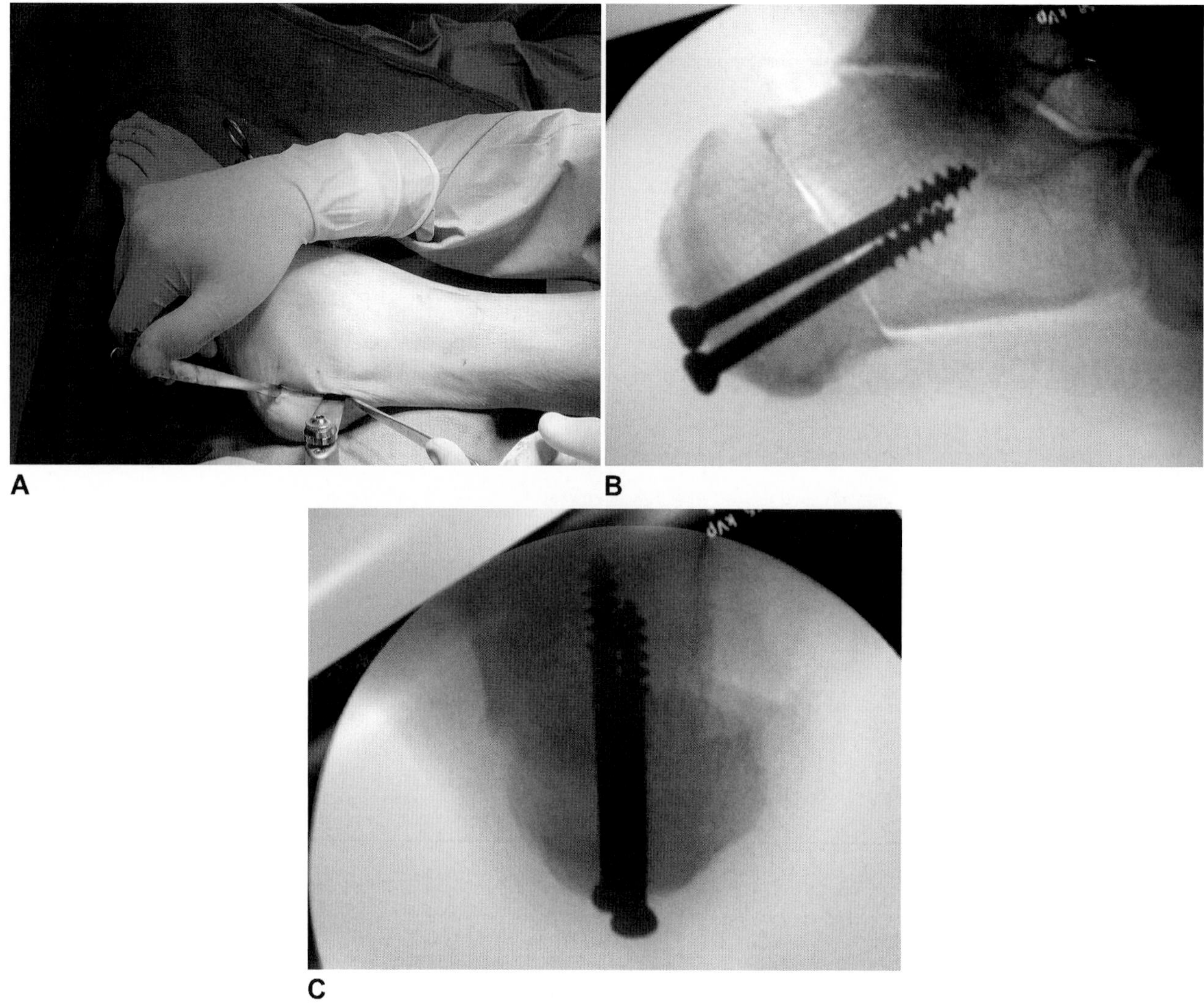

Figure 5–10: **A, Intraoperative lateralizing calcaneal osteotomy. Postoperative (B) axial and (C) lateral radiograph showing the lateralization of the calcaneus and internal fixation using two 6.5-mm screws.**

References

Beals TC, Manoli A. (1996) The "peek-a-boo" heel sign in the evaluation of hindfoot varus. Foot 6: 205-206.

One of the first discussions of how to identify the subtle cavus foot.

Brandes CB, Smith RW. (2000) Characterization of patients with primary peroneus longus tendinopathy: A review of twenty-two cases. Foot Ankle Int 21(6): 462-468.

An interesting discussion of the link between cavus foot shape and peroneal problems.

Coleman SS, Chesnut WJ. (1977) A simple test for hindfoot flexibility in the cavovarus foot. Clin Orthop 123: 60-62.

The original description of the classic Coleman block test.

Ledoux WR, Shofer JB, Ahroni JH et al. (2003) Biomechanical differences among pes cavus, neutrally aligned, and pes planus feet in subjects with diabetes. Foot Ankle Int 24(11): 845-850.

A very detailed study looking at foot shape and properties. The article is a bit cumbersome, with lots of data, but is the first thorough, modern assessment of foot shape.

Manoli AM, Graham B. (2005) The subtle cavus foot, "the underpronator," a review. Foot Ankle Int 26(3): 256-263.

A good discussion of the subtle cavus foot in the neurologically normal person.

Paulos L, Coleman SS, Samuelson KM (1980) Pes cavovarus. J Bone Joint Surg 62A: 942-953.

A surgical series of cavus feet, with focus on neuromuscular disease.

Sammarco GJ, Taylor R. (2001) Cavovarus foot treated with combined calcaneus and metatarsal osteotomies. Foot Ankle Int 22(1): 19-30.

Another series of surgical patients with cavus feet. All had neuromuscular disease. Unfortunately, there are no surgical series of cavus foot surgery in the neurologically normal patient.

CHAPTER 6

Neuromuscular Foot Deformity

Justin Greisberg*, Stefan Gerhard Hofstaetter§, and Hans-Jörg Trnka†

*M.D., Assistant Professor of Orthopaedic Surgery, Columbia University College of Physicians and Surgeons, New York, NY
§M.D., Foot and Ankle Center, Vienna, Austria
†M.D., Ph.D., Foot and Ankle Center, Vienna, Austria

- Much like the hand, the foot is a complex "machine" consisting of many bones and joints kept in a fine balance by many extrinsic (leg) and intrinsic (foot) muscles.
- Any disruption of the precise muscle balance leads to progressive deformity of the involved joints (Box 6–1).
- If the imbalance arises prior to skeletal maturity, growth of the bones will be abnormal and the bones and joints will become dysplastic.
- If the imbalance arises after skeletal maturity, the bones will have essentially normal shape, and any deformity will be through the joints.
  - With time, the joints can erode in response to deformity, leading to secondary 'dysplasia' of the bones.
- At the level of the ankle and hindfoot, there are several muscles pairs that balance each other.
  - The tibialis anterior dorsiflexes the first ray, while the peroneus longus plantar flexes it.
  - The posterior tibial muscle inverts the hindfoot, while the peroneus brevis everts.
  - The triceps surae is by far the strongest of the leg and foot muscles. The tibialis anterior and the extensor digitorum and hallucis longus all work in opposition to the triceps surae.
- In the forefoot, balance between intrinsic and extrinsic flexors and extensors keeps the toes straight at the metatarsophalangeal (MTP) and interphalangeal joints.
- Even when a muscle is weak, if there is no muscle to oppose it then the weak muscle will eventually cause a deformity.
- Although muscle imbalance theoretically could lead to any imaginable foot deformity, neuromuscular deformities are generally some form of cavus.
- The neuromuscular cavus foot appears with a high arch, variable amounts of hindfoot varus, plantar flexion of the first ray or entire midfoot, and clawing of the toes (Fig. 6–1).
- Although many neuromuscular feet will have the same general cavus shape, the specific components of the cavus will vary with the cause of the imbalance.

Box 6–1 Muscle Imbalance

"In the land of the blind, the one-eyed man is king"—quote from Michael Ehrlich, M.D., referring to the tendency for any muscle imbalance, even if the muscles are weaker than normal, to lead to deformity. An example might be a patient with an L4 level myelocele, where the only functional muscle in the leg would be the posterior tibialis. Even though the posterior tibialis might be weak, if it acts unopposed (no peroneus brevis) then the foot will be pulled into a varus deformity.

Causes of Neuromuscular Deformity

- Upper motor neuron lesions, such as a stroke or cerebral palsy (Box 6–2), lead to weakness with hyperreflexia and spasticity.

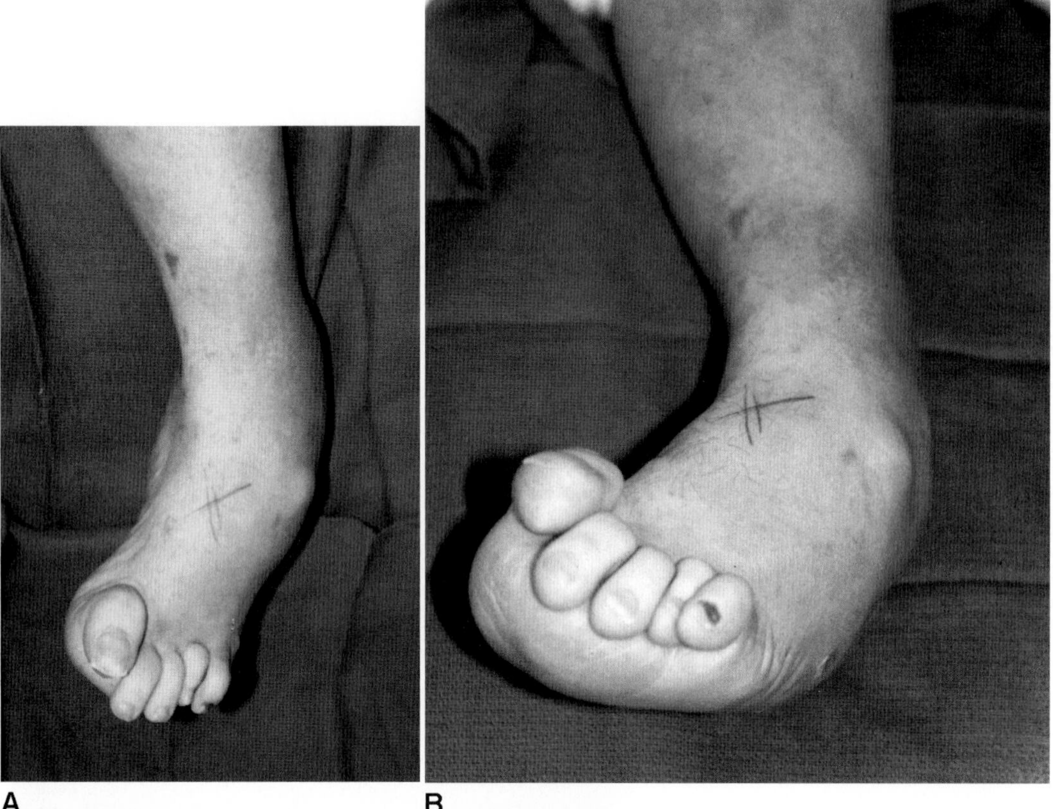

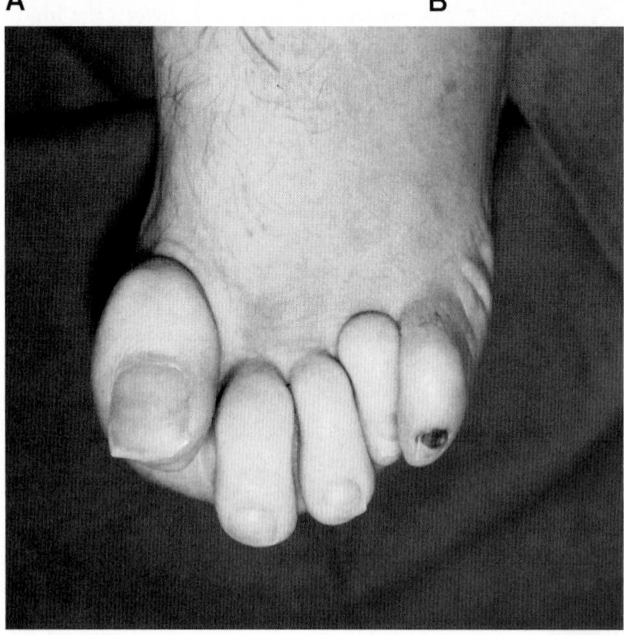

Figure 6–1: Photographs of the left foot of a patient with severe cavovarus deformity. **A,** The ankle and hindfoot varus. **B,** Severe clawing (extension at metatarsophalangeal joint and flexion at interphalangeal joints) of the toes is evident. **C,** The toe deformity has led to injury to the fifth toenail from improper shoe fit.

- Lower motor neuron lesions, such as poliomyelitis or traumatic nerve injury, lead to hyporeflexia.
- Muscle lesions—such as following untreated compartment syndrome or with myopathy, lead to weakness and hyporeflexia.
- A thorough classification of neuromuscular foot deformities is listed in Box 6–3.

Symptoms from the Neuromuscular Cavus Foot

- Neuromuscular imbalance leads to variably progressive deformity in the foot.
- Cavus or cavovarus deformity alters the distribution of pressure under the foot. Focusing weight-bearing forces on

Box 6–2 Cerebral Palsy

Cerebral palsy is a static neuromuscular disorder that frequently affects the feet. A tight heel cord (Achilles contracture) is seen in most involved limbs, but the hindfoot may be in varus (posterior tibial spasticity) or valgus. Perhaps 66% of patients will show planovalgus, and 34% cavovarus.

Box 6–3 Some Etiologies of Cavus Foot

Neuromuscular

- Myopathy: muscular dystrophy
- Peripheral neuropathy: Charcot-Marie-Tooth disease, polyneuritis
- Spinal cord/anterior horn cell disease: poliomyelitis, spinal dysraphism, diastematomyelia, syringomyelia, spinal cord tumor, spinal muscular atrophy
- Central nervous disease: Friedrich ataxia, Roussy-Levy syndrome, cerebral palsy

Congenital

- Clubfoot residual deformity
- Arthrogryposis

Traumatic

- Residual of compartment syndrome, crush injury, severe burn, malunion of fracture

Idiopathic

- Variant of normal (discussed in Ch. 5)

(After Ibrahim K. (1990) Pes cavus. In: Surgery of the Musculoskeletal System (Evarts CM, ed.). New York: Churchill Livingstone. pp. 4015-4034.)

smaller areas leads to higher pressures. The cavus foot will have higher pressures under the heel and metatarsal heads.
- Patients may complain of pain and/or callusing in these high-pressure spots.
- If the hindfoot is in varus, then pressure may be focused on the fifth metatarsal. This can cause pain and callusing, and in extreme cases fifth metatarsal stress fractures.
- The high arch may make shoe fitting problematic.
- Shoe-fitting problems may also arise if clawing of the toes occurs, with irritation over the dorsum of the interphalangeal joints.
- Clawing of the toes pulls the plantar metatarsal fat pad distally. This uncovers the metatarsal heads and can lead to metatarsalgia.
- A varus hindfoot predisposes to ankle sprains, which is even more of a problem when the peroneus brevis is weak.
- Muscle weakness may cause the patient to feel clumsy and fall.
- Severe deformity prevents the foot from being plantigrade. In severe cases, the patient will become non-ambulatory.
- If the neuromuscular disease also leads to sensory neuropathy, pressure sores may develop over high-pressure areas.

Evaluation of the Neuromuscular Patient

- A full history and physical is appropriate, but there are several areas that should be explored especially thoroughly.
- Family history should look for history of similar disease, because many neuromuscular diseases are inherited.
- Environmental exposures should be discussed, specifically looking for residence in an area where polio might be present.
- On examination, the overall shape and symmetry of both feet are assessed. Asymmetry is more common with acquired disorders (and some spinal cord abnormalities), while systemic diseases tend to create more symmetric deformity.
- The position of the hindfoot is assessed. While the patient is standing, the observer notes the position of the heel from behind. In the normal foot, the heel rests in slight valgus (just lateral to the long axis of the tibia). Most neuromuscular deformities pull the heel into varus.
  - As described in Chapters 2 and 5, if the heel is seen medial to the foot while looking at the patient from the front (the "peek-a-boo" heel), then it is in varus.
- The position of the forefoot can be assessed while the patient is seated, with the legs hanging over the edge of the table. With the heel straight, the metatarsal heads should be even. A plantar flexed first ray is commonly seen with neuromuscular cavus.
- The Coleman block test, as discussed in Chapter 5, is an important assessment of hindfoot flexibility when the hindfoot is in varus. With the patient standing with the heel and lateral metatarsal heads on a block, the first metatarsal is allowed to drop medial to the block. If the hindfoot is flexible in a cavus foot, the first metatarsal will drop lower than the foot, and the heel will fall into slight valgus (forefoot-driven hindfoot varus). If the hindfoot is rigid, the first metatarsal will not drop, and the heel will remain in varus.
- The alignment of the toes should be assessed, looking for the characteristic clawing (extension at MTP and flexion at interphalangeal joints).
- The flexibility of the hindfoot, ankle, and toes must be assessed initially and with time. Many diseases begin with a flexible deformity but become more rigid over time.
- The "quality" of the soft tissues should be assessed. With longstanding deformity, the tissues may become contracted on the "concave" side of the deformity (medial hindfoot in a varus deformity), so that realignment would put an unacceptable amount of stretch on these tissues.
- A full motor examination is performed, documenting the strength of each muscle group in both legs. A full sensory examination is listed either by dermatome or peripheral nerve, depending on the underlying pathology.
- The gait pattern must be observed. A foot drop may be visible during the swing phase.

- Weight-bearing radiographs are an important part of the deformity assessment.
- On the lateral view, calcaneal pitch more than 30° is typical of cavus.
- Lateral talometatarsal angle will show the first metatarsal to be plantar flexed. The first metatarsal may be plantar flexed much more than the other metatarsals in the cavus foot.
- Magnetic resonance imaging (MRI) of the foot is rarely needed, but MRI of the spine may be appropriate when the cause of deformity is not certain. It might be especially useful in the asymmetric cavus foot when there is a suspicion for spinal cord lesions.
- Unilateral progressive cavus deformity should prompt an MRI to search for intraspinal pathology.
- Cavus deformity, either unilateral or bilateral, in association with scoliosis should probably also be evaluated with an MRI of the spine.
- Electromyographic tests with nerve conduction velocities (EMG/NCV) are helpful in the initial evaluation of the patient to better define the neuromuscular lesion.
  - EMG in cases of neuropathy shows an increased amplitude and duration of response.
  - EMG in patients with myopathy shows a decreased amplitude and duration of response, with short polyphasic potentials.
  - Denervation or anterior horn cell loss demonstrates prolonged polyphasics, positive sharp waves, and fibrillations on EMG.
  - Abnormal NCV with prolonged latencies and minimal decrease in velocity suggests axonal degeneration.
- In rare cases, muscle or nerve biopsy may be needed to confirm a diagnosis.
- Finally, the vascular supply to the foot should be assessed.

Principles of Treatment of the Neuromuscular Cavus Foot

- The underlying disease must be controlled as best as possible, usually in conjunction with a neurologist.
- In cases of spasticity, medication may be helpful.
  - Common medications include baclofen, diazepam, and dantrolene.
- Specific muscle blocks with botulinum toxin may be helpful, especially if only one or two muscles are involved.
- Once a muscle imbalance in the foot has been identified, the goal is to prevent further deformity.
- Frequent stretching by the patient must be done, otherwise contracture will inevitably set in.
- Extradepth shoes will help accommodate a high arched foot with an orthotic, and a tall toe box will better fit claw toes.
- Custom accommodative orthotics can reduce peak pressures in the sole of the foot.
- Bracing of the weak or unstable ankle with a custom ankle-foot orthosis (AFO) can permit better ambulation and perhaps prevent further deformity.
  - In patients with sensory deficits, Plastizote (or other cushioned) linings are required in the brace, with frequent inspection of the skin for ulceration.

Surgery for the Neuromuscular Cavus Foot

- Surgery is indicated in certain situations. Of course, surgery is appropriate when non-operative treatment has failed, which most commonly means that the deformity is no longer braceable.
- Surgery is also indicated in situations where an obvious muscle imbalance is expected to lead to progressive deformity. If the muscle imbalance is corrected early, surgery may require only tendon transfers. If surgery is delayed, a later deformity will require fusions and/or osteotomies, making the recovery longer and the final function poorer.
- The basic principle of surgical treatment is to restore muscle balance and osseous alignment.
- Muscle balance is corrected through muscle transfers, lengthenings, and/or releases.
  - Lengthenings weaken a muscle.
  - Releases (tenotomies) remove the muscle entirely.
  - Muscle transfers remove the deforming force of the muscle and redirect it to another location.
- Muscle transfers can be in phase or out of phase.
  - In-phase transfers take a muscle and transfer it into another muscle that normally fires during the same part of the gait cycle. Example: transfer of the extensor digitorum longus to the tibialis anterior.
  - Out of phase transfers redirect a muscle to an insertion that is normally antagonistic. Example: posterior tibial tendon through the interosseous membrane to the tibialis anterior. Out of phase transfers are less likely to result in strong active motion in an adult.
- Osseous alignment can occasionally be corrected with capsulotomies in cases of mild deformity. Plantar fascia release (minimal incision or wide) can be used to "relax" the arch in some cavus feet.
- More severe deformity requires osteotomies or fusions.
- In adult patients with deformity secondary to brain injury, it may be appropriate to wait 18-24 months between injury and surgery to give enough time for any recovery.

Peroneal Nerve Palsy

- The common peroneal nerve (consisting of contributions from L4 to S1) courses over the posterior head of the fibula and around the lateral neck of the bone. This nerves

branches into the superficial and deep peroneal nerves in the anterolateral compartment of the leg. The course of the superficial peroneal nerve in the leg is variable.
- Injury to the peroneal nerves may occur as an entrapment neuropathy.
- More common, though, is direct or indirect trauma to the nerve, with neuropraxia or axonotmesis. The nerve is somewhat tethered at the level of the fibular neck, so any traction on the sciatic nerve can injure the nerve. The tibial nerve is not tethered about the knee, and is less vulnerable to injury.
- Peroneal nerve injury can occur during surgery, either from pressure on the nerve from poor positioning while anesthetized, or from traction during the procedure.
- Peroneal nerve injury is common in thin, non-ambulatory patients, and is related to a poorly fitting wheelchair or poor positioning while in bed.
- Inadequate padding about a short leg cast can injure the nerve.
- Diabetic neuropathy or entrapment neuropathy can lead to peroneal nerve dysfunction.
- Blunt or penetrating trauma can injure the nerve. A common example is a posterior hip dislocation.
- In contrast to other types of nerve palsies, peroneal nerve palsy may demonstrate a greater motor deficit than sensory deficit.

Symptoms of Peroneal Nerve Palsy

- The sensory loss is variable and rarely a problem.
- Motor loss of the anterior compartment results in a foot drop. At the minimum, patients may have a high stepping gait to avoid tripping over their foot. The foot may also slap the floor immediately after heel strike.

Treatment of Peroneal Palsy

- When the ankle remains flexible, these symptoms can be well controlled with an AFO. Patients must stretch the Achilles frequently to prevent contracture.
- If stretching is not performed, an equinus contracture will develop. Patients may partly compensate for this by obtaining an AFO with a heel lift, but this is usually not well tolerated.
- Surgery is indicated if an equinus contracture has developed, or if the patient cannot achieve good function with a brace.
- In some cases, surgery may be helpful for the patient who is not willing to wear a brace.
- The first step in surgery is to create an ankle dorsiflexor. In the typical case, no in-phase muscles are available, so the posterior tibial tendon can be transferred through the interosseous membrane to the dorsal midfoot.
- It is probably important to replace the posterior tibial tendon function by transferring the flexor digitorum longus into the stump of the tibial tendon on the navicular. Many surgeons feel that this step is not necessary.
- The second step is to weaken the Achilles tendon by lengthening.
- In some patients, the transferred posterior tibial tendon will adapt with time and become an ankle dorsiflexor.
- In most patients, the muscle acts more as a tenodesis, meaning that it balances the Achilles and keeps the ankle neutral, but does not provide much active dorsiflexion strength.

Deformity from Untreated Compartment Syndrome

- Although the standard treatment for acute compartment syndrome of the leg or foot is emergent fasciotomy, there are still many cases when that cannot be done.
- Untreated compartment syndrome leads to muscle necrosis and contracture.

Anterior Compartment

- If only the anterior compartment of the leg is involved, the patient will develop a clinical picture similar to peroneal nerve palsy, with foot drop.
- In these cases, stretching and bracing can be successful.
- If surgery is indicated, transfer of the posterior tibial tendon through the interosseous membrane will provide some dorsiflexion. Alternately, transfer of the peroneus longus or extensor digitorum longus to the midfoot may provide better function if those muscles are viable.
- In any case, Achilles lengthening is also required.

Four Compartments

- Often, the compartment syndrome involves all four compartments of the leg. This leads to contracture of the posterior compartments, with severe equinovarus deformity over time.
- If recognized early, bracing and stretching may prevent late contracture.
- When deformity is minimal, Achilles lengthening and bracing may be effective. (There are no viable muscles to transfer to regain active motion.)
- Once severe deformity has set in, more aggressive surgery is needed. The scarred remnants of the deep posterior muscles must be resected to prevent recurrent contracture. The Achilles must be lengthened or released as well.
- With fixed deformity, hindfoot and/or forefoot realignment and arthrodesis are necessary (Fig. 6–2).
- In many cases, the posterior tibial nerve, vessels, and overlying skin have contracted so that dorsiflexion of the ankle is not possible, even after complete release of muscles and capsules. Talectomy with tibiocalcaneal fusion is a viable option. Alternately, open capsulotomies and gradual stretching with an external fixator (Ilizarov device) may be successful.

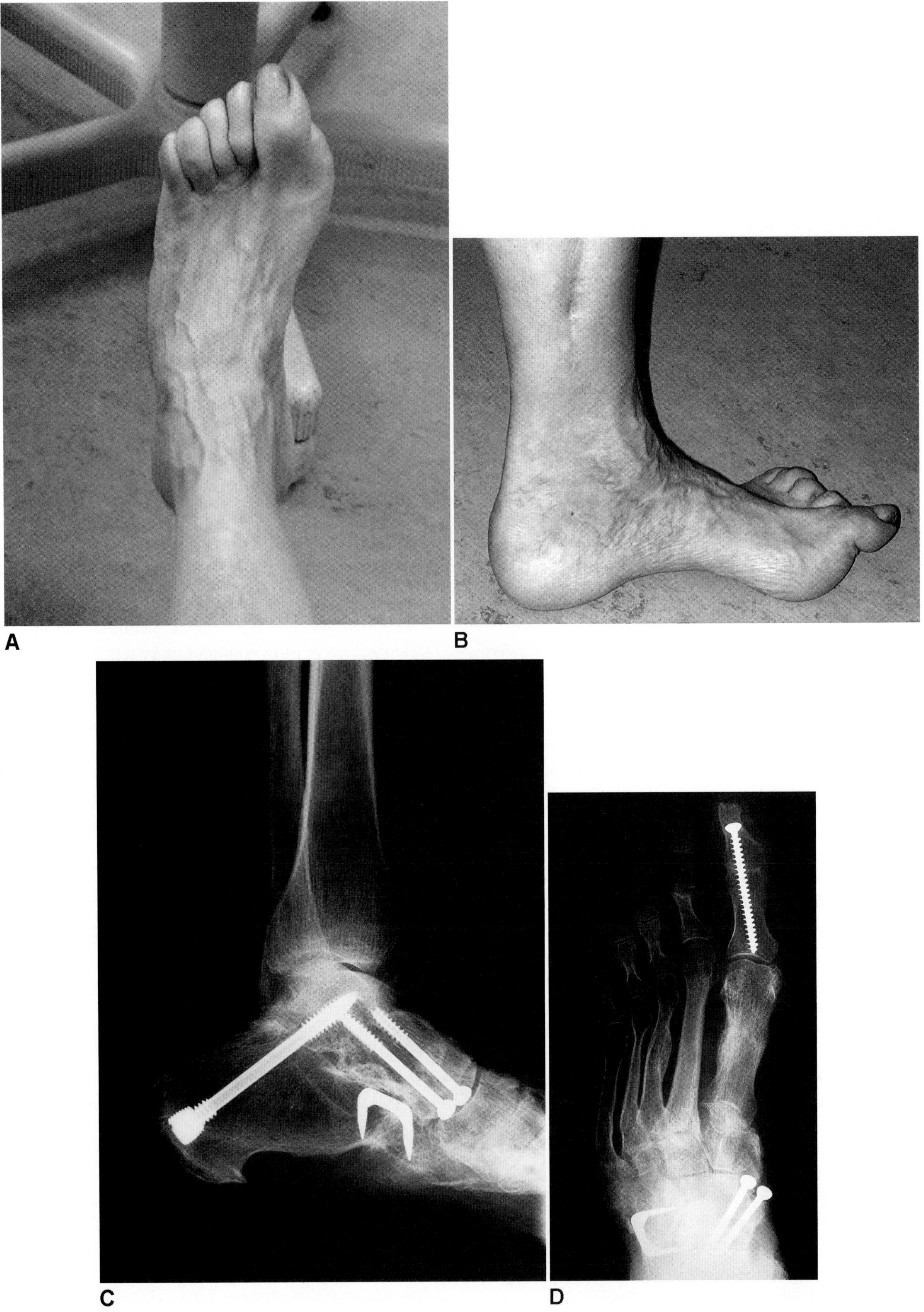

Figure 6–2: **A** and **B**, This patient with a compartment syndrome developed intrinsic muscle atrophy and fixed clawing of the hallux and lesser toes. **C** and **D**, The foot deformities were corrected with triple arthrodesis combined with an extensor digitorum longus transfer and a Jones procedure (fusion of the hallux interphalangeal joint with extensor hallucis longus transfer).

Foot Compartments

- Untreated compartment syndrome of the foot may result in claw toe deformities.
- When shoe modifications (tall toe box) cannot manage the deformity, surgical correction can be undertaken.
- Correction should include flexor tenotomy or transfer to the extensor (intrinsicplasty).
- Proximal interphalangeal arthroplasty or arthrodesis is usually necessary as well.
- Extensor lengthenings may be needed for correction of MTP dorsiflexion.

Charcot-Marie-Tooth Disease

- Charcot-Marie-Tooth, or CMT, is the most common inherited neurologic disorder, affecting approximately 15 per 100 000 people. The disease was described in the nineteenth century by Charcot and Marie in France, and independently by Tooth in England.
- CMT is actually a group of disorders better referred to as hereditary motor and sensory neuropathy, indicating that the disease affects both sensory and motor peripheral nerves.
- The disorder is inherited, with autosomal dominant, autosomal recessive, and X-linked recessive inheritance patterns, and is currently subdivided into type 1A, type 1B, type 2, and type X, based on the particular genetic defect involved (Box 6–4). There are at least 17 genetic variants of the disease, and probably many more. In some families, all the children develop the condition, and in others none inherit it. To determine the pattern of inheritance, each CMT patient should consult a genetic counsellor.
- CMT is slowly but variably progressive, and usually does not result in death. Most patients have normal life expectancy, with full and productive lives.
- The upper extremities can be involved, with distal motor weakness.
- As expected with a peripheral neuropathy, deep tendon reflexes are decreased.
- CMT often affects the foot in very consistent ways. Ninety-four percent of patients have foot involvement. There is characteristic weakness of the tibialis anterior and peroneus brevis.

Box 6–4 Charcot-Marie-Tooth Disease Variants

- Type 1: Autosomal dominant, with nerve biopsy revealing "onion" hypertrophy.
- Type 1A and 1B: Phenotypically similar but with different genetic defects.
- Type 2: Autosomal recessive, presenting during adolescence.
- X-linked: Presents during childhood.

- With tibialis anterior weakness, the peroneus longus is unopposed, resulting in plantar flexion of the first ray. This leads to a high arch (cavus).
- A weak peroneus brevis cannot oppose the posterior tibial muscle, with hindfoot varus. Thus a cavovarus foot will result.
- In some cases, an equinus deformity sets in, perhaps even prior to other deformities, because of imbalance between the tibialis anterior and the Achilles.
- Clawing of the toes may appear due to muscle imbalance in the toes, as well as "overactivity" of the long toe extensors (as they are substitutes for the tibialis anterior).
- Sensory loss is less severe than motor loss, but patients can demonstrate loss of two-point discrimination and vibratory sense.

Foot Symptoms in Charcot-Marie-Tooth Disease

- Weakness of the tibialis anterior can lead to a foot drop. Patients may feel clumsy or trip over their own feet while running.
- Patients may walk with a high steppage gait, or develop a foot slap.
- Claw toes can interfere with normal shoe wear.
- Lack of hindfoot eversion from the peroneus brevis can lead to ankle sprains and fractures.

Diagnosis of Charcot-Marie-Tooth Disease

- Family history is important.
- Nerve conduction tests show characteristics of peripheral neuropathy.
- Nerve biopsy may be helpful, especially in CMT type 1, where characteristic swelling is seen.
- Some subtypes of CMT are now detectable with blood tests.

Treatment of Charcot-Marie-Tooth Disease Foot Deformity

- Physical therapy, focusing on strengthening and stretching, is employed.
- Bracing with an AFO can be effective. A brace can reduce ankle sprains and reduce the energy requirement for gait.
- Extradepth shoes with a custom insert can be used, as well as shoes with a tall toe box for toe deformities.
- Surgery should be considered when the deformity is not braceable (the foot is not plantigrade). Surgery should also be considered early on if the disease is progressing despite bracing and stretching, because early surgery (tendon transfers) can be easier to recover from and leads to a better functional outcome than late surgery (fusions).

- In the earliest stages, prior to any fixed deformity, Achilles lengthening is performed. If the long toe extensors are strong, they are transferred to the dorsolateral midfoot to replace the weak tibialis anterior.
- If the extensor digitorum longus is weak, the tibialis posterior is transferred through the interosseous membrane to the dorsal midfoot.
- The peroneus longus is transferred into the peroneus brevis.
- These transfers remove the deforming forces and restore some dorsiflexion and eversion.
- Perhaps the earliest osseous deformity in CMT is plantar flexion of the first ray. If this has developed, the tendon transfers can be combined with dorsiflexion osteotomy of the first metatarsal, or dorsiflexion arthrodesis of the first metatarsocuneiform joint (Fig. 6–3).
- Lateral sliding calcaneal tuberosity osteotomy can be added if there is some heel varus.
- Once fixed hindfoot varus has set in, these motion-sparing procedures cannot be used. In these cases of advanced osseous deformity, triple joint realignment and arthrodesis is necessary (Fig. 6–4). If the ankle has begun to tilt into varus, ankle arthrodesis may be necessary as well. Obviously, major hindfoot fusions heal more slowly than tendon transfers, and result in less optimal functional outcomes.

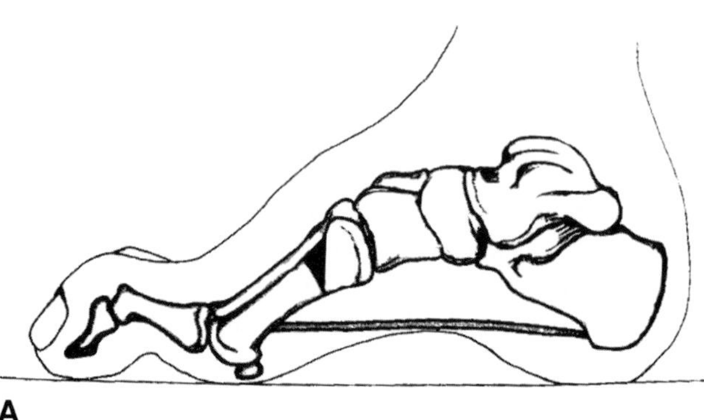
A

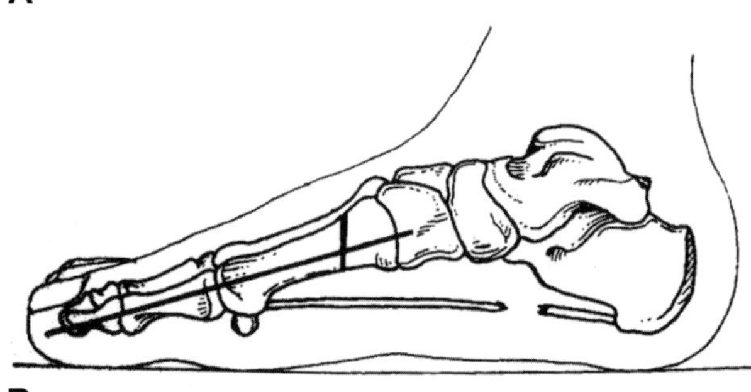
B

Figure 6–3: Illustration of the first metatarsal closing wedge osteotomy. A, Dorsally based wedge of bone is removed, approximately 1 cm distal to metatarsocuneiform joint. B, Postoperative illustration demonstrates dorsiflexed first metatarsal after proximal osteotomy. Plantar fascia release may be necessary. (From Coughlin MJ, Mann RA. (1999) Surgery of the Foot and Ankle, 7th edn. St. Louis: Mosby. p. 525.)

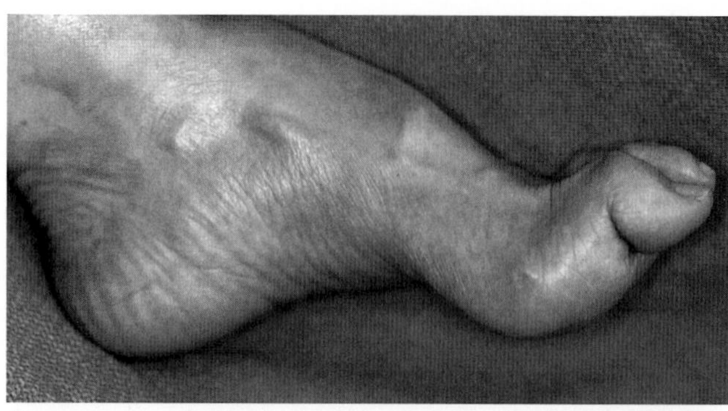
A

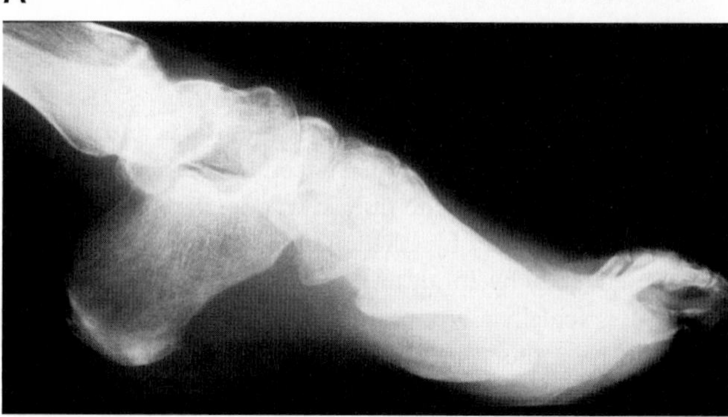
B

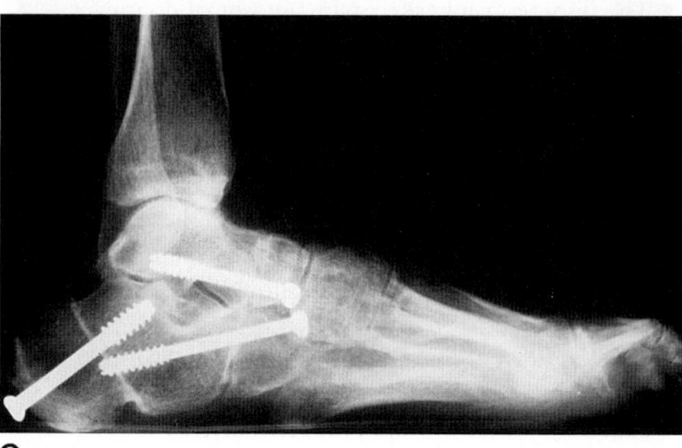
C

Figure 6–4: A, Photograph of a patient with Charcot-Marie-Tooth disease, with an equinus contracture, plantar flexion of the first ray, and claw toe deformities. B, Lateral radiograph shows the cavus deformity. C, Postoperative radiograph demonstrates the optimal correction after plantar fascia release, dorsal displacement of the calcaneus, and arthodesis.

Poliomyelitis

- Although polio is almost eradicated, it still appears in some less developed areas.
- The end result of polio virus infection is muscle weakness.

- The particular pattern of involved muscles varies between extremities and between patients, but certain characteristic patterns are seen.
- In the foot, it is common to see longstanding weakness of the Achilles. Absence of Achilles function leads to a calcaneus deformity. The foot is relatively dorsiflexed, with weight-bearing pressure focused on the heel pad (Fig. 6–5).
- Patients may complain of pain under the heel, sometimes with thick callusing.
- Custom insoles or AFO braces can be used to better distribute forces.
- When bracing fails to provide relief, surgery to restore strength in the Achilles can be undertaken.
- Depending on the strength of surrounding muscles, transfer of the flexor hallucis longus to the calcaneal tuberosity may be helpful.
- Because polio is often contracted during early childhood, the foot may have developed in the absence of Achilles strength. By maturity, the calcaneal pitch will be very high, with marked plantar flexion of the forefoot (very high arch). In such cases, consideration can be given to performing a dorsiflexion osteotomy of the midfoot, or calcaneal tuberosity osteotomy.

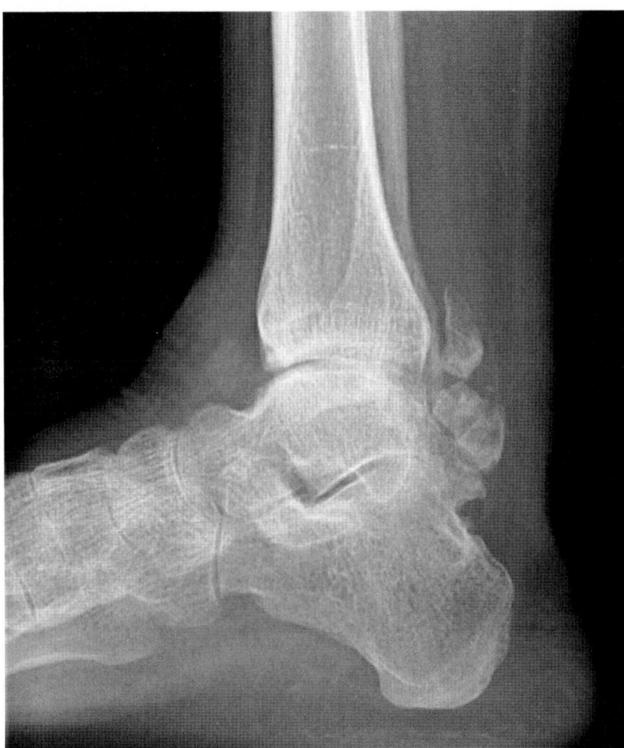

Figure 6–5: This woman had polio as a child. Note the increased calcaneal pitch, characteristic of patients with longstanding Achilles weakness. Because of the relative weakness of the Achilles, she bears most of her weight on the heel. She has suffered from plantar heel pain for years, with thick callusing of the skin. A custom orthosis has been only mildly helpful.

Procedures for the Clawed Hallux

- Many neuromuscular diseases result in severe clawing of the hallux, which interferes with shoe wear.
- When non-operative procedures have failed, surgical realignment can be helpful. A common procedure is to fuse the hallux interphalangeal joint and transfer the extensor hallucis longus to the first metatarsal or midfoot.

Summary of Cavus Foot Surgery

- Begin with muscle balancing: transfers, releases, lengthenings.
- Capsulotomies and plantar fascia release in some feet.
- Moderate cavus deformity will benefit from first metatarsal dorsiflexion osteotomy and/or lateral sliding calcaneal osteotomy.
- Ankle and/or hindfoot realignment and arthrodesis may be necessary in the most severe cases.

Surgical Procedures for the Severe Dysplastic Cavus Foot

- When the neuromuscular imbalance is severe and longstanding (especially when acquired during growth), the shape of the bones may not be normal. Joint realignment and arthrodesis may not restore a normal shape to the foot. In these more unusual cases, osteotomy(ies) with or without fusion are needed.
- For severe heel varus, a lateral closing wedge (Dwyer) osteotomy will help. A lateral sliding calcaneal osteotomy may preserve Achilles strength better and is technically easier to perform.
- With a very high calcaneal pitch, a dorsal sliding calcaneal tuberosity osteotomy will decrease pitch (Fig. 6–6).
- For severe equinovarus, Lambrinudi triple arthrodesis is indicated. In this procedure, wedges of bone are removed from the joints to allow better positioning during fusion (Fig. 6–7).
- For severe cavus deformity, dorsal closing wedge osteotomies across all metatarsals, or across the cuboid and cuneiforms, will decrease forefoot plantar flexion.
- In many of these cases, extensive plantar fascia release will be necessary, because the fascia is contracted in the severe cavus foot.

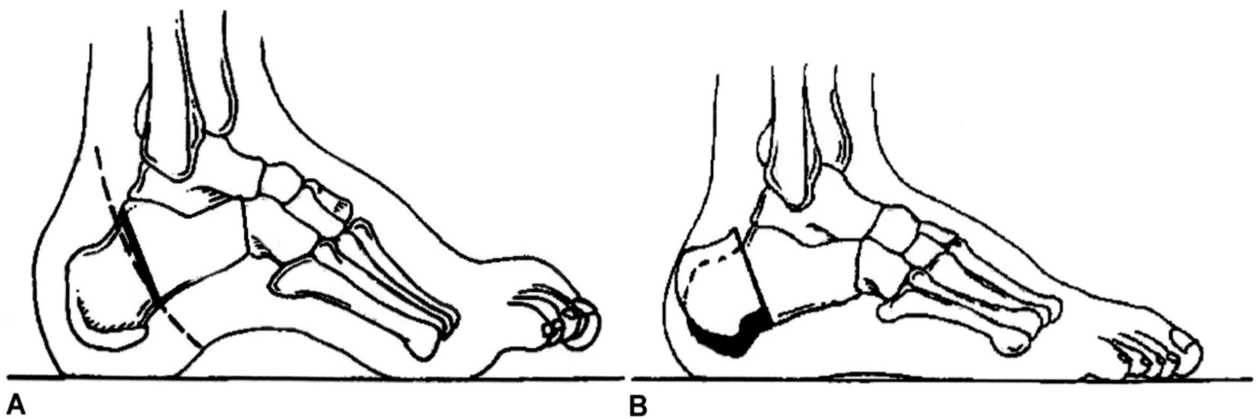

Figure 6–6: Calcaneal slide osteotomy. **A**, Neuromuscular disease can lead to abnormally high calcaneal pitch. **B**, Dorsal calcaneus displacement. Calcaneal tuberosity is moved dorsally to lower the longitudinal arch. (From Coughlin MJ, Mann RA. (1999) Surgery of the Foot and Ankle, 7th edn. St. Louis: Mosby. p. 525.)

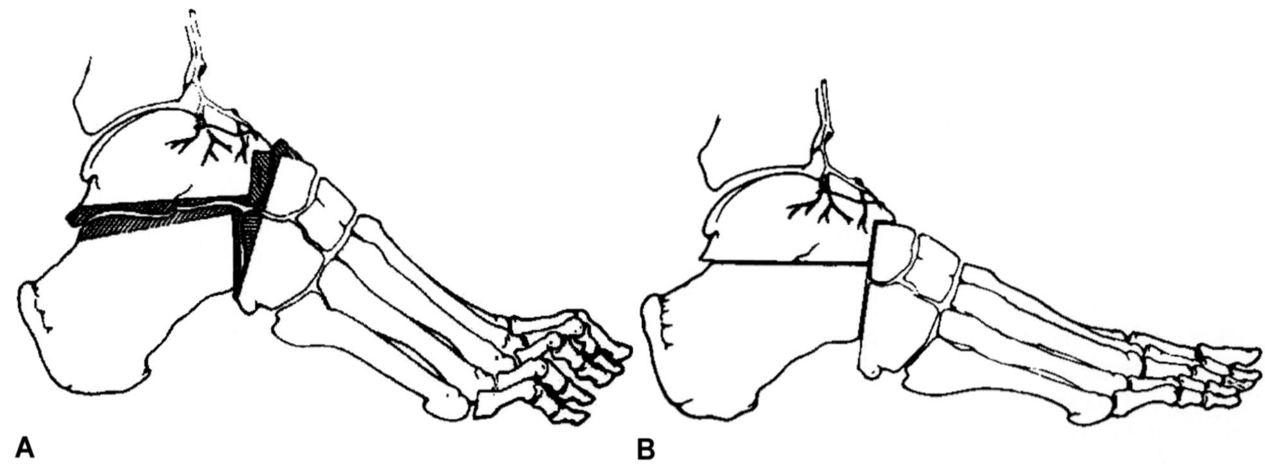

Figure 6–7: **A**, Triple arthodesis to correct severe cavovarus deformity may require resection of wedges of bone. Lateral closing in the subtalar joint is combined with mortising the navicular into the head of the talus. A lateral wedge is removed from calcaneocuboid joint to correct forefoot adduction. **B**, Position of foot postoperatively. Height reduction of longitudinal arch and forefoot adduction are the goals of this procedure. (From Coughlin MJ, Mann RA. (1999) Surgery of the Foot and Ankle, 7th edn. St. Louis: Mosby. p. 768.)

References

The challenge in cavus foot research is that the deformity is heterogeneous. There are many different etiologies of cavus foot, and there are many different manifestations. At least in part because of this heterogeneity, there are no studies providing objective outcome data on the natural history or treatment of the cavus foot.

Giannini S, Ceccarelli F, Benedetti MG et al. (2002) Surgical treatment of adult idiopathic cavus foot with plantar fasciotomy, naviculocuneiform arthrodesis, and cuboid osteotomy. A review of thirty-nine cases. J Bone Joint Surg 84-A(suppl 2): 62-69.

This paper presents a surgical series of cavus patients.

Ledoux WR, Shofer JB, Ahroni JH et al. (2003) Biomechanical differences among pes cavus, neutrally aligned, and pes planus feet in subjects with diabetes. Foot Ankle Int 24: 845-850.

Cavus feet were seen to have higher prevalences of claw toes, metatarsal head prominence, and bony prominences than other foot types. This is one of the few attempts to objectively define the cavus foot.

Sammarco GJ, Taylor R. (2001) Cavovarus foot treated with combined calcaneus and metatarsal osteotomies. Foot Ankle Int 22: 19-30.

In this small series of patients with varying etiologies for cavus foot, surgical correction with hindfoot and midfoot osteotomies led to improvements in non-validated outcome measures.

CHAPTER 7

Diabetic Foot Disorders

Dov Kolker* and Steven Weinfeld§

*M.D., Department of Orthopaedic Surgery, Mount Sinai School of Medicine, New York, NY
§M.D., Chief, Foot and Ankle Service, and Assistant Professor of Orthopaedic Surgery, Mount Sinai Medical Center, New York, NY

- Diabetes mellitus is a multisystem disease resulting from defects in insulin secretion and/or resistance to insulin action, with hyperglycemia.
- The total prevalence of diabetes in the USA was 18.2 million people (6.3% of the population) in 2002, with an incidence of 1.3 million new cases (people aged 20 years or older) diagnosed per year, and it is estimated that approximately 30% of all diabetics are undiagnosed.
- The socioeconomic costs (direct and indirect) of diabetes were approximately $132 billion in 2002, and an estimated 50% of the total costs for a diabetic hospital admission are due to diabetic foot complications.
- Diabetic foot complications are the most common cause of atraumatic lower extremity amputations, and are the leading cause of hospitalization among diabetics in the USA (Boulton et al. 2004). Foot complications have a negative impact on the health-related quality of life of a diabetic patient, with fear of ulceration, recurrent infection, and potential lifelong disability (Price 2004).
- There is currently no cure for diabetes, and treatment is based on preventing and managing the complications, requiring a multidisciplinary team approach and patient compliance.

Diabetic Vascular Disease

- Peripheral arterial occlusive disease is four times more prevalent in diabetics than in non-diabetics. It tends to occur at an earlier age in diabetics, and the risk of disease increases with the duration of diabetes.
- The calcification of atherosclerotic plaques in arteries of diabetic patients is more diffuse, and occurs within the tunica media of the arteries (Mönckeberg sclerosis), producing a "lead pipe" appearance on plain radiographs (as opposed to plaques in non-diabetic patients, which are patchy and occur in the tunica intima).
- The arterial occlusion of the proximal large vessels is similar to that in non-diabetics; however, the macrovascular disease is more diffuse in diabetics distal to the popliteal trifurcation. Distal vascular procedures have proven to be helpful in diabetic patients.
- Microvascular complications of diabetes (neuropathy, retinopathy, and nephropathy) and macrovascular complications (peripheral vascular disease, coronary artery disease, hypertension, hyperlipidemia, and cerebrovascular disease) together contribute to diabetic foot problems.

Evaluation

- A detailed history should be obtained, including a history of smoking, hypertension, and hyperlipidemia. Patients with advanced disease will complain of claudication.
- Pain due to vascular claudication is usually relieved with rest. However, ischemic foot pain can also occur at rest.
- On physical examination, absent popliteal or posterior tibial pulses, thin or shiny skin, absence of hair on the foot or leg, thickened nails, and dependent rubor are all

signs of vascular insufficiency. The clinical examination of diabetic patients is shown in Box 7–1.
- Any patient with signs of advanced vascular disease (such as a history of claudication, non-healing ulcers, or non-palpable pulses) should be evaluated by a vascular specialist.

Diagnostic Tests

- Non-invasive vascular tests include the ankle-brachial index (ABI) using Doppler ultrasound pressures, transcutaneous oxygen ($TcpO_2$) measurement (oximetry), the absolute toe systolic pressure (plethysmography), Doppler waveform analysis, and segmental Doppler limb pressures and pulse volume recordings (Teodorescu et al. 2004).
- Arterial pressure readings can be falsely elevated due to rigid arterial calcification in diabetics. This may artificially raise the ABI to greater than 1.
- An ABI of less than 0.80 is abnormal, and less than 0.45 in a diabetic patient is suggestive of limb-threatening ischemia.
- Absolute toe pressures may be more predictive of distal wound healing, with toe systolic pressure less than 45 mmHg indicating poor wound-healing potential, and less than 30 mmHg indicating critical limb ischemia.
- Transcutaneous oxygen measurement less than 20-30 mmHg represents poor wound-healing potential.
- When assessing Doppler waveform recordings, a triphasic waveform is normal. Biphasic (loss of reverse flow in early diastole) and monophasic waveforms suggest advanced occlusive disease.
- If lower extremity ischemia is strongly suspected, arteriography ("gold standard"), magnetic resonance angiography, or computed tomography angiography should be performed to assess the vascular flow.

Box 7–1 Clinical Examination of Diabetic Patients

- Examine both lower extremities.
- Observe gait.
- Inspect footwear for foreign objects.
- Record ulcer size (if present).
- Palpate pulses (patients without palpable pulses or who have a non-healing ulcer require vascular evaluation).
- Examine skin (feel for warmth, hair growth, examine between toes for blisters or ulceration, note skin and nail abnormalities).
- Note structural deformities and bony prominences (collapsed arch of Charcot foot or tall arch with claw toes of intrinsic muscle atrophy).
- Look for joint stiffness (patients with diabetes have more stiffness, less first ray mobility, and less ankle dorsiflexion compared with non-diabetics, which may contribute to neuropathic ulcer development).

Diabetic Neuropathy

- Peripheral neuropathy is the most common cause of diabetic foot complications.
- Diabetic neuropathy can involve the sensory, motor, and autonomic pathways.
- Diabetic neuropathy has been estimated to occur in 58% of patients with longstanding disease.
- Other common causes of peripheral neuropathy are listed in Box 7–2.
- Proposed causes of diabetic neuropathy are shown in Box 7–3.

Sensory Neuropathy

- The earliest finding in diabetic neuropathy is vibratory and proprioceptive loss.
- Signs and symptoms are variable but include paresthesias, burning sensations, hyperpathia, and dysesthesias, and usually reveal a symmetric sensory loss in a "stocking-glove" distribution.
- Because of the loss of protective (pain) sensation, foot ulceration generally occurs by repetitive trauma in areas of high mechanical pressure.
- The 5.07 (10-g monofilament) Semmes-Weinstein monofilament (SWM) test of 7-10 plantar foot sites is the recommended screening test for a patient at risk for ulcer formation due to loss of protective sensation.
- However, up to 10% of patients who pass the SWM test may still develop skin breakdown.
- A simplified screening test has been described recently. If a patient cannot sense the touch of a 4.5-g/4.65 SWM

Box 7–2 Possible Etiologies of Peripheral Neuropathy

- Diabetes mellitus
- Alcoholism
- Vitamin B_{12} deficiency
- Thyroid problems
- AIDS
- Uremia
- Lyme disease
- Medications (isoniazid, lithium, hydralazine, metronidazole, cimetidine, cisplatin, vincristine)
- Spinal pathology (cervical myelopathy)

Box 7–3 Proposed Causes of Diabetic Neuropathy

- Nerve ischemia from microvascular disease in vaso nervosum
- Accumulation of sorbitol or advanced products of glycosylation in neurons
- Deficiency of myoinositol, altering myelin synthesis
- Diminished sodium-potassium ATP (ATPase) activity
- Neural autoantibodies

when it is pressed under the first metatarsal head with just enough pressure to bend the filament, the patient should be considered at risk for ulceration (Saltzman et al. 2004a).

Autonomic Neuropathy

- Denervation of the eccrine and apocrine glands and arteries leads to abnormal thermoregulation and interference with the normal hyperemic response to infection.
- There is decreased sweating and loss of skin temperature regulation, causing dry, cracked skin and fissure formation, which predispose to infection by allowing a portal for bacterial entry.
- Autonomic neuropathy can also cause orthostatic hypotension; cardiovascular, urinary, and gastrointestinal problems; and erectile dysfunction. It may produce chronic venous swelling, usually requiring management with compression stockings.

Motor Neuropathy

- Motor neuropathy can cause muscle weakness and intrinsic muscle atrophy in the feet. The resulting muscle imbalance leads to claw toe and other forefoot deformities.
- Metatarsophalangeal hyperextension and a distally displaced fat pad accentuate pressure under the metatarsal heads, with risk for ulceration.
- Proximal interphalangeal flexion can cause pressure on the dorsum of the toe against the toe box of a shoe, and distal interphalangeal flexion can lead to increased pressure at the end of the toe. These are common areas for ulceration.
- Mononeuropathy and entrapment neuropathy can occur in diabetics. The most commonly involved nerve of the lower extremity is the common peroneal nerve, which can lead to a unilateral foot drop (Vinik et al. 2004).

Neuropathic Pain

- Although the etiology remains unclear, diabetic patients with decreased sensation may experience neuropathic pain resulting from small nerve fiber injury or from injury to the central or peripheral nervous system.
- Patients generally complain of burning or shooting pain that may be worse at night, and they may experience allodynia or anesthesia dolorosa.
- Neuropathic pain can be treated with low-dose antidepressants (amitriptyline, nortriptyline, desipramine, duloxetine hydrochloride [Cymbalta]), anticonvulsants (carbamazepine, phenytoin, lamotrigine, gabapentin [Neurontin], pregabalin), analgesics (tramadol), antiarrhythmics (mexiletine), or local topical agents (capsaicin cream, lidocaine).
- Surgical decompression of lower extremity peripheral nerves has been reported to relieve pain and restore sensation, but this approach is controversial and should be considered experimental (Dellon 2004).

Healing in Diabetes

- Delayed osseous and soft tissue healing is common in diabetics. Wound-healing potential is multifactorial, and is largely dependent on an individual's vascular and cardiopulmonary status; nutritional, endocrine, metabolic, and immune status; medication use (altered wound healing with corticosteroids and chemotherapeutic agents); and smoking history.
- Nutritional parameters suggested for successful wound healing include:
  - total lymphocyte count greater than 1500/μL
  - serum albumin greater than 3.5 g/dL
  - total protein greater than 6.2 g/dL.
- Wound healing also requires adequate wound oxygenation. This can be accomplished by optimizing the patient's cardiac, renal, and vascular status; edema reduction; and medication; and occasionally using hyperbaric oxygen therapy.
- Impaired fracture healing in diabetes has been linked to defects in type X collagen expression, abnormal chondrocyte maturation, and altered expression of genes that regulate osteoblast differentiation (Topping et al. 1994, Gooch et al. 2000).
- Poor glucose control and insulin deficiency will affect wound and fracture healing (Macey et al. 1989, Follak et al. 2005).
- Measurement of glycosylated hemoglobin (HbA1c) levels is the best method for medium- to long-term diabetic control monitoring (follows glycemic control over an 8- to 10-week period), with HbA1c levels of 7% or less yielding the best outcomes.

Gastrocnemius Contracture in Diabetes

- Many diabetic patients develop gastrocnemius tightness for uncertain reasons.
  - Gastrocnemius contracture is assessed by measuring passive ankle dorsiflexion with the knee flexed and then extended. Limited dorsiflexion (less than 5°) with the knee extended implies gastrocnemius tightness.
- Gastrocnemius tightness increases pressures across the arch and in the forefoot. This increased pressure may lead to ulceration, especially in the forefoot, and may be a contributing factor in the development of neuropathic degeneration (rocker bottom deformity).
- Gastrocnemius or Achilles tendon lengthening decreases forefoot pressures, and has been shown to decrease the incidence of forefoot reulceration in patients with previous ulcers (Mueller et al. 2003).

- Gastrocnemius lengthening should be considered for any "at risk" patient, which includes any patient with neuropathy. The exact role of gastrocnemius lengthening will be better defined in the future.

Diabetic Foot Care and Ulcer Prevention

- Foot ulcers are all too common in diabetics. Prevention of ulceration through foot-specific patient education, routine foot-screening examinations, routine (daily) nail and skin care (oils or creams with lanolin can be used for dry, cracked skin to help prevent skin breakdown), and use of appropriate footwear and orthoses are recommended.
- Inappropriate shoe wear can cause abnormal pressure to the skin, and hypertrophic nails can damage the soft tissues surrounding the nails. To help avoid an ingrown toenail, nails should be cut transversely (Pinzur et al. 2005).
- Smoking cessation and adequate glycemic control are also necessary.

Prescription Footwear

- An insensate foot in poorly fitting shoes is one of the most common causes for a diabetic ulcer.
- The optimal shoe is an extradepth shoe that will allow for a custom insole.
- Footwear options include a shoe with a padded heel counter and a wide and deep toe box, a Plastizote shoe, a Carville sandal (most accommodating for forefoot and hindfoot deformity), a deep walking shoe, a wide sneaker, or a custom-made shoe.
- Insoles are the mainstay of long-term non-operative management of the diabetic foot to decrease plantar pressure, and must be made out of accommodative material.
- Insoles are generally custom molded with dual layers; the upper layer should consist of a soft polyethylene foam (Plastizote or Pelite), which is most effective in "force distribution" to protect the plantar skin.
- As of April 1, 2004, the Medicare Therapeutic Shoe Bill covers one of the following for each diabetic individual (who qualifies under Medicare part B) in one calendar year: one pair of custom-molded shoes and two pairs of inserts, or one pair of extradepth shoes and three pairs of inserts.

Foot and Ankle Ulcers (mal perforans)

- Diabetic foot ulcers are the most common diabetic foot complication, and foot infection is the most common reason for a diabetic hospitalization in the USA. Fifteen percent of diabetic patients will develop a foot ulcer during their lifetime. Diabetic foot ulcers precede 85% of non-traumatic lower extremity amputations, and are generally preceded by the triad of neuropathy, deformity, and trauma (Boulton et al. 2004).

Pathophysiology

- The most common risk factor for developing a diabetic foot ulcer is peripheral neuropathy (Box 7–4) (Frykberg et al. 2000).
- Diabetic foot ulcers commonly occur in areas of structural deformity, and form over areas of bony prominences and high pressure.
- The area of maximum soft tissue damage secondary to vertical stress and shear occurs at the edge of pressure application ("edge effect").
- Ulcers can be neuropathic or ischemic.
- Neuropathic ulcers are caused by pressure or by shear forces, and generally have a healthy bed of granulation tissue beneath a necrotic cap.
- Ischemic ulcers with underlying vascular insufficiency are usually painful and generally have a necrotic base. Ischemic ulcers should be evaluated by a vascular surgeon for limb salvage.
- Diabetic individuals with sensory neuropathy generally lack sensation to deep pressure or pain. Loss of protective sensation due to peripheral sensory neuropathy, combined with unaccommodated structural foot deformities, commonly results in unrecognized acute or repetitive foot trauma (most commonly due to inappropriate footwear), leading to the development of ulcers with a risk of infection and possible amputation.

Pressure + neuropathy = ulceration

Classification of Diabetic Foot Ulcers

- Widely used classification systems are based on wound depth and appearance (Fig. 7–1, Table 7–1) (Wagner 1979, Brodsky 2003).

Box 7–4 Risk Factors for Ulceration

- Peripheral neuropathy
- Past history of ulceration or amputation
- Charcot neuroarthropathy
- Diabetic complications such as retinopathy and nephropathy
- Peripheral vascular disease
- Poor glycemic control
- Increased duration of diabetes
- Trauma
- Impaired visual acuity
- Edema
- Callus
- Limited joint mobility
- Structural foot deformity

(Data from Frykberg RG, Armstrong DG, Giurini J et al. (2000) Diabetic foot disorders: a clinical practice guideline. American College of Foot and Ankle Surgeons. J Foot Ankle Surg 39(5 suppl): S1-S60.)

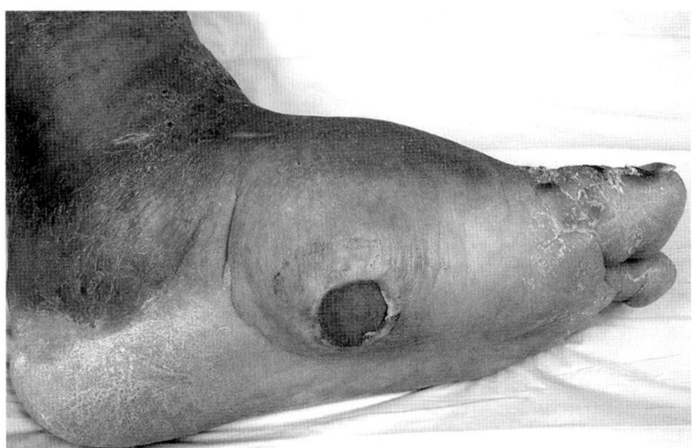

Figure 7–1: Grade 1 superficial ulcer with a granulating base in a patient with an acute Charcot foot.

- Neuropathic ulcers are generally not painful, whereas ischemic ulcers are often painful.
- Consider biopsy for a chronic non-healing ulcer to rule out the possibility of a Marjolin ulcer (squamous cell carcinoma arising from a chronic wound) or malignant melanoma.

Treatment

- Assuming appropriate medical management to optimize the systemic diabetes, treatment strategy includes ulcer bed preparation, local wound care with wound dressings, and protection and off-loading (Box 7–5).
- *Ulcer bed preparation* includes debridement of necrotic or infected tissue to viable margins and callus removal.
- *Local wound care: lotions and potions.* The most commonly used dressing is a normal saline moist to dry dressing, which acts to debride the superficial layer when removed. Absorbents (alginate or Hydrofiber) can be used for exudative wounds.
- Occlusive hydrocolloids, hydrogels, and debriding agents (including hypertonic saline gel) are appropriate for necrotic wounds.
- Foams can be used for exudative or necrotic wounds.
- Collagen dressings can be used for granulating or necrotic wounds.
- Transparent films (Opsite, Tegaderm) are helpful for dry granulating wounds without exudate.
- Antimicrobial dressings including iodine- and silver-impregnated dressings have also been used.
- Dressings with biologically active wound-healing agents may promote healing in wounds with reasonable healing potential, including those with a cellulose and collagen framework (Promogran), hyaluronic acid ester (Hyalofill), those that deliver platelet-derived growth factors (becaplermin gel [Regranex]), and those that apply living fetal foreskin cells (Apligraf, Dermagraft).

Table 7–1: Depth-Ischemia Classification of Diabetic Foot Lesions[a]

GRADE	DEFINITION	TREATMENT
Depth classification		
0	"At risk" foot: prior ulceration or underlying neuropathy with a deformity that may lead to ulceration	Patient education Regular clinical examination Accommodative footwear
1 (Wagner grade 1)	Superficial ulceration, not infected	Off-loading with total contact cast, walking brace, or accommodative footwear
2 (Wagner grade 2)	Deep ulceration with exposed tendons or joints (with or without infection)	Debridement Wound care Off-loading Antibiotics (if infection)
3 (Wagner grade 3)	Extensive ulceration with exposed bone, deep infection or abscess	Debridement ± partial foot amputation Off-loading Culture-specific antibiotics
Ischemia classification		
A	No ischemia	–
B	Ischemia without gangrene	Vascular evaluation/consultation Possible revascularization
C (Wagner grade 4)	Partial (forefoot) gangrene	Vascular evaluation/consultation Possible revascularization
D (Wagner grade 5)	Complete foot gangrene	Partial foot amputation Vascular evaluation/consultation Possible revascularization Major extremity amputation (below or above knee)

[a]A modification of the Wagner-Meggitt classification modified by Brodsky.
(After Brodsky J. (1999) The diabetic foot. In: Surgery of the Foot and Ankle (Coughlin MJ, Mann RA, eds.). St. Louis: Mosby. p. 911.)

Box 7–5 Ulcer Treatment Algorithm

1. Classify the wound.
2. Is there adequate vascularity to promote healing? (Is there ischemic pain, vascular claudication, non-palpable pulses, a non-healing or ischemic ulcer, or gangrene? If vascularity is in question, proceed with vascular consultation/non-invasive vascular examination).
3. Is it infected? (Cellulitis, osteomyelitis, or an abscess? If a sterile probe through the ulcer reaches bone, this is highly suggestive for the presence of osteomyelitis. Imaging studies include plain radiographs, bone scan/labeled white blood cell scan, or magnetic resonance imaging. If infected, admit patient to hospital; provide intravenous antibiotics and wound debridement; obtain vascular medicine and/or endocrine consult).
4. Wound debridement and local wound care.
5. Relief of pressure: external (postoperative shoe, Plastizote shoe, walking brace, bed rest, bivalved ankle-foot orthosis, total contact cast) versus internal (surgical reconstruction) with external postoperative support.

- A negative-pressure wound dressing (vacuum-assisted closure technique) has also been used to successfully treat non-healing diabetic wounds.
- *Protection and off-loading techniques* include casts, removable CAM walkers (which can be wrapped to ensure compliance), splints, or orthoses.
- Total contact casting (gold standard) is an effective method to heal plantar ulcers, with a reported mean healing time of approximately 39 days (Myerson et al. 1992, Matricali et al. 2003, Trepman et al. 2005).
  - Total contact casts may decrease plantar pressure at the ulcer site by distributing force over an increased weight-bearing area, may reduce shear forces and vertical plantar pressures, can protect from trauma, can immobilize the ulcer edges, and can reduce edema.
  - Initially, the total contact cast should be changed every 5-14 days due to the potential for extreme changes in soft tissue swelling, and a poorly fitted cast may lead to skin abrasion.
  - Initial non-weight-bearing status is preferred, although moderate early weight bearing only minimally reduces the time to healing of plantar ulcers and may improve patient compliance (Saltzman et al. 2004b).
  - The most common complication of total contact casting is recurrent ulceration.
  - Contraindications to total contact casting include active infection, arterial insufficiency, poor skin quality, and poor patient compliance.
- Treatment for the "at risk" foot (grade 0) involves patient education, regular clinical examination, accommodative footwear, and pressure-dissipating orthotics (Table 7–1).
- When a structural deformity or prominence is present that cannot be accommodated by external modalities, deformity correction or removal of the bony prominence is recommended to prevent ulceration.
- Grade 1 and 2 ulcers require debridement of the necrotic or infected tissue, local wound care, and off-loading/pressure relief techniques (external or surgical). Dressings and topical treatment abet the healing process.
- Once the ulcer has healed, patients should use off-loading devices to help prevent reulceration.
- Surgery is indicated when external accommodative modalities are not successful. Achilles tendon lengthening may help reduce the recurrence of neuropathic plantar forefoot ulcers in patients with limited ankle dorsiflexion by reducing peak plantar forefoot pressures (Mueller et al. 2003).
- A heel ulcer is the most difficult to manage, and most commonly requires surgery.
- Operative treatment is generally necessary for grade 3 ulcers and those with associated gangrene, which commonly require debridement of infected or gangrenous tissue with partial or whole foot amputation and culture-specific parenteral antibiotic therapy.

Infection

- Wound infections may occur as a result of abnormal white blood cell function, poor nutrition and glycemic control, and the presence of peripheral vascular disease.
- Antibiotics generally should not be used to treat a foot ulcer unless there are clinical signs of infection or underlying osteomyelitis.
- Infections related to superficial ulceration and cellulitis are most commonly caused by aerobic gram-positive cocci, or occasionally by enteric gram-negative bacilli, which can be safely treated by a first-generation cephalosporin or clindamycin.
- Diabetic deep wound infections with associated necrosis or gangrene are most commonly polymicrobial, with both aerobic and anaerobic ("fetid foot") organisms, and can be initially treated with broad-spectrum antibiotics.
- Swab cultures of the ulcer or sinus tract are generally not reliable.
- Unstable blood glucose control is commonly seen with infection.
- Whenever bone is exposed in an ulcer, it should be considered infected. Osteomyelitis in an ulcer should be treated by surgical resection of the infected bone, in whole or in part, with antibiotic therapy.
- Soft tissue gas in a diabetic is most commonly caused by aerobic organisms or by mixed gram-negative rods, but *Clostridium perfringes* and necrotizing fasciitis, which is a surgical emergency, must be ruled out.

Charcot Foot (Neuroarthropathy)

- Charcot arthropathy is a hypertrophic osteoarthropathy seen in patients with peripheral neuropathy.

- The first Charcot joint reported was due to syphilis; however, diabetes has become the leading cause of neuropathic arthropathy in the USA, primarily affecting the foot and ankle.
- Other causes of Charcot arthropathy include chronic alcoholism, chronic steroid use, syphilis, leprosy, infection, myelomeningocele, spinal cord injury/cord compression, syringomyelia (the most common cause of a Charcot joint in the upper extremity), poliomyelitis, renal dialysis, amyloidosis, pernicious anemia, spina bifida, multiple sclerosis, asymbolia, connective tissue disorders, adrenal hypercorticism, thalidomide embryopathy, paraneoplastic sensory neuropathy, and Klippel-Trenaunay-Weber syndrome.
- Diabetic Charcot arthropathy does not have a gender predilection, is more likely to occur with an increased duration of diabetes (usually greater than 10 years), and is bilateral in 30% of cases.

Pathophysiology

- Both neurotraumatic and neurovascular etiologies have been proposed.
- With repetitive trauma, the patient sustains a small fracture, perhaps microfracture, which worsens with persistent weight bearing in the absence of protective sensation.
- The neurovascular theory suggests that loss of vasomotor control leads to hyperemia, bony resorption, and weakening.
- Patients with Charcot arthropathy usually have good circulation.

Examination Findings

- Swelling, erythema, and warmth (skin temperature usually 3-6°C higher in the acute setting) of the foot and ankle are usually present.
- The patient may or may not have pain.
- An acute Charcot foot is commonly confused with cellulitis. In the Charcot foot, a decrease in erythema may be seen with foot elevation, as opposed to cellulitis, where the erythema will be unchanged with foot elevation.
- A subacute or chronic Charcot foot commonly presents with a structurally deformed foot with collapse of the medial longitudinal arch, a rocker bottom deformity, and bony prominences.

Diagnostic Evaluation

- Plain radiographs may not show any bony changes during the initial 3 weeks of acute Charcot arthropathy. Early radiographic changes include osteopenia and periarticular fragmentation.
- Later changes include bone resorption, bony proliferation with joint destruction, joint dislocation, and new bone formation. Osteolytic changes of Charcot arthropathy are commonly confused with infection. Surrounding osteopenia is generally not seen in a neuropathic fracture, as opposed to infection.
- Advanced imaging studies are generally not needed, because the clinical appearance usually is what distinguishes infection from acute Charcot foot. When needed, bone scintigraphy combined with indium-111 white blood cell scintigraphy is more specific but less sensitive than magnetic resonance imaging (without gadolinium) in distinguishing between osteomyelitis and Charcot arthropathy.
- Although rarely required, bone biopsy will show the characteristic findings of bone and cartilage debris embedded in synovium.

Classification

- The natural history of Charcot arthropathy can be described based on Eichenholtz stages, which incorporate clinical and radiographic evaluation (Table 7–2) (Eichenholtz 1966). Stage 1 is characterized by fragmentation, stage 2 by coalescence, and stage 3 by consolidation. Stage 0 has been added to the Eichenholtz classification in an effort to indicate the high risk of developing an acute Charcot arthropathy in a neuropathic individual with an acute traumatic event (Schon and Marks 1995).
- There is also an anatomical classification of Charcot arthropathy of the foot and ankle (Table 7–3) (Schon et al. 1998a). The most common anatomic site for the diabetic Charcot foot is the midfoot (tarsometatarsal region 60%) (Figs 7–2 and 7–3), followed by the hindfoot (20-30%). Charcot arthropathy of the forefoot is uncommon.
- Charcot involvement of the midfoot is usually stable and associated with bony prominences, primarily due to midfoot valgus and a rocker bottom deformity, whereas a Charcot hindfoot is usually associated with long-term instability (progressive deformity).
- Greater deformity is associated with an increased likelihood of requiring surgery (Schon types 1-4, stages A-C; Fig. 7–4, Tables 7–4 and 7–5).
- The Charcot ankle is the most unstable and is at high risk for ulceration. It typically falls into varus, with ulceration of the fibula through the skin.

Treatment

- Non-operative management is the mainstay for initial treatment of the Charcot foot or ankle. Treatment goals are to achieve clinical and osseous stability (consolidation), and to prevent and/or treat associated soft tissue problems (ulcer).
- Non-weight bearing is generally recommended for the acute Charcot foot; however, protected weight bearing in a cast may be done for patients who are unable to maintain non-weight-bearing status.

Table 7–2: Natural History of Charcot Arthropathy: Eichenholtz Stage

STAGE	CLINICAL	PLAIN RADIOGRAPHS	MANAGEMENT
0 ("at risk")	Neuropathic individual with an acute traumatic event	No destructive changes	Initial: foot elevation, protected off-loading in a cast or brace Long term: accommodative devices (therapeutic footwear, insoles, orthoses)
1 (fragmentation)	Erythema, swelling, warmth	Subchondral fragmentation, dissolution, subluxation, dislocation	Foot elevation Protected off-loading (non-weight bearing versus partial weight bearing) in a total contact cast or brace Rule out infection, gout, rheumatoid arthritis
2 (coalescence)	Decreased erythema, swelling, warmth	New bone formation Coalescence of larger bone fragments Sclerosis	Protected off-loading in a cast or brace/ Charcot restraint orthotic walker[a]
3 (consolidation)	Resolution of edema Residual deformity	Bone healing/remodeling Decreased sclerosis	Accommodative devices (therapeutic footwear, insoles, orthoses)[a]

[a]Surgical indications include acute dislocation, osteomyelitis, non-healing or recurrent ulcer, or deformity that cannot be accommodated by non-operative management.
(After Eichenholtz SN. (1966) Charcot Joints. Springfield: Charles C. Thomas. Stage 0 modified in Schon LC, Marks RM. (1995) The management of neuropathic fracture-dislocations in the diabetic patient. Orthop Clin North Am 26: 375.)

Table 7–3: Charcot Arthropathy: Anatomical Classification

TYPE	ANATOMICAL LOCATION	CLINICAL RELEVANCE
1	Midfoot (tarsometatarsal)	Most common Relatively stable deformity with development of rocker bottom deformity and plantar prominence
2	Hindfoot (subtalar/Chopart)	Unstable
3A	Ankle	Most unstable At risk for malleolar ulceration Longest time to heal
3B	Calcaneus	Fracture of the posterior tuberosity of the calcaneus may lead to pes planus
4	Multiple regions	More extensive pathology
5	Forefoot	Metatarsophalangeal joints usually involved, with infection

(After Brodsky J. (1999) The diabetic foot. In: Surgery of the Foot and Ankle (Coughlin MJ, Mann RA, eds.). St. Louis: Mosby. p. 948, and Trepman E et al. (2005) Charcot neuroarthropathy of the foot and ankle. Foot Ankle Int 26(1): 49.

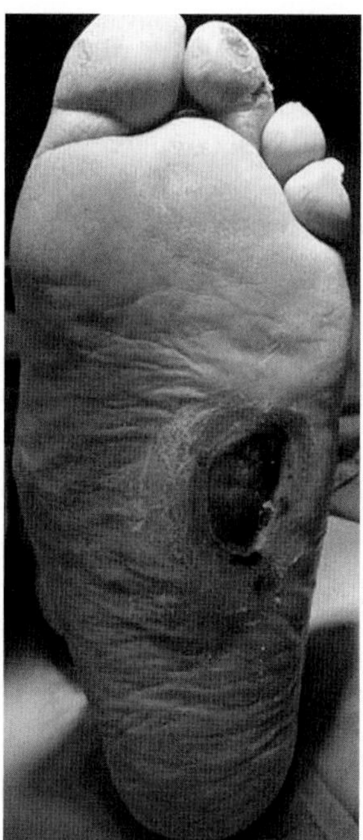

Figure 7–2: Grade 2 deep non-healing ulcer in a Charcot foot (seen again in Fig. 7–3) with a plantar lateral prominence under the fourth and fifth metatarsocuboid joints.

- Rest and limb elevation are recommended to decrease acute-phase swelling.
- Off-loading/immobilization methods include a total contact cast (gold standard), a well-padded bivalved cast or short leg cast, prefabricated removable walking braces, an ankle-foot orthosis, or a Charcot restraint orthotic walker after edema resolution.
- When the process has consolidated, treatment is accommodative, with therapeutic footwear and orthoses geared toward protecting the foot from ulceration over bony prominences.
- Bisphosphonates have also been used to heal Charcot arthropathy by inhibiting osteoclastic bone resorption (Jude et al. 2001).

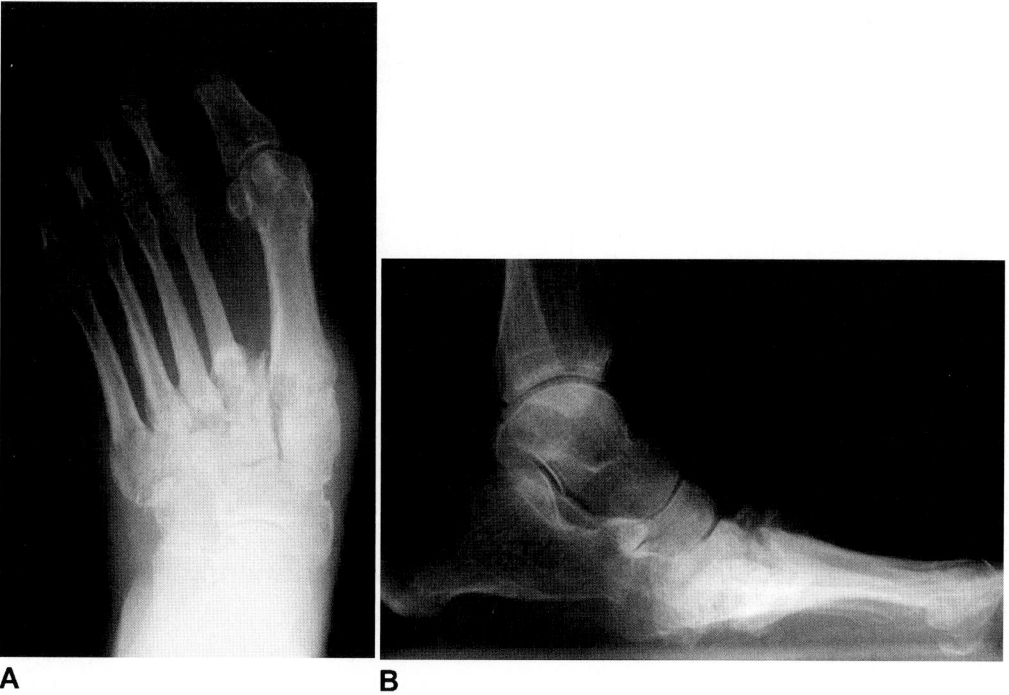

Figure 7–3: **A**, Anteroposterior and **B**, lateral radiographs showing Charcot involvement of the midfoot (Brodsky type 1, Schon type 2 midtarsus deformity) primarily involving the tarsometatarsal and naviculocuneiform joints.

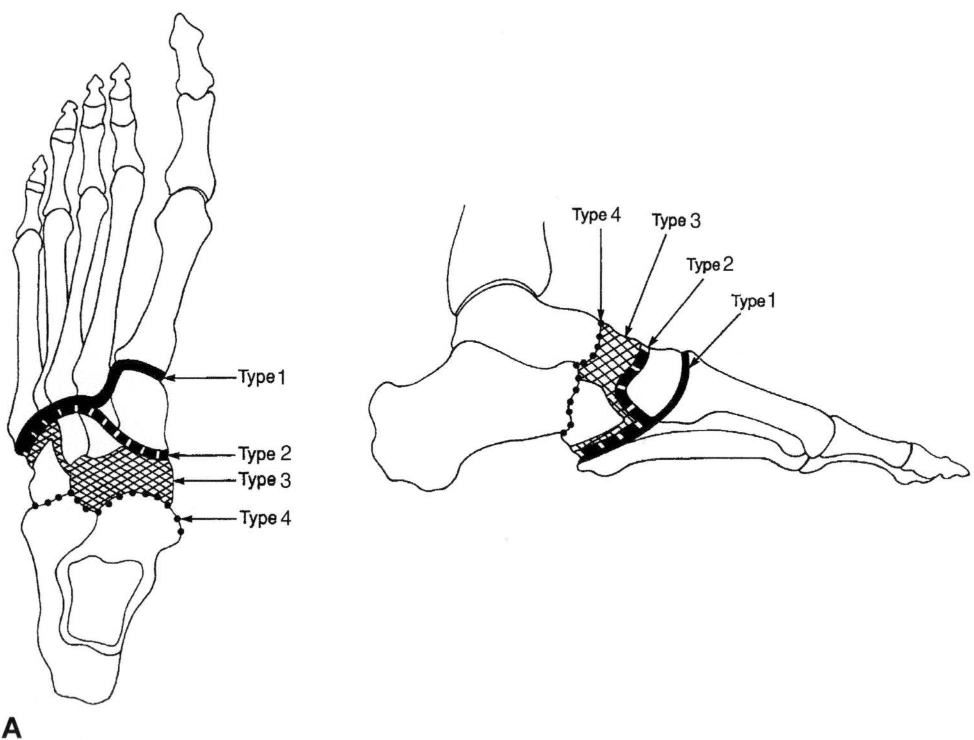

Figure 7–4: Illustration of the classification of midtarsus deformity based on **A**, anatomical location (type) and

Continued

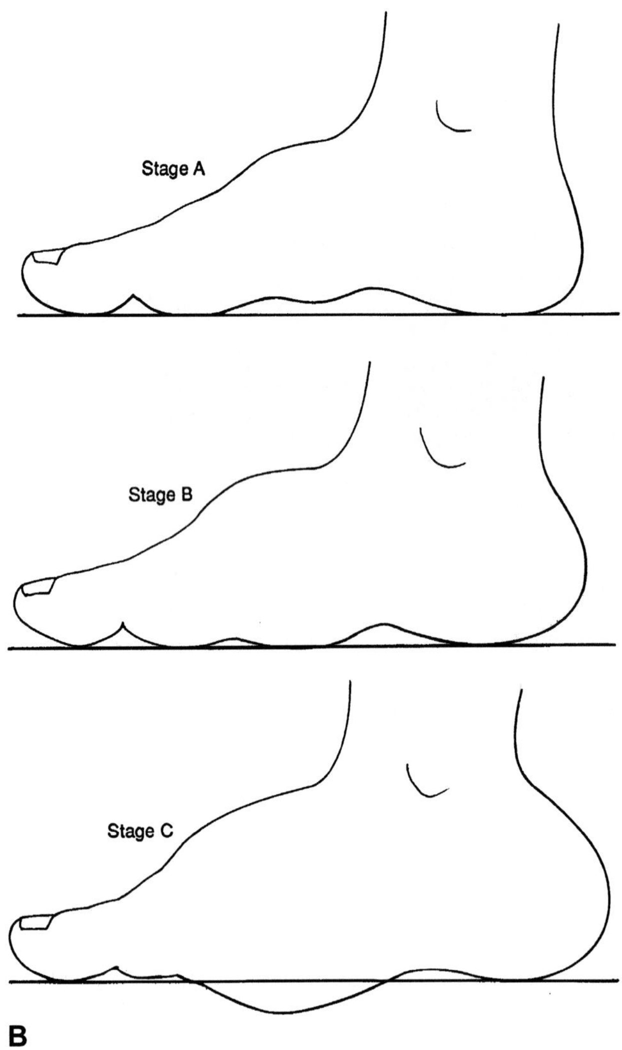

Figure 7–4: Cont'd **B, degree of collapse (stage). (From Schon LC, Weinfeld SB, Horton GA. (1998) Radiographic and clinical classification of acquired midtarsus deformities. Foot Ankle Int 19: 394-404.)**

Table 7–4: Classification of Midtarsus Deformity Based on Anatomical Location (Type)

TYPE	ANATOMICAL LOCATION
1	Midfoot: metatarsocuneiform joints
2	Midfoot: naviculocuneiform joints
3	Navicular
4	Transverse tarsal joint

(After Schon LC, Weinfeld SB, Horton GA. (1998) Radiographic and clinical classification of acquired midtarsus deformities. Foot Ankle Int 19: 394-404.)

- The main problem that may develop during non-operative treatment of a Charcot foot is ulceration. Increased contact pressure over a bony prominence or deformity can lead to ulceration, and then possibly infection or even amputation.

Table 7–5: Classification of Midtarsus Deformity Based on Degree of Collapse (Stage)

STAGE	DEFORMITY	CLINICAL RELEVANCE
A	Minimal deformity, with loss of arch height but no "rocker" or negative arch	Least likely to require surgery
B	Loss of medial or lateral arch to the plantar level, with a plantar prominence	–
C	Collapse of both the medial and lateral arches, and a midfoot prominence more plantar than the heel or ball of the foot	Most likely to require surgery

(After Schon LC, Weinfeld SB, Horton GA. (1998) Radiographic and clinical classification of acquired midtarsus deformities. Foot Ankle Int 19: 394-404.)

Surgical Treatment

- Reconstructive surgery is recommended for non-healing or recurrent ulcers (including those that are infected), or marked instability/deformity that cannot be accommodated by non-operative modalities. The goals of surgery are to produce a functionally stable, "braceable" plantigrade foot without soft tissue breakdown.
- For a foot that is already braceable or "shoeable," ostectomy and ulcer debridement may be all that is necessary. This is particularly true when the foot is well aligned and stable but with an osteophyte causing local pressure.
  - This situation may arise after previous Charcot reconstructive surgery, when osteophyte may develop in an otherwise braceable foot.
- Realignment and fusion is needed for the unbraceable foot with or without infection.
- Displaced ankle fractures in the neuropathic patient should also generally be treated with surgery (open reduction and internal fixation) (Fig. 7–5).
- Amputation is necessary when extensive infection makes reconstruction not feasible.

Principles of Charcot Reconstruction

- The key to reconstructing neuropathic deformity (or an acute fracture) is more fixation and longer non-weight-bearing time. This is because patients with neuropathy cannot tell when they are putting too much pressure on the foot (Fig. 7–6).
- Reconstructive surgery includes realignment and fusion. The goal is not to restore normal anatomy, but rather have the foot straight, with no focal pressure points (shoeable).
- In the absence of infection, most surgeons prefer internal fixation to maintain alignment.
- External fixators, especially when using thin wire frames, may be helpful in cases with active infection, or as an adjunct when there is significant bone loss compromising the strength of internal fixation.

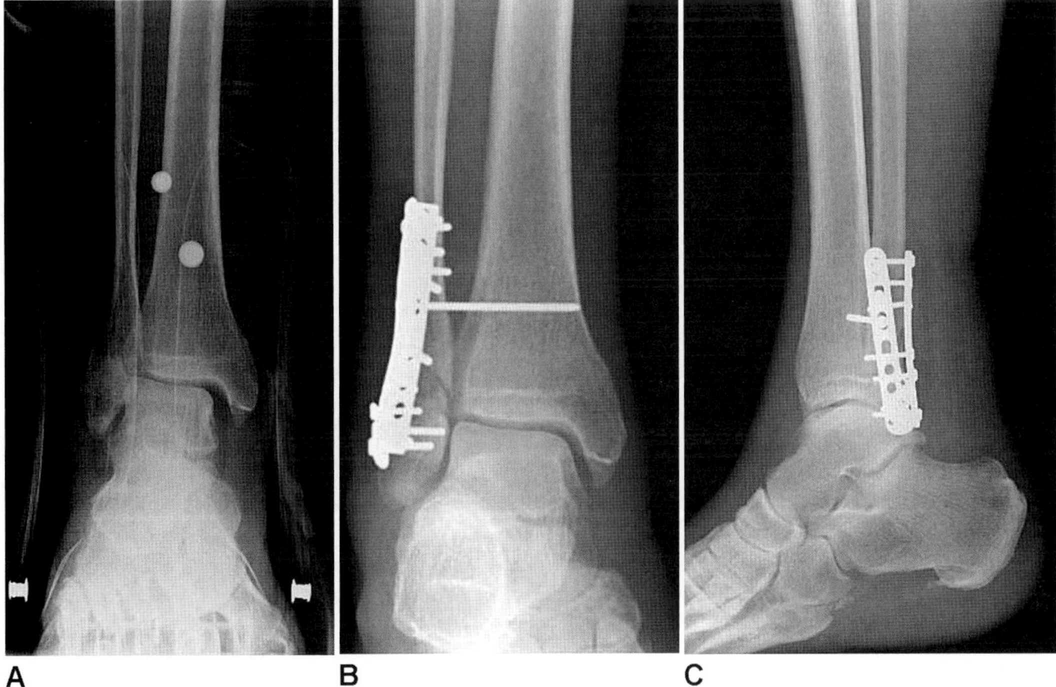

Figure 7–5: **A,** This 65-year-old diabetic man presented days after a minor ankle twisting. He had no pain but noticeable swelling. He was initially treated in a cast, which led to ulceration over the lateral malleolus. **B** and **C,** To prevent further ulceration, open reduction and internal fixation with two plates was performed. After 3 months of strict non-weight bearing, he resumed a normal life. (Radiographs courtesy of J. Greisberg, M.D.)

- In a foot with midfoot deformity, realignment often requires resecting one or more dislocated midfoot bones. Fixation can be accomplished with multiple screws and/or plates. In some cases, it may be necessary to span uninvolved joints to get adequate purchase.
- In the hindfoot, realignment is followed by fixation with multiple screws. Realignment may require resection of all or part of the navicular or cuboid.
- The neuropathic ankle is difficult to manage, as much of the talus may be missing. Internal fixation can be

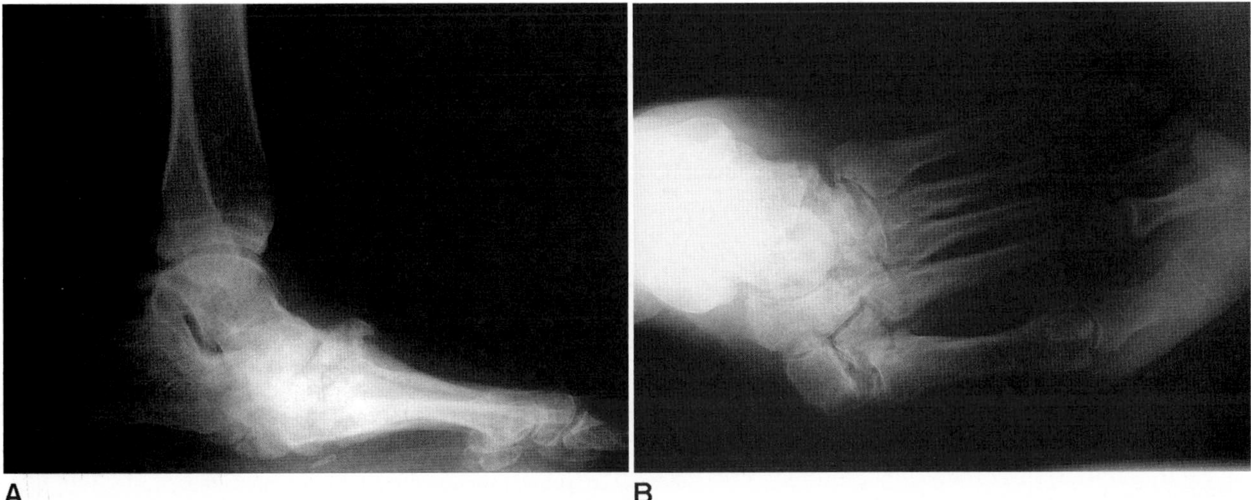

Figure 7–6: **A** and **B,** This woman had a long history of diabetes and can no longer fit into any shoe. Her foot shows Charcot degeneration of the hindfoot and forefoot, with marked deformity.

Continued

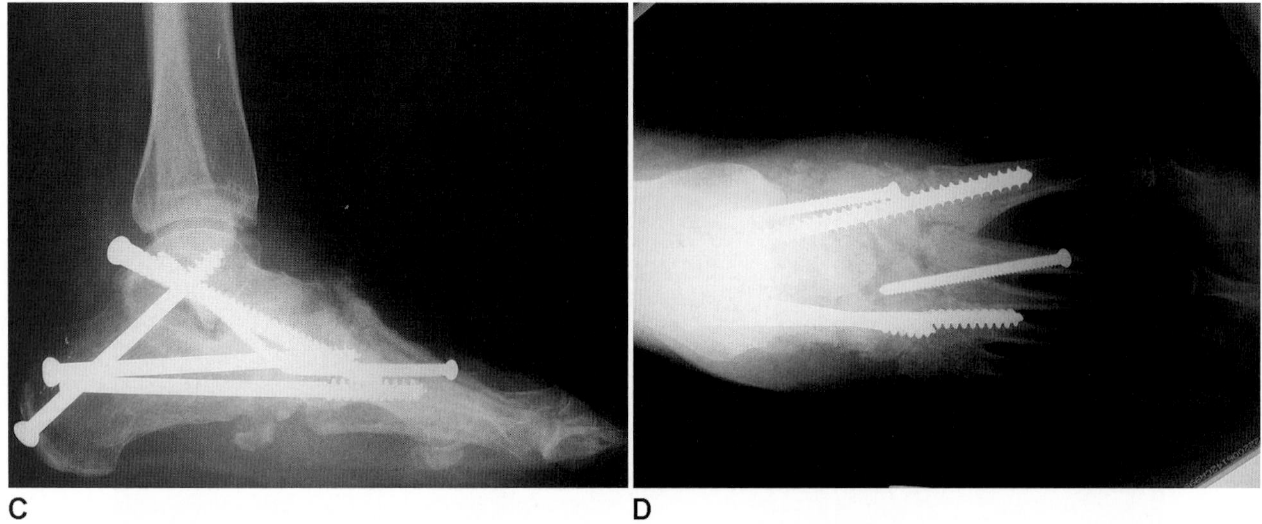

Figure 7–6: Cont'd **C and D, Realignment and fusion were performed through two incisions. Use of long, strong screws plus 3 months of non-weight bearing helped her heal without complication. (Radiographs courtesy of J. Greisberg, M.D.)**

accomplished with a retrograde intramedullary nail or a blade plate. In some cases, multiple lag screws or an external fixator may be best.

- The complication rates for Charcot reconstruction are higher than with other foot arthrodeses. Because the alternative in most cases is amputation, the extra risk is usually worth taking.
- Following reconstruction, prolonged limb immobilization is generally recommended for at least 3 months, followed by bracing for at least 12 months or perhaps indefinitely for the Charcot ankle or hindfoot. As a general rule, treatment of a fracture in the neuropathic patient should include immobilization for double the normal period of time.

Amputations

- Amputations in the diabetic patient do not carry a good prognosis. After a lower limb amputation, there is a 68% 5-year mortality rate and a 50% incidence of contralateral lower limb amputation within 5 years (Larsson et al. 1998).
- Preoperative vascular evaluation and vascular reconstruction should be performed prior to amputation. This may permit a lower level of amputation.

Forefoot Deformity

- Motor neuropathy leads to loss of intrinsic function, with subsequent muscle imbalance.
  - The intrinsic muscles normally flex the metatarsophalangeal and extend the interphalangeal joints.
- Loss of intrinsic motor function results in claw toe deformities.
- Ulceration commonly occurs beneath the lesser metatarsal heads, but can also occur at the dorsal aspect of the proximal or distal interphalangeal joints, at the tip of the toe, or between the toes.
- When the deformity cannot be accommodated by external modalities (shoes with tall toe box), deformity correction or removal of the bony prominence is recommended to prevent ulceration.
- In a foot with good vascular supply, forefoot realignment surgery is appropriate.
  - When a vascular surgeon cannot restore adequate distal perfusion, amputation is necessary.
- An ulcerated and infected metatarsal head should be excised.
- In the absence of infection, surgery can be reconstructive.
  - Proximal interphalangeal resection arthroplasty with muscle balancing (flexor release or transfer to the extensor, and extensor lengthening).
- A metatarsal-shortening osteotomy may be helpful in some cases (such as with metatarsophalangeal dislocations).

References

Brodsky JW. (2003) The diabetic foot. In: Surgery of the Foot and Ankle (Coughlin MJ, Mann RA, eds.). St. Louis: Mosby. pp. 895-969.
A thorough discussion of diabetic foot disease.

Frykberg RG, Armstrong DG, Giurini J et al. (2000) Diabetic foot disorders: a clinical practice guideline. American College of Foot and Ankle Surgeons. J Foot Ankle Surg 39(5 suppl): S1-S60.

Larsson J, Agardh CD, Apelqvist J et al. (1998) Long-term prognosis after healed amputation in patients with diabetes. Clin Orthop Relat Res 350: 149-158.
Outcomes for diabetic amputees are quite different than for young patients with traumatic amputations.

Pinzur MS, Slovenkai MP, Trepman E et al. (2005) Guidelines for diabetic foot care. Recommendations endorsed by the Diabetes

Committee of the American Orthopaedic Foot and Ankle Society. Foot Ankle Int 26(1):113-119.

Price P. (2004) The diabetic foot: quality of life. Clin Infect Dis 39(suppl 2): S129-S131.

Teodorescu VJ, Chen C, Morrissey N et al. (2004) Detailed protocol of ischemia and the use of noninvasive vascular laboratory testing in diabetic foot ulcers. Am J Surg 187(5A): 75S-80S.

A thorough discussion of diabetic vascular assessment.

Basic Science of Diabetes

Follak N, Kloting I, Merk H. (2005) Influence of diabetic metabolic state on fracture healing in spontaneously diabetic rats. Diabetes Metab Res Rev 21(3): 288-296.

One of several studies showing impaired healing in an animal model of diabetes.

Gooch HL, Hale JE, Fujioka H. (2000) Alterations of cartilage and collagen expression during fracture healing in experimental diabetes. Connect Tissue Res 41(2): 81-91.

Macey LR, Kana SM, Jingushi S et al. (1989) Defects of early fracture-healing in experimental diabetes. J Bone Joint Surg 71A(5): 722-733.

Topping RE, Bolander ME, Balian G. (1994) Type X collagen in fracture callus and the effects of experimental diabetes. Clin Orthop Relat Res 308: 220-228.

Neuropathy

Dellon AL. (2004) Diabetic neuropathy: Review of a surgical approach to restore sensation, relieve pain, and prevent ulceration and amputation. Foot Ankle Int 25(10): 749-755.

One surgeon's experience with nerve decompression in diabetes. The results have been questioned by many other experts, and have not been reproduced by others.

Kapur D. (2003) Neuropathic pain and diabetes. Diabetes Metab Res Rev 19(suppl 1): S9-S15.

Saltzman CL, Rashid R, Hayes A et al. (2004a) 4.5-Gram monofilament sensation beneath both first metatarsal heads indicates protective foot sensation in diabetic patients. J Bone Joint Surg 86A(4): 717-723.

Describes a simple screening test for neuropathy.

Vinik A, Mehrabyan A, Colen L et al. (2004) Focal entrapment neuropathies in diabetes. Diabetes Care 27(7): 1783-1788.

Ulcers

Boulton AJ, Kirsner RS, Vileikyte L. (2004) Clinical practice. Neuropathic diabetic foot ulcers. N Engl J Med 351(1): 48-55.

Jeffcoate WJ, Price P, Harding KG, International Working Group on Wound Healing and Treatments for People with Diabetic Foot Ulcers. (2004) Wound healing and treatments for people with diabetic foot ulcers. Diabetes Metab Res Rev 20(suppl 1): S78-S89.

Matricali GA, Deroo K, Dereymaeker G. (2003) Outcome and recurrence rate of diabetic foot ulcers treated by a total contact cast: Short-term follow-up. Foot Ankle Int 24(9): 680-684.

Mueller MJ, Sinacore DR, Hastings MK et al. (2003) Effect of Achilles tendon lengthening on neuropathic plantar ulcers. A randomized clinical trial. J Bone Joint Surg 85A(8): 1436-1445.

Achilles lengthening dramatically reduced reulceration rate in this series.

Myerson M, Papa J, Eaton K et al. (1992) The total-contact cast for management of neuropathic plantar ulceration of the foot. J Bone Joint Surg Am 74(2): 261-269.

Saltzman CL, Zimmerman MB, Holdsworth RL et al. (2004b) Effect of initial weight-bearing in a total contact cast on healing of diabetic foot ulcers. J Bone Joint Surg Am 86-A(12): 2714-2719.

Although it is commonly recommended that patients wait at least a day before walking on a cast, immediate weight bearing seems to be an acceptable alternative.

Trepman E, Pinzur MS, Shields NN (2005). Application of the total contact cast. Foot Ankle Int 26(1): 108-112.

An up-to-date description of total contact casting technique.

Charcot Disease

Eichenholtz SN. (1966) Charcot Joints. Springfield: Charles C. Thomas.

A classic discussion of neuropathic deformity.

Jude EB, Selby PL, Burgess J et al. (2001) Bisphosphonates in the treatment of Charcot neuroarthropathy: A double-blind randomised controlled trial. Diabetologia 44(11): 2032-2037.

The role of bisphosphonates in Charcot disease is discussed.

Marks RM, Parks BG, Schon LC. (1998) Midfoot fusion technique for neuroarthropathic feet: Biomechanical analysis and rationale. Foot Ankle Int 19(8): 507-510.

Myerson MS, Henderson MR, Saxby T et al. (1994) Management of midfoot diabetic neuroarthropathy. Foot Ankle Int 15(5): 233-241.

Pinzur M. (2004) Surgical versus accommodative treatment for Charcot arthropathy of the midfoot. Foot Ankle Int 25(8): 545-549.

With appropriate footwear, more than half of patients with midfoot disease (not hindfoot or ankle) can be treated without surgery.

Schon LC, Easley ME, Weinfeld SB. (1998a) Charcot neuroarthropathy of the foot and ankle. Clin Orthop Relat Res 349: 116-131.

Schon LC, Marks RM. (1995) The management of neuropathic fracture-dislocations in the diabetic patient. Orthop Clin North Am 26: 375.

Schon LC, Weinfeld SB, Horton GA et al. (1998b) Radiographic and clinical classification of acquired midtarsus deformities. Foot Ankle Int 19(6): 394-404.

Wagner FW Jr. (1979) Management of the diabetic neurotrophic foot. Part II. A classification and treatment program for diabetic, neuropathic, and dysvascular foot problems. In: Instructional Course Lectures: The American Academy of Orthopaedic Surgeons, vol. 28. St. Louis: Mosby. pp. 143-165.

CHAPTER 8

Rheumatoid Arthritis and Inflammatory Disorders

Lew C. Schon* and Kevin J. Logel§

*M.D., Director of Foot and Ankle Services, Department of Orthopaedic Surgery, Union Memorial Hospital, Baltimore, MD
§M.D., Department of Orthopaedic Surgery, Union Memorial Hospital, Baltimore, MD

Rheumatoid Arthritis

Epidemiology

- The prevalence of rheumatoid arthritis (RA) in the USA ranges from 0.3 to 1.5%; it affects women about three times more frequently than men. Foot and ankle complaints are often the heralding sign in RA and are present in about 90% of patients with RA (Jaakola and Mann 2004).

Pathophysiology

- Gender and immune susceptibility are major determinants in the development of RA. RA is associated strongly with certain class 2 major histocompatibility complexes (specifically human leukocyte antigen [HLA] DR4) (Box 8–1) (Smyth and Janson 1997).
- The inflammation can affect joints, tendons, and ligaments.
- Joint inflammation leads to arthritis (degeneration or erosion of the articular cartilage and subchondral bone).
- Ligament inflammation results in stretching or tearing, with eventual deformity. In the hindfoot, this might appear as planovalgus (flatfoot), while in the forefoot there may be hallux valgus.
- Tendon involvement can be seen as well, such as posterior tibial tendinitis.

Box 8–1 Cascade of Events in Rheumatoid Arthritis

- Endothelial cell expression of adhesion molecules in response to cytokines.
- Migration of monocytes/lymphocytes into synovium, where chemotactic factors attract polymorphonuclear leukocytes to synovial fluid.
- Activated synovial macrophages produce interleukin-1, tumor necrosis factor-α, and growth factors that act on chondrocytes and fibroblasts.
- Proteinases, prostaglandins, leukotrienes, and reactive oxidases released cause cartilage degradation and bone resorption.

(After Smyth CJ, Janson RW. (1997) Rheumatologic view of the rheumatoid foot. Clin Orthop 340: 7-17.)

Diagnosis

- Three clinical patterns of RA prevail.
  - The progressive pattern (10%) follows a progressively destructive course without remission.
  - The monocyclic pattern (20%) typically involves a single episode of non-destructive synovitis that dissipates after several months.
  - The polycyclic pattern (70%) has multiple recurrent episodes of synovitis with eventual joint destruction.
- Early signs of RA include symmetric swelling of small joints of the hands or feet. This is usually associated with joint stiffness in the morning that lasts at least 1 hour, later improves, and has been present for at least 6 weeks. The American Rheumatism Association diagnostic criteria for RA are seen in Box 8–2.
- In the foot and ankle, RA most commonly affects the metatarsophalangeal (MTP) joints. Early on in the disease,

Box 8–2 1987 Revised American Rheumatism Association Criteria for Rheumatoid Arthritis[a]

- Morning stiffness for at least 1 h and present for at least 6 weeks
- Swelling of three or more joints for at least 6 weeks
- Swelling of the wrist, metacarpophalangeal, or proximal interphalangeal joints for 6 or more weeks
- Symmetric joint swelling
- Hand radiograph changes typical of rheumatoid arthritis (RA) that must include erosions or unequivocal bony decalcification
- Rheumatoid nodules
- Serum rheumatoid factor by a method positive in less than 5% of normals

[a] Four or more of the criteria must be present for greater than 6 weeks to diagnose RA.)

patients complain of MTP stiffness and fullness. The radiographs may show juxtaarticular osteopenia.

- Extraarticular manifestations of RA may also be present. These include rheumatoid nodules (20-30%), local nerve compression or neuroma (5-25%), pes planus deformity (40%), and local tendinitis.
- Although most patients referred to an orthopedist may already carry a diagnosis of RA, occasionally an undiagnosed patient will present to the orthopedist primarily. If RA is suspected, basic laboratory values that should be obtained include complete blood cell count with differential, erythrocyte sedimentation rate, C-reactive protein, antinuclear antibodies, and rheumatoid factor.

Clinical Evaluation

- A thorough history including the onset of the various symptoms (i.e. swelling, pain, warmth, stiffness, weakness, redness, and numbness) should be obtained. The nature/character/location of the pain should be noted, along with exacerbating and ameliorating factors. In addition, an assessment of the patient's activity level, living situation, and working status is important in generating a treatment plan.
- An up-to-date list of the patient's medications, such as corticosteroids, immunosuppressive medications, and non-steroidal antiinflammatory drugs (NSAIDs), is useful. Other comorbidities—such as diabetes; vascular disease; and gastrointestinal, renal, hepatic, cardiac, and pulmonary disease—should be taken into consideration.
- Physical examination should include a thorough assessment of the entire patient. Cervical spine instability directly correlates with the severity of hand and foot involvement. Upper extremity involvement may affect the ability to comply with postoperative weight-bearing restrictions (i.e. crutches, walkers) or the donning and doffing of immobilization devices (i.e. braces).
- A focal examination of both lower extremities should include observation of gait, range of motion of all joints, motor strength testing, sensory examination, and vascular examination. Any sign of coexistent vasculitis (toe ischemia, leg ulcers) should be worked up before surgery is contemplated. Examination of shoe wear patterns may also provide clues as to the deformity and areas of increased pressure.
- Some rheumatoid patients may have unrecognized peripheral neuropathy, with all the potential complications. Charcot arthropathy may be present in some cases.
- Radiographic evaluation of patients with RA typically involves bilateral weight-bearing anteroposterior, lateral, and oblique views of the foot, and an anterior and mortise view of the ankle.

Treatment Modalities

- Pharmacotherapy is the mainstay of treatment in RA.
  - A wide variety of antiinflammatories are available, including non-steroidals as well as glucocorticoids.
  - Disease-modifying antirheumatic drugs (DMARDs) commonly used include hydroxychloroquine, methotrexate, gold, and penicillamine.
  - Immune-modifying drugs have recently been introduced and may be effective for use in both early and recalcitrant cases of RA.
- The side effect profiles of these therapies are well known, and may include gastric intolerance (NSAIDs), renal toxicity (NSAIDs), secondary adrenal insufficiency, osteopenia (corticosteroids), and the potential for increased risk of perioperative infection (immunomodulating drugs, especially interleukin-1 antagonists and tumor necrosis factor-α antagonists). Limited data exist regarding the true rate of postoperative infection in patients taking these drugs, but early reports suggest there is no difference in healing or infection rates compared with patients not on the drugs.
- Non-operative management of RA in the foot may include:
  - lambs' wool or felt padding placed over or around prominences
  - extrawidth/extradepth shoes
  - stretching shoes strategically to accommodate bony protrusions
  - orthotic devices (custom inserts or custom ankle-foot orthoses [AFOs])
  - appropriately placed pads (e.g. removable adhesive-backed felt pads) to unload skin over areas of deformity.
- A working knowledge of the foot orthotic devices available (soft accommodative, semirigid, and rigid) or the ankle-foot orthotic devices (plastic molded posterior AFO, stirrup-style AFO, and composite AFO—Arizona brace) and open lines of communication with both the patient and the orthotist are crucial to the successful use of these non-operative measures.
- When non-operative management has failed to alleviate symptoms, or deformity has become progressive or "unbraceable", surgical intervention becomes necessary (Fig. 8–1).

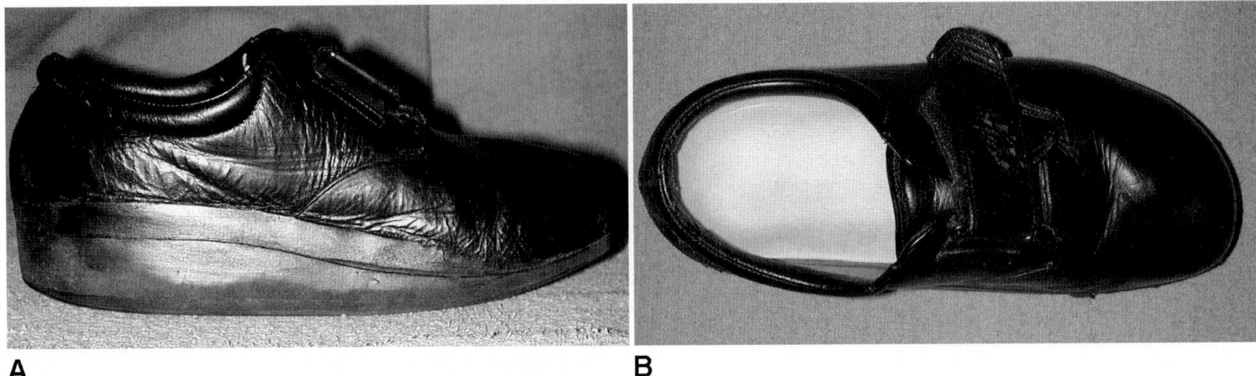

Figure 8–1: **A, Orthopedic shoe with Velcro strap, extradepth toe box, and a rocker bottom sole. B, Accommodative Plastizote insole that cushions and deforms to decrease pain from bony prominences.**

Forefoot

- Early in the course of RA, the most common site of involvement in the lower extremity is the forefoot. Usually, the deformities seen in the RA forefoot are progressive hallux valgus, dorsal subluxation of the lesser MTP joints with varus angulation, and flexion deformities at the interphalangeal joints (Fig. 8–2).
- The mechanism leading to deformity involves inflammation of the MTP joint synovium that causes capsular distension, loss of passive joint stabilizers (collateral ligaments and plantar plate), and subsequent destruction of articular cartilage.
- MTP synovitis leads to dorsal subluxation or dislocation of the proximal phalanx on the metatarsal head in the lesser rays. The extension at the MTP joints pulls the plantar fat pad from under the metatarsal head into a location distal to it. Displacement of the fat pad leads to pain under the forefoot, or metatarsalgia (Fig. 8–3).
- Early in the course of the disease, accommodative shoe wear and appropriate semirigid or accommodative orthotic devices may alleviate symptoms adequately. For example, metatarsalgia from fat pad migration can be treated with a metatarsal pad.
- Operative intervention should be reserved for pain or deformity that is not remedied by non-operative modalities.
- When considering surgery for any inflammatory arthritis, the physician needs to assess the entire foot as a whole. Frequently, there are multiple deformities in the hindfoot and forefoot. It is important to identify which deformities are contributing to the clinical symptoms.

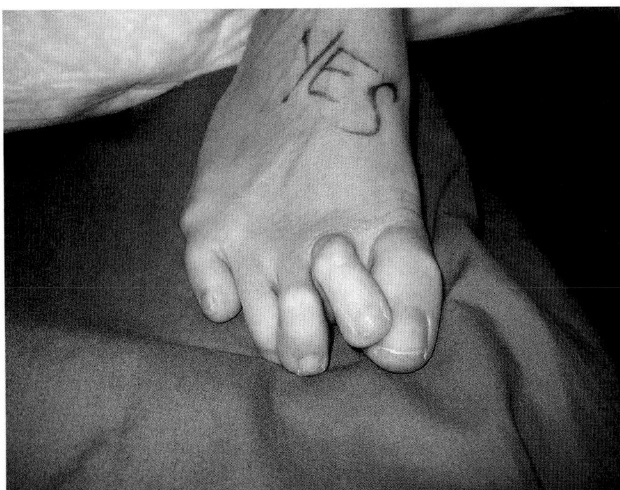

Figure 8–2: **Dorsal subluxation and varus angulation of the second metatarsophalangeal joint. Hallux valgus is also present in this patient with early rheumatoid arthritis.**

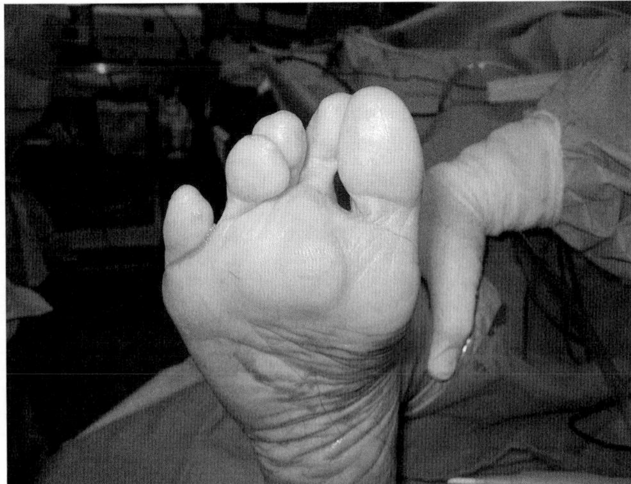

Figure 8–3: **Plantar view of patient in Figure 8–2, showing migration of distal plantar fat pad as a result of dorsal subluxation of lesser metatarsophalangeal joints. The prominence plantarly represents a plantarly deviated metatarsal head compounded by a shifted fat pad and plantar hyperkeratosis.**

The Hallux

- The mainstay of hallux valgus treatment in the setting of RA is arthrodesis of the first MTP joint. This procedure addresses a hallux that lacks viable cartilage or bony surfaces, adequate ligaments, or functional tendons by fusing the proximal phalanx to the metatarsal head. In this way, pain, deformity, and instability are corrected. Traditional hallux valgus procedures (distal metatarsal osteotomies) may be performed in early disease states with some limited success, but a 2-year follow-up study demonstrated high failure rates due to progression of the disease (Thordarson et al. 2002).
- Progression of hallux interphalangeal arthritis has been reported following arthrodesis of the first MTP joint. In most cases, the interphalangeal arthritis is asymptomatic and does not require further treatment. If symptomatic, treatment is typically arthrodesis of the interphalangeal joint.
- Resection arthroplasty (Keller) involves removal of all or a portion of the base of the proximal phalanx and shaving of the medial prominence of the first metatarsal head. Early success rates were high, but first MTP joint instability, recurrence of the hallux valgus deformity, transfer metatarsalgia, and plantar callosity formation have tempered its use.
- Swanson introduced silicone arthroplasty to address the shortcomings of resection arthroplasty in low-demand RA patients (Swanson et al. 1979). Silastic and metallic implants have been used for treatment of hallux valgus and the degenerative changes associated with RA. High rates of osteolysis and implant failure have been reported (Fig. 8–4). Newer designs of silastic implants with titanium grommets have shown improved wear rates, but few long-term studies are available.
- Many, if not most, patients with inflammatory arthritis and hallux valgus deformity have marked instability of the first metatarsocuneiform joint. While most surgeons use first MTP arthrodesis for inflammatory hallux valgus, others have found success with the Lapidus procedure (metatarsocuneiform realignment and arthrodesis with distal soft tissue realignment). In theory, this preserves more normal hallux function in active patients.

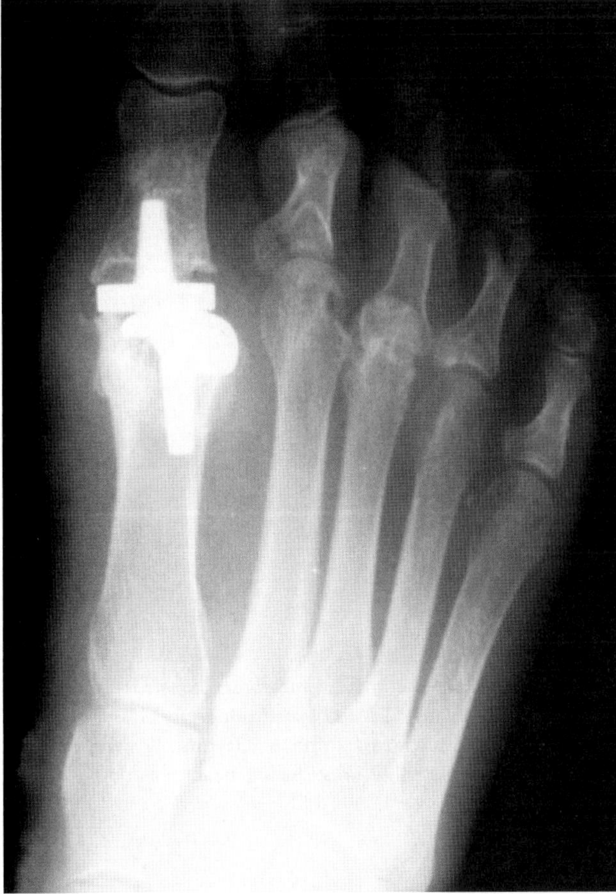

Figure 8–4: **Arthroplasty of first metatarsophalangeal joint with metallic implant. Note lucency of implant in proximal phalanx. This implant was removed for painful loosening and converted to an arthrodesis.**

Lesser Metatarsophalangeals/Toes

- Non-operative management of lesser MTP and toe involvement in the early stages of RA can be attempted using metatarsal pads, toe sleeves, accommodative orthotics, and shoe wear modification (extradepth shoe).
- In 1912, Hoffman first described resection of the metatarsal heads through a plantar incision for severe dorsiflexion deformities (clawing) of the lesser MTP joints. This removes the prominent metatarsal head, relieving the pain from metatarsalgia.
- Clayton (1960) later modified the Hoffman procedure to include resection of the base of the proximal phalanx as well as the metatarsal head through a dorsal approach. Current methods use a combination of the Hoffman-Clayton procedure with metatarsal head resection and preservation of the base of the proximal phalanx.
  - A percutaneous pin is used to stabilize the MTP joint for 4-6 weeks after surgery to minimize the incidence of recurrent angular deformities (Fig. 8–5).
- As is often the case in RA, deformities are severe, and correction of the interphalangeal flexion deformities as well as the lesser MTP deformities is required.
- Rigid toe deformities involving the distal or proximal interphalangeal joints typically require fusion to achieve adequate correction. However, flexible deformities of the distal or proximal interphalangeal joints may be treated with closed manipulation (osteoclasis) or flexor tenotomy.
- High rates of success have been reported using lesser metatarsal head resection and hammertoe correction, such as osteoclasis (manipulation of the proximal interphalangeal joint) or proximal interphalangeal joint fusion, in conjunction with first MTP fusion in RA patients.

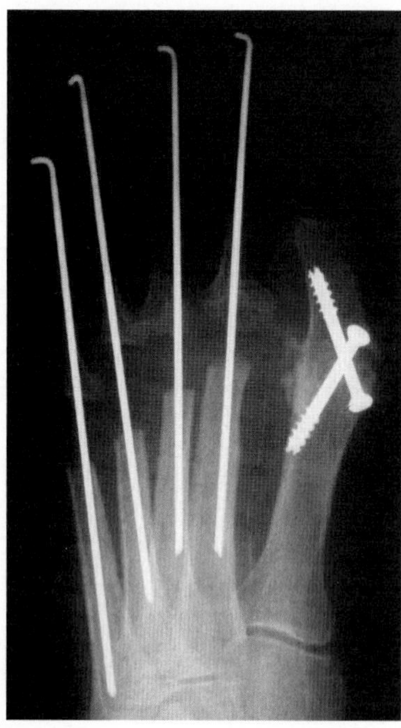

Figure 8–5: Classic rheumatoid forefoot reconstruction with first metatarsophalangeal (MTP) arthrodesis and lesser metatarsal head resections (Hoffman-Clayton). K wires are used to stabilize the MTP joint during healing.

- A typical "package" for a severe rheumatoid deformity thus includes:
  - first MTP realignment and fusion, with internal or percutaneous fixation
  - second through fifth metatarsal head resection
  - second through fifth proximal interphalangeal joint resection/fusion, with percutaneous pinning across the interphalangeal and MTP joints (Fig. 8–5).
- Of course, it is important to remember that the foot with a fused hallux and lesser metatarsal head resections will not function normally. Generally good results have been reported with these procedures, at least in part because the preoperative deformity is so disabling.
  - Some surgeons have referred to this multiple metatarsal head resection as an "internal amputation" of the forefoot.
- In some patients, preservation of the lesser MTP joint(s) can be accomplished with a combination of metatarsal-shortening osteotomies, synovectomy, and flexor to extensor tendon transfers (Girdlestone-Taylor) in the toes.
- In cases of MTP dislocation where the MTP joint is to be preserved, the ray must be shortened to allow reduction. The digital vessels will not stretch enough to allow MTP reduction without shortening.

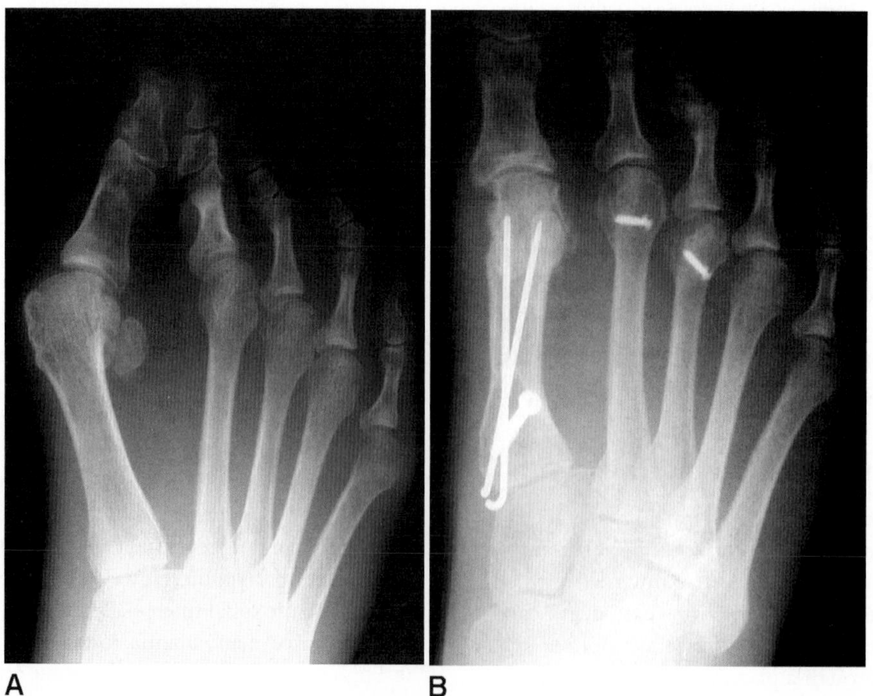

Figure 8–6: **A**, Preoperative radiograph of a patient with mild first metatarsophalangeal (MTP) arthritis, symptomatic hallux valgus, and MTP subluxation. Given the minimal pain at the hallux MTP joint, a joint-sparing procedure was performed to correct the wide intermetatarsal angle and reduce the subluxated lesser MTPs. **B**, Shortening metatarsal osteotomies may be used in conjunction with joint-sparing procedures of the hallux MTP joint to reduce milder deformities of the lesser metatarsophalangeal joints.

- In some cases, metatarsal-shortening osteotomy will relax the vessels enough to allow MTP reduction.
- In other cases, the ray can be shortened by resecting the distal half of the proximal phalanx.
- When combined with tendon balancing (extensor lengthening and flexor tenotomy or flexor to extensor transfer), the toe will remain reduced and may achieve better function than with metatarsal head resection.
- For an active patient, Lapidus procedure (or perhaps a proximal metatarsal osteotomy) in the first ray can be combined with lesser MTP-preserving surgery to achieve a foot with more normal function. The recovery is much longer than with Hoffman-Clayton-type procedures, and outcome studies are needed to prove that the theoretic benefits of such surgery can justify the increased recovery time (Fig. 8–6).

Midfoot

- Roughly two-thirds of patients with RA will have radiographic evidence of midfoot involvement. However, symptomatic arthritis of the midfoot in RA patients is uncommon as a primary complaint.
- Midfoot pain, often involving the first tarsometatarsal joint, may be related to stresses across that area rather than actual tarsometatarsal joint synovitis or articular cartilage destruction. Increased stresses can occur as a result of hindfoot valgus and/or hallux valgus deformities, or as a result of posterior tibial tendon insufficiency.
- Subsequent development of arthritis in the lesser tarsometatarsal joints may also occur as a result of increased stresses transferred from the medial column laterally. Isolated synovitis or RA of the tarsometatarsal joints is uncommon.
- Non-operative measures directed at midfoot involvement in RA can typically be successful. When there is a rigid deformity with a rocker bottom or abduction, bracing may be difficult. AFOs may be more beneficial to aid in delaying disease progression when more flexible deformity of the midfoot exists.
- In severe midfoot deformities treated with orthotics or bracing, careful surveillance of skin over plantar prominences is imperative.
- Operative intervention is considered when pain or deformity has progressed or when the deformity is severe and rigid. Arthrodesis of the involved joint(s) is favored, with realignment of the foot deformity (correction of forefoot abduction, longitudinal arch flattening) (Fig. 8–7).
- Localization of the involved midfoot joints can be difficult. In some cases, a computed tomography, magnetic resonance imaging, or bone scan may be useful in determining which joint(s) to fuse.

Hindfoot

- Hindfoot involvement usually occurs later in the disease process. In a study of patients with RA, patients with disease duration of less than 3 years had 8% hindfoot involvement; with disease duration of greater than 5 years, 25% had hindfoot involvement (Spiegel and Spiegel 1982).
- Radiographically, the talonavicular joint is involved 40% of the time, the subtalar joint 30%, and the calcaneocuboid joint 25%.
- Clinically, the hindfoot deformity is valgus (varus is rare). The underlying pathophysiology relates to the progressive destruction of capsular/ligamentous supports of the subtalar joint, which is intimately associated with transverse tarsal joint function. The resultant deformity is a progressive collapse of the medial longitudinal arch and subsequent planovalgus deformity.
- Associated posterior tibial tendon insufficiency in the setting of RA may lead to a more progressive unilateral planovalgus deformity. Controversy exists as to whether the planovalgus deformity of RA is a result of progressive joint laxity from RA synovitis or associated posterior tibial tendon involvement in the inflammatory process.
  - A gait analysis/electromyographic study by Keenan et al. (1991) looked at the activity of the posterior tibial muscle in patients with RA and pes planovalgus. They found an *increase* in the activity of the posterior tibialis during the stance phase, suggestive of an attempt to stabilize the unstable foot.
- Non-operative treatment of hindfoot involvement in RA includes rest, limited weight bearing, and casting/immobilization for acutely swollen/inflamed joints. Orthotics, custom shoes, and AFOs may be used to stabilize a flexible deformity or provide temporary relief.
- Surgical treatment of the hindfoot is indicated when deformity is progressive and unresponsive to conservative measures. The goal is to define the specific joint(s) involved with regard to pain and deformity. The overall objective of surgery is to achieve a stable plantigrade foot.
- The mainstay of hindfoot surgery in the setting of RA is arthrodesis. Isolated arthrodesis of the talonavicular or subtalar joints may rarely be indicated in early disease before significant deformity has occurred.
- Biomechanically, isolated fusion of the talonavicular joint essentially eliminates hindfoot motion, whereas isolated arthrodesis of the calcaneocuboid or subtalar joints will still allow a small amount of hindfoot motion.
- Non-union rates of isolated talonavicular arthrodesis in patients with inflammatory arthritis range from 3 to 37%. Rigid internal fixation with screws or possibly staples, and careful technique, can achieve high fusion rates (Chiodo et al. 2000).
- Triple arthrodesis is indicated when all three hindfoot joints are involved or when a fixed hindfoot deformity exists. The ideal position of the hindfoot is 5° valgus of the heel and neutral position of the forefoot (no pronation or supination) (Fig. 8–8).
  - Good results with high patient satisfaction and union rates (90%) have been reported.

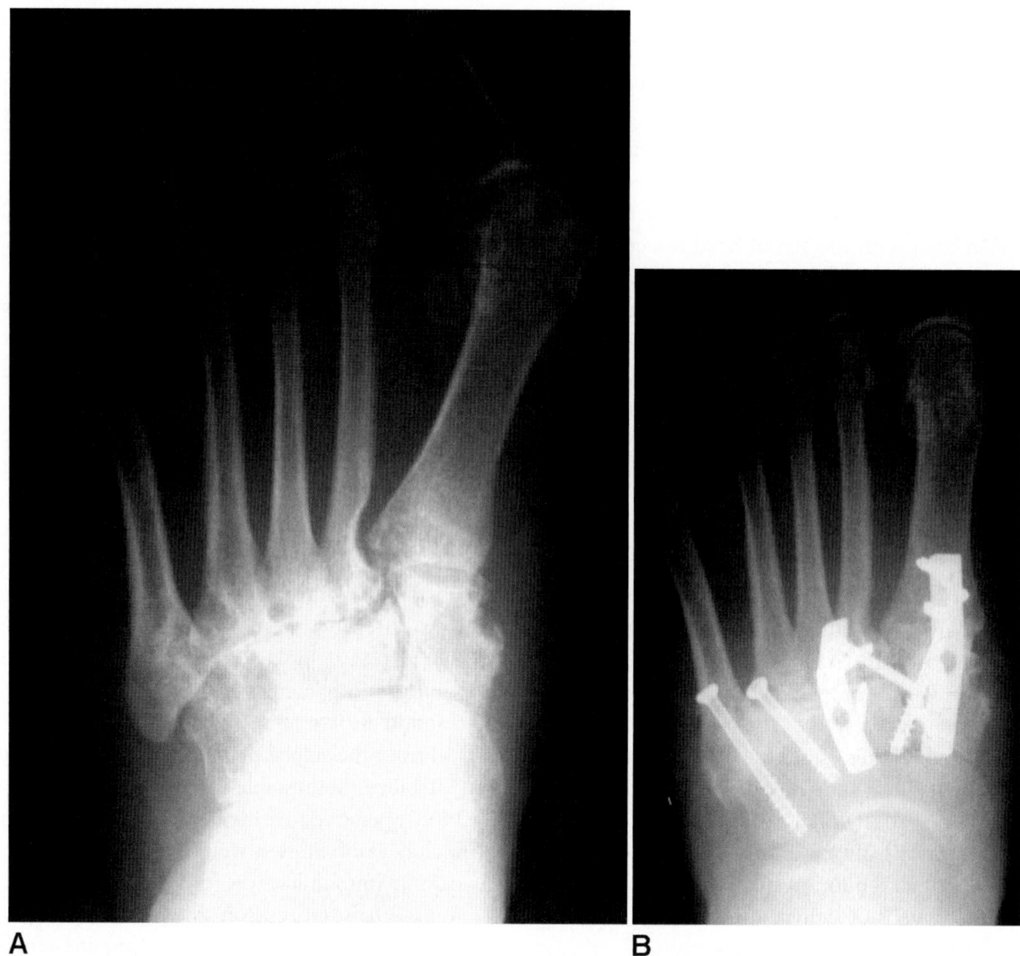

Figure 8–7: **A, Radiograph of patient with involvement of the entire midfoot. This patient had severe pain at the fourth and fifth metatarsal-cuboid joints. B, The same patient after fusion of the tarsometatarsal joints. Correction of deformity should be performed with arthrodesis as needed. If no deformity exists, in situ fusion is indicated.**

- The talonavicular joint is the most common joint in a triple arthrodesis to go on to non-union.

Ankle

- Ankle involvement in RA increases with duration of the disease. The earliest manifestation is typically synovitis. The incidence of ankle involvement has been reported to be much less frequent than hindfoot joints. Significant deformity at the ankle joint as a result of RA is uncommon (Fig. 8–9).
- Non-operative treatments for ankle involvement in RA include pharmacotherapy (NSAIDs, corticosteroids, and DMARDs), rest/immobilization, and custom orthotics/bracing. An AFO is often required to improve alignment or to immobilize an involved ankle joint.
- Painful or disabling ankle synovitis, when present early in the disease process, may be amenable to limited arthroscopic debridement with synovectomy. In most cases, by the time the ankle has become involved, the extent of articular cartilage damage may preclude the use of simple arthroscopic debridement.
- The "gold standard" for surgical treatment of the ankle in RA is arthrodesis. Ankle arthrodesis has typically had reliable results, with high patient satisfaction and fusion rates (60-100%). Techniques described include internal fixation, external fixation, or arthroscopically assisted, and should be chosen on a patient to patient basis (Fig. 8–10).
- Ideal position of arthrodesis should be neutral dorsiflexion, 0-5° valgus, and rotation to match the contralateral side.
- Even with successful fusion, patients may continue to have difficulty walking or may develop arthritis in nearby hindfoot joints, requiring the use of orthotics/braces or assistive devices (canes).
- Stress fractures of the distal tibia and/or fibula may occur following ankle arthrodesis, especially if varus or valgus malalignment of the ankle or hindfoot is present. Patients with inflammatory arthropathy tend to have long disease histories, diverse medications, and osteoporosis that predispose them to stress fractures.
- In some cases, RA patients may have severe deformity with involvement of both the ankle and hindfoot joints

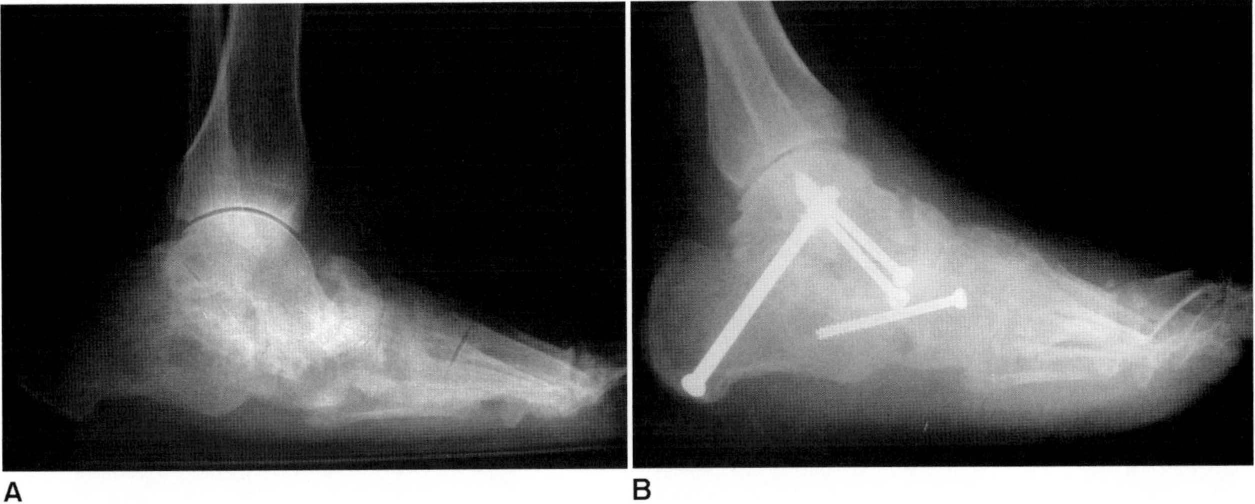

Figure 8–8: **A**, The contralateral side. Note the severe involvement of all hindfoot joints and the collapse at the talonavicular joint, leading to a rocker bottom deformity. Extensive forefoot disease is also present. **B**, Triple arthrodesis performed on the same patient. Note correction of the rocker bottom deformity.

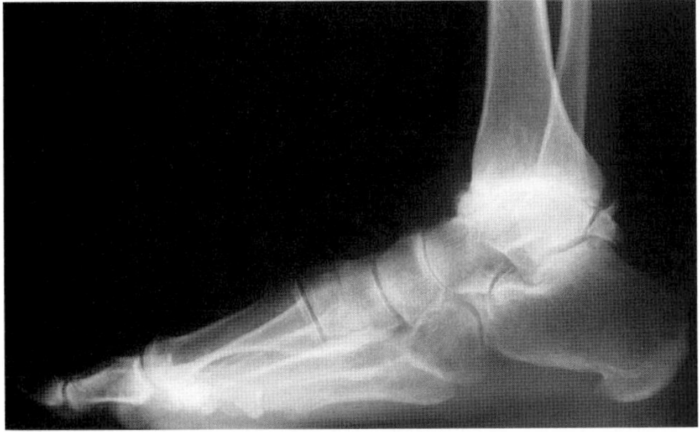

Figure 8–9: Radiograph showing primary involvement of the ankle joint. In this case, minimal deformity is seen.

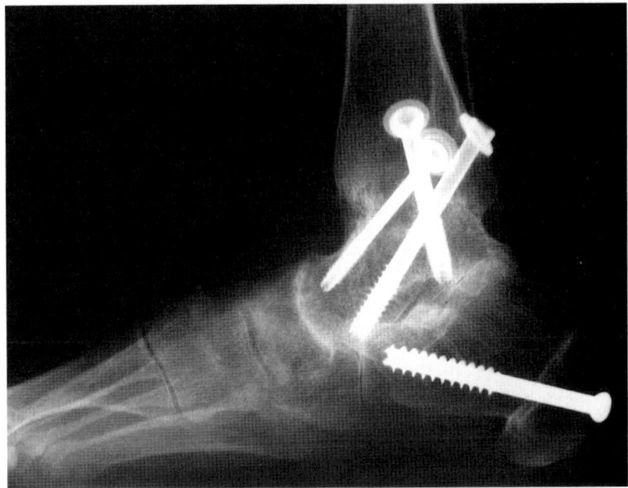

Figure 8–10: Radiograph showing solidly healed ankle fusion (2 years postoperatively) performed for progressive ankle arthritis. A previous medial displacement calcaneal osteotomy and flexor digitorum longus tendon transfer had been performed for pes planovalgus caused by posterior tibial tendon insufficiency. Note the progression of disease to all three hindfoot joints.

simultaneously. A tibiotalocalcaneal, tibiocalcaneal, or pantalar arthrodesis may be required to correct the deformity. A pantalar arthrodesis involves the fusion of the ankle, subtalar, calcaneocuboid, and talonavicular joints (Fig. 8–11).

- Rates of union in these extensive hindfoot and ankle procedures are similar to those of ankle or hindfoot arthrodesis alone. However, complications are increased and overall functional outcomes are decreased after these extensive hindfoot arthrodeses. These procedures are technically difficult and should be reserved as a salvage option (Acosta et al. 2000).
- Total ankle replacement (TAR) may be a viable alternative to ankle arthrodesis in patients with advanced RA. Preservation of the tibiotalar articulation may be advantageous given the high frequency of concomitant involvement of the ankle and hindfoot, and these patients' limited ability to compensate for a fused ankle joint.
- First-generation TARs were designed in the 1970s; they were implanted with cement and designed to be constrained or semiconstrained. High rates of loosening were noted at early and intermediate follow-up in both RA and osteoarthritis patients, raising the question of durability.
- Second-generation TARs were designed to be uncemented and less constrained to deal with the problem of loosening.

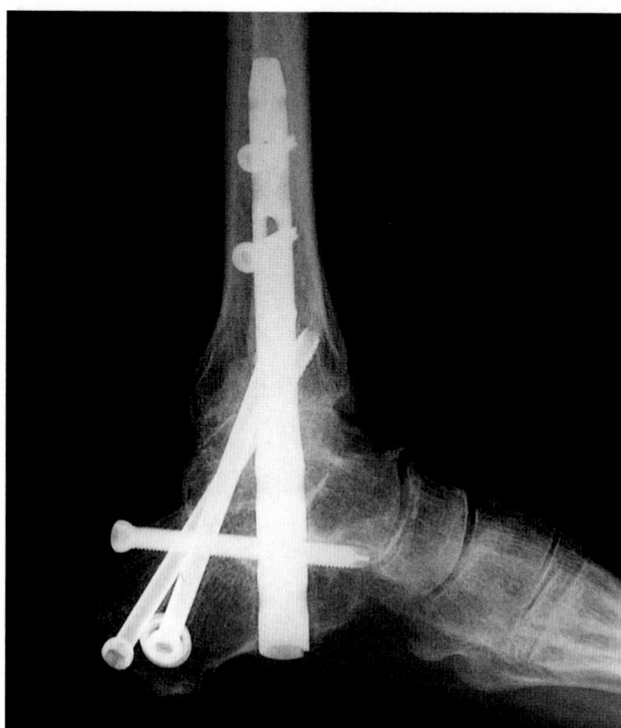

Figure 8–11: **Radiograph showing tibiotalocalcaneal arthrodesis for involvement of the ankle and subtalar joints performed with an intramedullary device and augmented with screw fixation.**

- Intermediate results were promising, with 94% survival of the Agility (DePuy) implant at 5-year follow-up, but an increase in the revision rate to11% at average of 9-year follow-up is concerning (Knecht et al. 2004). Ninety-three percent survival of the Buechel-Pappas low-contact stress implant at 10 years (Buechel et al. 2002) and 75% survival of the cemented Scandinavian total ankle replacement (STAR) were seen in RA patients at 14 years' follow-up (Kofoed and Sorensen 1998). More recent data from the STAR prosthesis suggest improved survival (95%) of the uncemented design at a mean follow-up of 9.4 years.
- A more recent study, evaluating two different types of second-generation implants used in RA patients, reported 88.5% survival (no radiographic evidence of loosening) at an average of 6.3 years. Osteolysis was present around the tibial component in nearly 12% of the ankles (Su et al. 2004).

- The typically lower demand RA patient coupled with the improvement in TAR design and implantation techniques may make TAR in RA a more appealing alternative in the future. Although improved results have been reported with the second-generation implants, the procedure remains technically challenging, and long-term follow-up is needed.
- Complications of TAR include infection, fracture during implantation (malleolar), component loosening, nerve injury, wound complications, and continued pain. Salvage procedures for failed TAR include revision TAR, conversion to ankle arthrodesis (often requiring a bulk allograft to compensate for extensive bone loss), soft tissue coverage procedures for skin slough or infection, and occasionally amputation for chronic infection or intractable pain (Fig. 8–12).

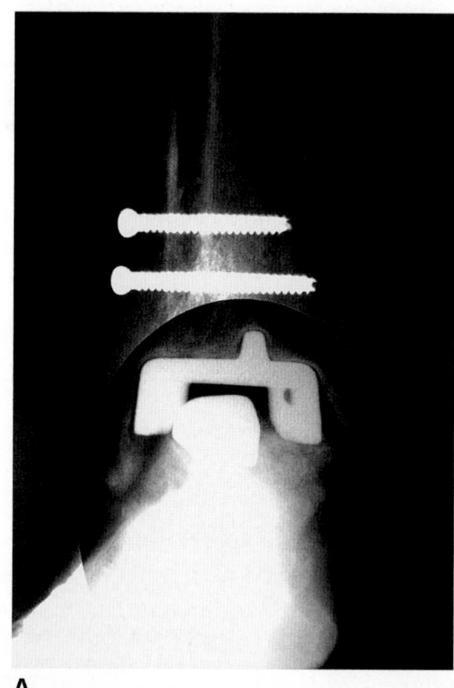

A

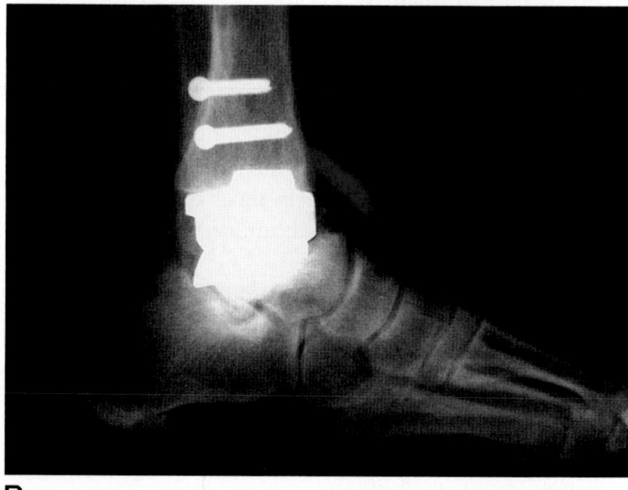

B

Figure 8–12: **A, Radiograph of a total ankle arthroplasty (Agility-DePuy) with osteolysis around the tibial component despite a solidly healed syndesmosis fusion. This component was loose, and the ankle was revised to an arthrodesis. B, Lateral radiograph of the same patient, showing subsidence of the talar component at 3 years.**

Extraosseous Manifestations of Rheumatoid Arthritis

- The inflammatory process can lead to attenuation and occasionally failure of ligaments and tendons. The posterior tibial tendon and peroneal tendons are the most frequently involved. Actual rupture of tendons is rare but may occur in areas where a tendon passes over a bony prominence, or where steroid injections have inadvertently been applied to the tendon.
- Pes planovalgus is the most common foot deformity seen in association with RA, and may occur in up to 46% of patients. The underlying pathophysiology of the flatfoot deformity is highly controversial but may involve attenuation of the medial longitudinal arch supporting structures, failure of the posterior tibial tendon, or erosive arthritis of the ankle and subtalar joints.
- Rheumatoid nodules appear in 20-30% of patients with RA. They generally occur over the extensor surfaces of joints and adjacent long bones. Symptomatic nodules are typically found over bony prominences such as the malleoli, or on the plantar surfaces of the heel or metatarsal heads. The exact cause of rheumatoid nodule formation is unclear, but it seems to involve an immune complex-mediated vasculitis. The presence of rheumatoid nodules generally indicates a more aggressive form of RA (Figs 8–13 and 8–14).
- Vasculitis is an immune complex-mediated destruction of blood vessels. The effects of vasculitis may range from benign nail fold infarcts to more malignant systemic necrotizing arteritis. Rheumatoid vasculitis generally occurs late in the disease and in patients with high rheumatoid factor titers. In the foot, vasculitis can result in digital infarcts, ulcers, or diffuse rashes. These may be the earliest signs of more severe systemic involvement.

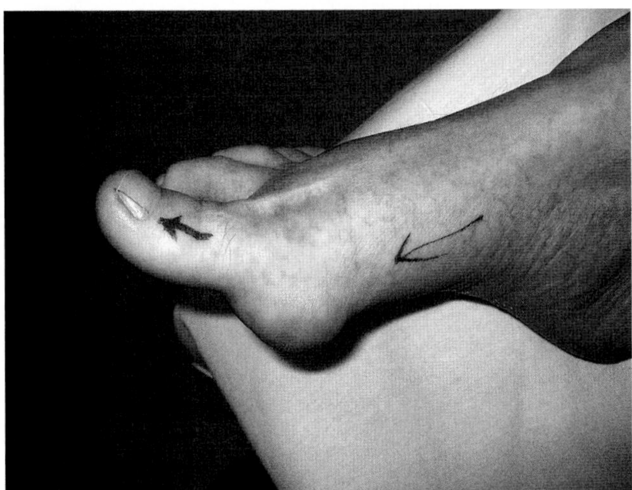

Figure 8–13: **Photograph of large rheumatoid nodule. The nodule was symptomatic and was removed. The presence of a nodule may herald a more aggressive form of the disease.**

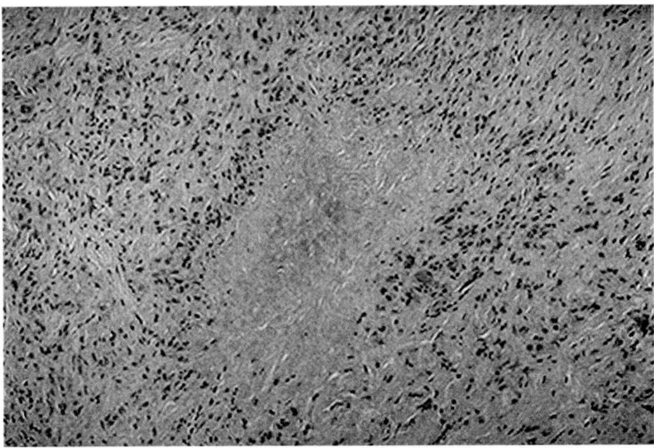

Figure 8–14: **Photomicrograph of a rheumatoid nodule showing a central area of fibrinoid necrosis surrounded by pallisading epithelioid macrophages and mononuclear cells. (Courtesy of Sherman S. Coleman, M.D., University of Utah, UT.)**

- Mild forms of vasculitis may be treated by rheumatologists with antiinflammatory drugs such as NSAIDs or steroids. Appropriate surgical debridement or excision of cutaneous lesions or nodules and gangrenous digits is indicated.
- Neurologic involvement in RA may occur as a result of spinal column disease (especially atlantoaxial), compression of peripheral nerves (rheumatoid nodule or synovitis in a closed space tarsal tunnel), or severe foot deformity causing neuropathy. Treatment consists of nerve decompression, often in conjunction with a bony procedure (such as a hindfoot fusion) when appropriate non-operative modalities have failed.

Seronegative Inflammatory Arthropathies

- The seronegative spondyloarthropathies describe a group of inflammatory arthritides that involve the sacroiliac joints or the vertebral column, have similar extraarticular manifestations, and lack the rheumatoid factor.
- The typical extraarticular features include lesions of the skin (psoriasis), lesions of the eye (conjunctivitis, iritis, uveitis), and inflammation of the bowel or genitourinary system (colitis, urethritis).
- Musculoskeletal manifestations include an asymmetric oligoarthritis of the lower extremity joints and associated enthesopathies. Enthesitis is the inflammation of a tendon at its insertion site and typically involves the Achilles tendon or pelvic tendons in the spondyloarthropathies.
- The four diagnostic groups of seronegative spondyloarthropathies include ankylosing spondylitis, psoriatic arthritis, Reiter syndrome, and the arthritis of inflammatory bowel disease.

- There is a strong association between the spondyloarthropathies and the presence of HLA B27. Over 90% of patients with ankylosing spondylitis are HLA B27-positive. HLA B27 is thought to play a role in the pathogenesis of spondyloarthropathies, as well as serving as a marker.

Ankylosing Spondylitis

- Foot and ankle manifestations of ankylosing spondylitis include the enthesopathies, especially at the insertion of the Achilles tendon. It may present in a teenage boy who is very active in sports as the first clinical sign of ankylosing spondylitis.
- A complete physical examination looking for other sites of involvement should be performed. Common sites include insertion sites of tendons or ligaments (spinous processes, the iliac crest, costosternal borders, and ischial tuberosities), the lumbar spine, and the sacroiliac joints (symmetric sacroiliitis).
- Stretching to maintain flexibility of joints and inflamed tendons is important. NSAIDs are the pharmacologic mainstay of treatment. The objectives of therapy are pain control, the preservation of good body mechanics, and stamina.

Psoriatic Arthritis

- Psoriasis occurs in about 2% of the population in the USA. Of those with psoriasis, about 5-10% develop arthritis. There is usually asymmetric joint involvement of the small joints of the upper and lower extremities, the presence of skin lesions, and the absence of rheumatoid factor.
- Classic radiographic findings of psoriatic arthritis include:
  - lack of juxtaarticular osteoporosis
  - the presence of periostitis and proliferative new bone formation
  - osteolysis, marginal erosions, and "pencil in cup" deformities
  - asymmetric involvement of distal joints (Fig. 8–15).
- Typical presentation (70%) is oligoasymmetric involvement of the small joints of the hands and feet. Uniform swelling of the involved digit(s) may be present and is referred to as dactylitis or the "sausage digit."
- Predominant involvement of the distal interphalangeal joints with associated dactylitis is another variant of psoriatic arthritis. There are also characteristic nail changes (pitting, keratoses, and onycholysis) that are highly associated with the presence of arthritis.
- In all forms of psoriatic arthritis, enthesopathies and tendinitis may be present. The Achilles tendon, retrocalcaneal bursa, metatarsalgia, base of the fifth metatarsal (peroneal enthesitis), and posterior tibial tendon are potential sites of involvement in the foot.
- First-line treatment involves NSAIDs for peripheral arthritis and enthesitis. Psoriatic arthritis unresponsive to NSAIDs may require the addition of disease-modifying medications (methotrexate, sulfasalazine, azathioprine, or cyclosporine).

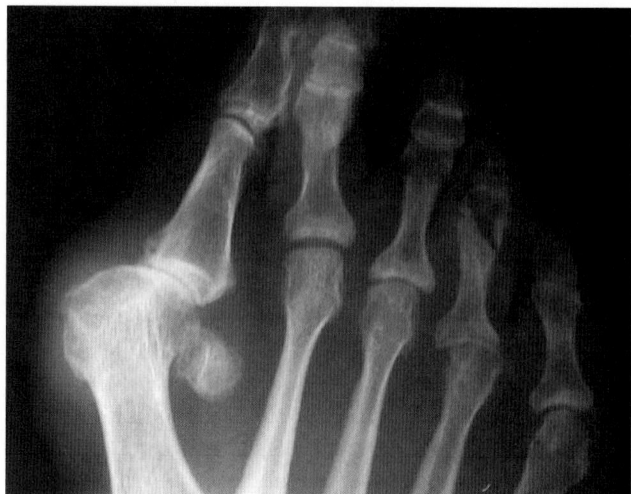

Figure 8–15: Radiograph showing marginal erosions of the third and fourth toes in this patient with psoriatic arthritis.

- In the foot specifically, the use of orthotics to help support the Achilles tendon/posterior tibial tendon may be beneficial. Surgical intervention is indicated when deformity/pain is progressive. Reconstructive procedures similar to those used in RA are often effective (Hoffman procedure).

Reiter Syndrome and Reactive Arthritis

- The classic triad of urethritis, conjunctivitis, and arthritis is present in only 33% of cases. Arthritis symptoms usually occur within a month of the onset of a urogenital or gastrointestinal illness.
- Lower extremity joints are most likely to be involved (knees, ankles, and feet) and are typically worse with rest, better with exercise. Intensity of inflammation resembles septic arthritis or gouty arthritis. Enthesopathies, dactylitis, and bursitis are common findings in the lower extremity.
- Radiographic findings are significant for soft tissue swelling in the lower extremities. Bony proliferation and periostitis may be seen, but osteolysis is typically absent. The changes of enthesitis are often found at the calcaneus, ischial tuberosity, tibial tuberosity, and greater trochanter.
- NSAID therapy remains the initial treatment for reactive arthritis and Reiter syndrome. Ice, wrapping, and rest followed by stretching, and range of motion, are also mainstays of treatment. Orthotics may be useful in relieving off-loading the posterior tibial tendon, metatarsal heads, or Achilles tendon.

Gout

- Gout is an inflammatory arthritis caused by the deposition of monosodium urate crystals in the joint and surrounding soft tissues. The classic triad of rubor, dolor, and calor (redness, pain, and heat) are typically found at the joint(s) involved.
- Hyperuricemia is a prerequisite for developing gout. The causes may be primary hyperuricemia (overproduction or under-excretion) or secondary hyperuricemia (in the setting of another disease or as a result of drug intake). The true incidence of gout is unclear, as it is a self-limited condition.
- Gout typically occurs in men over the age of 40. There are genetic, dietary, and environmental influences on the occurrence of gout.
- Diagnosis of gout is made by both clinical history and laboratory evaluation. Acute-onset pain, swelling, and redness usually in the first MTP joint (subtalar or ankle joint may also be involved) may occur. In about 90% of cases, the first joint involved is the first MTP.
- Laboratory diagnosis involves examination of the synovial fluid from the affected joint for negatively birefringent monosodium urate crystals under a polarizing light microscope. The synovial fluid may also contain a high number of inflammatory cells (usually polymorphonuclear neutrophilic leukocytes), often greater than 50 000/mm^3. Serum urate levels greater than 7 mg/dL in men and 6 mg/dL in women are considered hyperuricemia. The incidence of gout rises significantly when serum urate levels exceed 8 mg/dL.
- Radiographic changes of gout typically depend on the duration of the disease. Early on, there is soft tissue swelling with little or no evidence of joint involvement. Gouty tophi, or deposits of urate crystals in the soft tissues, may be visible. In chronic disease, there may be periarticular bony erosions with characteristic punched-out appearance and overhanging edges. There is usually no juxtaarticular osteoporosis or joint space narrowing until very late in the disease process.
- The first-line treatment of gout is to reduce inflammation during an acute attack. NSAIDs and colchicine may be used. These drugs do not lower the serum uric acid levels.
- Treatment of hyperuricemia is necessary to prevent future attacks. Occasionally, cessation of certain dietary items (alcohol, red meat) or medications known to raise uric acid levels (thiazides) will reduce serum uric acid levels.
- Antihyperuricemic medications may be necessary to lower serum uric acid levels. These drugs work by either increasing the renal excretion of urate (uricosurics—probenecid) or by inhibiting the production of urate (xanthine oxidase inhibitors—allopurinol).
- Surgical management of gout is uncommon. In the acute setting, there is little indication for surgical intervention. In chronic tophaceous gout, resection of prominent or painful tophi may be warranted, but close wound surveillance should be undertaken postoperatively because the incidence of wound complication is increased. The concern is not for primary postoperative wound infection but rather for a triggering of an acute attack of gout with wound dehiscence and secondary infection (Fig. 8–16).
- In the presence of significant deformity involving the hallux or lesser MTP joints, resection arthroplasty or arthrodesis may be indicated. Excessive tophi or active drainage should be handled carefully, with the associated wound complications in mind.

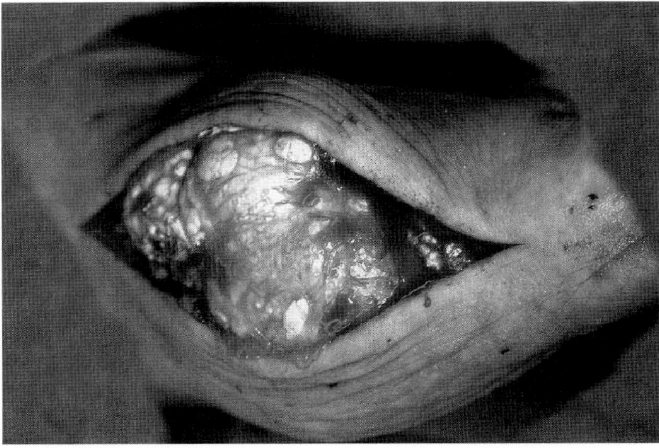

Figure 8–16: **Intraoperative findings of gouty tophus at the first metatarsophalangeal joint. Resection of tophi can sometimes precipitate an attack of gout. Postoperative wound complications may also be seen in the setting of large collections of tophi lying subcutaneously.**

References

Acosta R, Ushiba J, Cracchiolo A. (2000) The results of primary and staged pantalar arthrodesis and tibiocalcaneal arthrodesis in adult patients. Foot Ankle Int 21: 182-194.

Retrospective clinical review of 27 feet (18 with RA) that underwent either primary or staged pantalar arthrodesis or tibiotalocalcaneal arthrodesis. Nine of the 27 had prior surgery on the joint(s) involved. Successful arthrodesis was achieved in 23 of 27 by an average of 23 weeks. The four non-unions occurred in a single joint, and all were in the pantalar arthrodesis group. The authors caution that pantalar or tibiotalocalcaneal arthrodesis is technically challenging and should be used for salvage purposes only.

Buechel Sr FF, Beuchel Jr FF, Pappas MJ. (2002) Eighteen year evaluation of cementless meniscal bearing total ankle replacements. Instr Course Lect 51: 143-151.

Review of two designs of the rotationally unconstrained Buechel-Pappas cementless TAR reported survivorship of the shallow sulcus design (40 ankles) of 74.2% at 18 years, and 93.5% of the deep sulcus (50 ankles) design at 10 years. The authors also noted significant improvement in the talar component stability (fewer cases of subsidence) in the deep sulcus design as compared with the shallow sulcus design. Patient satisfaction at a mean of 10 years' follow-up in the shallow sulcus design was good/excellent in 70%, and at a mean of 5 years' follow-up the deep sulcus design had 88% good/excellent results.

Chiodo CP, Martin T, Wilson MG. (2000) Technique for isolated arthrodesis for inflammatory arthritis of the talonavicular joint. Foot Ankle Int 21: 307-310.
A retrospective review of 20 isolated talonavicular arthrodeses performed for inflammatory arthritis using screws and staples. Radiographic evidence of fusion was reached in 19 of 20 feet by an average of 11 weeks. The authors concluded that isolated talonavicular arthrodesis is an effective and reliable procedure for the treatment of inflammatory arthritis of the talonavicular joint.

Clayton ML. (1960) Surgery of the forefoot in rheumatoid arthritis. Clin Orthop 16: 136-140.
The author describes his experience with 25 rheumatoid feet, in which he performed resection arthroplasties of the lesser MTP joints. He described a modification of the Hoffman lesser metatarsal head resection in which a portion of the base of the proximal phalanx is also resected. This modification was intended to prevent recurrence of the contracted or clawed toe.

Coughlin MJ. (2000) Rheumatoid forefoot reconstruction. J Bone Joint Surg 82-A(3): 322-341.
Retrospective review of 47 rheumatoid feet undergoing first MTP joint arthrodesis, lesser metatarsal head resection, and hammertoe correction, with an average of 6 years' follow-up. Forty-five of 47 feet had good or excellent outcomes. Thirty percent (14 feet) required secondary procedures for hardware removal (7), hallux interphalangeal arthrodesis (2), or additional procedures on the lesser MTP joints (5). A thorough discussion section describes rationale for operative techniques, a review of the literature, and potential pitfalls in the treatment of rheumatoid forefoot disease.

Gerber LH. (2000) Spondyloarthropathies and gout. In: Foot and Ankle Disorders (Myerson MS, ed.). Philadelphia: Saunders. pp. 1205-1222.

Jaakola JI, Mann RA. (2004) A review of rheumatoid arthritis in the foot and ankle. Foot Ankle Int 25(12): 866-874.
A thorough review of the clinical presentation, evaluation, and treatment of RA in the foot and ankle. This article emphasizes the high incidence of foot and ankle involvement in RA, and the importance of the orthopaedic surgeon in managing the sequelae.

Keenan MA et al. (1991) Valgus deformities of the feet and characteristics of gait in patients who have rheumatoid arthritis. J Bone Joint Surg 72-A: 237-247.
Two groups of rheumatoid patients were evaluated, one with normal alignment of the feet and the other with valgus deformity of the hindfoot. The group with hindfoot valgus had no evidence of posterior tibial tendon insufficiency, and showed an increase in the intensity and duration of activity on quantitated electromyography during stance phase. These findings suggest that posterior tibial tendon insufficiency may not be the lone driving force for pes planovalgus deformity in rheumatoid patients.

Knecht SI, Estin M, Callaghan JJ et al. (2004) The Agility total ankle arthroplasty: Seven to sixteen-year follow-up. J Bone Joint Surg 86-A: 1161-1171.
Longer term results (mean 9 years) of the TAR (Agility-DePuy) in 132 ankles (36 implants deceased). Of the 96 ankles evaluated, 14 (11%) required revision or conversion to fusion. Of 117 ankles with radiographs at minimum 2 years' follow-up, 89 (76%) had periimplant lucency, 19% had progressive subtalar arthritis, 15% had progressive talonavicular arthritis, and 8% had syndesmosis non-union. However, 90% of the 69 ankles followed clinically had pain relief and satisfactory outcomes. The authors acknowledge that while patient satisfaction was high, the importance of achieving syndesmosis stability and the prevention of component subsidence are paramount to good outcomes.

Kofoed H, Sorensen TS. (1998) Ankle arthroplasty for rheumatoid arthritis and osteoarthritis: Prospective, long-term study of cemented replacements. J Bone Joint Surg 80-B: 323-332.
Prospective long-term study looking at 52 cemented TARs using the STAR. Survivorship of the prosthesis in patients with osteoarthritis (72.7%) and with RA (75.5%) at 14 years was noted. The authors reported only one deep infection, five revisions, and five conversions to arthrodesis. There was no development of secondary osteoarthritis in the subtalar joints in patients with ankle osteoarthritis after arthroplasty. Five out of 27 of the RA patients went on to subsequent arthritis in the subtalar joint after arthroplasty.

Mann RA, Beaman DN, Horton GA. (1998) Isolated subtalar arthrodesis. Foot Ankle Int 19: 511-519.
Retrospective review of 48 isolated subtalar arthrodeses for varying diagnoses, with mean follow-up of 56 months. All had successful arthrodesis. Ninety-three percent were very satisfied with the surgery. Of note, transverse tarsal motion was diminished by 40%, dorsiflexion by 30%, and plantar flexion by 9% with an isolated subtalar fusion.

Mann RA, Schakel ME. (1995) Surgical correction of rheumatoid forefoot deformities. Foot Ankle Int 16: 1-6.
A review of long-term results in rheumatoid patients who underwent hallux MTP arthrodesis and resection arthroplasties of the lesser MTP joints. At average follow-up of 3.7 years, 90% of patients were satisfied with their improvement in the ability to walk, wear shoes, and have diminished pain. The authors add a technical note in recommending the preservation of the bases of the proximal phalanges and temporary K-wire fixation of the lesser MTP arthroplasties to improve cosmetic result and prevent recurrent deformity.

O'Brien TS, Hart TS, Gould JS. (1997) Extraosseous manifestations of rheumatoid arthritis in the foot and ankle. Clin Orthop 340: 26-33.
This review discusses the extraosseous and extraarticular manifestations of RA commonly encountered in the foot and ankle. The article attempts to define the pathophysiology of these extraosseous manifestations, as well as offer treatment modalities, both non-operative and operative.

Smyth CJ, Janson RW. (1997) Rheumatologic view of the rheumatoid foot. Clin Orthop 340: 7-17.
A review of RA and its effects on the foot and ankle from a rheumatologist's perspective. Good background on the

pathophysiology of disease, mechanism of joint destruction, diagnostic criteria, and medical therapies available. This review emphasizes the benefits of early diagnosis and non-operative treatment of RA in the foot and ankle.

Spiegel JM, Spiegel JS. (1982) Rheumatoid arthritis in the foot and ankle: Diagnosis, pathology, and treatment. Foot Ankle 2: 318-324.

A review of RA in the foot and ankle, describing clinical findings; the incidence of ankle, hindfoot, midfoot, and forefoot involvement; and general treatment strategies.

Su EP, Kahn B, Figgie MP. (2004) Total ankle replacement in patients with rheumatoid arthritis. Clin Orthop 424: 32-38.

The authors performed a retrospective review of two (Hospital for Special Surgery custom total ankle and Buechel-Pappas) second-generation TARs. In 26 rheumatoid ankles with an average follow-up of 6.4 years, 88.5% of components were radiographically stable (no evidence of loosening or subsidence). Tibial osteolysis was seen in 11.5% of Buechel-Pappas total ankles. The authors conclude that second-generation implants can provide reliable relief for RA patients at intermediate follow-up, but that the high incidence of osteolysis warrants close evaluation.

Swanson AB, Lumsden RM, Swanson GD. (1979) Silicone implant arthroplasty of the great toe. A review of single stem and flexible hinge implants. Clin Orthop Relat Res 142: 30–43.

A review of the use of first MTP joint implant arthroplasty as an alternative to resection arthroplasty or arthrodesis in the treatment of hallux rigidus. Ninety-five arthroplasties were performed on rheumatoid feet, with 24 requiring a secondary procedure on the foot. Nine of these secondary procedures involved revision of the hallux arthroplasty. Other complications noted include infection (2), inflammatory reaction to implant (1), implant damage (1), avascular necrosis of metatarsal head (1), bone overproduction (2), cock-up toe deformity (7), varus overcorrection (6), and a recurrence of hallux valgus deformity in the rheumatoid patients (25). The authors advocate careful selection of patients and strict adherence to suggested indications, surgical technique, and follow-up care.

Thordarson DB, Aval S, Kreiger L. (2002) Failure of hallux preservation surgery for rheumatoid arthritis. Foot Ankle Int 23: 486-490.

The authors reviewed 13 feet in patients with RA who underwent procedures to correct hallux valgus to preserve the hallux MTP joint. No radiographic evidence of hallux MTP arthritis was present at index procedure. In 11/13 feet, subsequent valgus deformity recurred or radiographically apparent erosions at the hallux MTP joint appeared by an average of 24 months postoperatively. Only 5/11 of these feet went on to have fusion due to deformity or severe pain. The remaining six had symptoms but wanted no surgery.

Hallux Valgus

Heather E. Hensl[*] and Andrew K. Sands[§]

[*]R.P.A.-C., Physician Assistant, Department of Orthopedic Surgery, Saint Vincent's Hospital, New York, NY
[§]M.D., Chief, Foot and Ankle Surgery, and Director, Foot and Ankle Institute, Department of Orthopedic Surgery, Saint Vincent's Medical Center, New York, NY

- Hallux valgus is a painful deformity of the forefoot at the level of the first metatarsophalangeal (MTP) joint, in which there is medial angulation of the first metatarsal and lateral deviation of the hallux.
- Hallux valgus deformity is often referred to as a bunion. For most patients, the term *bunion* refers to the medial prominence or bump.

The Natural History of a Bunion

- A bunion deformity begins as a normal or slightly angulated MTP joint. However, the MTP joint, through intrinsic or extrinsic causes, becomes vulnerable to longstanding valgus pressures. The result is valgus angulation of the hallux.
- The causes could stem from improper footwear or be secondary to congenital predisposition.
- This valgus angulation progresses over time due to pulling forces exerted on the proximal phalanx by both the adductor hallucis and the extensor hallucis longus tendons.
- In response to these valgus forces, an opposing force is applied to the first metatarsal head, producing a varus angulation of the first metatarsal shaft. As a result, the deformity increases.
- The MTP joint is enclosed by a joint capsule, which is also vulnerable to prolonged exposure to the bunion deformity. The medial aspect stretches out, and the lateral capsule becomes contracted.
- The sesamoids remain in place during this medial movement of the metatarsal head, culminating in the lateral subluxation of the sesamoids under the metatarsal head (which is more accurately described as medial subluxation of the first metatarsal away from the sesamoids) (Fig. 9–1).
- Although the deformity primarily involves the first MTP joint, there must be angulation at the first metatarsocuneiform (MTC) joint for the metatarsal to angle medially.

Etiology of the Deformity

Genetic Basis

- Studies originating out of African countries where indigenous populations often do not wear shoes have demonstrated occurrence of hallux valgus deformities. Interestingly enough, deformities in these populations are often asymptomatic.
- In the juvenile and adolescent hallux valgus, heredity seems to play a major role. Coughlin (1995) found a 72% rate of maternal transmission in juvenile hallux valgus patients.
- Many have drawn links between the formation of hallux valgus and the presence of other foot/ankle abnormalities. These include flatfoot deformity, hypermobility of the first ray, equinus contracture, and hindfoot deformity secondary to rheumatoid arthritis or posterior tibial tendon dysfunction.

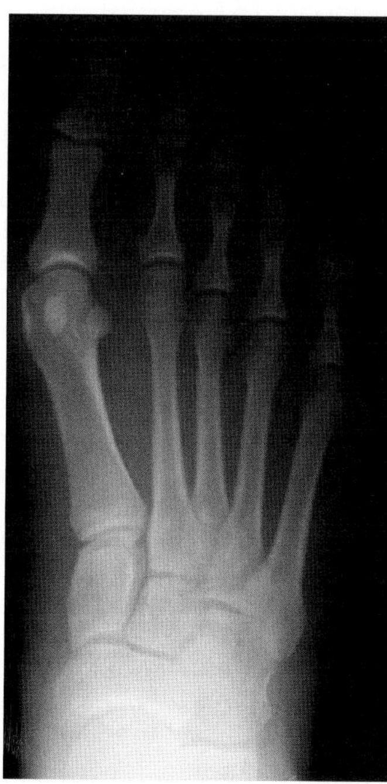

Figure 9–1: This anteroposterior view of a foot with mild hallux valgus shows the medial deviation of the first metatarsal away from the lesser rays. In this early stage, the first toe remains relatively straight. The sesamoids are normally centered under the metatarsal head in grooves called cristae. As the first metatarsal drifts medially away from the foot, the sesamoids will appear lateral to the head. In fact, the sesamoids remain in their normal position, but the metatarsal is drifting away.

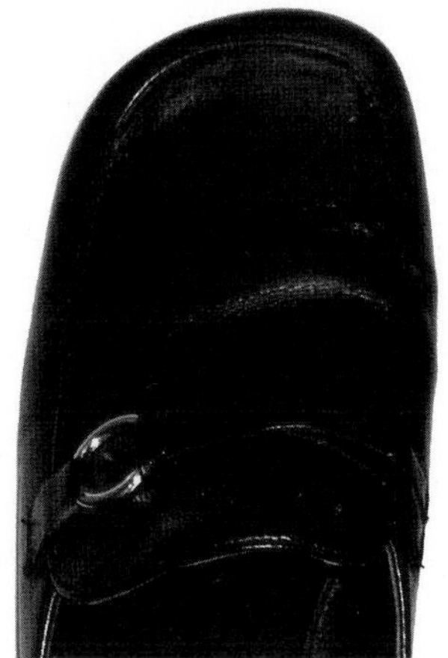

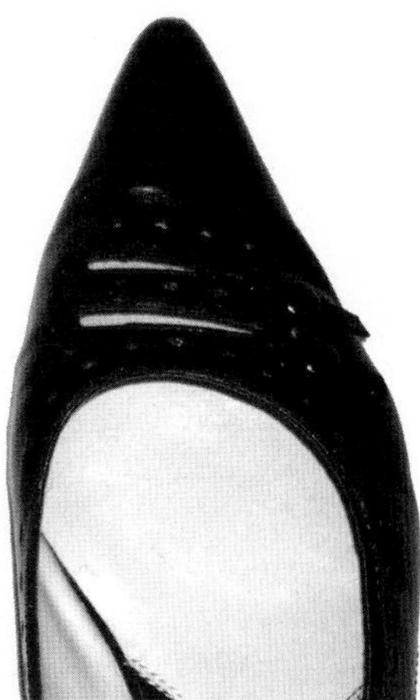

Figure 9–2: The shoe on the right is representative of a shoe with a narrow toe box that may contribute to forefoot deformity. The shoe on the left has a wider toe box and is more accommodative of the deformed forefoot.

Gender

- Ferrari et al. (2004) performed a study introducing a new technique to measure bone size and shape via three-dimensional laser scanning. Males were found to have overall larger bones than females. Based on measurements of articular surfaces, female bones demonstrated a greater potential for movement in the medial direction. This could result in the first metatarsal being more adducted, and therefore predispose the female foot to developing a bunion.
- Others explain the 9:1 incidence of bunions in females versus males as being due to use of high heels with pointed toe boxes. Prolonged wearing of shoes that constrict the forefoot place abnormal pressure on the hallux (Fig. 9–2).
- Although hallux valgus occurs in populations that do not wear shoes, it is 15 times more prevalent in populations that wear shoes. It is in shoe-wearing populations that we typically are confronted with the painful bunion.

Association with Deformities and Disease

- The association with flatfoot is controversial, with many authors noting that pronated feet have a tendency to develop bunion deformities.
- A generalized ligamentous laxity can exist, which commonly results in excessive pronation and hindfoot valgus deformity. This renders the foot unstable and can allow for hypermobility and hallux valgus.
- Metatarsus primus varus (MPV) is often thought to be an associated condition, although it can be argued that MPV is an essential component of the hallux valgus deformity.
- Systemic inflammatory diseases, such as rheumatoid arthritis and psoriasis, have been linked to bunions. In such disorders, the synovitis results in erosion of the joint capsule, with MTP joint deformity.
- The shape of the first metatarsal head may play a role in bunion formation. The more round the metatarsal head, the less stable the MTP joint. Thus there is a greater inclination for angulation to ensue.
- Patients with a contracted Achilles/gastrocnemius are more susceptible to bunion development. The equinus contracture forces the hindfoot into greater than normal plantar flexion.
  - Hansen (2000) has suggested that this contracture may be the most common primary cause of forefoot dysfunction, a basic abnormality that propagates a succession of both anatomical and functional failures in the foot.
  - The contracture, in turn, causes breakdown of the medial column and the foot's weight-bearing tripod, ultimately leading to increased hypermobility of the first ray and bunion formation.

Hypermobility of the First Ray

- The precise role of first metatarsal hypermobility (instability at the first MTC joint) is controversial. Some surgeons feel that excess mobility is a rare cause of hallux valgus.
- However, others feel hypermobility of the first metatarsal is the basic defect in all hallux valgus.

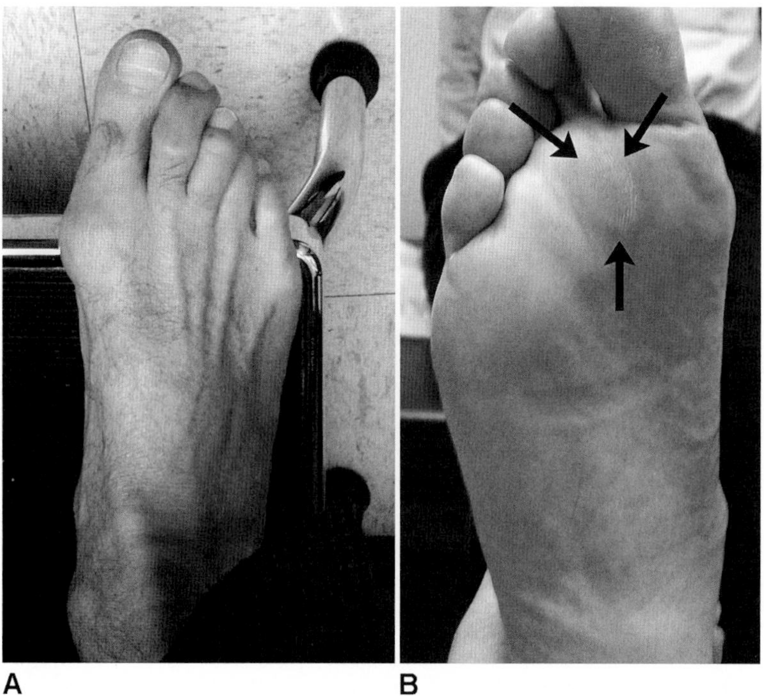

Figure 9–3: **A,** The man with hallux valgus is not bothered too much by the medial "bunion" bump. **B,** He is bothered by the large callus under the second metatarsal head (indicated by the arrows), which is the result of transfer metatarsalgia. His symptoms were not adequately relieved by a metatarsal pad, and he went on to have surgical realignment with a Lapidus fusion, which relieved his pain completely.

- Despite this ongoing controversy, there is no doubting that deformity or instability at the first MTC joint must be present to some degree if the first metatarsal is to drift medially away from the rest of the foot.
- Hypermobility of the first ray is three-dimensional, so that dorsal subluxation of the metatarsal on the midfoot may occur. Clinically, this appears as arch sag or collapse. This offers a reasonable explanation why hallux valgus is often associated with a flatfoot.
- Dorsal elevation of the first ray will lead to transfer loading of the second ray, with transfer metatarsalgia and second MTP overload. These disorders are frequently seen with hallux valgus (Fig. 9–3).
- The transfer of load to the second metatarsal may lead to hypertrophy on radiographs (Fig. 9–4 and Box 9–1).

Measuring First Ray Mobility

- Many external measuring devices have been developed over the years in an attempt to actually quantify the sagittal mobility of the first ray during physical examination. However, there is still no proven, reliable, universally recognized instrument.
- Such devices usually consist of a structure that applies a dorsiflexing force to the first metatarsal head, and then measures the resultant amount of vertical displacement.
- The value of an examination with such a device versus a standard manual examination has yet to be determined.
- One study found that the position of the ankle during a manual examination influences the degree of first ray

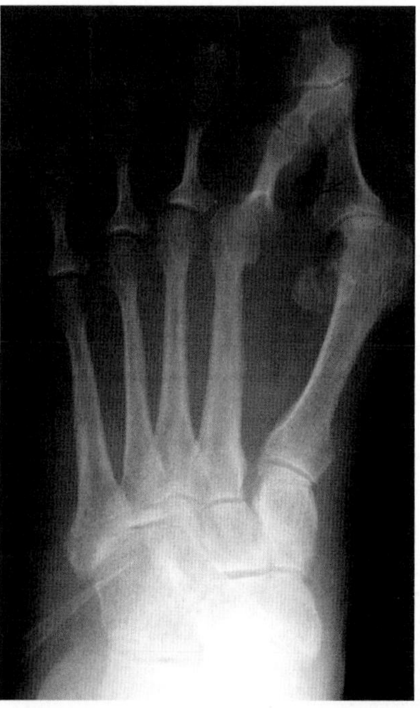

Figure 9–4: This radiograph shows a foot with a large hallux valgus deformity. Transfer of loads to the second ray has led to a "crossover" second toe, with clawing. Careful observation of the radiograph shows thickening of the second metatarsal cortex, consistent with hypertrophy from transfer of loads from the unstable first metatarsal. Although many surgeons feel that this second metatarsal hypertrophy is a sign of first metatarsal instability (hypermobility), others think there is no relationship.

Box 9–1 Morton Foot

- Morton described a foot disorder where the first metatarsal was much shorter than the second, with transfer metatarsalgia and thickening of the medial second metatarsal cortex.
- Grebing and Coughlin (2004) measured this radiographically but failed to find a link between second metatarsal thickness and hypermobility.

mobility, and therefore discrepancies will probably exist between the standard manual examination and an examination with an external device (Grebing and Coughlin 2004).

- Glasoe et al. (2000) tested one such device but found that at high forces, unwanted second metatarsal movement resulted in the device's overestimation of the first ray's displacement.
- Coughlin et al. (2004) performed a study on cadaver specimens to evaluate for changes in hypermobility of the first ray after surgical correction of hallux valgus. The specimens underwent proximal crescentic osteotomies with distal soft tissue reconstructions. The first ray sagittal motion was measured with a Klaue device both before and after the correction. Mobility of the first ray was decreased immediately following osteotomy.

Pathogenesis of Hallux Valgus

Anatomical Considerations of the Hallux and First MTP Joint

- This joint is a "ball and socket" joint, with motion in both dorsal (40-100°) and plantar (3-43°) directions.
- There are fan-shaped ligaments originating from the medial and lateral aspects of the first metatarsal head, which make up the medial and lateral collateral ligaments. These ligaments allow for very limited abduction and adduction when the joint undergoes varus and valgus stresses.
- Along the plantar aspect of the hallux and first MTP joint, there is a fibrous structure known as the plantar plate.
- The sesamoids, which normally lie beneath the first metatarsal head, are held in place by the thick intersesamoid ligament, the intermetatarsal ligament, and the adductor hallucis muscle.
- All the above structures, together with the abductor and adductor hallucis, the extensor digitorum brevis, and the flexor hallucis brevis, converge to form the joint capsule.

Pain in Hallux Valgus

- Pain in hallux valgus typically stems from one of four origins: the medial eminence of the bunion, the MTP joint, the lesser metatarsals, and the sesamoids.

Medial Eminence Pain

- This is the most common chief complaint in patients with hallux valgus.
- As the hallux is forced laterally, the medial portion of the first metatarsal head becomes "uncovered," and the bunion deformity emerges.
- The eminence encounters pressure and friction with shoe wear, resulting in pain. Pain may be from irritation of the cutaneous nerves.
- A bunion bursa can form over the medial aspect, causing swelling and tenderness over the deformity. It is unnecessary to surgically excise such bursae, as they commonly resolve on surgical correction of the deformity.

Metatarsophalangeal Joint Pain

- When the MTP joint has a flat articular surface, it is generally stable, and the joint surfaces will be congruent.
- If there is a rounded metatarsal head and the joint is incongruent, it can be unstable or subluxed. It is in this setting that *progressive* hallux valgus formation can ensue, along with other associated deformities.
- The proximal phalanx moves laterally and the metatarsal head migrates medially, with progressive weakening in the medial joint capsule and increasing contracture of the lateral joint capsule.
- Pain can develop as a result of the changes in capsule integrity.
- Clinical and radiographic evidence of osteoarthritic changes at the joint can eventually develop as the deformity advances. There may be progressive painful stiffening of the MTP joint.

Transfer Metatarsalgia and Lesser Toe Pain

- Metatarsalgia is typically much more painful than the hallux valgus deformity but tends to occur later in the course of bunion development.
- Increasing hallux valgus deformity leads to transfer of loads to the second metatarsal head (see Fig. 9–3). This initially causes synovitis of the second MTP joint.
- Subsequently, the hallux will move under the second toe, causing it to dorsally sublux and deform. Alterations in muscle balance lead to a hammertoe or, more precisely, a claw toe.
- Because the toes are being forced dorsally, the metatarsal heads are concomitantly pushed in a plantar direction.
- These factors result in a further lateral shift in weight bearing, and the lesser metatarsal heads become overloaded and painful.
- Ultimately, the second and occasionally the third toe will dislocate dorsally at the MTP joint.
- The cock-up deformity of the hammertoe can also be a source of discomfort; if a shoe's toe box is not high enough, friction will occur.

- The end result is pain under the lesser metatarsal heads, and pain over the dorsum of the lesser toes.

Sesamoid-derived Pain

- The sesamoids do not shift as the first metatarsal head deviates medially with worsening deformity, because of the strong ligamentous connections to the lateral forefoot.
- But, over time, a portion of the medial joint capsule gives way to the excessive pressure of the metatarsal head. With this development, the abductor hallucis muscle begins to slip under the metatarsal head, creating further malalignment of the sesamoids with the first metatarsal.
- The first metatarsal head subluxes away from the sesamoids, and the sesamoid-stabilizing "grooves" on the plantar surface of the metatarsal head, called *cristae*, undergo atrophy (Fig. 9–5).
- Over time, the abductor hallucis muscle slips completely under the metatarsal head. There is a reversal of roles; the intrinsic muscles that once acted to stabilize the MTP joint will now force the joint into further deformity.
- Pronation of the proximal phalanx can also occur at this stage of the deformity.

Examination

History

- While diagnosing hallux valgus is relatively straightforward, a good history can reveal important information regarding etiology and patient expectations.
- Be sure to get a detailed general history, including age, gender, occupation, footwear preference, and athletic inclinations.
- When inquiring about medical history, look for medically related disorders (gout, diabetes, collagen diseases, psoriasis, osteoarthritis or rheumatoid arthritis, or peripheral vascular disease).
- The most common chief complaint with this condition will be a deformity at the first MTP joint, with associated pain over the medial aspect.
- Patients may also complain of pain over the dorsal aspect of the joint, beneath the sesamoids, from lesser toe deformities, or from metatarsalgia.
- Other symptoms include difficulty with shoe wear, limitations of physical activities, callosities (especially plantar aspect of the second metatarsal head), corns, lesser toe deformities, and neuromas.
- With respect to foot and ankle history, inquire about previous foot problems and prior surgeries.
- Question patients as to their expectations regarding pain, activities, and shoe wear; patients need forewarning of possible limitations.
- Forefoot surgery usually leads to improved but not perfectly normal alignment. Surgery also leads to visible scars, prolonged swelling, and some stiffness. When patients' expectations are more cosmetic than functional, they will generally be disappointed.

Physical Examination

- Start with observation of gait.
- Next, inspect the feet while the patient is standing/weight bearing. Assess the degree of hallux valgus, any lesser toe deformities present, and position of the arch.
- Have the patient sit, with legs dangling, and perform a comprehensive hindfoot and forefoot examination.
- Examine the first MTP joint for medial skin breakdown, callus, erythema, inflammation, or dorsal exostosis. Feel for tenderness secondary to neuritic pain or a painful bursa, and also feel for sesamoid tenderness.
- The lesser toes should be assessed for associated deformities, such as claw toes, hammertoes, or corns. Check for MTP joint instability.
- Look at the plantar foot for distribution and degree of callosities, most frequently at the second metatarsal head

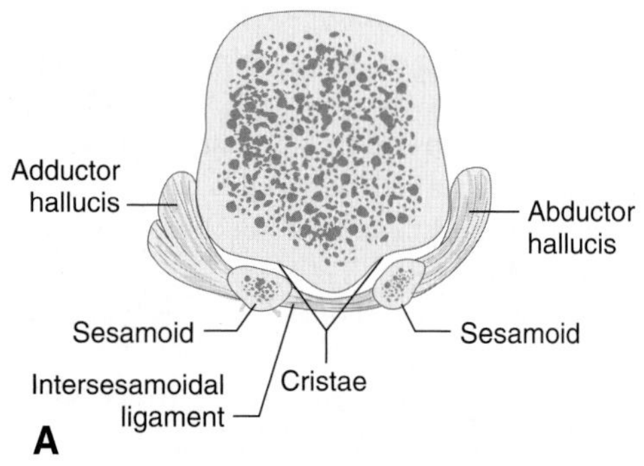

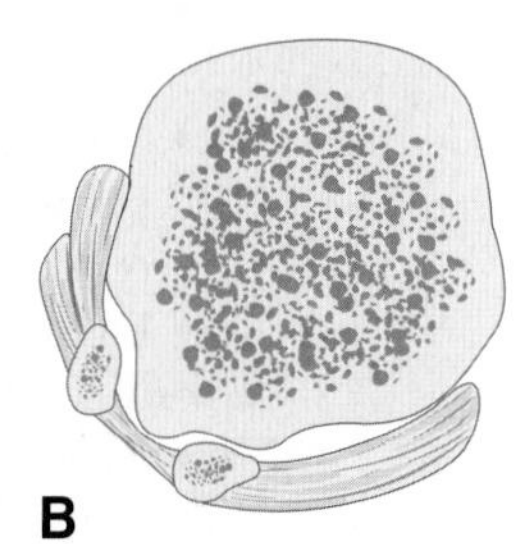

Figure 9–5: **A,** Normally, the sesamoids reside in shallow grooves called cristae. **B,** With hallux valgus (and medial subluxation of the first metatarsal), the sesamoids slide out of the grooves and the cristae atrophy. MT, metatarsal.

but also common over the tibial sesamoid. Also assess the condition of metatarsal fat pad for atrophy.

- Attempt to elicit neuroma symptoms at the intermetatarsal spaces.
- Assess ankle, subtalar, and transverse tarsal motion.
- Test active and passive dorsiflexion and plantar flexion of the first MTP joint. With longstanding hallux valgus, there may be limited dorsiflexion when the great toe is brought out of lateral deviation; this limitation is not likely to improve with surgery.
- Examine for hypermobility of the first ray. Have one hand holding firmly around the patient's second MTP joint. Hold the first MTP joint in the other hand, and toggle the first metatarsal back and forth, dorsomedially and plantar laterally, observing for laxity.
- Excessive laxity could be defined as elevation of the first metatarsal above the level of the second with dorsal pressure.
- Examine also for equinus contracture. With the knee extended, check passive ankle dorsiflexion. Check again with the knee flexed. The ankle should dorsiflex 10° past neutral in both situations.
- Vascular assessment is important as well. Test for capillary refill at toes, and palpate the dorsalis pedis and posterior tibial pulses. Evaluate the skin and hair on the lower extremity.
- For a neurologic assessment, test sensation over the lower extremity. Determine if there is any preexisting peripheral cutaneous nerve damage, which can be associated with larger bunion deformities. Careful assessment is essential, because injury to the dorsomedial cutaneous nerve can occur during surgical correction.
- One study found that while only 21% of patients participating in the study complained of sensory symptoms, an additional 44% were subsequently found to have measurable reduction in sensation on examination (Herron et al. 2004).

Radiographic Evaluation

- It is essential to have weight-bearing radiographs when assessing the deformity, specifically an anteroposterior and a lateral view.
- Fuhrmann et al. (2003) studied the influence of weight bearing on forefoot geometry, and found both hallux valgus and intermetatarsal angles to have statistically significant changes in value with non-weight bearing versus weight bearing.
- The lateral x-ray will serve to reveal lesser toe deformities, including claw toes and hammertoes, as well as the angle of declination that the first metatarsal makes with the floor.
- It is important to note any arthritic changes present, such as narrowing of the first MTP joint.
- Subluxation or dislocation of the lesser MTP joints may be seen.
- Current treatment may be affected by prior surgical interventions and their results, including hardware, excessive removal of medial eminence, and avascular necrosis of the metatarsal head.

What to Do About Angles?

- There are various angles associated with radiographic hallux valgus evaluation. Much controversy surrounds the importance of these angles. Some surgeons advocate careful measurement of these angles on x-rays in order to aid in appropriate treatment planning. Others do not rely on the measurements at all.
- Hallux valgus angle (HV angle): The angle between lines bisecting the proximal phalanx and the first metatarsal shaft. Normal is less than 15°.
- The axis of the first metatarsal is described in Box 9–2.
- Intermetatarsal angle (IM angle): The angle between the lines of the first and second metatarsal shafts. Normal is less than 9°.
- There are differing opinions on how to go about measuring this angle, with multiple common methods currently in use. The most consistent method for the IM angle is to measure the angle formed by the intersection of the first and second metatarsal shaft axes.
- Distal metatarsal articular angle (DMAA): The relationship between the distal articular surface of the first metatarsal head and the long axis of the first metatarsal. Normal is less than 10° of lateral deviation.
- Some feel that the DMAA measurement is extremely important in hallux valgus evaluation, and use it to guide the choice of operative procedure.
- Chi et al. (2002) questioned whether the DMAA can be measured reliably. After finding that the DMAA varied with examiner and with the HV angle, they concluded it to be of limited value as a clinical measurement.
- Coughlin and Freund (2001) conducted a study on the reliability of physicians in making angular measurements of hallux valgus deformities, and also determined that the DMAA could not be measured with consistency. The evaluation included the HV angle, the 1-2 IM angle, and the DMAA. While physicians were very reliable with their HV angle and 1-2 IM angle, the DMAA had much

Box 9–2 The Axis of the First Metatarsal

The axis of the first metatarsal has been defined by some as a line connecting the midpoint of the metatarsal base and the head. Thus a resection of the medial eminence (true bunionectomy) with no other correction will improve the hallux valgus angle (because the midpoint of the head has been shifted by the eminence resection), even though no real realignment has occurred. Others define the axis of the metatarsal to be a line connecting the midpoints of the proximal and distal metaphyses. Obviously, this definition would not be affected by eminence resection.

inconsistency. Coughlin attributed this to the fact that reference points can vary depending on hindfoot position and hallux valgus procedure, both of which can alter alignment or rotation of the first metatarsal.
- Interphalangeal angle: The angle created by the line that bisects the base of the proximal phalanx and the long axis of the proximal phalanx. Normal is considered less than 10°.
- MTC angle: Normal is considered less than 10° of medial angulation. If the obliquity is greater, the joint could be considered unstable.
- Brage et al. (1994) set out to determine the influence of x-ray beam orientation on the first MTC angle. There proved to be significant difference in the angle as the x-ray beam's orientation changed, and the authors deemed that this angular measurement should not be used as an indication for MTC fusion in hallux valgus surgery.
- While there is no set standard of classification, bunions are sometimes categorized as follows.
  - Mild: HV angle less than 30°, IM angle less than 13°.
  - Moderate: HV angle between 30 and 40°, IM angle between 13 and 20°.
  - Severe: HV angle greater than 40°, IM angle greater than 20°.

Determination of Joint Congruency

- On x-ray, assess the base of the proximal phalanx and compare it with the articular surface of the first metatarsal head. When these two entities are parallel, the joint is considered to be "congruent". If the surfaces are subluxed, the joint margins will be offset, or "incongruent".

New Technology: Computerized Measurements

- With the vast developments in computers and technology, new software has emerged that is designed to measure radiographic angles in the foot.
- Many facilities are moving away from standard x-ray films and acquiring digital workstations that utilize high-resolution monitors for image evaluation.
- One study set out to assess the differences between goniometric measurements and computer-assisted angle measurements in hallux valgus. Overall, the authors found better reliability with computerized measurements, and elimination of the inherent error with goniometer use (Farber et al. 2005).

Non-operative Treatment

- The mainstay of non-operative treatment is accommodative, wide box shoe wear, with or without orthotics.
- Surgery in an asymptomatic patient, or for cosmesis, is contraindicated.

Shoe Modifications

- Optimal shoe wear for patients with hallux valgus consists of a soft sole with a wide toe box (see Fig. 9–2). The shoe's shape must be comparable with the widened forefoot seen in hallux valgus.
- A widened toe box serves to minimize rubbing over the medial eminence. There must also be sufficient height in the shoe's toe box to allow for the common associated lesser toe deformities.
- In the past, the option was limited to "old lady" orthopaedic shoes. Now, there are many new, more acceptable variations available for patients.
- While there are various other over the counter products available, including bunion pads, night splints, and toe spacers, they do not appear to be any more beneficial in improving outcomes than no treatment at all. These devices can be used to alleviate symptoms, but they do not change the natural history.

Orthotics

- Who should get them? Possibly patients with hypermobility and flatfoot deformity. Individuals suffering from sesamoid pain or metatarsalgia may benefit from an orthotic with a metatarsal pad. Concavities over the metatarsal heads, combined with cushioning just proximal to the metatarsal head prominences, serve to alleviate pressure and redistribute weight bearing.
- Custom or off the shelf? Custom-molded orthotics are more specific to the individual patient's ailments and efficient, as they can be transferred from shoe to shoe. The desired orthotic is soft and cushioned, not hard and rigid.
- Orthotics do not prevent deformity progression.

Custom-made Shoes

- Patients with severe deformities, combined with advanced metatarsal fat pad atrophy, may find the greatest comfort from custom-made shoes. However, these tend to be costly.

Surgery

- Removing pain is the primary goal. Obtaining a foot that is "shoeable" is a secondary goal. Getting back into "fashionable," narrow shoes is not a realistic goal.
- In addition to removing pain, another goal should be to redistribute weight bearing among the metatarsal heads and to the toes.
- As there are various types of bunions, with different underlying causes, there is not one single perfect operative procedure for bunion correction. In fact, there are over 100 surgeries for hallux valgus deformity described in the literature.

Considerations

- Is there arthritis or severe stiffness at the MTP joint? More consideration to fusion of the MTP joint.
- Is there hypermobility of the metatarsal on examination, or is there transfer metatarsalgia? These factors are predictably relieved by MTC fusion.
- Is the patient very young, with a large deformity and a strong family history? More "aggressive" procedures, such as the Lapidus fusion, minimize the chance for recurrence.
- Is the deformity "large"? Distal osteotomies are not good for large deformities.
- Contraindications for surgery include poor vascular inflow, non-compliant patients, and unrealistic expectations. Smoking probably increases chances for non-union.
- The specific treatment must be dependent on the underlying cause of the deformity.

Distal Soft Tissue Realignment

- All the procedures include realignment and balancing of soft tissues around the first MTP joint.
- On the medial side, the capsule is tightened (capsulorraphy), and any adhesions between the sesamoids and the metatarsal head are freed up.
- Laterally, it is essential to free (cut) the capsule between the lateral sesamoid and the metatarsal head. This will allow the head to move laterally back on top of the sesamoids.
- In some cases, a lateral release of the MTP capsule between the metatarsal and proximal phalanx may be helpful. Some surgeons also release the adductor hallucis tendon as it attaches to the proximal phalanx.
- It is important to bring the metatarsal head back over the sesamoid complex. Doing so will avoid any unnecessary stress to the joint capsule, and eliminate the possibility of the abductor hallucis sliding underneath the metatarsal head.
- When sufficient lateral shift of the first metatarsal is performed with any procedure, sesamoid reduction is achieved, making a lateral sesamoid adductor tendon release unnecessary.
- Esemenli et al. (2003) determined that distal metatarsal osteotomy with lateral shifting of the first metatarsal head greater than 7.2 mm adequately reduces the sesamoids in a majority of patients.

Bunionectomy

- In the simplest procedure, the distal soft tissue balancing is performed along with medial eminence resection. The Silver procedure is an example of this.
- The McBride procedure also includes an incision at the dorsal aspect of the first web space for the release of constricted lateral structures, excision of the lateral sesamoid, and adductor release. Then, the great toe is held in alignment by plication of the medial joint capsule.
- Excision of the lateral sesamoid can lead to hallux varus. A modification of the McBride procedure without excising the lateral sesamoid has resulted in a decrease in the incidence of hallux varus formation.
- These bunionectomies are most useful for the patient with a large medial eminence and small HV angle, and also for the elderly patient with a large bunion prominence and reasonable expectations.
- The postoperative recovery requires little compliance from the patient. The recovery is relatively quick.

Distal Osteotomies

- The classic procedure is the chevron, which combines a distal metaphyseal osteotomy (with lateral translation of the distal fragment) with the soft tissue release/ rebalancing. The amount of correction obtained is limited by how far the distal fragment can be translated. Large deformities are not correctable with this procedure.
- In the chevron procedure, a "sideways V" cut is made in the distal aspect of the first metatarsal, and the metatarsal head is shifted laterally approximately 3-4 mm on the proximal metatarsal. If a new bony prominence on the medial side of the metatarsal shaft results, it may be removed.
- The angle of the cut should be approximately 60° and extend through the lateral cortex, but no further. This is done in an effort to avoid damaging lateral tissues and the vital circulatory structures housed within.
- The lateral shift at the osteotomy site should be no greater than one-third the total metatarsal shaft width. Fixation is achieved with a pin, a screw, or a bioabsorbable tack.
- Schneider et al. (2004) studied postoperative chevron patients with a minimum follow-up of 10 years, and found that the excellent clinical results of chevron osteotomy are consistent and improve over time.
- Potential complications include recurrence, transfer metatarsalgia, peripheral nerve entrapment, metatarsal head avascular necrosis, and arthrofibrosis.
- Avascular necrosis of the first metatarsal head can occur after the chevron procedure, and is usually the result of over-stripping the soft tissue. Many cases may be subclinical. To avoid avascular necrosis, soft tissue preservation is essential, and caution must be used when performing the osteotomy.
- Perhaps the most significant complication is under-correction of the deformity. This is most likely when the procedure is "overextended." Distal procedures should not be used in the presence of large deformities, or with metatarsal hypermobility.
- Some surgeons have advocated combining a metatarsal shortening with the osteotomy. The Mitchell procedure includes such a shortening. It is a double step-cut

osteotomy performed at the first metatarsal neck, where the distal fragment is translated laterally and the amount of shift is dependent on the degree of deformity being corrected.

- The shortening does loosen the distal tissues, improving realignment of the toe, but can result in a Morton foot with transfer metatarsalgia.

Proximal Osteotomies

- Because the correction occurs close to the center of rotational angulation (the center is usually at the MTC joint), proximal osteotomies can realign large deformities well.
- There are many variations. Some use short cuts at the base of the metatarsal, such as the proximal chevron and the crescentic osteotomies. Others use long oblique cuts, such as the Ludloff, the Mau, and the Scarf osteotomies.
- All have much less intrinsic stability than the distal osteotomies and require more rigid internal fixation. While the distal osteotomies can tolerate immediate weight bearing well, the proximal procedures require limited weight bearing for roughly 1 month. In some cases, this may be non-weight bearing, while others can be managed with weight bearing through the heel (Fig. 9–6).
- These procedures generally heal well, and non-union is unlikely. Dorsal malunion (elevation of the distal fragment), probably from early weight bearing, is common and can lead to transfer metatarsalgia.

Metatarsocuneiform Arthrodesis: The Lapidus Procedure and its Variations

- If one accepts that the deformity of hallux valgus arises primarily from the first MTP joint, and secondarily from the first MTC joint, then the Lapidus procedure makes the most sense.
- The original procedure described by Lapidus was realignment of the first metatarsal, with fusion of the base of the first metatarsal to the base of the second. Lapidus secured the correction with sutures. As might be expected, there were problems with recurrent angulation.
- The modern procedure, sometimes called the modified Lapidus, achieves correction through the first MTC joint. Realignment of the first metatarsal and fusion to the medial cuneiform is emphasized, but in cases of severe instability of the first ray, fusion of the base of the first metatarsal to the second may be added as well. In rare cases, instability will best be cured by fusion of the medial to the middle cuneiform (Fig. 9–7).
- The procedure can be used for any hallux valgus deformity, but the longer period of non-weight bearing and the slower overall recovery make it less ideal for the smallest deformities. Certainly, a foot with first ray instability or a patient with a high risk of recurrence is a good candidate. It can be argued that the Lapidus fusion is the best choice for a foot with transfer metatarsalgia as well.
- The modified Lapidus is an effective technique for revision procedures.

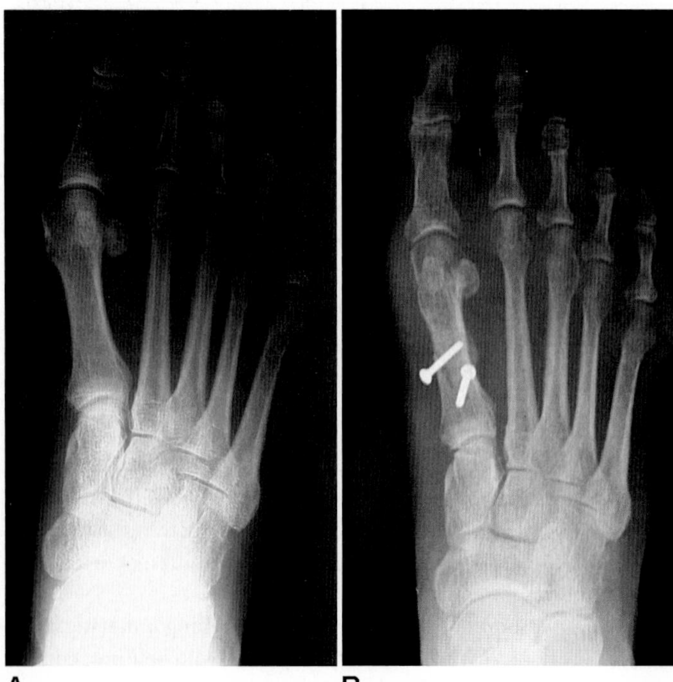

Figure 9–6: **A,** This 50-year-old woman was bothered by a moderate hallux valgus deformity. Symptoms were entirely around the first metatarsophalangeal joint, especially over the medial "bump." **B,** She was treated with a proximal oblique osteotomy (Ludloff). Although she reported compliance with heel touch weight bearing, the screws backed out in the first month after surgery. (Further discussion confirmed non-compliance.) Although the first ray alignment is much improved, the sesamoids remain incompletely reduced.

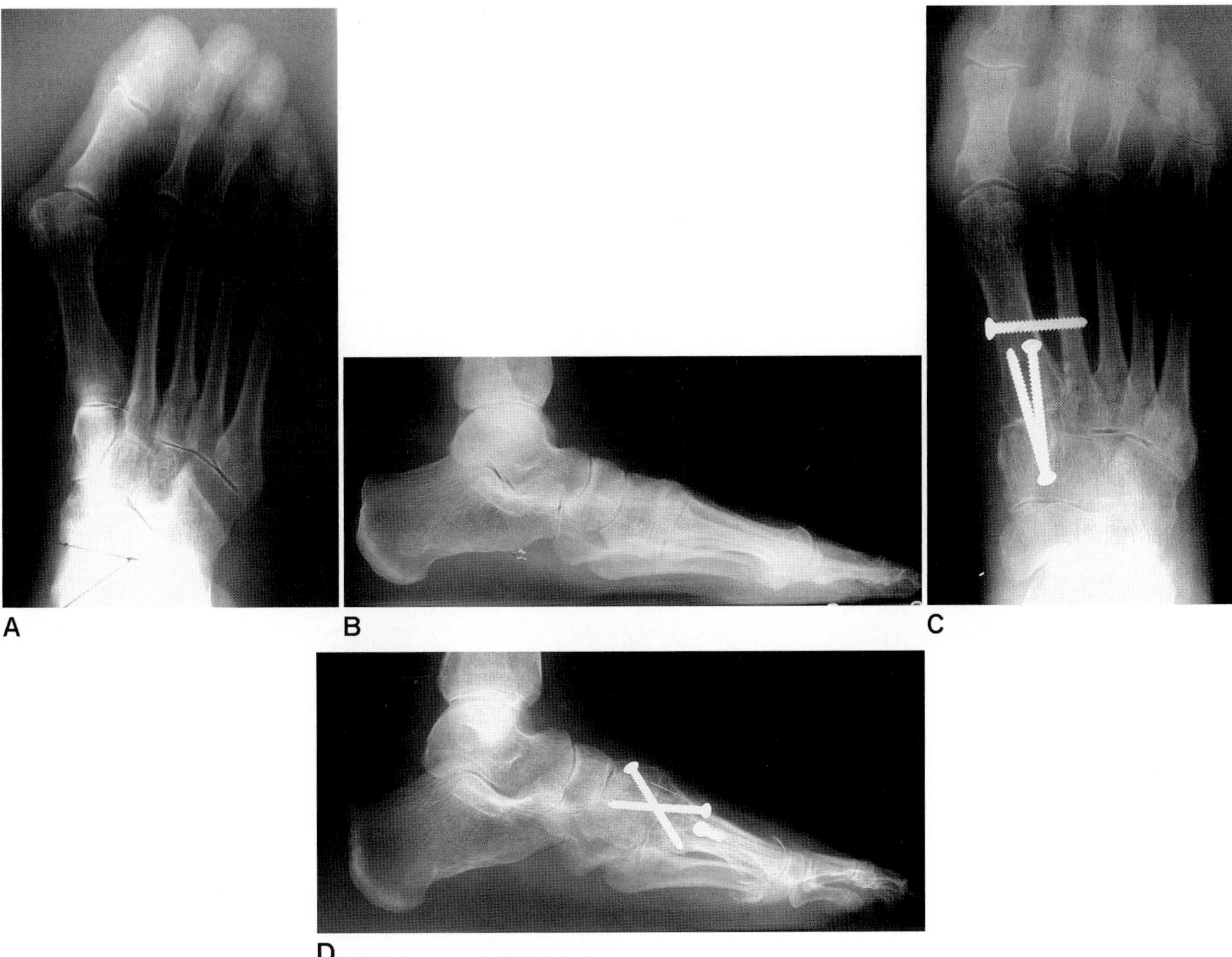

Figure 9–7: **A**, This patient suffered from hallux valgus with transfer metatarsalgia. **B**, The lateral view shows a low arched foot, with low calcaneal pitch, and some plantar flexion of the talus. **C**, After a successful modified Lapidus fusion, the first ray is well aligned, and the sesamoids are reduced back under the metatarsal head. **D**, With only a gastrocnemius recession and the Lapidus procedure, arch height is quite improved. Calcaneal pitch is up, and the talus is well aligned with the first metatarsal. These radiographs support the notion that collapse of the medial column in the midfoot from an unstable first metatarsal can lead to secondary arch collapse (discussed further in Ch. 1).

- Some surgeons consider the young athlete a poor choice for this procedure because of the potential for midfoot stiffness. However, the midfoot is not a site of motion for the normal foot, and other surgeons would argue that this is the best candidate for the procedure, because the young athlete with a symptomatic deformity is most likely to have hypermobility.
- As with all hallux valgus surgeries, distal soft tissue realignment is important.
- The MTC joint is exposed through a dorsal incision, and the joint surfaces are completely denuded of articular cartilage. Sometimes a saw is used to resect a laterally based wedge of bone from the medial cuneiform to facilitate realignment.
- After the distal soft tissues are balanced, the first metatarsal can be translated laterally, back on top of the sesamoids.
- Some have advocated the use of an iliac crest bone block in joint positioning, especially if lengthening is needed, while others have noted that this serves only to complicate the procedure.
- Preliminary fixation can be provided by K wires or a pointed reduction clamp. A solid screw is placed across the first MTC joint, distal to proximal, placed with a pocket hole technique to prevent dorsal cutout. A second screw is next placed; this time proximal to distal, for added compression and rotational stability. In cases of extreme hypermobility, a third screw can be added from the first metatarsal into the base of the second metatarsal.
- Non-union rates have averaged 5-15% in various series. The use of autologous cancellous bone graft at the fusion site has decreased the rate. Most surgeons require non-weight bearing for 6 weeks after surgery (Fig. 9–8).

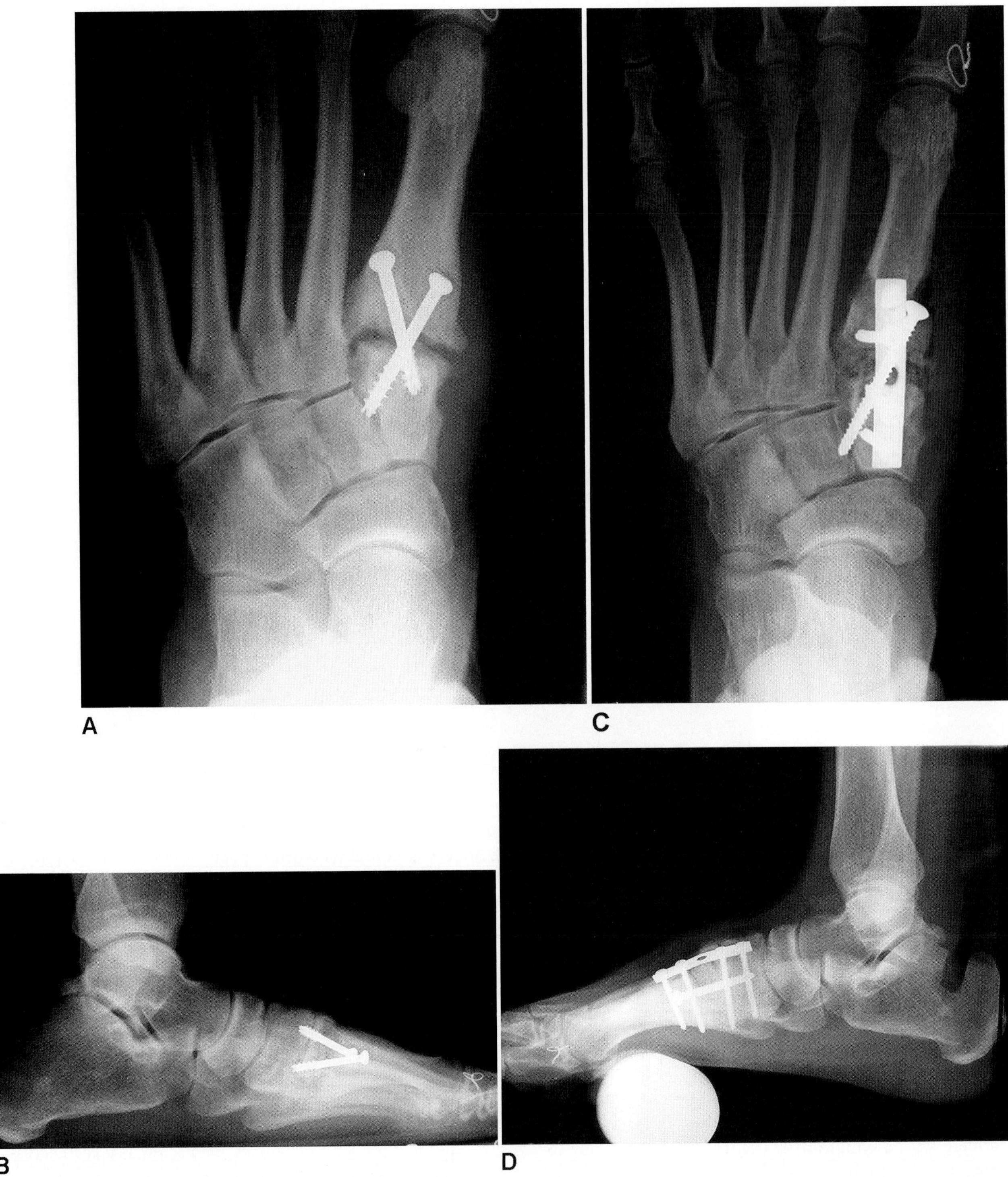

Figure 9–8: **A,** This attempted Lapidus fusion went on to a non-union. The screws were short, partially threaded, and cannulated. Partially threaded screws have only a short segment of threads; fully threaded ones provide better purchase and can be lagged by over-drilling proximally. Cannulated screws tend to have shallow thread depth. Better fixation will be achieved with long, solid screws. **B,** There is obviously room for longer screws in the bones. **C,** The fusion was revised with structural bone graft to regain length. One long screw with a dorsal plate provide rigid fixation. **D,** The structural bone graft was harvested from the calcaneal tuberosity. The fusion went on to heal after 2 months of strict non-weight bearing.

- This procedure is technically difficult to perform. If the first metatarsal is not plantar flexed enough, transfer metatarsalgia will result. If it is plantar flexed too much, pain under the first metatarsal head will develop.
- The technical difficulty, slow recovery, and higher non-union rate make this procedure less desirable to some surgeons and patients. However, the ability to best correct the deformity makes it an attractive choice. Other powerful procedures have their own disadvantages, such as the risk for dorsal malunion in proximal osteotomies (Box 9–3).

Resection Arthroplasty

- The Keller procedure is a resection arthroplasty, with removal of one-third of the proximal phalanx. This decompresses the MTP joint. The resection is combined with removal of the medial eminence.
- There is no osteotomy to heal, so recovery is quick and there are no postoperative weight-bearing limitations. Resection arthroplasty should be reserved for elderly patients with low functional requirements.
- This procedure has been associated with an 80% patient satisfaction rate, with a noted decrease in pain.
- An older variation, with resection of the metatarsal head, is no longer performed, because of relatively high incidence of transfer metatarsalgia.

First Metatarsophalangeal Joint Arthrodesis

- In cases of severe first MTP arthritis or stiffness, fusion may be best. First MTP fusion is often used in patients with rheumatoid arthritis, and sometimes in revision surgery.
- During the fusion, the hallux is placed into a dorsiflexed (relative to the metatarsal not the ground) and slightly valgus position.
- The joint is stabilized with two crossed lag screws or a dorsal plate and screws.
- In one study, 88% of patients rated their result as excellent or good (Taylor et al. 2004).
- Non-union can occur but is often not addressed unless accompanied by pain. Some patients experience painful hardware, with some authors noting as much as 10% of cases later requiring removal of hardware.

Box 9–3 Which Procedure is the Best?

Hallux valgus deformity arises from angulation at the first metatarsophalangeal and metatarsocuneiform (MTC) joints, not from angulation in the first metatarsal. The modified Lapidus procedure is the only procedure to address these sites of deformity definitively. Metatarsal osteotomies create a new deformity in the first metatarsal to "realign" the deformity in the MTC joint.

Akin Procedure

- The Akin procedure is a medial closing wedge osteotomy of the first toe proximal phalanx. It can be combined with soft tissue realignment and medial eminence resection.
- It is the perfect procedure for the rare case of hallux valgus interphalangeus, where the angulation is in the proximal phalanx, not at the MTP joint.
- The procedure can also be used as an aid with other procedures, to increase the correction obtained during surgery.
- The osteotomy is fixed with a suture, wire, or miniscrew.

Gastrocnemius Lengthening

- In the young patient with hypermobile first ray and low or flat arch, there is usually gastrocnemius equinus. In these cases, gastrocnemius lengthening should be considered. These are patients with higher chances for later development of other problems, such as flatfoot with posterior tibial tendonitis. A simple gastrocnemius slide now may decrease the chance for trouble in the future.
- Gastrocnemius slide is particularly useful in cases of forefoot pain, such as with metatarsalgia.
- The incision is made over the medial aspect of the lower leg, between the mid and distal third. The deep fascia is opened, and the sural nerve is protected posterior to the muscle.
- The gastrocnemius aponeurosis is then cut completely, but the soleus is left intact. Because the soleus limits proximal retraction of the muscle, this procedure has no postoperative weight-bearing restrictions.
- Recurrence is common, so night splinting and frequent stretching are recommended.

Review of Complications

- Typical surgical complications, such as infection, first MTP stiffness, and nerve injury (classically injury to dorsal medial sensory nerve), may occur.
- Under-correction is a complication often related to choosing a "small" procedure (such as a distal chevron osteotomy) for a "big" problem (large bunion with instability).
- Recurrence can develop years after the procedure, and probably relates to unresolved metatarsal instability. A Lapidus fusion, if well healed, should eliminate or prevent this complication. Of course, a return to improper shoes may make the complication unavoidable.
- Transfer metatarsalgia can develop with a dorsal malunion of an osteotomy or fusion, or with shortening of the first ray.
- Avascular necrosis of the metatarsal head is a potential complication of distal osteotomies.
- Overcorrection can lead to hallux varus.

Hallux Varus

- Hallux varus is a *medial* deviation of the proximal phalanx on the first metatarsal head.
- The deformity is most frequently *acquired*. In rare cases, hallux varus may develop after trauma, or can be a result of congenital soft tissue defects, but it most commonly occurs after a surgical procedure, especially bunion correction (Fig. 9–9).
- Release of the adductor tendon can create a muscle imbalance, which in turn leads to a new deformity of hallux varus.
- There can be an additional cock-up component of this deformity if the surgical procedure included excision of the fibular sesamoid (a procedure no longer advised).

Pathogenesis

- Most frequently associated with distal osteotomies but can be a complication of any first MTP surgery.
- Most common contributing factors:
  - over-plication of the medial capsule structures
  - medial displacement of the tibial sesamoid
  - overcorrection with postoperative dressing
  - excessive medial eminence resection (maybe the most important cause)
  - over-translation of the metatarsal head laterally in proximal or distal osteotomies, resulting in malalignment.
- Excessive bone resection can leave the MTP joint unstable, even if the toe appears to be in a corrected position at the time of surgery. To avoid taking too much of the medial eminence, resection should be in line with the medial border of the metatarsal shaft.
- Destabilization of the MTP joint can also occur if a metatarsal osteotomy is overcorrected, with the metatarsal head translated too far laterally; this is most common with proximal osteotomies.

Diagnosis and Treatment

- The deformity is obvious clinically.
- Treatment is dependent on severity of deformity and pain level.
- A mild varus deformity is considered to be 7-10° and is usually flexible. If mild, flexible, and noted early in the postoperative period, aggressive dressing changes to pull the toe into valgus and reestablish alignment of the MTP joint are advocated. Otherwise, a medial capsule release may be attempted to correct the deformity.
- If longstanding or severe, the deformity can become fixed. This becomes problematic as the great toe then rubs up against shoes. In this situation, releasing the

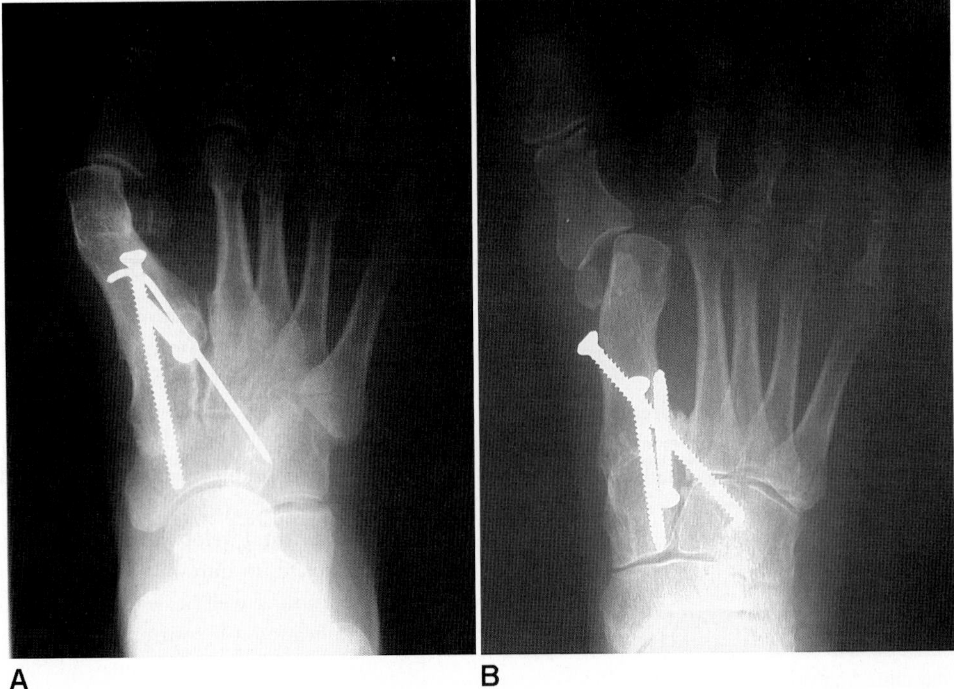

Figure 9–9: **A,** This patient with Down syndrome has ligamentous laxity and a large hallux valgus. Previous Lapidus fusion resulted in a residual deformity (under-correction). Note the large resection of the medial metatarsal head. **B,** Revision fusion achieved better alignment of the metatarsal but resulted in severe hallux varus. The first toe drifted medially because of the previous large metatarsal head resection, combined with the ligamentous laxity of Down syndrome. The deformity was finally corrected at a later surgery with syndactylization of the first toe to the second. Although not cosmetically pleasing, syndactylization does not rely on ligament reconstruction, which might be a problem in this patient with laxity.

capsule and taping the toe into lateral deviation are rarely effective at correcting the deformity.

- There are two common corrective procedures for hallux varus; the choice is dependent on whether or not degenerative joint disease has developed at the first MTP joint.
- Extensor hallucis longus transfer preserves adequate motion for normal foot function.
- First MTP fusion is done when degenerative changes are present.
- If the hallux varus deformity arises from over-translation of the metatarsal head laterally from an osteotomy, a further, corrective osteotomy may be required to translate the metatarsal head back into a stable position.

Adolescent Hallux Valgus

Etiology

- Bunion development can be seen in teenaged or even preteen patients.
- Heredity seems to play a major role. Coughlin (1995) found a 72% rate of maternal transmission in juvenile hallux valgus patients. Tight shoes are probably not a contributing factor in this population.
- It is crucial to recognize concomitant abnormalities, such as a flatfoot. There usually is an obvious MPV—medial deviation of the first metatarsal at the MTC joint.
- Juvenile and adolescent cases of hallux valgus frequently demonstrate joint hyperlaxity, with a hypermobile first MTC joint.
- One study observed metatarsus adductus (an inward twisting of the forefoot relative to the hindfoot) in 22% of adolescent hallux valgus patients, a rate much higher than that of the general population.

Treatment

- The treatment of choice is non-operative management. It may be better to delay surgery until closure of the growth plates.
- While there are not many published studies on surgical results in this population, there has been an extremely high rate of recurrence noted in comparison with the adult population. In one study of juvenile hallux valgus, 6 out of 45 patients who underwent a multiprocedure approach at surgical correction ended up with recurrences of the deformity (Coughlin 1995).
- If operative treatment is pursued, commonly used options include basilar concentric osteotomy and the modified Lapidus procedure. Good correction can also be achieved with medial cuneiform wedge osteotomy, usually combined with first metatarsal base fusion. This very proximal procedure provides excellent correction of MPV.
- Another option is a first metatarsal double osteotomy, described as an effective and reliable technique in the treatment of severe adolescent hallux valgus deformity. The procedure is said to have low rates of recurrence and complications. In one study of first metatarsal double osteotomy, 90% of patients reported good to excellent results (Johnson et al. 2004). Patient satisfaction was mainly determined by the amount of stiffness at the first MTP joint.

References

Hypermobility of the First Ray

Coughlin MJ, Jones CP, Viladot R et al. (2004) Hallux valgus and first ray mobility: A cadaveric study. Foot Ankle Int 25: 537-544.

Proponents of the Lapidus procedure fear that first ray hypermobility will not be corrected with osteotomies. In a cadaver model, the authors showed that first ray mobility decreases immediately following proximal metatarsal osteotomy, suggesting that first ray hypermobility may be the result of the deformity, not the cause. This study raises more questions than answers.

Glasoe WM, Yack J, Saltzman CL. (2000) The reliability and validity of a first ray measuring device. Foot Ankle Int 21: 240-246.

Although the concept of first metatarsal hypermobility is well established, there is no consistent method for assessing first ray mobility. These authors describe a device that measures dorsal translation of the metatarsal. They found that pressure above 55 N leads to unwanted second metatarsal motion, which can confound the measure.

Hansen ST Jr. (2000) Functional Reconstruction of the Foot and Ankle. Philadelphia: Lippincott Williams & Wilkins.

Several of the chapters in this text provide an interesting summary of Morton's theories and the possible role of first ray hypermobility/instability.

Pathogenesis

Ferrari J, Hopkinson DA, Linney AD. (2004) Size and shape differences between male and female foot bones: Is the female foot predisposed to hallux abductovalgus deformity? J Am Podiatr Med Assoc 94: 434-452.

An analysis of skeletons found that first metatarsals in females had the potential for more movement to occur in the direction of adduction, possibly resulting in the female first metatarsal being more adducted than that in the male skeleton. Such differences may underlie the predisposition of the female foot to develop hallux valgus deformity.

Grebing BR, Coughlin MJ. (2004) Evaluation of Morton's theory of second metatarsal hypertrophy. J Bone Joint Surg Am 86: 1375-1386.

The authors found increased first ray dorsal mobility in patients with hallux valgus, but did not find evidence for second metatarsal hypertrophy in those patients.

Radiographs in Hallux Valgus

Brage ME, Holmes JR, Sangeorzan BJ. (1994) The influence of x-ray orientation on the first metatarsocuneiform joint angle. Foot Ankle Int 15: 495-497.

In another study of experienced foot surgeons, there was good agreement in measurement of the IM angle and the MTC angle, but the MTC angle varied with slight changes in x-ray projection. Because of this potential variability, the authors recommend against using this measure in clinical practice.

Chi TD, Davitt J, Younger A et al. (2002) A radiographic study of the relationship between metatarsus adductus and hallux valgus. Foot Ankle Int 23: 722-726.

A study of three experienced foot surgeons found poor correlation when measuring the DMAA. Other measures, such as the IM angle, showed good correlation. This questions the utility of the DMAA in regular practice.

Coughlin MJ, Freund E. (2001) The reliability of angular measurements in hallux valgus deformities. Foot Ankle Int 22: 369-379.

Another study of foot surgeons again found poor agreement with the DMAA, and better agreement with the IM angle.

Farber DC, Deorio JK, Steel MW III. (2005) Goniometric versus computerized angle measurement in assessing hallux valgus. Foot Ankle Int 26: 234-238.

In yet another study of radiographic measures in hallux valgus, the use of computer workstations improved agreement between observers for these measures.

Fuhrmann RA, Layher F, Wetzel WD. (2003) Radiographic changes in forefoot geometry with weight-bearing. Foot Ankle Int 24: 326-331.

This study documents the dramatic difference in alignment with and without weight bearing.

Surgery for Hallux Valgus

Edwards WH. (2005) Avascular necrosis of the first metatarsal head. Foot Ankle Clin 10: 117-127.

Avascular necrosis is reviewed in this article. It is most commonly seen following distal osteotomy with excessive soft tissue dissection.

Esemenli T, Yildirim Y, Bezer M. (2003) Lateral shifting of the first metatarsal head in hallux valgus surgery: Effect on sesamoid reduction. Foot Ankle Int 24: 922-926.

In this study looking at the radiographic results of distal metatarsal osteotomy, more than 7 mm of lateral shift of the distal fragment was needed to reduce the sesamoids under the metatarsal head with large hallux valgus deformities.

Herron ML, Kar S, Beard D et al. (2004) Sensory dysfunction in the great toe in hallux valgus. J Bone Joint Surg Br 86: 54-57.

Sensory nerve abnormalities are quite common in patients with hallux valgus, even before surgery.

Schneider W, Aigner N, Pinggera O, et al. (2004) Chevron osteotomy in hallux valgus: Ten year results in 112 cases. J Bone Joint Surg Br 86: 1016-1020.

Long-term follow-up of 112 feet in 73 patients found that correction was maintained in most patients. Degenerative changes slowly progressed on radiographs, with uncertain clinical significance.

Taylor DT, Sage RA, Pinzur MS. (2004) Arthrodesis of the first metatarsophalangeal joint. Am J Orthop 33: 285-288.

In a short-term, retrospective review of patients undergoing fusion of the first MTP joint, all patients had union with generally good results. Other studies have shown similarly good outcomes.

Adolescent Hallux Valgus

Coughlin MJ. (1995) Juvenile hallux valgus: Etiology and treatment. Foot Ankle Int 16: 682-697.

In a retrospective review of 60 feet in 45 patients, results of surgery were generally good using a "multiprocedural" approach. There were six recurrences and eight major complications (mostly under- or overcorrection).

Johnson AE, Georgopoulos G, Erickson MA et al. (2004) Treatment of adolescent hallux valgus with the first metatarsal double osteotomy. J Pediatr Orthop 24: 358-362.

Using a double osteotomy, these surgeons achieved 90% good or excellent results.

CHAPTER 10

First Metatarsophalangeal Disorders

Aaron Colman* and Gregory C. Pomeroy§

*M.D., Sports Medicine Atlantic Orthopaedics, Portsmouth, NH
§M.D., Clinical Associate Professor, University of New England, and Director, Portland Orthopaedic Foot and Ankle Center, South Portland, ME

Hallux Rigidus

General

- *Hallux rigidus* is currently the term most commonly used to describe stiffness at the first metatarsophalangeal (MTP) joint. In the vast majority of cases, the underlying pathology is degenerative arthritis.
- The stiffness in hallux rigidus is typically from a limitation in dorsiflexion, while the plantar flexion is relatively well maintained. Pain, degeneration of the joint, and a characteristic dorsal osteophyte of the first metatarsal head are often associated with the stiffness.
- Hallux rigidus is a local degenerative process and is not a precursor of future arthritic changes in other joints. Unfortunately, once hallux rigidus occurs, it is often progressive.
- Whether stiffness leads to arthritis, or arthritis leads to stiffness, is a matter of debate. Multiple etiologies have been suggested (see Table 10–1) that could support either concept.
- Hallux rigidus is the second most common condition affecting the first MTP joint, second only to hallux valgus. After age 30, more than 1% of the population is affected by hallux rigidus. The age of onset is broad, ranging from adolescents to the elderly.

Table 10–1: Etiologies of Hallux Rigidus

CATEGORY	SPECIFIC CAUSE
Traumatic	Single-event trauma Microtrauma
Iatrogenic	Post bunion surgery Elevation of first ray
Inflammatory disorders	Rheumatoid Gout Seronegative arthritis
Congenital	Long first ray Irregular "ball and socket" of the first metatarsophalangeal joint Long and narrow foot Pronated foot Hallux elevatus primus
Vascular	Avascular necrosis of the first metatarsal head
Acquired	Obesity Shoe wear

Etiology

- There is no unifying theory as to the cause of hallux rigidus. Some authors believe that adolescent hallux ridigus is different from that which presents later in life, while others believe that it is a continuation of the same disease.
- Hallux rigidus has been attributed to a variety of causes, such as acute trauma (turf toe), repetitive microtrauma, avascular necrosis, an abnormally long first ray that places additional stress on to the first MTP joint, and spasms of the toe flexors.
- The most common presented theory has been hallux elevatus primus (metatarsus primus elevatus). *Hallux*

elevatus primus is a term used to describe the elevation of the first ray in relation to the second ray. The role of hallux elevatus primus in initiating hallux rigidus has been a topic of debate in the literature.

- The mechanism proposed is that the elevation of the first ray allows the flexor hallucis brevis to sublux the proximal phalanx of the great toe plantarward during heel rise phase of gait as the flexor hallucis brevis contracts. When the first MTP joint is subluxed plantarward, joint mechanics are altered. The joint cannot completely dorsiflex as the dorsal lip of the proximal phalanx will impinge on the dorsal metatarsal head. This repetitive microtrauma is the theory believed by some for the development of hallux rigidus.
- When the first ray is not elevated, the proximal phalanx stays reduced because the contraction of the flexor hallucis brevis is balanced by the force exerted back from the floor.
- Alternately, elevation of the first ray may tighten the plantar fascia to the first toe. With plantar fascia tightening, attempted dorsiflexion of the first toe will be limited, and the dorsal articular surface of the phalanx will impinge on the metatarsal head.
- Despite these interesting theories, the role of an elevated first ray in the disease remains unproven. One recent study could identify no relation between first metatarsal mobility and hallux rigidus (Coughlin and Shurnas 2003).

History

- Patients will often complain of limitation of activities secondary to pain in the first MTP joint. Use of high-heeled shoes, sprinting, cross-country skiing, and lunging forward motion such as occurs in tennis are often provoking activities. Patients often will have loss of dorsiflexion and pain pronounced during heel rise just before toe-off.
- Less commonly, patients may also complain of burning or paresthesias of the great toe. This can be caused by traction or compression of the dorsal digital nerve over the dorsal spur. Pain with plantar flexion of the MTP joint can also occur when synovium or the extensor hallucis longus tendon is stretched over dorsal spur.
- Pain and tenderness with shoe wear from mechanical impingement of the dorsal exostosis against the toe box can also occur. Softer sole shoes and harder playing surfaces tend to aggravate symptoms by magnifying the stress across the MTP joint. Patients who walk on the lateral aspect of their foot to avoid rolling off the great toe may develop transfer metarsalgia and complain of pain in the lesser metatarsophalangeal joints.

Physical Examination

- Inspection commonly demonstrates swelling and erythema of the skin over the first MTP joint and a dorsal exostosis. Mild tenderness to palpation is often localized to the joint line.
- The normal passive range of motion of the first MTP joint is 3-43° of plantar flexion and 40-100° of dorsiflexion. During active push-off such as in running or jumping, the first MTP joint dorsiflexes up to 100°. Loss of this normal range of motion can lead to first MTP joint pain, changes in gait, and a limitation of activities.
- Evaluation of gait might reveal a limp, shifting of weight laterally on to the lesser metatarsals, or internal rotation of hip to prevent rolling off of the first MTP joint at toe push-off. These changes in gait can lead to transfer metatarsalgia.

Radiographs

- Two-view standing radiographs of the foot should be obtained. The lateral radiograph will often demonstrate a dorsal osteophyte of the first metatarsal head. The anteroposterior radiograph can easily demonstrate any joint space narrowing, squaring of the metatarsal head, and subchondral sclerosis or cysts (Figs 10–1 to 10–3).
- Mild to moderate dorsal osteophyte with good preservation of joint space is grade 1 disease. Moderate osteophyte with mild loss of joint space is grade 2, and grade 3 disease has severe loss of joint space.

Treatment

- In general, non-operative treatment is the initial treatment for hallux rigidus. A stiff shank shoe or boot, or an orthotic with a Morton extension (Fig. 10–4), may decrease painful range of motion and decrease joint inflammation with time. Activity modification,

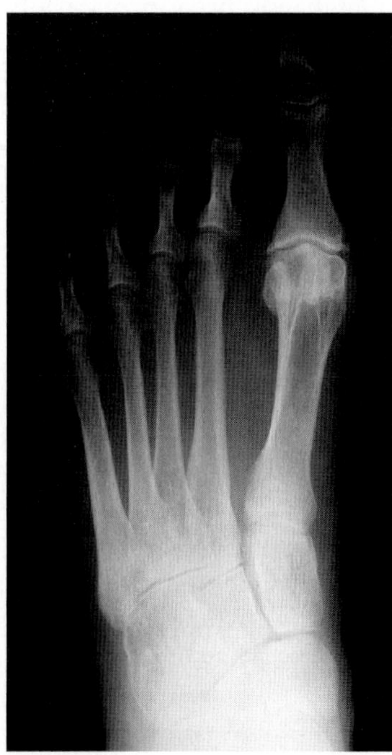

Figure 10–1: Mild hallux rigidus. Small osteophytes with minimal joint space narrowing.

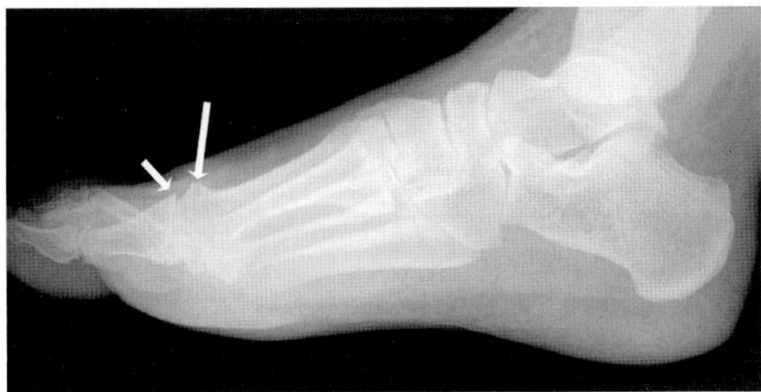

A

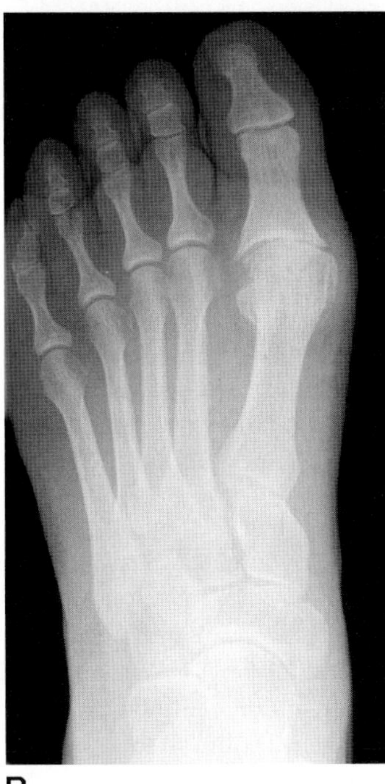

B

Figure 10–2: Mild hallux rigidus. **A**, On the lateral view, the characteristic dorsal osteophyte is visible. **B**, The anteroposterior view reveals mild joint space narrowing.

antiinflammatory medications, a greater depth toe box, and/or the addition of a rocker sole may also help to relieve symptoms.

- Over time, nearly all patients will have radiographic evidence of progressive joint deterioration. However, only approximately 25% will have worsening of their symptoms.
- Surgery is considered when conservative therapy has failed. Multiple surgical procedures have been described (Figs 10–5 to 10–7).
- Cheilectomy is derived from the Greek word *cheilos*, meaning "lip." A cheilectomy is the excision of the dorsal one-quarter to one-third of the metatarsal head along with its dorsal osteophyte. The procedure also includes mobilization of periarticular fibrosis to increase motion. The goal of decompression is to achieve 60–80° of dorsiflexion intraoperatively (Fig. 10–8).

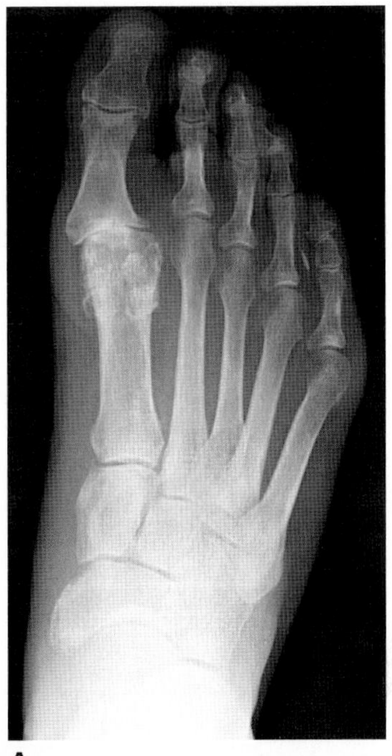

A

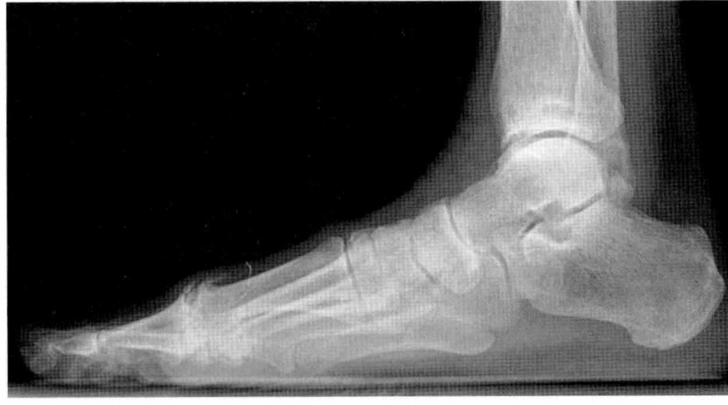

B

Figure 10–3: Severe hallux rigidus. **A**, The anteroposterior view shows complete loss of joint space and even mild subluxation. **B**, On the lateral x-ray, there is complete loss of joint space and dorsal osteophyte.

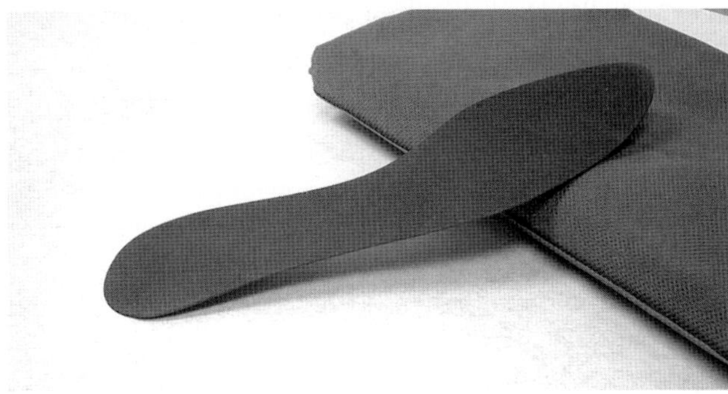

Figure 10–4: This thin, full-length orthotic is made of a rigid material and can be placed inside a shoe to stiffen the forefoot. By limiting metatarsophalangeal joint dorsiflexion, symptoms of hallux rigidus can be improved.

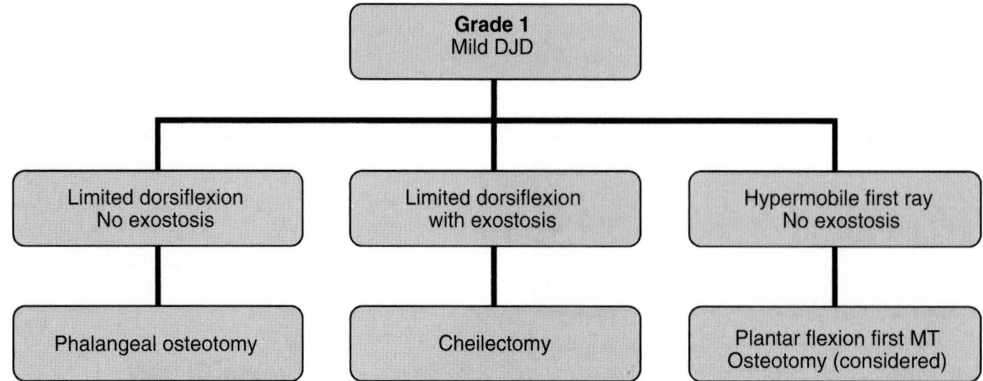

Figure 10–5: **Surgical treatment for grade 1 hallux rigidus. DJD, degenerative joint disease; MT, metatarsal.**

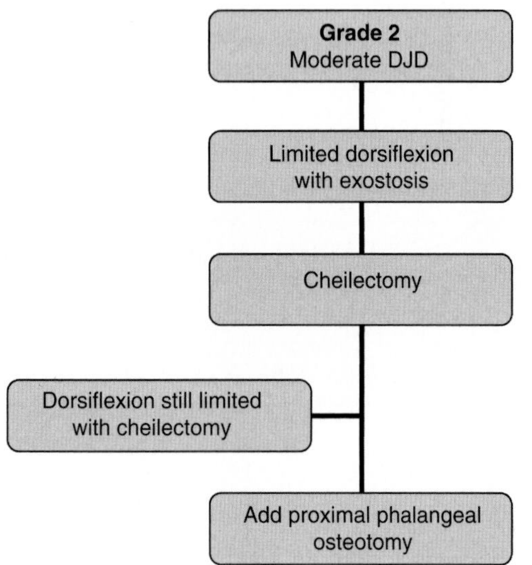

Figure 10–6: **Surgical treatment for grade 2 hallux rigidus. DJD, degenerative joint disease.**

- It is important to resect enough metatarsal head, but too aggressive a resection may lead to joint instability and possible hallux valgus and transfer metatarsalgia. Too little resection will often result in failure because of persistent dorsal impingement.
- If 50% or more of the metatarsal head cartilage is lost, cheilectomy is contraindicated. In this situation, cheilectomy will not provide consistent pain relief.
- The ideal patient for a cheilectomy is an active patient with restricted dorsiflexion and localized pain during toe push-off, but with minimal arthritis on radiographs. Patients undergoing cheilectomy with a preoperative grade 1 hallux rigidus have better satisfaction than those with grade 3 changes (Hattrup and Johnson 1988).
- Although there will be a significant increase in dorsiflexion intraoperatively, motion at follow-up typically improves only 15-30°.
- Pain relief is usually excellent, and satisfaction rates have been reported to be 72-90% approximately 3-5 years postoperatively.
- Cheilectomy with a Moberg closing wedge osteotomy (a proximal phalanx dorsal closing wedge osteotomy) borrows range of motion from typically unaffected plantar flexion to enable a greater arc in dorsiflexion. The proximal phalanx is angled up to provide more dorsiflexion.
- A comparison between cheilectomy and cheilectomy with Moberg osteotomy demonstrated a 73% satisfaction rate with cheilectomy versus a 96% satisfaction rate with cheilectomy and osteotomy. Cheilectomy with osteotomy adds a risk of non-union and increases recovery time.
- A metatarsal plantar flexion osteotomy or metatarsocuneiform fusion to treat hallux rigidus in feet with hallux elevatus primus is controversial. For an osteotomy even to be considered, the MTP joint must be without significant dorsal osteophytes. Currently, no study has demonstrated the effectiveness of this surgery to prevent disease progression.
- Metatarsophalangeal arthrodesis is considered the "gold standard" for those with an active lifestyle and inflammatory arthritis or grade 3 hallux rigidus (Fig. 10–9). Long-term studies have shown greater than 95% satisfaction rates beyond 10 years.
- Proper positioning of the arthrodesis is critical for success. Current recommendation is to position the toe with 15° valgus and 25° of dorsiflexion in relation to the shaft of the first metatarsal. Excessive dorsiflexion can lead to interphalangeal joint impingement against the toe box. Excessive plantar flexion of the MTP joint or less than 20° of valgus can lead to interphalangeal joint arthrosis or pain on toe push-off.
- Current debate in MTP arthrodesis centers on fixation. In the past, threaded pins were used, but internal fixation with two or three lag screws generally provides more rigid fixation.

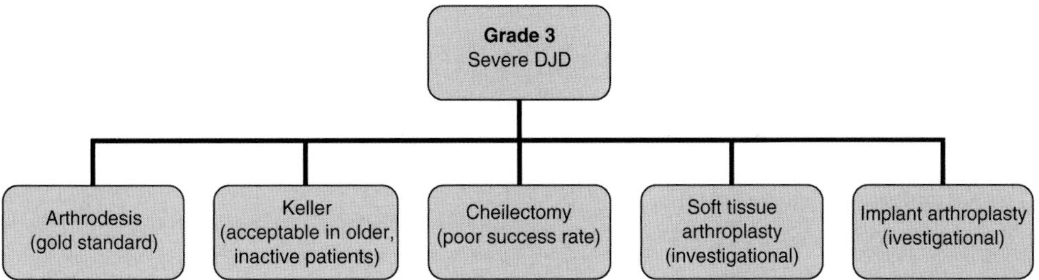

Figure 10–7: Surgical treatment for grade 3 hallux rigidus. DJD, degenerative joint disease.

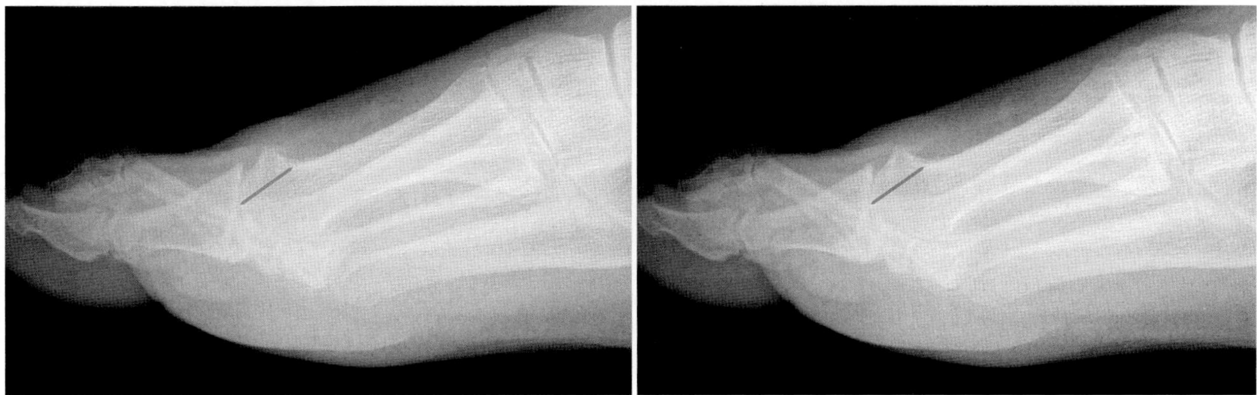

Figure 10–8: When performing a cheilectomy, the dorsal 25% of the metatarsal head should be resected, indicated by the gray line.

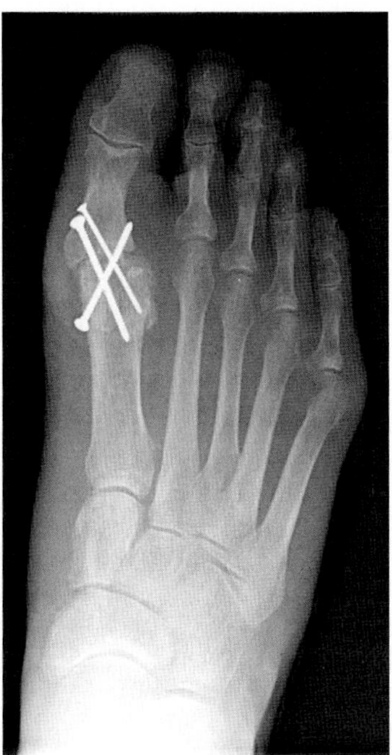

Figure 10–9: The patient from Figure 10–3 was treated with arthrodesis, using miniscrews.

- Plate fixation has been problematic in the past because of the lack of soft tissue to cover a plate. Recent contoured, low-profile plates may be better. Biomechanical studies show a lag screw combined with a plate to offer the strongest fixation, but no clinical studies have demonstrated any benefit of a plate over lag screws.
- Keller resection arthroplasty is a resection of the proximal one-third of the proximal phalanx. Potential candidates are older patients with a less active lifestyle. Weight bearing is allowed shortly after surgery, which is an advantage over arthrodesis. Resection arthroplasty will also help the patient get into high-heeled shoes more readily than with arthrodesis.
- Complications include decreased power of the great toe, transfer metatarsalgia, and cock-up deformity of the hallux. This procedure is contraindicated in patients less than 60 or with an active lifestyle. It probably should be reserved for the more sedentary patient who cannot comply with the postoperative requirements for fusion.
- After fusion, most agree that patients should be non-weight bearing for 4-6 weeks or until there is some evidence of early radiographic union. In an older patient with inadequate upper extremity strength to manage crutches or a front-wheel walker, a first MTP fusion may

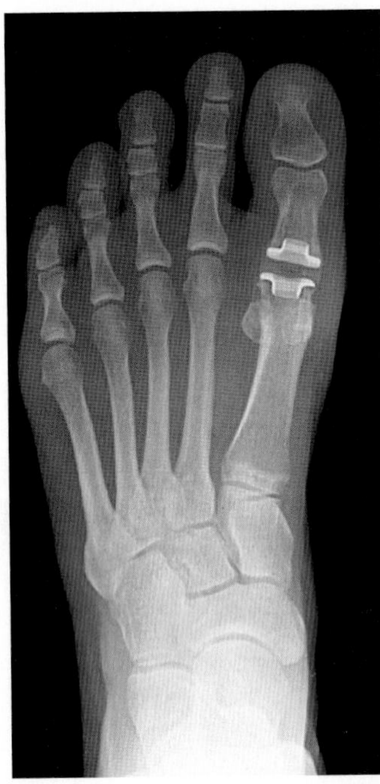

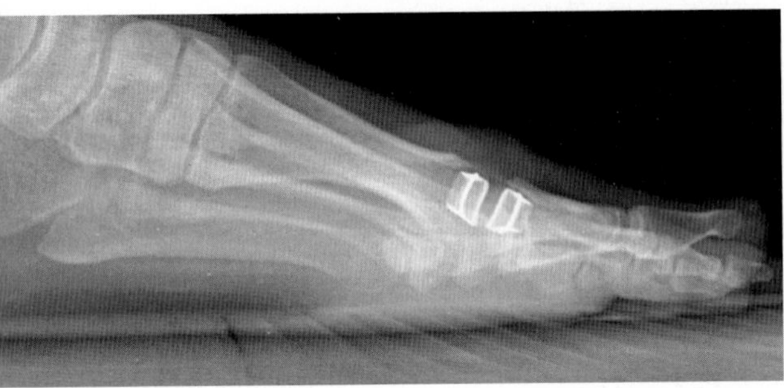

Figure 10–10: Implant arthroplasty is an unproven option for hallux rigidus. This patient had her implant removed 6 months after surgery for persistent pain. She was satisfied with the resultant fusion.

result in prolonged confinement to a wheelchair. If the patient elects to undergo the Keller procedure, these patients should be counseled preoperatively about the potential complications of transfer metatarsalgia, cock-up, and weakness in the push-off phase of gait.

- Total joint arthroplasty of the MTP joint with Silastic or Vitallium have shown variable results and a decreased satisfaction with time (Fig. 10–10). A recent small prospective study showed increased complications with total joint arthroplasty compared with fusion (Gibson and Thomson 2005).
- A failed implant arthroplasty can be converted to a fusion, but the loss in bone stock will lead to marked first ray shortening, with transfer metatarsalgia. The arthrodesis can be performed with structural bone graft (usually iliac crest), bridged by a plate.

Turf Toe

General

- *Turf toe* is a sprain of the soft tissue plantar structures of the first MTP joint from extreme dorsiflexion. The term was coined by Bowers and Martin in 1976, when an increased incidence of first MTP joint sprains were attributed to a hard artificial playing surface and the use of flexible shoe wear.
- The injured plantar structures in turf toe, also called the capsular-ligamentous-sesamoid complex, comprise the plantar plate, flexor hallucis brevis, collateral ligaments, abductor and adductor hallucis tendons, and sesamoids. These soft tissue structures are the primary stabilizers of the first MTP joint because the shallow "ball and socket" of the first MTP joint has minimal inherent bony stability (Figs 10–11 and 10–12). An intact and functioning capsular-ligamentous-sesamoid complex is critical for high-performance athletes who must drive off their foot, run, or jump.
- Pain and lack of push-off strength from turf toe can result in significant functional disability, especially in the professional athlete. On the US National Football League injury roster, turf toe is a common sprain preventing these athletes from returning to play. The injury not only causes short-term morbidity, but carries a high incidence of long-term morbidity that may be devastating to some athletes' careers.

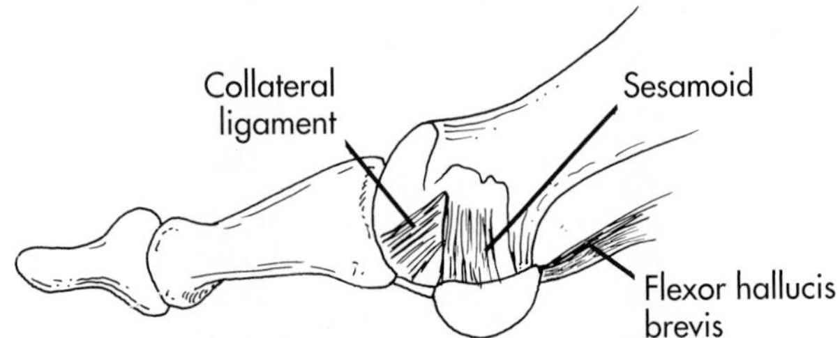

Figure 10–11: Medial and lateral collateral ligaments, plantar plate, and flexor hallucis brevis stabilize the first metatarsophalangeal joint. (From Coughlin MJ, Mann RA. (1999) Surgery of the Foot and Ankle, 7th edn. St. Louis: Mosby. pp. 439.)

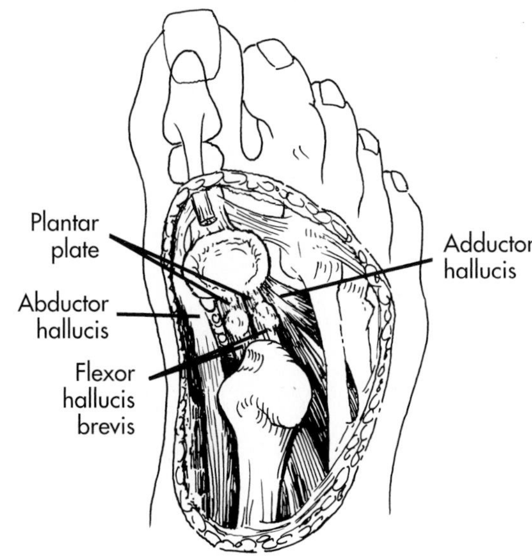

Figure 10–12: The sesamoids are held in position by the adductor and abductor hallucis, flexor hallucis brevis, and plantar plate. (From Coughlin MJ, Mann RA. (1999) Surgery of the Foot and Ankle, 7th edn. St. Louis: Mosby. pp. 439.)

- Turf toe entails a wide spectrum of severity, from a mild sprain of the plantar plate to a possible first MTP dislocation that spontaneously reduces. An accurate examination with an understanding of the anatomy is necessary to grade, predict prognosis, and treat the patient, with the goal of minimizing the high prevalence for long-term morbidity.

Etiology

- Many factors have been implicated in having a role in turf toe. Artificial playing surfaces and more flexible shoes are the most commonly discussed factors in the development of turf toe. The artificial playing surfaces are typically harder and allow for greater traction, enabling a greater force to be generated across the MTP joint by the athlete, such as when a football lineman drives off the stance with his back foot. Flexible shoes allow for greater hyperextension of the MTP joint that can strain the plantar structures. This is in comparison with the older grass shoe cleat with a steel plate that was more rigid, limiting hyperextension and protecting the forefoot.
- As the hallux MTP joint extends, the sesamoids are drawn distally, the plantar plate and collateral ligaments are placed on stretch by the cam effect of the metatarsal head, and the dorsal articular surface of the MTP joint is compressed. The plantar plate will typically tear from the metatarsal neck, where it is weaker. A combined valgus load could additionally rupture the medial collateral ligament; conversely, a rare varus load can tear the lateral collateral ligament.
- There is a high incidence of American football players sustaining turf toe injuries, while the incidence in soccer and lacrosse players has not been as high. In one group of 80 active football players, 45% sustained a first MTP joint sprain in just one season. The mechanism is typically an axial load on a foot fixed in equinus. The increased incidence in football over soccer may be from tackles or pileups that load the posterior heel, driving the hallux into severe hyperextension.
- Other suggested causative factors were increased ankle dorsiflexion, heavier weight, age, pes planus, and interphalangeal arthritis. Most of these factors have limited data supporting their role in turf toe.

History and Physical Examination

- Description of the events causing the injury, level of pain with ambulation, and amount of swelling and ecchymosis can help determine the severity of the injury.
- On physical examination, palpate the dorsal capsule, medial and lateral collateral ligaments, plantar sesamoids, and flexor hallucis brevis. Compare the range of motion, joint stability, and plantar flex/dorsiflexion strength to those of the contralateral side. A dorsal-plantar drawer test of the MTP joint can test the integrity of the plantar capsular-ligamentous complex. The examination can be difficult to perform in acute tears secondary to pain and swelling.
- Weight-bearing anteroposterior, lateral, and sesamoid axial radiographs should be obtained for all hyperextension injuries to assess for capsular avulsions, sesamoid fractures, impaction fractures, or diastasis of sesamoids.
- Proximal migration of the sesamoids may indicate rupture of the plantar plate. Sesamoids migrate proximally secondary to the pull of flexor hallucis brevis. If the distance from the distal pole of the sesamoids and the MTP joint line is greater than 3 mm on the tibial side and 2.7 mm on the fibular side, there is a 99.7% chance of a plantar plate rupture (Watson et al. 2000).

Grading

- Clanton and Ford (1994) described three grades of injury. Grade 1 is considered a stretching of the capsulo-ligamentous complex about the first MTP joint. There is often tenderness plantar and medially, with only minimal swelling and no ecchymosis.
- A grade 2 injury is a partial tear of the capsulo-ligamentous complex about the first MTP joint. This is often accompanied with more intense tenderness, swelling, and the presence of ecchymosis.
- A grade 3 injury is a complete tear of the plantar plate, often with impaction of the proximal phalanx into the metatarsal head dorsally. Severe pain, swelling, and ecchymosis at the MTP joint are characteristic. An associated sesamoid fracture is possible. Players are unable to bear weight on medial portion of forefoot without significant pain.

- Grading should be reassessed after 3-5 days of rest to help better determine prognosis.

Treatment

- Treatment is predominantly non-surgical.
- Grade 1 injuries can typically be treated with a custom insole to limit hyperextension of the forefoot, or with taping. The mild tenderness usually resolves within a few days, and the patient can often return to play within a few days.
- Grade 2 injuries need 1-2 weeks of rest before the moderate tenderness and ecchymosis resolve. The use of a custom rigid insole and return to play in 7-14 days are reasonable.
- Grade 3 injuries typically need crutches to facilitate ambulation. A short leg cast with a toe spica in slight plantar flexion for 3-6 weeks is sometimes beneficial to promote rest and elevation. After ecchymosis and painful range of motion resolve, return to play is reasonable with a custom rigid insole around 4-6 weeks postinjury.
- Surgical treatment is seldom necessary but would be considered in spontaneously reduced MTP dislocation with trapped soft tissue, a progressive diastasis of a multipartite sesamoid, or the presence of fragments in the joint.
- Long-term sequelae of a turf toe injury can be prevalent and disabling. One study found 50% of 20 patients with turf toe to have residual symptoms 5 years after injury. Most common symptoms are joint stiffness and pain in MTP joint with running and cutting maneuvers. Diminished flexor strength, joint synovitis, clawing of the great toe, hallux rigidus, and hallux valgus have also been described.

Disorders of the Sesamoids

General

- Sesamoids of the first MTP joint are embedded in the tendons of the flexor hallucis brevis. They increase the mechanical leverage of the flexor hallucis brevis, which is the primary plantar flexor of the first MTP joint. They absorb the majority of the weight of the first ray, especially when standing on toes, and protect the flexor hallucis longus tendon, which lies between the two sesamoids. Sesamoids are connected to the plantar plate, which is an extension of the flexor hallucis brevis tendon. The sesamoids are stabilized by the medial and lateral collateral ligaments and the adductor and abductor hallucis tendons.
- Vascular supply enters the sesamoid from proximal and plantar, and a minor blood supply exists through the distal pole. The two blood supplies might account for bipartite sesamoids.
- Bipartite sesamoids are common (Fig. 10–13). Prevalence as high as 30% has been reported, and approximately 80% are bilateral. Most bipartite sesamoids occur in the more load-bearing tibial sesamoid versus the fibular sesamoid. Sesamoids can be divided into three and four parts, and this does not necessarily signify a fracture.

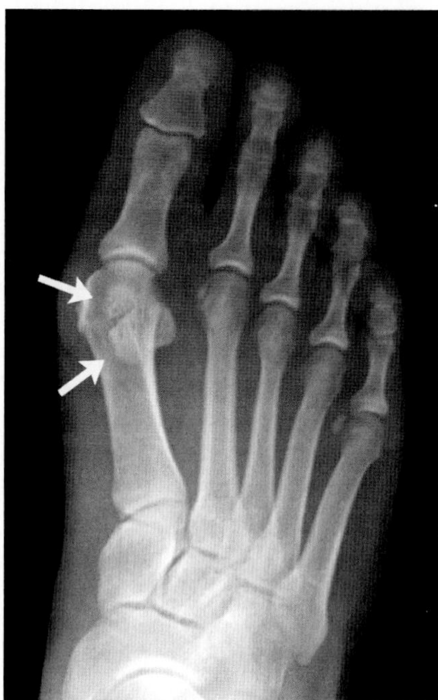

Figure 10–13: A bipartite medial sesamoid (marked by arrows) is a common finding. This patient had no problems with her sesamoid but is bothered by plantar fasciitis.

Fracture

- Differentiating a bipartite sesamoid from a fractured sesamoid can be difficult. Fractured sesamoids have point tenderness localized to the sesamoid. Typically sharp radiolucent lines indicate a fracture versus a smoother rounded contour typically seen in bipartite sesamoids. Bone scan or computed tomography scan may aid in the diagnosis of a fracture. The appearance of callus formation on plain film is definitive for the diagnosis, although it is not always visible. Stress dorsiflexion radiographs may show gapping, indicating a fracture rather than a bipartite sesamoid.
- Treatment for a non-displaced sesamoid fracture is a non-weight-bearing short leg cast until healed. This typically requires 6-8 weeks. If 6 months of conservative treatment fails, consider bone grafting, partial excision, or complete excision of sesamoid.
- Fractures that are displaced can be treated with excision of the distal fragment or entire sesamoid, and repair of the flexor hallucis brevis tendon mechanism. Although repair of a fracture with miniscrews can be done, the screws are often prominent, and anecdotal reports of results are mixed.
- Excision of a single sesamoid, if done with repair of the tendon, can lead to good outcomes. In one small case

series, excision of the proximal pole of the medial sesamoid stress fracture led to excellent results in five of six patients (Biedert and Hintermann 2003).

Arthritis

- Arthritis of the metatarsal-sesamoid joint is often associated with mechanical malalignments. A complaint of diffuse aching on the plantar forefoot is common. Symptoms are more subtle than in sesamoiditis. Radiographs typically demonstrate the involved sesamoid being enlarged with spurs compared with normal sesamoids.
- Initial treatment is a stiff shank and custom orthotic with a metatarsal relief pad. If symptoms are associated with sesamoid subluxation, a soft tissue release to correct subluxation may improve symptoms. If conservative treatment fails, excision of the sesamoid should be considered.

Sesamoiditis

- Some consider sesamoiditis a diagnosis of exclusion. It has been described as a "stress reaction" of the bone prior to a stress fracture, an inflammation and swelling of the peritendinous structures of the sesamoid, and sesamoid chondromalacia. A positive bone scan or magnetic resonance imaging and negative plain radiographs are typical. Physical examination shows sharp tenderness to palpation at the involved sesamoid, pain with weight bearing, and dorsiflexion.
- Treatment starts with activity modification; changes in shoe wear, such as lowering the heels; adding orthotics with metatarsal relief; and trying anti-inflammatory agents. If conservative treatment fails, excision of the sesamoid can be performed. In theory, bone grafting without excision should work, but results of sesamoid preservation have been disappointing anecdotally.
- Resection of a single sesamoid has historically led to complications such as transfer metatarsalgia, hallux valgus or varus, or cock-up toe. With repair of the flexor hallucis brevis muscles, better results have been achieved.
- In one recent series, about 90% of active patients with medial sesamoidectomy were able to return to their preinjury level of activity (Lee et al. 2005).

Intractable Plantar Keratosis

- Intractable plantar keratosis can often be associated with a prominent tibial sesamoid with a plantar flexed first ray (as part of a cavus deformity), or with forefoot fat pad atrophy.
- Conservative treatment entails unweighting the first metatarsal head with orthotics, paring the callus, and the use of flat sole shoes.
- Surgical options for failed conservative treatment include planing (shaving) down of the sesamoid, sesamoidectomy, or reconstruction of foot malalignment (dorsiflexion osteotomy of the first metatarsal as part of a cavus realignment).

Complications

- One complication of sesamoid surgery is persistent pain. This is probably due to incomplete understanding of the pathology, and may occur more commonly with sesamoid-preserving surgery than with excision.
- Loss of the medial flexor hallucis brevis complex (medial sesamoid excision without repair of flexor hallucis brevis tendon) leads to hallux valgus. Loss of the lateral flexor hallucis brevis will encourage hallux varus. Loss of both sesamoids or flexor hallucis brevis tendons will result in a cock-up toe. Repair any defect created by the excision of a sesamoid to maintain the intrinsic muscular balance.
- Place incisions either medial or between the first and second metatarsal heads to limit incisional pain in high weight-concentrated areas.

References

Biedert R, Hintermann B. (2003) Stress fracture of the medial great toe sesamoid in athletes. Foot Ankle Int 24(2): 137-141.

A small series of patients with medial sesamoid stress fractures had generally good results with excision of the proximal fragment only.

Brage ME, Ball ST. (2002) Surgical options for salvage of end-stage hallux rigidus. Foot Ankle Clin 7(1): 49-73.

The article is an in-depth review of multiple surgical options for end-stage hallux rigidus. Concludes that MTP joint arthrodesis is the gold standard for young or old active patients, and either arthrodesis or a Keller for old inactive patients. Biologic or prosthetic interpositional arthroplasties are still in investigational stages.

Clanton TO, Ford JJ. (1994) Turf toe injury. Clin Sports Med 13(4): 731-741.

This article is a well-organized, extensive review of turf toe injury. Discusses the anatomy and biomechanics of the capsuloligamentous complex, etiology and mechanism of injury, work-up, and algorithm for treatment. Stresses the time needed for healing for different grades of injury before returning to play.

Coughlin MJ, Shurnas PS. (2003) Hallux rigidus. Grading and long-term results of operative treatment. J Bone Joint Surg Am 85-A(11): 2072-2088.

Long-term follow-up of 114 patients with hallux rigidus treated surgically. The authors noted no association with first metatarsal elevation, but did note good results with both cheilectomy and arthrodesis for appropriate patients.

Giannini S, Ceccarelli F, Faldini C et al. (2004) What's new in surgical options for hallux rigidus? J Bone Joint Surg Am 86-A(suppl 2): 72-83.

Article is a retrospective study of 111 feet using a variety of surgical techniques to maintain range of motion of the first MTP joint. Depending on the grade of hallux rigidus, a capsular release, decompressive osteotomy, cheilectomy, bioabsorble spacer, or fusion was performed. The study makes an attempt to assess less traditional surgical techniques.

Gibson JNA, Thomson CE. (2005) Arthrodesis or total replacement arthroplasty for hallux rigidus: A randomized controlled trial. Foot Ankle Int 26(9): 680-690.

A randomized controlled trial, with patient outcomes clearly favoring fusion at 2 years. Six of the 39 arthroplasties underwent revision surgery for painful loosening.

Haddad SL. (2000) The use of osteotomies in the treatment of hallux limitus and hallux rigidus. Foot Ankle Clin 5(3): 629-661.

The article reviews historical concepts for the development of hallux rigidus, and describes prior proposed treatments. The concepts are explained well with helpful diagrams.

Hamilton WG, Hubbard CE. (2000) Hallux rigidus. Excisional arthroplasty. Foot Ankle Clin 5(3): 663-671.

The article describes a capsular arthroplasty of the first MTP joint as an alternative to a first MTP fusion. The procedure is a modification of a Keller procedure that uses interposed dorsal capsule and plantar plate.

Hattrup SJ, Johnson KA. (1988) Subjective results of hallux rigidus following treatment with cheilectomy. Clin Orthop Relat Res 226: 182-191.

A retrospective review of 58 patients treated with cheilectomy demonstrated increased failure rates in those with a higher grade hallux rigidus.

Horton GA. (2000) Hallux rigidus. In: Principles of Foot and Ankle Surgery (Myerson MS, ed.). Philadelphia: Saunders. pp. 289-307.

The chapter reviews the etiology, biomechanics, work-up, and treatment of hallux rigidus. Multiple surgical procedures and techniques are discussed. The author promotes cheilectomy for mild hallux rigidus, with possible proximal phalanx osteotomy when dorsiflexion is less than 70°, and fusion for severe hallux rigidus.

Lee S, James WC, Cohen BE et al. (2005) Evaluation of hallux alignment and functional outcome after isolated tibial sesamoidectomy. Foot Ankle Int 26(10): 803-809.

Another small series, with no cases of hallux valgus at an average of 5 years' follow-up. Ninety percent of patients returned to high levels of activity, with little or no symptoms.

Mann RA, Coughlin M. (1999) Surgery of the Foot and Ankle, 7th edn. St. Louis: Mosby. pp. 438-462.

The chapter is an extensive overview of multiple disorders that occur to the sesamoids. Stresses the significance of the sesamoids, and suggests multiple sesamoid-sparing surgical techniques such as realignment or planing of prominent sesamoids versus sesamoid excision.

Mann RA, Coughlin M. (1999) Surgery of the Foot and Ankle, 7th edn. St. Louis: Mosby. pp. 604-633.

This chapter is an extensive review of the history, physical examination, radiographic findings, and treatment strategies for the management of hallux rigidus. Surgical technique for phalangeal osteotomy, cheilectomy, excisional arthroplasty, first metatarsal osteotomy, and arthrodesis are described in detail.

Shereff MJ, Baumhauer JF. (1998) Hallux rigidus and osteoarthrosis of the first metatarsophalangeal joint. J Bone Joint Surg Am 80(6): 898-908.

Critically reviews multiple published studies for the treatment of hallux rigidus. Authors conclude that cheilectomy and fusions are effective and time-tested treatments for hallux rigidus.

Trevino SG. (2000) Disorders of the hallucal sesamoids. In: Principles of Foot and Ankle Surgery (Myerson MS, ed.). Philadelphia: Saunders. pp. 379-398.

The chapter reviews the embryology, anatomy, biomechanics, work-up, and treatment of multiple disorders of the hallucal sesamoids. The effectiveness of surgical approaches and potential complications are detailed. Excision of sesamoids can be an effective solution in patients who fail conservative measures.

Watson TS, Anderson RB, Davis WH. (2000) Periarticular injuries to the hallux metatarsophalangeal joint in athletes. Foot Ankle Clin 5(3): 687-713.

The article provides a useful overview of the anatomy of the first metatarsal phalangeal joint, mechanics, and treatment strategies for turf toe. The article is one of the few that discusses surgical repair or reconstruction for turf toe injuries that failed conservative treatment.

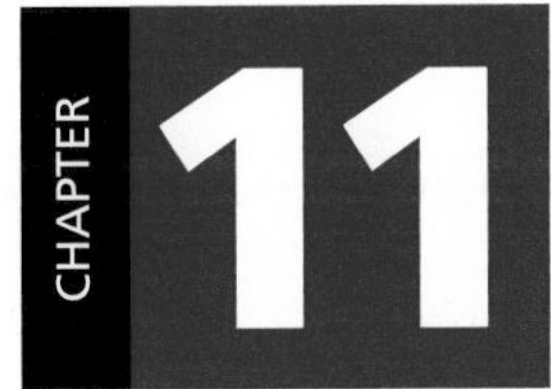

Lesser Toe Disorders

Lloyd C. Briggs Jr.*

*M.D., M.S., Orthopaedic Institute of Ohio, Lima, OH

Overview

- Although small in relation to the rest of the limb, the lesser toes perform a relatively large role in normal lower extremity function.
- The lesser toes help with balance, but more importantly they aid in dissipating forefoot pressures while standing or walking as well as contribute significantly to maintaining arch stability via the windlass mechanism, through their attachments to the plantar aponeurosis.
- An interdependent system of dynamic, static, and bony restraints is responsible for the maintenance of normal toe alignment and stability.
- Given the relatively small size of the lesser toes in proportion to the relatively large repetitive stresses they experience during normal gait, failure of one of these restraints can lead to a domino-like failure of the others, leading to deformity and dysfunction.
- Optimal treatment of lesser toe deformities necessitates not only examining the presenting deformities, but also understanding the problems of etiology and contributing mechanical factors to determine the most appropriate non-operative or operative treatment.
- To further complicate treatment of toe problems, many systemic conditions, most notably peripheral vascular disease and peripheral neuropathy, will often first manifest themselves in the feet and toes, adding the consideration of non-mechanical sources of foot pain to the physician's differential diagnosis.
  - These systemic conditions as well as the foot's dependent nature can produce challenges in treatment of these disorders, in that vascular embarrassment and healing difficulties can accompany toe surgery, adding importance to understanding optimal non-operative treatment modalities.
- Toe surgery, while often correcting the underlying deformity, has significant limitations and will predictably lead to stiffness, loss of toe voluntary motion, prolonged and sometimes permanent swelling, and scar formation.
  - These complications, while usually well tolerated by patients, necessitate thorough understanding and realistic expectations by both the physician and the patient in order to maximize both the perceived and the objective surgical outcomes.

Hammertoes, Mallet Toes, and Claw Toes

Introduction

- *Hammertoes*, *mallet toes*, and *claw toes* are sagittal plane deformities of the lesser toes (toes 2-5). They are extremely prevalent in the population and run the gamut from asymptomatic minor deformities to very disabling ones.
- Medical consultation is generally sought because of shoe wear difficulties (impingement of the toes on the shoe box) or problems generated by mechanical dysfunction of the forefoot, especially metatarsalgia (pain under the metatarsal head). The problem can involve isolated or several toes.
- The etiologies of lesser toe deformities are multifactorial, including traumatic, congenital, neuromuscular, rheumatologic, and mechanical disorders.

- The most common cause is simple wear and tear produced by ill-fitting shoes.
- These many different precipitating factors can lead to almost identical end resultant deformities, making determination of the exact etiology of a particular deformity a challenge in many cases.

- The majority of the time, the observed toe deformity falls into one classification, but the definitions of these various deformities have some overlap, making an understanding of the anatomy, common precipitating factors, and natural history of these disorders important in determining the appropriate treatment.

Definitions

- Note: There is some overlap in the classification of these deformities. Below are the currently agreed definitions of these deformities. However, when reviewing the literature, the terms *hammertoe* and *claw toe* often are used somewhat interchangeably.
- *Mallet toe deformity* is generally defined as a flexion deformity at the distal interphalangeal (DIP) joint of the toe (Fig. 11–1). Mallet toes most commonly involve the longest lesser toe, and may be the result of trauma or impingement of the toe on the shoe box.
- *Curly toe deformity* is similar to a mallet toe but much less commonly seen. It involves a flexion deformity at the proximal interphalangeal (PIP) joint and DIP joint (greater than 5°) without deformity at the metatarsophalangeal (MTP) joint.
- *Hammertoe deformity* is defined as primarily a flexion deformity at the PIP joint (Fig. 11–2). It may be accompanied by a slight MTP joint extension deformity, but this is not the primary deformity.
  - A hammertoe may involve several toes or just one toe, and most commonly has a mechanical cause such as flexion of the toe from an ill-fitting shoe, MTP joint synovitis, or crowding from a significant hallux valgus deformity.
- *Crossover toe deformity* is often confused with a hammertoe deformity, as they both have a PIP joint flexion deformity.
  - The differentiating feature is that, like claw toes and mallet toes, a hammertoe is a purely sagittal plane deformity. A crossover toe has a sagittal plane deformity as well as an axial plane deformity (it crosses over the other toes) secondary to MTP joint instability.
- *Claw toe deformity* is defined as a toe where the primary deformity is a hyperextension deformity at the MTP joint (Fig. 11–3).
  - There is often a PIP joint flexion deformity as in hammertoes, but this is thought to be a secondary deformity. Unlike hammertoes, claw toes commonly will have a DIP joint flexion deformity.
- The primary disagreement with regard to classification of these deformities is the confusion between claw toes and hammertoes. Although it is not always the case, claw toes will more commonly be neurologic in nature (e.g. Charcot-Marie-Tooth, peripheral neuropathy, compartment syndrome) and rheumatologic in nature (e.g. rheumatoid arthritis) than will hammertoes. Claw toes will more commonly involve several toes, whereas hammertoes more commonly involve one or two toes.
- All the toe deformities are further classified as "rigid" or "flexible" deformities, depending on whether the deformity is passively correctable.

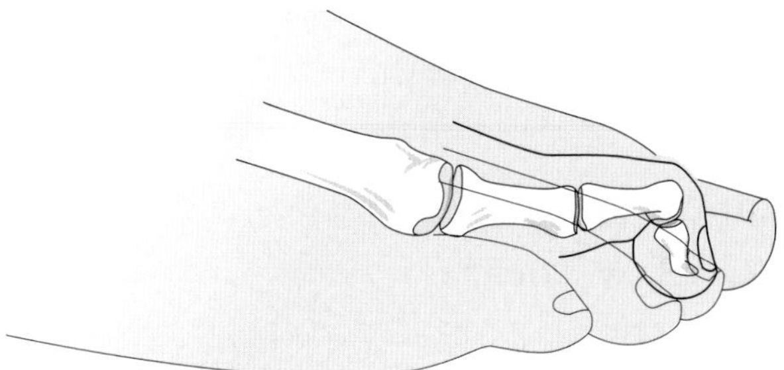

Figure 11–1: Mallet toe deformity.

Anatomy

- Lesser toe alignment and stability are maintained by both dynamic and static components.
- The bony anatomy of the lesser toes is made up of three phalanges (occasionally the fifth toe will have two), each articulating with the phalanx next to it, and the concave surface of the base of the proximal phalanx articulating with the convex metatarsal head. This arrangement

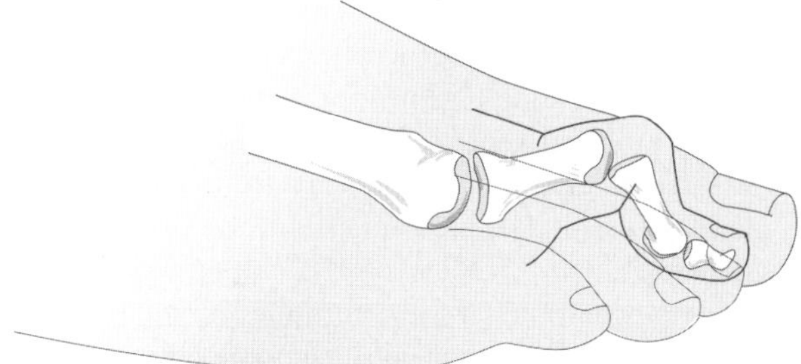

Figure 11–2: Hammertoe deformity.

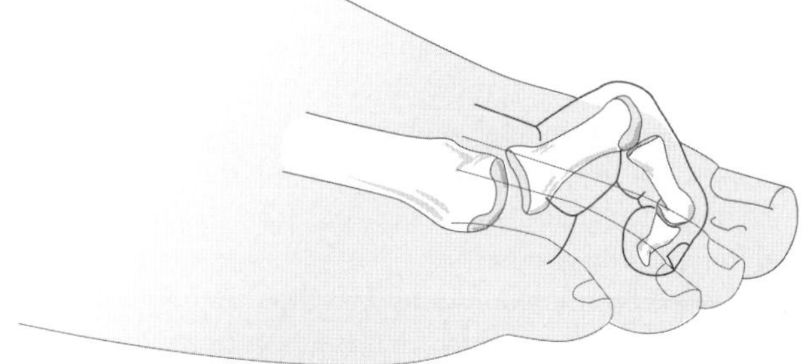

Figure 11–3: Claw toe deformity.

provides for sagittal plane motion but provides little inherent stability.

- The primary static restraints of the toe are the thick plantar plate, the plantar aponeurosis, the joint capsule, and the collateral ligaments. These structures allow the DIP joint and PIP joint to flex but block extension past neutral while they allow the MTP joint to flex and extend during the normal gait cycle.
- The dynamic stabilizers of the toes can be divided into intrinsic (originating in the foot) and extrinsic (originating in the leg) muscles. The tibial nerve innervates all the intrinsic muscles as well as the extrinsic flexor muscles, while the peroneal nerve innervates the extrinsic extensor muscles.
- The extrinsic muscles terminating at the lesser toes are the extensor digitorum longus (EDL) and the flexor digitorum longus (FDL). The intrinsic muscles terminating at the lesser toes comprise the seven interosseus muscles, the four lumbricals, and the abductor digiti minimi, as well as the extensor digitorum brevis (EDB) and the flexor digitorum brevis (FDB).

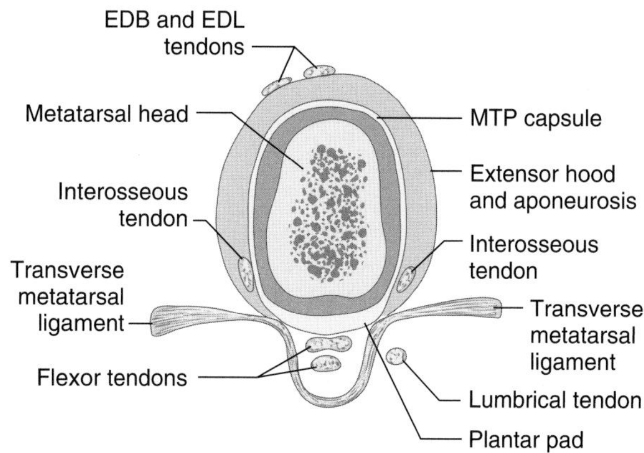

Figure 11–4: Cross-section through the metatarsal head of the lesser toe. Note that the interossei tendons travel dorsal to the transverse metatarsal ligament, whereas the lumbrical tendon travels plantar to it. (From Coughlin MJ, Mann RA. (1999) Lesser toe deformities. In: Surgery of the Foot and Ankle, 7th edn (Coughlin MJ, Mann RA, eds). St. Louis: Mosby. p. 326.)

Extrinsic Muscles

- The EDL runs over the dorsal aspect of the MTP joint and invests the extensor hood over the proximal phalanx before inserting on both the middle and distal phalanx.
- These multiple insertions make the EDL a strong extensor at the MTP joint through its attachments at the extensor hood. However, it can extend the PIP and DIP joints only when the intrinsic muscles hold the proximal phalanx in a neutral or flexed position at the MTP joint.
- The FDL runs under the metatarsal head deep to (dorsal to) the FDB and inserts on the distal phalanx. As a result of having no direct connection to the proximal phalanx, the FDL serves as a strong flexor of the DIP joint but is a weak flexor of the MTP joint.

Intrinsic Muscles

- The EDB is an intrinsic muscle that sends a slip to the second, third, and fourth toe. The EDB tendon inserts into the lateral aspect of the EDL tendon and weakly extends the PIP joint.
- The FDB runs plantar to the FDL tendon through most of its course, splitting into two terminal slips at the level of the proximal phalanx, and traveling over either side of the FDL before inserting on the middle phalanx. The FDB is a weak flexor of the MTP joint.
- The four lumbricals, one unipennate and the rest bipennate, originate from the FDL tendon, run under the intermetatarsal ligament, and insert on the tibial side of the plantar plate and the extensor hood at the level of the MTP joint (Fig. 11–4). They are strong flexors of the MTP joint when the joint is in neutral, but quickly lose their mechanical advantage at the joint as the joint is extended.
- Prior to inserting on the extensor hood, the seven interosseus muscles of the foot, four dorsal bipennate interossei, and three plantar unipennate interossei run dorsal to the intermetatarsal ligament but plantar to the axis of rotation of the metatarsal head when the toe is in a neutral position.
  - As the dorsiflexion at the MTP joint increases, the tendons of the interossei will travel dorsally with the extensor hood closer to the axis of rotation of the joint, and then eventually dorsal to the axis of rotation, converting them from flexors to extensors of the joint (Fig. 11–5).

Flexion and Extension Forces at the Joints (Fig. 11–6)

- At the DIP joint, the FDL provides a strong flexion force while the EDL provides a relatively weak extension force, and then only if the intrinsic muscles are able to hold the proximal phalanx in a neutral alignment.
- At the PIP joint, the FDL provides weak flexion, while the FDB provides strong flexion through its direct insertion on the middle phalanx. As at the DIP joint, the EDL provides a relatively weak extension force if the intrinsic muscles are able to hold the proximal phalanx in a neutral alignment.
- At the MTP joint, the EDL is a strong extensor. The FDL and FDB, with no direct insertions on the proximal phalanx, provide weak flexion power while intrinsic muscles, the lumbricals and the interossei muscles, provide the majority of the flexion power to oppose the EDL.
  - The strong pull of the intrinsic muscles is dependent on the position of the proximal phalanx. With MTP joint

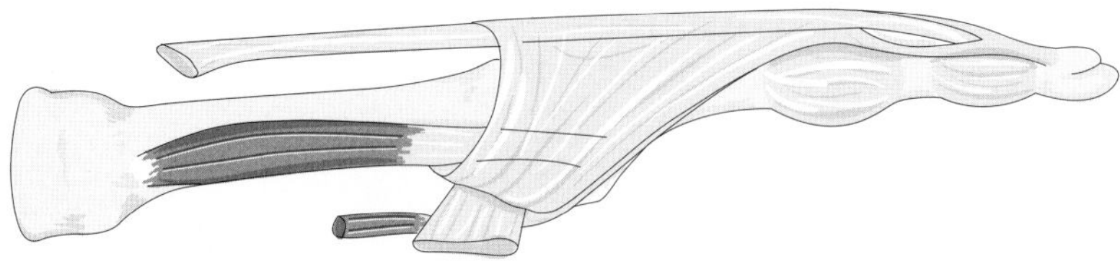

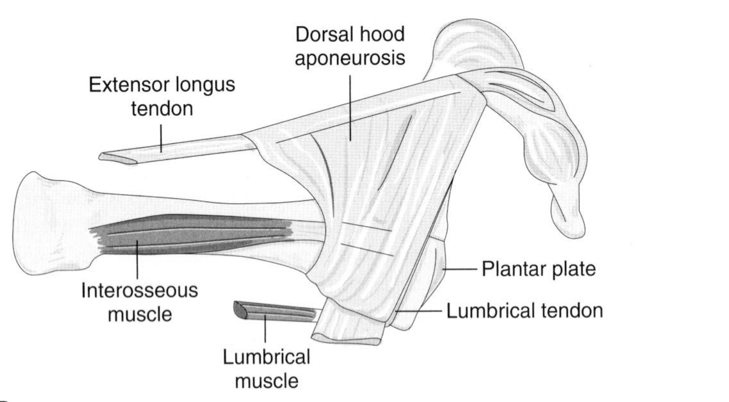

Figure 11–5: Anatomy of the intrinsic and extrinsic musculature of the normal toe **A**, and in a claw toe deformity **B**.

extension, the flexion power is greatly diminished, as the interossei muscles become extensors of the joint as their mobile tendons travel dorsally and the lumbrical muscles lose their mechanical advantage.

Pathophysiology

- A *mallet toe* by definition is a flexion deformity at the DIP joint.
  - While there may be many etiologies for mallet toes, one theory is that through trauma or impingement of tight shoes, the EDL tendon at the DIP joint attenuates or ruptures, creating a strong unopposed flexion by the FDL tendon at the DIP joint, resulting in deformity.

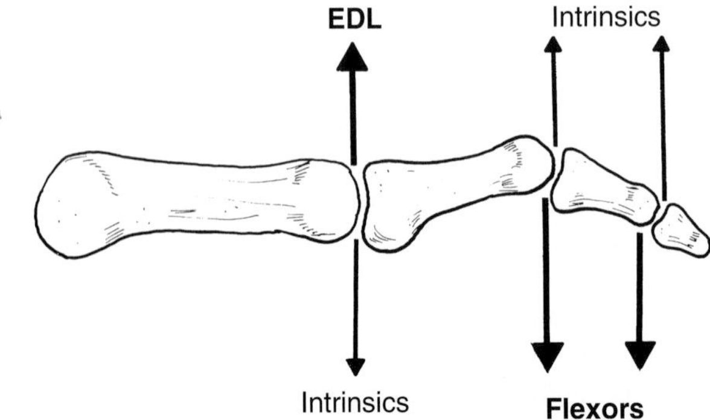

Figure 11–6: Intrinsic and extrinsic muscle forces about the lesser toe. The smaller intrinsic muscles are overpowered by the extrinsic muscles, leading to a hammertoe or claw toe deformity. (From Coughlin MJ, Mann RA. (1999) Lesser toe deformities. In: Surgery of the Foot and Ankle, 7th edn (Coughlin MJ, Mann RA, eds). St. Louis: Mosby. p. 328.)

- A *hammertoe* (a flexion deformity at the PIP joint) is thought to occur as the result of impingement of the end of the toe against the shoe, or MTP joint synovitis causing the MTP joint to dorsiflex.
  - This results in the FDB and FDL strongly flexing the PIP joint without the EDL being able to oppose the flexion, because it can extend the joint only when the proximal phalanx is neutrally aligned.
  - This is one theory why wearing a significant heel (dorsiflexing the MTP joint) or wearing shoes with a tight toe box may lead to hammertoe deformity.
- A *claw toe* with its dorsiflexion deformity at the MTP joint and flexion deformity at the PIP joint and DIP joint is thought to commonly occur as the result of an imbalance of the intrinsic and extrinsic foot musculature. It can often involve more than one toe, and can commonly have a neurologic origin.
- A claw toe can develop as the extrinsic muscles overpower the intrinsic muscles of the foot; the EDL overpowers the lumbrical and interossei muscles, creating dorsiflexion at the MTP joint. As the dorsiflexion deformity increases, the lumbricals lose their ability to flex the MTP joint, and as the interossei tendons pass dorsal to the axis of rotation and function as extensors. This leaves the FDL and FDB, both weak flexors of the joint, overwhelmed by the EDL extension force at the MTP joint, leading to a MTP joint extension deformity (Fig. 11–5). With the resultant MTP dorsiflexion deformity, the FDL and FDB flex the PIP joint and the FDL flexes the DIP joint without the counterbalancing extension by the EDL, which cannot extend these joints with the MTP joint dorsiflexed.

Diagnostic Evaluation for Lesser Toe Disorders

- Radiographs are important in the work-up of lesser toe disorders to rule out other mechanical sources of pain (i.e. stress fracture, arthritis).
  - This is particularly important because patients will often seek treatment for hammertoe deformities merely because the only visible abnormality they observe is a toe deformity, and they assume that the toe is the source of their discomfort.
- Three views of the foot (standing anteroposterior, standing lateral, and oblique radiographs of the foot) are the standard and should be evaluated for metatarsal stress fractures, hallux valgus deformity, or MTP joint arthritis.
  - When evaluating MTP joint arthritis by determining the narrowing of the joint as seen on the anteroposterior radiograph, be aware that significant flexion, subluxation, or even dislocation at the MTP joint can give the appearance of a greatly reduced or absent MTP joint space, and can be unreliable in evaluating the cartilage integrity.
- The *gun barrel sign* describes the appearance of the proximal phalanx when viewed end on. If the proximal phalanx is sufficiently extended at the MTP joint, the anteroposterior foot view of the proximal phalanx will appear as a circle, a cylinder viewed end on. It will give the appearance of looking down the barrel of a gun.

History for Lesser Toe Disorders

- A history should elicit as precisely as possible the patients' problem as they see it (i.e. shoe wear, pain, cosmetic appearance). If they are complaining primarily of pain, the exact location as well as the degree and frequency of discomfort should be recorded.
- Generally, lesser toe deformities will be aggravated by activity. It often will be partially relieved with attempts to switch to a more comfortable shoe. Global foot pain, pain that radiates up the leg, and night pain can be indicators of a non-mechanical pain such as peripheral neuropathy, radiculopathy, or vascular insufficiency.
- Patients should be questioned regarding what treatments they may have tried in the past and the degree of improvement. A history of ulceration or infection of the toes should be specifically elicited to help determine if the patient is at risk for future ulceration.
- The shoe wear requirements for the patient's occupation (i.e. steel-toed shoes) as well as the patient's shoe wear desires are important to understand, because successful non-operative treatment will usually require shoe wear modification.
- Review of systems should include questions concerning systemic arthritis, neuromuscular conditions, orthopaedic problems, diabetes, gout, and peripheral vascular disease. The review is important to not only assess possible contributing factors to the development of the lesser toe deformities, but also help determine if any of the patient's pain may be non-mechanical in origin.

Physical Examination for Lesser Toe Disorders

- The goal of the physical examination is to not only evaluate the toe deformity but also to evaluate the global function of the foot and ankle, which may give clues as to the deformity's mechanical etiology.
- As with most foot examinations, gait examination is performed along with a standing examination of both legs uncovered from the knees to the toes. The alignment is observed from both the anterior and the posterior, followed by a non-weight-bearing examination. A planovalgus or cavus posture of the foot, both associated with claw toe deformity, should be noted.
- A planovalgus foot deformity secondary to a posterior tibial tendon dysfunction will over time create clawing of the toes secondary to the recruitment or "over-pull" of the FDL tendon.
  - The FDL is recruited by the body to help indirectly stabilize the medial aspect of the ankle to compensate for the ineffective posterior tibial tendon and muscle function.
- Initially, the sensation and pulses should be evaluated along with the skin integrity, which should be inspected for old surgical and non-surgical scars or areas of swelling.
  - Old compartment syndrome can result in claw toe deformity because of the development of an intrinsic and extrinsic muscle imbalance, and the foot should be examined for muscle wasting.
- Lesser toe deformities usually present with toe complaints in one of three areas: the tip of the toe, the dorsal aspect of the PIP joint, or under the foot at the MTP joint. These areas should be evaluated for evidence of callus or corn formation.
- The pain at the tip of the toe results from the shoe rubbing on the toe, or the relatively unpadded toe tip resting on the ground or grabbing the ground as the patient walks.
  - The PIP joint pain occurs from the shoes rubbing on the toe box. This rubbing may be exacerbated if patients are recruiting their toe extensor tendons to help dorsiflex their ankle during gait, as is commonly the case in patients with an equinus (gastrocnemius) contracture.
- A second area of common complaint is pain under the metatarsal heads, which accompanies the drawing up of the toe.
  - As the proximal phalanx dorsiflexes on the metatarsal head, the weight-bearing surface area of the forefoot decreases, increasing the plantar pressures on the metatarsal head. In addition, as the proximal phalanx

dorsiflexes it takes the plantar fat pad with it, uncovering the metatarsal head.

- Checking the ankle range of motion and strength is an important part of the examination. Equinus deformity or weakness of the anterior tibial muscle will result in the recruitment and over-pull of the EDL tendon to compensate for the restricted or weak ankle dorsiflexion. Over time, this over-pull will lead to a claw toe deformity.
- The toes should be examined for range of motion at each of the various joints, and the exact deformity at each toe should be determined.
  - The deformity should then be categorized as fixed or flexible.
  - The *push-up test* involves passively pushing up under the metatarsal heads on the non-weight-bearing foot until the ankle is brought to neutral (Fig. 11–7). In the case of a flexible toe deformity, the toes should correct to a neutral alignment, whereas in a rigid deformity they will not.

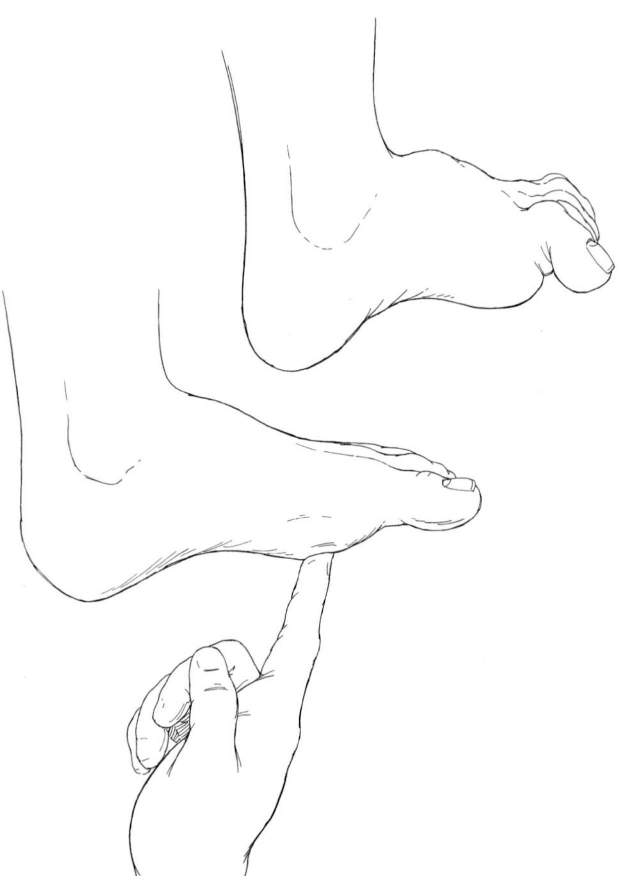

Figure 11–7: The push-up test is used to assess the flexibility of the lesser toe deformity. (From Cooper PS. (2000) Disorders and deformities of the lesser toes. In: Foot and Ankle Disorders (Myerson M, ed.). Philadelphia: Saunders. p. 311.)

Non-operative Treatment

- While it is always best to tailor non-operative care to a particular deformity, most lesser toe deformity problems will improve with the general recommendation of shoe wear modification, specifically switching to a shoe with a wider and/or higher toe box. Occasionally, a patient's existing leather shoe can be stretched to provide more forefoot room.
- Patients as they age will tend to buy the same size shoe they have always bought, unaware that their shoe size may have changed with time. Often, the need for shoe modification can be made clear to the patient by tracing the outline of their bare foot as they stand on a piece of paper, then superimposing a tracing of the outline of their shoe over that, giving the patient a visual demonstration as to the need for a bigger shoe.
- A shoe with a sufficiently large toe box will have the advantages of exerting less pressure over the PIP joints and less pressure on the tips of the toes, as well as allowing the toes to move within the shoe. This motion may prevent the intrinsic muscle atrophy that can occur with the chronic restriction of toes.
- Other non-operative treatments target the specific area of discomfort. Pain under the metatarsal heads can be improved with a metatarsal pad. A custom orthosis can provide similar or improved metatarsal support but can also lead to crowding of the toe box as it "fills" the shoe.
- PIP joint discomfort can be treated with various toe pads, especially in the flexible deformity, but tend not to be as useful in the case of the rigid deformity, as they can have the paradoxical effect of "stuffing" the toe box.
- Discomfort at the tip of the toe can often be improved with a soft toe cap or a toe crest that fits under the toes and helps relieve the pressure on the tip of the toe.
- As a rule, most flexible toe deformities tend to respond much better to conservative care than do rigid deformities. In addition to the various pads, taping of the toes or toe straps can be used, and daily toe stretching may help slow the progression of the deformity, although this is difficult to maintain long term.

Operative Treatment

- Claw toe, hammertoe, and mallet toe deformities tend to progress with time, starting initially as a flexible deformity and then becoming fixed. As they become fixed, they are more and more difficult to accommodate in a shoe; surgery may be required.
- The number one predictor of patient satisfaction *after* toe surgery is realistic *preoperative* expectations.
  - Toe surgery will generally lead to a toe that is shorter and more swollen, with less motion and less volitional control. This is the surgical trade-off for a toe that is less painful, straighter, and "shoeable." The toe is not "normal." If a patient is unable to accept this inevitable

postoperative outcome, this is a strong contraindication to surgery.

- Toe surgery also carries significant neurovascular risk, especially if the patient has peripheral vascular disease, has had previous toe surgery, or is in need of an extensive toe procedure.
  - Peripheral vascular status must be very carefully investigated (arterial Doppler studies or transcutaneous oxygen perfusion measurements when necessary) prior to toe surgery. Loss of a toe is a rare but possible complication.
- Another common complication of surgery is recurrence of deformity. Especially in the situation where ill-fitting shoes have clearly contributed to the deformity, postoperative return to the same ill-fitting shoes can easily ruin an initially good surgical outcome.
  - Patients need to be counseled preoperatively about the role their shoes may have played in the development of their problem.
- Choice of surgical procedure depends on the nature of the deformity (claw toe, mallet toe, or hammertoe), as well as whether the deformity is rigid or flexible, with flexible deformities generally requiring a soft tissue procedure while rigid deformities require a bony procedure (Table 11–1).
- A bony procedure is recommended in the cases of fixed deformity to prevent damage to the plantar neurovascular structures, which invariably have become contracted with time and may be embarrassed by correction of the deformity and the accompanying lengthening of the toe.
  - Bony resection will allow the toe to straighten without stretching and injuring the plantar neurovascular structures.
- A *flexible mallet toe* is generally treated with a simple flexor tenotomy from a plantar approach, with pinning of the DIP joint for 3 weeks. In the case in which a disproportionately long toe ("proud toe") was felt to be the underlying etiology, shortening of the toe as with a fixed mallet toe procedure would be recommended to prevent recurrence.

Table 11–1: Lesser Toe Deformity Correction

DEFORMITY	GENERAL OPERATIVE TREATMENT
Mallet toe (flexible)	FDL tenotomy
Mallet toe (fixed)	Resect middle phalanx distal condyles ± FDL tenotomy
Hammertoe (flexible)	FDL flexor to extensor tendon transfer at the level of the proximal phalanx
Hammertoe (fixed)	Resect proximal phalanx distal condyles ± FDL tenotomy
Claw toe (flexible)	FDL flexor to extensor tendon transfer with EDL lengthening, EDB tenotomy, and MTP capsular release
Claw toe (fixed)	Resect proximal phalanx distal condyles with EDL lengthening, EDB tenotomy, MTP capsular release, and possible shortening osteotomy

EDB, extensor digitorum brevis; EDL, extensor digitorum longus; FDL, flexor digitorum longus; MTP, metatarsophalangeal.

- A *fixed mallet toe deformity* is generally treated with a resection of a portion of the distal condyles of the middle phalanx, followed by pinning of the DIP joint for 3 weeks with or without a flexor tenotomy, depending on the degree of correction obtained with the bony resection.
- A *flexible hammertoe deformity* can be treated with a Girdlestone-Taylor flexor to extensor tendon transfer. The FDL tendon is released from its insertion at the distal phalanx through a plantar approach. The tendon is then split in two and passed at the level of the proximal phalanx along the periosteum from plantar to distal. The two limbs are reunited on the dorsal aspect of the toe and secured to one another.
- This FDL transfer removes the deforming flexion force of the FDL tendon at the DIP joint and the PIP joint, and establishes a secure attachment to the FDL to the proximal phalanx, making the FDL a strong flexor at the MTP joint. While theoretically this operation directly addresses the anatomical pathology, the operation is rather extensive and has the tendency to make the toe extremely stiff.
- A *fixed hammertoe deformity* is treated with a dorsal approach to the PIP joint, with either a resection arthroplasty or an arthrodesis. The proximal phalanx distal condyles are resected, and the toe is usually pinned in extension for 3 weeks. An FDL tentomy is sometimes performed as well.
- There is no clear advantage of arthrodesis over arthroplasty except in specific cases. Several clinical series have shown good results with both procedures, although slight misalignment is not unusual. Arthroplasty is technically somewhat easier to perform, but there can be late loss of alignment.
- Arthrodesis has the advantage of not needing a pin extending from the toe if an internal implant is used making the post-operative course easier. Arthrodesis is less likely to have a recurrence of the deformity so it may be a good choice for situations in which recurrence is likely such as revision toe surgery and severe deformity.
- Although rotational deformities are less common with arthodesis, a "cock-up" toe may be seen after surgery. The toe is straight at the interphalangeal joints but slightly dorsiflexed at the MTP, so that the pulp of the toe does not touch the ground. This may be more cosmetic than functional concern for most patients.
- A *flexible claw toe deformity* is generally treated similarly to a flexible hammertoe deformity, with a FDL flexor to extensor tendon transfer and an extensor tendon lengthening at the MTP joint if necessary.
- A *fixed claw toe deformity* is generally treated in a stepwise fashion from proximal to distal, attempting to correct the deformity. At each stage, if there is a question as to whether an appropriate amount of correction has been

obtained a *push-up test* is performed with the goal being to have the toe sit in a neutral alignment when the ankle is passively brought to neutral (Fig. 11–7).

- The MTP deformity is addressed with an EDL tendon Z-lengthening and EDB tenotomy. If the deformity remains, sequentially the MTP joint capsule is released, followed by the dorsal third of the medial and lateral collateral ligaments. Further correction may necessitate a metatarsal shortening osteotomy and/or Girdlestone-Taylor FDL tendon transfer.
- The *fixed claw toe deformity* at the PIP joint is treated with a PIP joint resection similar to a fixed hammertoe deformity.

Second Metatarsophalangeal Joint Instability

Introduction

- Second MTP joint instability is a painful condition arising as a result of the static and passive restraints of the MTP joint being overcome, resulting in a dorsal subluxation of the proximal phalanx on the metatarsal head during gait.
- Although acute rupture of the plantar plate can cause spontaneous second MTP joint instability, the more common situation is gradual attenuation of the plantar plate as the result of mechanical overload.
- This subluxation during the toe-off portion of gait causes irritation of the joint, which leads to pain and synovitis, which further stresses the static restraints of the joint, leading to further subluxation and a predictable pattern of toe deformity if left untreated.
- The most common cause of MTP joint instability is mechanical overload or abnormally concentrated pressure on the MTP joint. Predisposing factors need to be evaluated in the patient presenting with this problem, because oftentimes they need to be addressed to successfully treat the problem.
- A long second metatarsal, hypermobile first ray, hallux valgus deformity, equinus deformity, hallux rigidus, and hammertoe and claw toe deformities can all lead to increases in the second MTP joint pressures and begin the cycle of synovitis, static restraint compromise, and joint subluxation.
- Rheumatologic causes can also lead to synovitis in the joint with stretching or attenuation of the collateral ligaments of the joint, making the second toe less able to resist the second metatarsal mechanical overload during the gait cycle.

Anatomy and Pathophysiology

- The second toe is firmly attached at the proximal phalanx to the metatarsal through a thick plantar plate as well as medial and lateral collateral ligaments. The plantar plate acts to block dorsal translation of the MTP joint as it is loaded, but the collateral ligaments have been shown to provide up to 50% of the restraint of dorsal subluxation (Bhatia et al. 1994).
- The second metatarsal joint tends to be the longest in the foot, so increased forefoot pressures from any etiology will often present as second toe pathology, but if left unaddressed these same pressures can result in a third, then fourth, then fifth toe overload.
- As the second MTP joint becomes overloaded, the joint will begin to sublux, resulting in inflammation and swelling of the joint synovium. The synovitis will erode or stretch the collateral ligaments and plantar plate, which normally hold the toe in a reduced position throughout the gait cycle.
- The plantar plate is stronger at its insertion into the proximal phalanx and weaker at its insertion on the plantar metatarsal neck. An acute rupture will generally occur at the insertion at the metatarsal neck, but by far the more common situation will be a gradual attenuation of the plantar plate.
- As the static restraints of the toe are weakened, the toe will begin to sublux to a greater degree with less force exerted on it. At the MTP joint, the increased subluxation will mechanically make it difficult for the dynamic restraints (FDL, FDB, intrinsic muscles, and lumbricals) to resist subluxation of the toe, just as with a progressive claw toe deformity.
- As the toe continues to sublux with gait, the swelling and synovitis within the joint will increase and the static supports will be further compromised, causing the toe to drift up, and a flexible and then fixed hammertoe deformity will develop. With time as the collateral ligaments attenuate, a medial deviation may develop as well (crossover toe deformity).
- In the case of MTP joint instability, the patients will complain of pain secondary to the synovitis and swelling within the MTP joint; however, toe subluxation can cause a neuritic type of pain through two mechanisms.
    - The swelling of the MTP joint may put pressure on the neighboring nerves as they run out to the toe. As the toe subluxes out of the joint, the plantar nerves, tethered as they run under the intermetatarsal ligaments, are functionally stretched. This stretching may give neuritic symptoms in the first and second web space similar to a neuroma.

Diagnostic Evaluation

- Standing radiographs should be obtained similar to the evaluation of claw toes, hammertoes, and mallet toes to rule out other pathologies (i.e. stress fracture, MTP joint arthritis) that might account for the patient's pain.
- Radiographs should also be reviewed for predisposing causes of second MTP joint overload: hallux valgus, hallux rigidus, a long second metatarsal (> 4 mm longer than the adjacent metatarsals), or a disproportionately short first metatarsal (Morton foot).
- Radiographs that show loss of joint space at the MTP joint on an anteroposterior view of the foot need to be looked at with a lateral x-ray to see if this indicates joint subluxation, an arthritic joint, or a joint dislocation.

- The second metatarsal length can be classified as an index plus type (the first metatarsal is longer than the second), index plus-minus-type position (the first is equal to the second), or index minus type (the second metatarsal is longer than the first). Cortical hypertrophy of the second metatarsal seen on the anteroposterior radiograph may also give clues as to the relative weight bearing of the metatarsals.
- Bone scans will commonly show uptake in the area of the MTP joint, and will commonly be misread as a metatarsal stress fracture. A magnetic resonance imaging (MRI) scan is rarely needed to help make the diagnosis but will better delineate swelling in the joint and reactive bony changes from a distal metatarsal stress fracture.

History

- The history and examination are similar to those for hammertoe and claw toe deformities, with specific attention paid to those factors that may increase forefoot pressures, such as high heel shoe wear.
- With second MTP joint synovitis, patients will give a history of pain centered over the area of the second MTP joint. The pain will be worse with walking and better with rest. Many patients give the history that as they take longer strides the pain will get worse.
- A history of shooting pain into the toes or burning in the forefoot may indicate a traction neuritis or pressure along the nerve, but also may indicate the existence of a neuroma, which can accompany this condition.
- Acute second MTP joint instability will present with a patient giving the history of a "pop" in their foot after running or walking. The pop will be accompanied by swelling and pain in the area of the second MTP joint. With swelling in the forefoot, a rheumatologic history as well as a history of gout should be obtained.

Physical Examination

- With second MTP joint instability, subtle swelling on the dorsal aspect of the foot should be noted.
  - Occasionally, a separation of the second and the third toe can be seen. This is referred to as a *Y-toe deformity* and can indicate second MTP joint synovitis and chronic forefoot overload.
- The appearance of the foot should be noted, making special note of any coexisting hallux valgus deformity. The first ray should be examined for hypermobility (greater than 1 cm dorsal excursion of the first metatarsal head beyond the plane of the second and third metatarsal heads, when the first is passively pushed dorsally with one hand while the other hand stabilizes the second, third, fourth, and fifth metatarsal heads).
- Palpation of the foot should be performed, with particular attention paid over the metatarsals to rule out a stress fracture. Palpation of the intermetatarsal web spaces with attempts to elicit a Mulder click is important to rule out a coexistent Morton neuroma.
- Range of motion of the MTP joints, ankle joint, and first MTP joint is important.
  - Restricted range of motion of the ankle joint will lead to increased forefoot pressures, most commonly in the second MTP joint.
  - Restricted range of motion of the first MTP joint will tend to lead to a compensatory loading of the second MTP joint as the body passes over the foot in the stance phase of gait.
- The ankle should be checked for a heel cord contracture with the knee extended and flexed.
  - The *Silfverskiold test* performed with moderate dorsiflexion pressure on the ankle, and with the talonavicular joint held in a neutral position, should allow 10° of dorsiflexion of the ankle with the knee flexed and at least 5° with the knee extended (DiGiovanni et al. 2002).
- Evaluating the anterior drawer of the MTP joint is the critical test for establishing the diagnosis of second MTP joint instability. The maneuver should not only demonstrate instability of the second MTP joint, but should largely reproduce the patient's symptoms. Both sides should be compared to account for baseline or physiologic laxity.
- The anterior drawer test is performed as one hand grasps the foot along the MTP joints while the other grasps the proximal phalanx and gently applies pressure in a dorsal direction, attempting to sublux the joint (Fig. 11–8). The instability is graded 1, slight; 2, marked (50% subluxable); or 3, dislocateable (Thompson and Hamilton 1987).

Non-operative Treatment

- Non-operative treatment involves two parts: alleviating the patient's pain and then addressing the predisposing factors that may lead to recurrence.
- The non-operative treatment course is based on the severity of the symptoms. The patient should be counseled that the treatment goal is to decrease pain, and

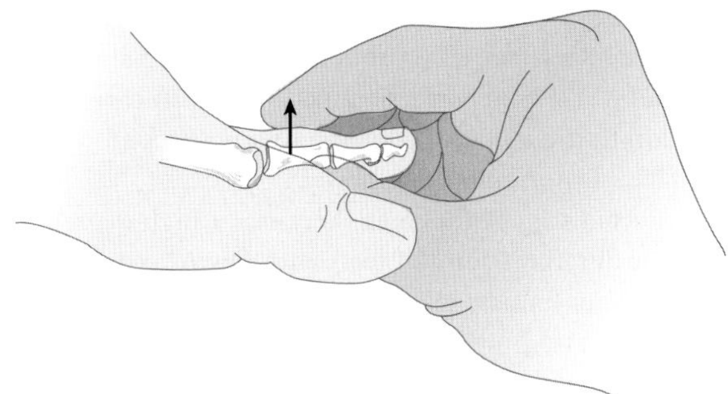

Figure 11–8: The "Lachman test" of the metatarsophalangeal joint to test for instability.

that any toe deformity that has occurred to this point most likely will remain without operative care.

- Mild discomfort can be treated with splinting or taping of the toe for several weeks to months, with unloading of the metatarsal head with a metatarsal pad or an orthosis. Symptoms will tend to resolve with strapping or taping of the toe, but symptoms will tend to recur once the taping or splinting is stopped.
- Severe discomfort and swelling can be treated with a stiff-soled rocker bottom modification of the shoe or rocker bar, or even a walking boot.
- A single steroid injection into the MTP joint can occasionally be helpful in ameliorating symptoms, but the mechanical factors that may have contributed to the forefoot overload should be addressed first (i.e. orthosis, or shoe modifications).
  - As by the very nature of the problem the capsular structures are diseased and weakened, a steroid injection may further weaken the structures. A steroid injection should only be used judiciously, and the MTP joint should be protected for at least 2 weeks after the injection.
- Addressing the patient's equinus deformity with a daily stretching program can be initiated after the initial acute phase has resolved. In the acute phase, stretching will tend to exacerbate the forefoot discomfort.

Surgical Treatment

- Surgical treatment for second MTP joint instability is reserved for the patient who has failed conservative treatment and has adequate vascular supply to heal a forefoot surgery.
- Second MTP joint instability can be addressed in one of three ways: FDL Girdlestone-Taylor flexor to extensor tendon transfer, plantar condylectomy and pinning, or metatarsal osteotomy.
- FDL Girdlestone-Taylor flexor to extensor tendon transfer has the advantages of allowing concomitant correction of angular deformity of the toe, as well as providing stability at the MTP joint. The major disadvantage of this procedure is that it can lead to extreme stiffness of the joint, which may be poorly tolerated.
- Although the transfer will correct the deformity well, if the second metatarsal is too long, there will be continued second MTP pain and inflammation. In this case, the tendon transfer can be combined with a second metatarsal shortening osteotomy.
- In a recent series of 64 feet, there was a high degree of patient dissatisfaction (14 feet) with flexor to extensor transfer, due in part to residual stiffness and swelling (Myerson and Jung 2005).
- Plantar condylectomy and pinning of the toe involve lengthening of the extensor tendons through a dorsal approach to the MTP joint, followed by release of the capsule and dorsal portion of the collateral ligaments. The toe is then plantar flexed, and a portion of the plantar metatarsal head is removed (one-quarter). The toe is reduced, plantar flexed slightly (10°), and pinned for 3 weeks, followed by a course of taping for another 3 weeks.
- Plantar condylectomy has the advantages of reducing the metatarsal functional length to a small degree and unloading the metatarsal. The toe maintains more flexibility than the tendon transfer and will allow athletic participation. The disadvantage is that the toe will still have some residual subluxation, but it usually is not symptomatic.
- A shortening metatarsal osteotomy as a treatment involves a dorsal approach to the MTP joint and extensor tendon lengthening, followed by an EDB tenotomy and a capsular release. A shortening osteotomy of the second metatarsal is then performed, which can be done in a number of different ways, most commonly in a long oblique manner or as a horizontal osteotomy (Fig. 11–9).
- The horizontal osteotomy (also known as a Weil osteotomy) is made parallel to the plantar surface of the foot through the dorsal aspect of the metatarsal head or just superior to the cartilage of the metatarsal head. The toe is shortened until it falls into the normal cascade between the first and third metatarsal heads, and then fixed with a screw. Pinning of the MTP joint is optional.
- Because the plane of the osteotomy is not parallel to the plantar surface of the foot, shortening with a horizontal (Weil) osteotomy displaces the metatarsal head plantarly. This can actually worsen metatarsal head pain.
- In theory, the ideal osteotomy is to excise a cylindric segment of the metatarsal shaft, such as an osteotomy is very unstable, requires, more rigid fixation, and has a higher non-union rate.
- A metatarsal osteotomy has the advantage of addressing uneven weight-bearing surface on the plantar aspect of the foot, but can lead to some MTP joint stiffness and an MTP joint dorsiflexion contracture.
- *Crossover toe deformity* is a lesser toe deformity that has a sagittal plane deformity as well as an axial plane deformity because of advanced instability at the MTP joint (Fig. 11–10).
  - This is a much more difficult deformity to correct compared with a purely sagittal plane deformity.
  - Surgical treatment depends on the degree of deformity, and often requires collateral ligament release with tightening of the opposing collateral ligament, an EDB tendon transfer, or a FDL flexor to extensor tendon transfer often combined with a metatarsal osteotomy.
- *Dislocation of the MTP joint* is treated with extensive soft tissue release and usually requires an FDL flexor to extensor tendon transfer, a metatarsal osteotomy, or a combination of both.

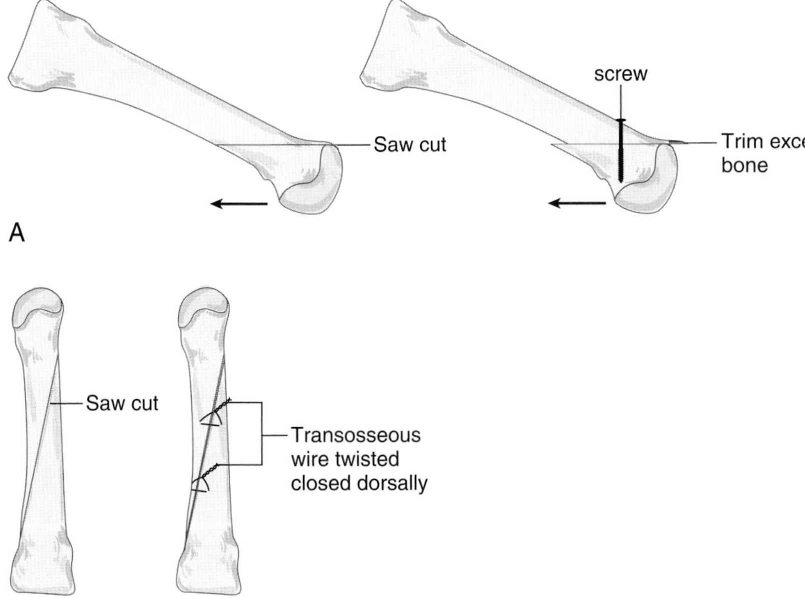

Figure 11–9: Distal horizontal metatarsal osteotomy **A**, and a long oblique vertical osteotomy **B**.

Additional Procedures

- A careful history and physical should attempt to detect predisposing factors that may lead to increased forefoot pressures, manifesting as second MTP joint instability. At the time of surgery, consideration of correcting these underlying deformities must be given in light of the degree of deformity present and the increased morbidity of the additional surgical procedures.

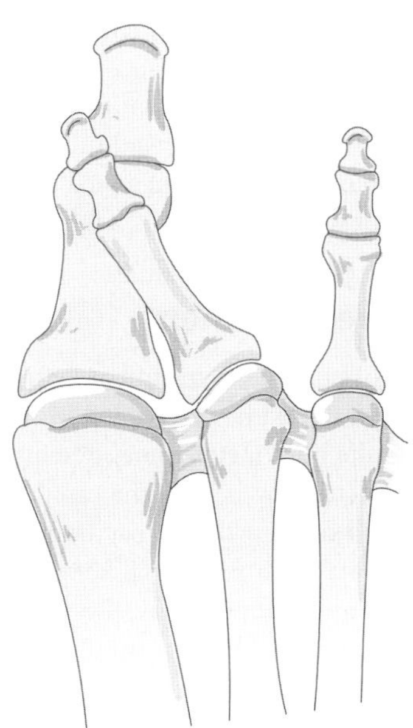

Figure 11–10: A crossover toe deformity resulting from a rupture of the lateral collateral ligament and plantar plate, and contracture of the medial collateral ligament.

- Hallux valgus deformity if severe should be addressed, especially if the lateral deviation of the great toe crowds out the space for the second toe with the foot weight bearing. If physical examination indicates a hypermobile first ray, the bunion deformity should be addressed with a Lapidus procedure (first MTC joint arthrodesis) at the time of the second toe procedure.
- Hallux rigidus can also contribute to second MTP joint instability by shifting the plantar pressures laterally during toe-off to compensate for an inability to roll over the great toe.
  - Severe hallux rigidus is generally addressed with an arthrodesis of the first MTP joint.
  - Moderate hallux rigidus can be addressed with a cheilectomy.
  - The pain relief produced by either procedure, and restoration of the MTP joint motion with a cheilectomy, will generally allow the normal toe-off gait to be restored.
- A heel cord contracture should generally be treated with either a heel cord lengthening or a gastrocnemius lengthening (Strayer procedure). Heel cord contracture will restrict the dorsiflexion of the ankle, increasing the forefoot pressures. Occasionally, anterior ankle osteophytes will similarly restrict ankle dorsiflexion and need to be resected to diminish forefoot stresses.

Bunionette Deformity

Introduction

- A bunionette deformity is the rough equivalent of hallux valgus deformity of the fifth toe. The prominence of the

lateral aspect of the fifth metatarsal head and/or a medial drift of the fifth toe proximal phalanx at the MTP joint results in a symptomatic protrusion on the lateral aspect of the foot.
- The bunionette deformity is also historically known as a tailor's bunion because of the tailor's crossed leg sitting position, which made the lateral aspect of the foot particularly prone to developing this problem.

Anatomy

- As the most lateral metatarsal, the fifth metatarsal is exposed laterally to pressure from ill-fitting shoe wear. The lateral aspect of the fifth metatarsal head is the lateral eminence, analogous to the medial eminence of the first metatarsal.
- The fifth toe shares similar anatomy with the other lesser toes, but with two differences. It does not receive a slip from EDB as do the other toes, and has an additional muscle, abductor digiti minimi, inserting on the lateral aspect of the proximal phalanx of the fifth toe. This muscle is analogous to the abductor hallucis of the great toe.

Pathophysiology

- Bunionette deformity will occur as a result of medially directed pressure on the fifth toe as a result of shoe wear. A small toe box will push the fifth toe over (adduction force) and exacerbate the prominence of the fifth metatarsal as well as provide pressure against the lateral eminence itself.
- Widening of the forefoot, secondary to hallux valgus deformity, may indirectly increase pressure on the lesser fifth toe and lead to the fifth toe mirroring the deformity of the great toe.

History

- A symptomatic bunionette deformity will present with pain with restrictive shoe wear, which resolves when the shoes are removed. The deformity will usually progress slowly, and the symptoms are usually gradual in onset.
- A history is taken similar to that for other lesser toe deformities. The patient should be questioned as to whether erythema or swelling has occurred over the lateral aspect of the foot. Episodes of skin breakdown should be elicited from the patient as well.
- Symptoms of low back pain or sciatica should be inquired about. The S1 nerve root, the most common nerve impingement in the lumbar spine, will often give symptoms of pain over the lateral aspect of the foot.
- A rheumatologic history should be obtained, as rheumatoid arthritis can result in the development of a bunionette deformity.

Physical Examination

- The overall standing posture of the foot should be examined for a concomitant hallux valgus deformity. The widening of the forefoot that accompanies a hallux valgus deformity will result in an exacerbation of lateral eminence pressure with shoe wear.
- The lateral aspect of the foot should be palpated, especially over the fifth metatarsal, for signs of a stress fracture. The palpation of the lateral eminence should reproduce the patient's symptoms.
- Strictly speaking, a bunionette deformity refers to the hyperkeratosis or bursitis that occurs over the lateral eminence of the fifth metatarsal, but occasionally an intractable plantar keratosis (IPK) may accompany the bunionette deformity, and this should be looked for under the metatarsal head and noted.
- If a fifth metatarsal plantar keratosis is found, then careful inspection of the foot posture is important to assess for a *varus forefoot* position. A varus or supinated foot will increase loading on the lateral column, including the fifth metatarsal. Treatment is then directed at realignment of the entire foot, not just the fifth metatarsal.

Diagnostic Tests

- Evaluation of a bunionette deformity necessitates standing radiographs of the foot to evaluate the deformity. Joint space narrowing and arthritis of the fifth MTP joint should be evaluated, as should the congruence of the proximal phalanx and the fifth metatarsal joint.
- There are two radiographic parameters that are useful in bunionette evaluation: the fourth-fifth intermetatarsal angle (IMA) (abnormal $> 8°$) and the fifth MTP angle (normal $< 10°$).
- A foot with a concomitant hallux valgus as a result of an increased first-second IMA, and a bunionette deformity with an increased fourth-fifth IMA, is referred to as a *splayfoot*.
- Based on the shape of the fifth metatarsal, the bunionette deformity is graded (Fig. 11–11).
  - A type 1 bunionette has a prominent lateral eminence.
  - A type 2 bunionette has a bowed metatarsal shaft.
  - A type 3 bunionette has an increased IMA.
- Classification of the bunionette is helpful in determining the appropriate surgical treatment.

Non-operative Treatment

- The mainstay of bunionette treatment is shoe modification. A wider toe box should be recommended to help accommodate the bunionette. Shoe stretching in the area over the bunionette may help in the case of leather shoes.
- A metatarsal pad or an orthosis may be helpful to relieve pain from a plantar fifth metatarsal keratosis. An orthosis with medial column support may also be helpful if the bunionette is aggravated by a planovalgus posture of the foot.

Operative Treatment

- Operative treatments for bunionette deformities are generally predicated on which type of bunionette

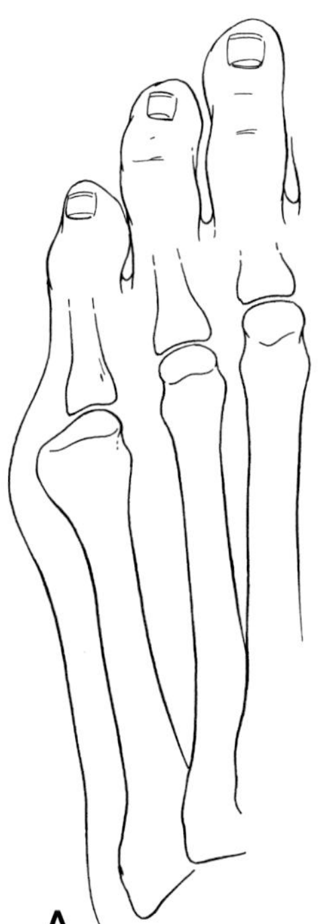

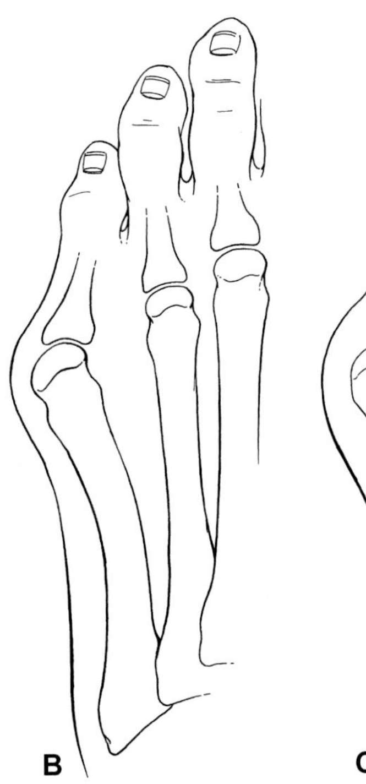

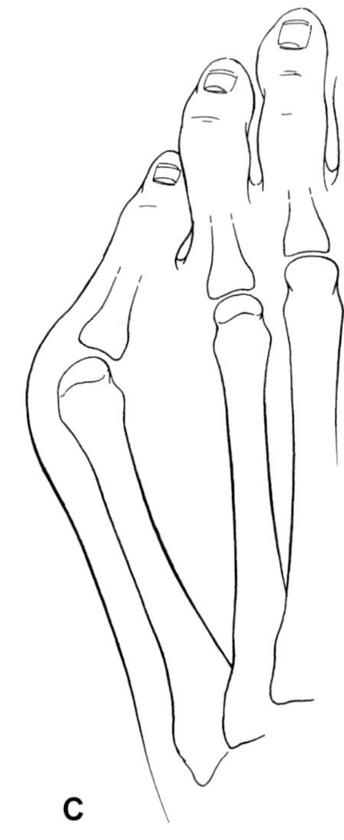

Figure 11–11: Types of bunionette deformities. **A,** Type 1 is associated with an enlarged lateral eminence. **B,** Type 2 is associated with a lateral bowing of the diaphysis. **C,** Type 3 is associated with an increase in the fourth-fifth intermetatarsal angle. (From Cooper PS. (2000) Disorders and deformities of the lesser toes. In: Foot and Ankle Disorders (Myerson M, ed.). Philadelphia: Saunders. p. 336.)

deformity exists and whether a plantar keratosis accompanies the deformity.

- Type 1 bunionettes are treated with a lateral eminence excision. The lateral portion of the metatarsal head is excised up to the border of the articular cartilage, in line with the lateral aspect of the foot, to produce a smooth lateral border. The lateral capsule is reefed and the medial capsule can be released if necessary, but unlike hallux valgus surgery—in which capsular tightening can potentially add some permanent correction to the deformity—over time the fifth toe will tend to be pushed back medially to its original position by the toe box once shoe wear is resumed.
- Because the soft tissues of the fifth toe allow little permanent correction of the toe angulation and the foot will not be significantly narrowed after the procedure, a pure lateral eminence excision procedure should be reserved for true type 1 bunionettes.
- Type 2 bunionettes with a bowed fifth metatarsal can be treated with a distal chevron osteotomy or a metatarsal shaft osteotomy.
- The distal chevron involves a lateral approach to the fifth metatarsal head, with a capsular incision through the lateral capsule and abductor digiti minimi tendon. The lateral eminence is exposed and resected in line with the lateral border of the foot.
- A chevron cut is then made in the metatarsal head/neck and the metatarsal head is shifted medially 3 mm, the proximal metatarsal prominence is resected, the osteotomy is fixed, and the capsule is tightened and closed.
- A chevron osteotomy gives good, stable correction for the mild deformity, but the correction (shifting of the head) is limited by the inherent narrowness of the metatarsal and the need to maintain sufficient bony contact at the osteotomy site. The complication associated with a chevron osteotomy is avascular necrosis of the metatarsal head, but this can be lessened by minimizing medial metatarsal dissection.
- The type 3 bunionettes and severe type 2 bunionettes can be treated with a metatarsal shaft osteotomy and lateral eminence excision. A long oblique osteotomy is favored with stable internal fixation, and the lateral eminence is resected in line with the metatarsal shaft.
- Many different shaft osteotomies have been described for bunionette deformity. The critical factor for selecting a shaft osteotomy is to avoid a metatarsal osteotomy through the proximal metatarsal diaphyseal junction. This area, because of its tenuous blood supply, has a poor healing potential.
- A plantar keratosis under the fifth metatarsal often accompanies bunionette deformity, although it in itself is not, in the strictest sense, a bunionette deformity. The keratosis indicates an overly prominent metatarsal head fibular condyle or a varus forefoot posture. It is recommended that this keratosis be addressed at the time of surgery either with a plantar condylectomy or with an elevation component to the metatarsal osteotomy. This may help relieve the problem, but it can also lead to a transfer lesion to the fourth metatarsal, especially if the underlying problem is a forefoot varus position.
- Metatarsal head resection for bunionette deformity is a good option in the rheumatoid arthritis patient if combined with resection of multiple metatarsal heads, but is not otherwise generally recommended because of its high complication rate of toe instability and transfer lesions.

- As with hallux valgus surgery, bunionette surgery complications include recurrence, incomplete relief of pain, painful scars, MTP joint subluxation, toe dislocation, and avascular necrosis in the case of the distal osteotomies. As with hallux valgus surgery, return to tight or ill-fitting shoe wear needs to be strongly discouraged.

Freiberg Infraction

Introduction

- Freiberg infraction is an osteochondrosis of the lesser metatarsal head. First described in 1914 and attributed to a traumatic etiology, current theory suggests that the condition results from a vascular insult to the subchondral bone.
- Freiberg infraction is most commonly seen in the second metatarsal but can occur in the third or fourth as well. It is seen predominantly in women in the age group of 11-17 years.
- This avascular necrosis of the metatarsal head initially leads to swelling and stiffness of the joint, and in its later stages leads to various degrees of subchondral collapse and arthritic changes of the MTP joint.

Diagnostic Tests

- Radiographs are reviewed to check for degenerative changes of the MTP joint and evaluate the second metatarsal length, which has been implicated as a predisposing factor in development of this condition.
- A high index of suspicion is necessary to make the diagnosis in its early stages, as Freiberg disease will often present with no significant radiographic findings. Bone scan or MRI may be helpful in diagnosis but will not generally alter clinical treatment.
- In its later stages, radiographs may demonstrate joint collapse, flattening of the metatarsal head, osteophytes, and joint narrowing.

Classifications

- The Hamilton and Thompson (1987) classification of Freiberg disease has four subgroups:
  - type 1—no articular cartilage lesion
  - type 2—peripheral osteophytes but no joint collapse
  - type 3—peripheral osteophytes and joint collapse, with articular destruction.
  - a rare type 4—described for multiple metatarsal involvement and attributed to an epiphyseal dysplasia.
- The Katcherian (1998) classification breaks down the first three Hamilton and Thompson subgroups into five levels
  - level A—partial fracture of the subchondral bone
  - level B—early subchondral collapse
  - level C—advanced subchondral collapse
  - level D—peripheral osteophytes and loose bodies
  - level E—severe degenerative changes, metatarsal head flattening, and loss of joint space.

Non-operative Treatment

- In the early stages of Freiberg infraction, the patient will present with a stiff, swollen joint, which is painful to flex or extend. The initial treatment is centered on restricting the motion at the MTP joint and decreasing swelling.
- During the acute inflammatory period, strapping or taping the toe to restrict dorsiflexion may be useful. Based on the degree of symptoms, a carbon fiber plate orthosis, a metatarsal pad, a rocker bar or a rigid rocker bottom sole modification to the shoe, or even a walker boot or cast can be used as well.
- A judicious use of a steroid injection into the MTP joint can be a useful adjunct to help alleviate pain but may make the arthritis component worse. Following an injection, the toe needs to be protected to avoid iatrogenic ligament injury.

Operative Intervention

- Freiberg infraction surgery needs to be tailored to the patient's particular symptoms, the degree of degeneration of the joint, and the area of joint involvement. All the surgical procedures are intended to alleviate symptoms, and the patient should be advised that progression of arthritic change of the joint may continue despite appropriate surgical care.
- If the cartilage injury is limited to the dorsal aspect of the joint, cheilectomy (debridement of the dorsal aspect of the metatarsal head) and debridement of the joint will help restore motion and give good symptomatic relief.
- If a larger portion of the metatarsal head is involved, but a significant plantar portion of the head is preserved, a closing wedge osteotomy through the metatarsal head and neck is recommended, although this procedure has the theoretic risk of further compromising the metatarsal head's blood supply and/or producing a transfer lesion. This procedure effectively dorsally rotates the portion of the head with intact cartilage so that it can articulate with the proximal phalanx.
- In the case of complete degeneration of the articular surface, two salvage operations can be considered: excision of the metatarsal head or proximal phalanx resection and capsular interposition arthroplasty.
  - Because both procedures can produce an unstable joint, significant transfer lesions, and a poor cosmetic appearance, they are not recommended if another reasonable surgical option is available.

Intractable Plantar Keratosis

Introduction

- An IPK forms on the sole of the foot under the metatarsal heads as a result of pressure on the underlying skin. The mechanical pressure causes an increase in activity of the skin's keratinocytes, which produces one of two types of IPK: discrete and diffuse (Fig. 11–12.).

- *Diffuse IPK*, often referred to as calluses, appears as relatively large areas of thickened skin, are rarely symptomatic, and are the result of the skin's response to pressure or shear forces exerted by the entire metatarsal head. While usually the result of mechanical overload of the forefoot, rheumatologic conditions or fat pad atrophy can contribute to its development.
- *Discrete IPK*, often referred to as corns, appears as small (2-3 mm), well-defined areas on the sole of the foot, and is the result of plantar pressure exerted on the skin overlying the metatarsal head fibular condyle.

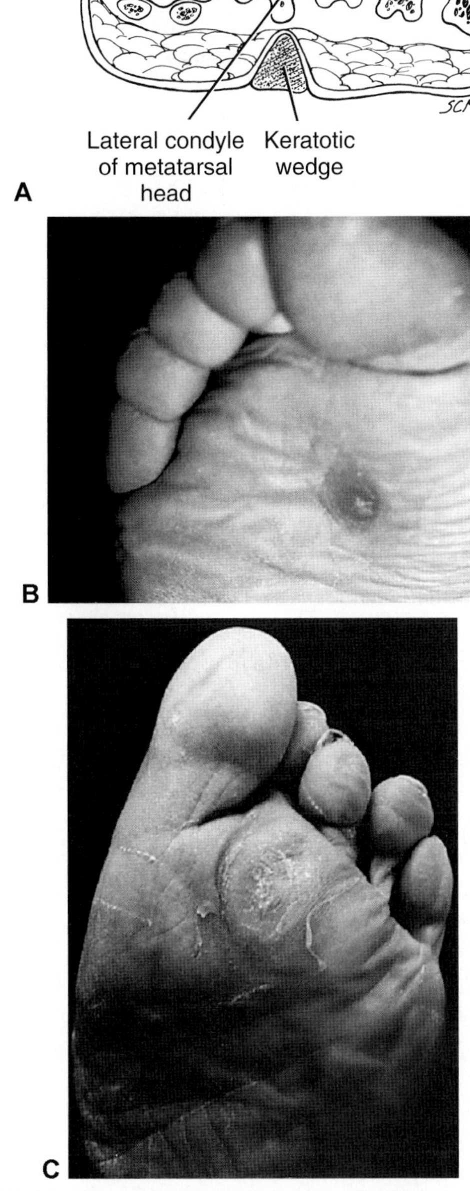

Figure 11–12: **Plantar keratosis. A, Prominent fibular condyle of the metatarsal head resulting in an intractable plantar keratosis (IPK). B, IPK beneath the second metatarsal head. C, Diffuse IPK or callus under the second metatarsal head in hammertoe deformity. (From Murphy GA. (2003) Lesser toe abnormalities. In: Campbell's Operative Orthopaedics, 10th edn. (Canale, ST, ed.). Philadelphia: Mosby. p. 4066.)**

History and Physical Examination

- Diffuse IPK will rarely be symptomatic, but the symptomatic patient will complain of pain under the metatarsal head that is worse in bare feet and better with shoe wear.
- Mechanical sources of increased pressure on the forefoot should be sought, including an equinus deformity, restricted ankle motion, varus forefoot deformity, cavus foot deformity, a Morton's foot, a hypermobile first ray, lengthened second metatarsal, history of high heel shoe wear, and claw toe deformities.
- Discrete IPK will present with patients complaining that they feel like they are walking with a pebble in their shoe. The pain is of a progressive nature, will be activity related, and will often times seem to be out of proportion to the size of the lesion.
- Discrete IPK can be confused with certain dermatologic conditions, most commonly a plantar wart. A discrete IPK should appear as a 2- to 3-mm area with the skin lines coursing through it. It should be centered over the fibular condyle of a metatarsal head, and it should be painful with direct pressure but not with moderate side to side pinching.
- A plantar wart can appear on any area of the foot, and it can be of any size. After it is pared down, it will have a punctate or stippled appearance secondary to the pattern of the wart's blood vessels as they travel to the surface of the lesion. Generally, it will be tender with direct as well as side to side pressure.
  - When evaluating a suspected IPK, multiple areas of involvement, areas of involvement other than under the metatarsal heads, and areas in which the skin lines do not travel through the "corn" suggest a wart rather than an IPK.

Diagnostic Tests

- Radiographs are primarily useful in evaluating underlying foot abnormalities, which may be contributing to the formation of increased pressure on the metatarsal and the formation of an IPK (such as a Morton foot or a long second metatarsal).
  - A sesamoid view of the foot can be useful to demonstrate the relative prominence of the metatarsal heads and their corresponding fibular condyles.
- A paper clip or other marker can be taped to the foot over the area of the IPK prior to obtaining the radiographs in order to demonstrate the exact location of the IPK in relation to the osseous anatomy.

Non-operative Treatment

- Non-operative treatment for discrete IPK involves trimming the corn and surrounding callus with a scalpel. This should lead to instant improvement in weight-bearing symptoms, and will help confirm that the area is not a plantar wart, which will demonstrate a diagnostic punctate bleeding pattern with trimming, not easily confused with the avascular corn's appearance.
- Patients with an IPK can use a pumice stone after showering or bathing to slowly reduce the thickness of the callus.
- Over the counter salicylic acid patches or topical liquid may be useful in softening up the corn so that the patient can more easily manually remove it. A metatarsal pad appropriately placed in the shoe proximal to the area of discomfort may help reduce pressure on the metatarsal head, as can a custom-molded insert.

Operative Treatment

- Operative treatment is aimed at removing the underlying bony prominence and addressing the mechanical factors leading to the formation of the IPK. Elipsing the IPK and its surrounding skin should not be done, as this will simply replace the IPK with a painful scar.
- In cases where an IPK is due to an elevated adjacent metatarsal (fracture malunion) or a hypermobile first metatarsal (so the IPK is under the second metatarsal head), treatment should include realignment of the adjacent metatarsal.
- A discrete IPK can be treated with a plantar condylectomy with pinning of the involved metatarsal. The MTP joint is approached dorsally, and the EDB tendon is cut while the EDL is Z lengthened. The joint is plantar flexed, and the dorsal portion of the collateral ligaments is released. The plantar condyles are exposed with a metatarsal head retractor, and the plantar condyles are resected parallel to the plantar surface of the foot.
- A plantar condylectomy will remove approximately one-third to one-quarter of the plantar metatarsal head. To avoid recurrence, it is important not to leave any residual bony prominences on the plantar aspect of the metatarsal head.
- A diffuse IPK is treated with a metatarsal osteotomy to unload some of the weight-bearing pressure on the metatarsal. The osteotomy can be performed at the proximal base of the metatarsal with a dorsal closing wedge osteotomy; at the diaphysis by either removing a section of the diaphysis or making a long, oblique osteotomy to shorten the metatarsal; or at the distal aspect of the metatarsal with a horizontal osteotomy.
- Complications from surgical correction of an IPK are primarily recurrence and transfer lesions. The patient should be advised that, post correction, a custom orthosis may be necessary to further compensate for pressure variations of the forefoot.

Interdigital Corns

Introduction

- Corns are discrete areas of dense hyperkeratinization that form as the result of external pressure on the skin overlying a bony prominence. Two types of corns form on the toes: hard corns and soft corns.
- Hard corns commonly occur over the exposed surface of the fifth toe in response to pressure from a shoe box. Hard corns will typically form over the lateral aspect of the PIP or DIP joint of the fifth toe.
- Soft corns are lesions similar to hard corns, but soft corns form between the toes and have a unique macerated appearance because they are kept moist from opposition of the neighboring toes (Fig. 11–13). Soft corns most commonly occur between the fourth and fifth toes but can occur between other toes.
- Soft corns are produced by the impingement of the bony prominences of adjacent toes, and as such are often given the term "kissing corns." A tight toe box plays a role in increasing the pressure between the toes, but once the corn forms it often becomes a self-perpetuating problem as the hard keratin core of the corn acts as a constant mechanical irritant.

History

- The patient will often present with other forefoot complaints as well as the interdigital corns. Often, the patients will be somewhat embarrassed by the degree of pain associated with this small area.
  - Although ill-fitting shoes often contribute to the problem, by the time the patient seeks medical care a change in shoe wear alone usually will not solve the problem.
- Patients with diabetes may present unaware of the formation of these corns, as they often are hidden from view. The soft corns in a diabetic patient represent a preulcerative state, and they need to be addressed. Breaks in skin continuity can lead to infection under the callus and abscess in the web space.

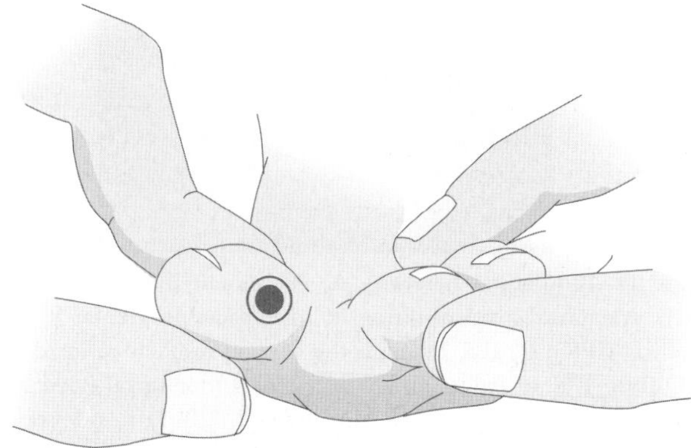

Figure 11–13: Soft interdigital corn on the medial aspect of the small toe.

Physical Examination

- The key to the physical examination is identifying the area of the corn and the bony prominences responsible for the corns. In the case of interdigital corns, the contributions of both toes to the impingement must be identified.
- Unstable interphalangeal joints need to be identified. The constant rubbing of adjacent condyles can lead to attrition of the collateral ligaments, and angular deformity can occur, which leads to a greater joint and condyle prominence as the toe bows. Previous lesser toe surgery can also lead to instability of the toes.
- Hallux valgus deformity should be evaluated, as it can result in stuffing of the toe box causing the lesser toes to impinge on one another.

Diagnostic Tests

- Radiographs are the standard method to visualize the bony osteophytes or prominences that are invariably underlying the corns. Radiographic markers or cut portions of paper clips can be taped to the areas of the corns to help visualize the exact structures involved.

Non-operative Treatment

- Non-operative treatment begins with toe sponge spacers, silicon toe pads, or oval sponge rubber corn pads, but patients need to understand that they need a wider toe box to accommodate the toes—even more so with the spacer inserted between the toes, because it will further stuff the toe box.
- Hard corns on the outside of the fifth toe can often be treated by trimming of the corn and application of salicylic acid corn pads combined with routine callus debridement after showering or bathing with a punnice store.
- Soft corns are best treated with removing the callus with a scalpel, and then allowing the toes to dry with a wisp of lamb's wool placed between the toes to allow the moisture to wick out from between the toes. Diabetic patients and other patients who lotion their feet for dry skin should be instructed not to apply lotion between the toes. Using drying agents between the toes, such as rubbing alcohol or carbolfuchsin, has also been advocated.

Operative Treatment

- The chief principle of operative care for hard and soft corns is to remove the bony prominences responsible for the corn formation without trading the corn for a painful scar. The incisions need to be full thickness and be in areas where the residual scar will not impinge.
- One way to address both hard and soft corns is to remove the underlying osteophytes. An incision is made dorsally, centered over the area of the corn. Full-thickness flaps are made down on to the bone and then the bony prominences are removed. The osteophytes on both adjacent toes need to be removed in line with the shaft of the toe.
- The goals of surgery are to create a smooth bony surface for the digit, and not to over-resect an area of prominence and create other areas of impingement.
  - If too much of the joint is removed, it can be destabilized, which will lead to recurrence. Resection should be limited to one-third or less of the joint. If the joint is unstable after the prominences are removed, it should be temporarily pinned.
- A second way to address the soft corn when the corn is located at the skin fold of the web space is to perform a partial syndactylization and eliminate the area of skin irritation altogether.
- A partial syndactylization to the PIP joint is preferred, because it still allows a space between the toes and is fairly cosmetic. A skin marker is used to mark the area of skin resection on the one toe, and then the toes are pressed together to make an imprint on the neighboring toe. The skin is then incised and the two adjacent skin flaps are sewn together.
- Rarely, the soft corn is partially the result of an unstable interphalangeal joint and the joint prominence that is created as the toe books medially or laterally. In these rare instances, in addition to removing bony prominences the interphalangeal joint of the toe needs to be fused to prevent recurrence of the deformity.
- Complications of treatment of interdigital corns include persistent swelling (6-9 months) and recurrence, especially if the patient returns to wearing poor-fitting shoes.

References

Bhatia D, Myerson MS, Curtis MJ et al. (1994) Anatomical restraints to dislocation of the second metatarsophalangeal joint and assessment of repair technique. J Bone Joint Surg Am 76: 1371-1375.

The forces required to dislocate the MTP joint were examined in 15 cadaver feet in which the long tendons were preserved and tensioned and the plantar plate and collateral ligaments were divided in different combinations.

Coughlin MJ, Mann RA. (1993) Lesser toe deformities. In: Surgery of the Foot and Ankle, 6th edn (Coughlin MJ, Mann RA, eds.) St. Louis: Mosby-Year Book. pp. 341-465.

The chapter discusses the current knowledge concerning lesser toe deformities, including the anatomy, etiology, diagnosis, and operative and non-operative treatments.

DiGiovanni CW, Kuo R, Tejwani N et al. (2002) Isolated gastrocnemius tightness. J Bone Joint Surg Am 84: 962-970.

A prospective comparison of ankle dorsiflexion and gastrocnemius tightness in a patient population with forefoot and/or midfoot symptoms compared with a control group.

Katcherian DA. (1998) The treatment of Freiberg's disease. In: Foot and Ankle Clinics: Lesser Toe Deformities (Richardson EG, Myerson MS, eds.). Philadelphia: Saunders. pp. 323-344.

A detailed review of the current literature with regard to Freiberg disease, including a discussion of the author's own classification system and surgical treatment techniques.

Morton DJ. (1935) The Human Foot: Its Evolution, Physiology and Functional Disorders. New York: Columbia University Press.

This text discusses the phylogeny of the foot and how its structure contributes to various foot pathologies.

Myerson MS, Jung HG. (2005) The role of flexor-to-extensor transfer in correcting metatarsophalangeal joint instability of the second toe. Foot Ankle Int 26(9): 675-679.

A series of patients treated with flexor-to-extensor tendor transfer for second MTP instability are reviewed. The results were confounded by additional procedures performed for related problems in a majority of the feet. Although the majority of toes were quite improved in alignment and stability, patient's reported dissatisfaction with stiffness and residual axial and sagittal plane deformity.

Thompson F, Hamilton W. (1987) Problems of the second metatarsophalangeal joint. Orthopaedics 10: 83-89.

Second MTP joint problems are reviewed. Second MTP joint instability is discussed, a grading system is proposed, and an anterior drawer test ("positive Lachman") for the second MTP joint is described. A classification of Freiberg disease is also presented.

Common Pediatric Foot and Ankle Conditions

Craig P. Eberson[*] and Jonathan Schiller[§]

[*]M.D., Assistant Professor, Department of Orthopaedics, Division of Pediatric Orthopaedics and Scoliosis, Brown Medical School, Hasbro Children's Hospital, Providence, RI
[§]M.D., Department of Orthopaedics, Brown Medical School/Rhode Island Hospital, Providence, RI

Clubfoot

Introduction

- Talipes equinovarus (TEV), or clubfoot, is a common disorder seen in roughly 1 in 1000 live births.
- Forty percent are bilateral.
- TEV may result from intrauterine molding and be completely passively correctable, the so-called positional clubfoot, or it may be rigid.
- Clubfeet may be associated with underlying disorders such as myelomeningocele, Larsen syndrome, and Streeter dysplasia (constriction band syndrome), as well as other inherited conditions. It may be seen as an isolated condition (idiopathic).
- Initial treatment consists of ruling out associated conditions, followed by a course of non-operative treatment, with surgery reserved for recalcitrant cases.

Etiology

- The etiology of TEV is probably multifactorial.
- Theories have included an arrested stage of normal fetal development, abnormal connective tissue, or a neurologic etiology.
- Involvement of the entire lower limb (the calf is often significantly smaller than the contralateral side in a unilateral deformity) points to a dysplasia involving more than simply the foot.
- Positional clubfeet may be caused by intrauterine crowding seen with oligohydramnios, large birth weight, and multiple births.

Clinical Presentation

- Examination of a baby with TEV requires a thorough evaluation to rule out associated conditions.
- The spine, hips, and upper extremities should be closely inspected, as should the remainder of the lower extremity.
- A neurologic examination should be performed to rule out a paralytic clubfoot, as seen in spina bifida.
- Concomitant lower extremity contractures suggest arthrogryposis or Beal's syndrome.
- The absence of hip dysplasia should be confirmed.
- Examination of the foot entails evaluation of the forefoot (adduction), the midfoot (cavus), the hindfoot (varus and equinus), and the amount of internal rotation of the foot. The degree of deformity and its correctability should be determined. The presence of medial and posterior creases should be noted, as well as the general condition of the leg musculature (Fig. 12–1).
- Further evaluation, such as magnetic resonance imaging (MRI) of the neural axis, may be required, depending on clinical findings.

Radiologic Imaging

- Kite angles are most commonly used. These are the talocalcaneal angle measured on the anteroposterior and

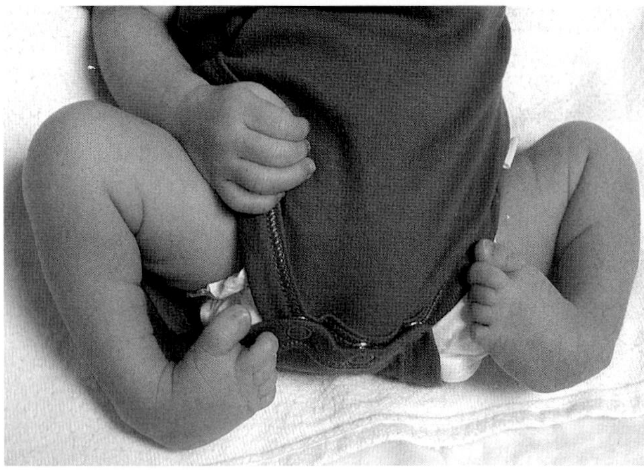

Figure 12–1: Child with bilateral clubfeet. Note the extreme internal rotation. This child's condition was diagnosed antenatally by ultrasound. After successful correction using the Ponseti method of clubfoot manipulation, the condition recurred due to non-compliance with the brace. His parents elected not to try an additional trial of casting, and he underwent bilateral posteromedial releases.

lateral radiographs. Because of the deformity of the foot, these radiographs should be taken with the beam aligned relative to the hindfoot.

- In a clubfoot, the Kite angle is usually less than 20° on the anteroposterior view, and less than 25° on the lateral view. In essence, the talus and the calcaneus are parallel rather than convergent.
- While radiographs can be used to follow treatment results, there is significant variability in the measurements due to difficulty in positioning the foot, incomplete ossification of the bones of the foot, and difficulty determining the axis of the talus and calcaneus. Clinical examination of the foot must also be used to make treatment decisions.

Non-operative Treatment

- The initial treatment of TEV is non-operative. While many descriptions of manipulative treatment exist, that of Ignacio Ponseti, M.D., of Iowa is the method most commonly used (Ponseti 1996). While the details of his method may be reviewed in detail in his book, the general concepts bear mentioning. A firm understanding of the pathologic anatomy is necessary to properly manipulate the foot.
- Casts are applied every 5-7 days until the foot is corrected. First, the forefoot is supinated by dorsiflexing the first ray in order to eliminate the cavus deformity. Although the foot appears supinated in a clubfoot deformity, the first ray is actually *pronated* with respect to the hindfoot. Rather than pronating the foot, which is the basis of other treatment methods, supinating the foot allows the forefoot to align with the hindfoot. With a thumb applying pressure to the talus (*not* the calcaneus), the foot is externally rotated and then gradually allowed to pronate in order to correct the varus. Finally, the foot is dorsiflexed. Applying a dorsally directed force without sufficient hindfoot flexibility may result in a break in the midfoot, the so-called rocker bottom deformity.
- Often, a percutaneous Achilles tenotomy is performed in the office to allow the foot to dorsiflex properly. When the foot is in the corrected position, the final cast is left in place for 3 weeks (Fig. 12–2). Straight last shoes connected to a Dennis Brown bar are then used full time for 3 months, followed by nighttime use until after walking age.

Surgical Treatment: Primary Procedures

- An understanding of the pertinent normal anatomy is crucial. While the details are beyond the scope of this chapter, it is important to know the relationship between the bony anatomy and neurovascular structures in the

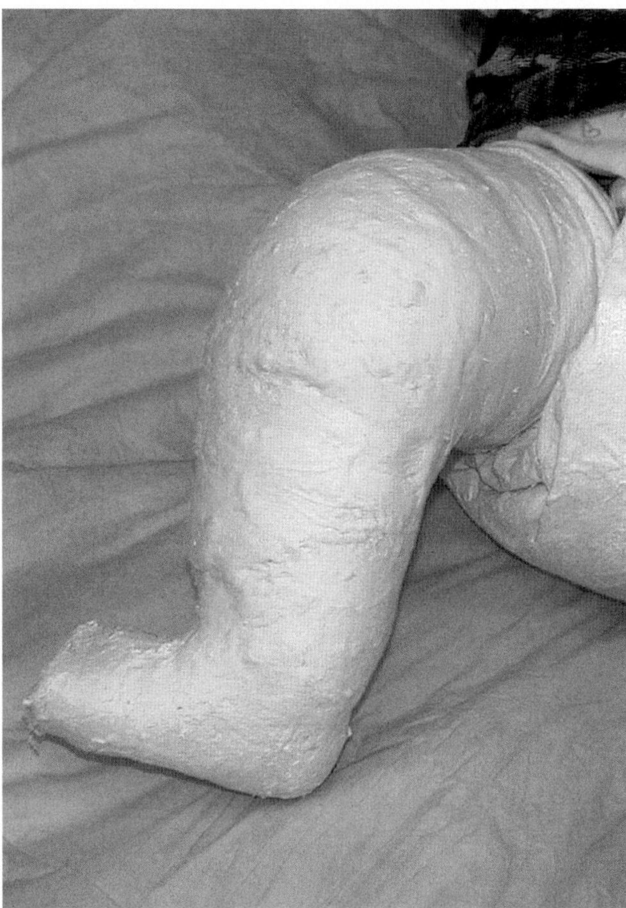

Figure 12–2: The last cast applied to a patient undergoing serial casting for congenital clubfoot. The foot is dorsiflexed 15°, having just undergone a percutaneous Achilles tenotomy. Note the significant external rotation necessary to avoid recurrence.

normal foot to understand how they relate in a clubfoot (Cummings et al. 2002).

- The approach will vary depending on age of patient, prior treatment, and degree of deformity.
- Surgery is best performed between 9 and 12 months of age. This allows proper visualization of anatomical structures, prevents extensive scarring seen with neonatal surgery, and allows the child to be weight bearing soon after surgery, which helps to maintain a plantigrade foot.
- Release involves systematic release of all involved structures until deformity is corrected.
- Our preferred technique is to begin with a Cincinnati incision and to identify and protect the neurovascular bundle, followed by a release of the posterior ankle and subtalar joints. The foot is then assessed, and the medial portions of the joints released as well, taking care not to cut the deep deltoid ligament. Again, the foot is reassessed, and if needed the talonavicular joint is opened, the spring ligament sectioned, and the navicular reduced. If significant cavus still exists, the plantar fascia is released as well. Finally, if a bean shape is still present in the foot, a calcaneocuboid release can be performed by working plantar and lateral to the talonavicular joint. Occasionally, the Cincinnati incision can be continued laterally to perform this release.
- Also included may be lengthening of the following tendons: flexor hallucis longus, flexor digitorum longus, tibialis posterior, and Achilles. *Care should be taken not to over-lengthen the Achilles tendon.*
- Pinning of the talonavicular and subtalar joints may be required to maintain position in addition to casting. These are usually removed at 6 weeks, followed by an additional 6 weeks of walking casts. An ankle-foot orthosis may be used following casting in selected patients.

Surgical Treatment: Secondary Procedures and Revision Surgery

- Recurrence of a clubfoot should prompt further investigation to rule out an underlying cause (i.e. tethered spinal cord).
- The choice of procedure depends on the nature of the residual deformity. These secondary procedures are also often needed in the treatment of patients who present for treatment at an older age.
- The specific components of the recurrent clubfoot should be evaluated to design a surgical plan. Residual forefoot supination, hindfoot varus, internal rotation, equinus, or muscle weakness may all need to be addressed. As in any foot deformity, the surgical plan should be to correct flexible deformities through tendon balancing, and correct rigid deformities with soft tissue release (if applicable) or osteotomy.
- If the first procedure involved a less than complete release, and the child is young (i.e. less than 4 years), a repeat release may be attempted, although the surgeon should weigh this against the likelihood of increased scarring from repeat surgery.
- Transfer of the anterior tibial tendon to the midfoot may be helpful in addressing a dynamic supination deformity that is causing overload of the lateral column of the foot. Ponseti and colleagues routinely perform this procedure in patients who have undergone casting and have a residual dynamic supination deformity.
- Weakness of the triceps surae from over-lengthening of the Achilles tendon is difficult to overcome. Transfer of local tendons to augment plantar flexion, such as the posterior tibialis, flexor hallucis longus, or peroneals, has been described. Unfortunately, normal strength is usually not realized, emphasizing the importance of the primary repair.
- Osteotomy is also a valuable tool. A residual bean shape of the foot can often be corrected via a lateral column shortening. This may be done in the form of a distal calcaneal resection (Lichtblau procedure), a calcaneocuboid fusion (Evans procedure), or a cuboid decancellation.
- Residual heel varus may be addressed with a calcaneal osteotomy. A Dwyer closing wedge osteotomy or a sliding osteotomy will allow the weight-bearing line to move more laterally. This is often combined with other procedures.
- Occasionally, patients will have a plantigrade foot with significant residual medial rotation, leading to a severe intoeing gait. A supramalleolar derotational osteotomy is helpful in these patients.
- For severe residual deformity, gradually correcting the deformity using an external fixator may be helpful in avoiding neurovascular or skin compromise associated with rapid surgical correction.
- After the age of 10, triple arthrodesis is often the procedure of choice.

Complications of Surgical Treatment

- Complications may include inadequate correction of the initial deformity, infection, ischemia with soft tissue loss, and others. The vascularity of the clubfoot is not normal, and failure to protect the medial neurovascular bundle, and/or postoperative swelling, may compromise the foot. Often, the anterior tibial artery is hypoplastic or absent. Infection that requires removal of fixation invites loss of position and may lead to a worse deformity than seen preoperatively.
- Aggressive release, including sectioning of the talocalcaneal interosseous ligament, may lead to a valgus overcorrection if care is not taken. This deformity is difficult to treat, often requiring an opening wedge triple arthrodesis. A lateral column lengthening, combined with a medial column shortening, is also an option. For this reason, most authors do not recommend a complete release of this structure.

- A dorsal bunion is seen when the peroneus longus is weakened or cut, leading to unopposed pull of the anterior tibialis combined with "over-pull" of the toe flexors. Treatment involves realignment of the first ray through tendon release or transfer and osteotomy.
- Subluxation of the navicular can be seen as well, arising from incomplete release or reduction of the navicular, or loss of fixation. Re-reduction can be attempted in young children (i.e. less than 6) if treatment for the resulting foot deformity is required.

Flatfeet

Introduction

- Flatfeet are a common cause for concern for parents but usually require no treatment. Of primary importance is distinguishing painless, flexible flatfeet from painful or rigid feet.
- A rigid flatfoot suggests the presence of a tarsal coalition, congenital vertical talus (CVT), or neurogenic flatfoot from Achilles contracture. A painful flatfoot may be due to the above, as well as due to an accessory navicular, an inflamed subtalar joint from inflammatory arthritis, or a hypermobile foot associated with increased ligamentous laxity. Most of these conditions will be covered in other parts of this chapter (Box 12–1).

Etiology of Flexible Flatfoot

- The primary issue is one of "sag" of the midfoot, which results from ligamentous laxity. This may be laxity typical of a young child or associated with a collagen vascular disorder.
- Also contributory is a tight heel cord; in order for the heel to strike the ground during gait, the foot everts, thus unlocking the subtalar joint. This causes a collapse at the level of the midfoot and a flatfooted appearance.

History

- As always, a good history is paramount. It is important to determine the reason for the visit (i.e. pain, deformity, grandmother's insistence). If painful, the location of the pain is important. The onset of the deformity (i.e. congenital or recent onset), a family history, and review of symptoms should also be obtained. Prior treatment and/or surgery should be noted.

Box 12–1 Differential Diagnosis of Flatfeet

Congenital

- Tarsal coalition
- Congenital vertical talus
- Calcaneovalgus foot
- Infantile benign (flexible) flatfeet
- Accessory navicular

Acquired

- Achilles contracture
- Spastic flatfoot
- Inflammatory subtalar arthritis
- Collagen vascular disorder

Physical Examination (Fig. 12–3)

- Causes of increased ligamentous laxity should be sought (i.e. Marfan syndrome).
- Angular deformity of the lower extremity should be noted. Young children with physiologic valgus at the knee (age 3-5 years) will often appear flat-footed due to collapse at the ankle joint. This condition usually resolves as the valgus corrects spontaneously.
- A neurologic examination should be done to rule out increased muscle tone (i.e. spastic flatfoot) or other neuromuscular condition.
- The examination of the foot should include:
  - Heel cord flexibility. With the knee extended and the foot inverted, the amount of dorsiflexion is noted.
  - Callus pattern. Normally, there should be callus on the plantar heel and the first metatarsal head, as well as diffusely over the remaining metatarsals. Presence of increased callus, redness, or skin breakdown over the arch or the medial great toe indicates a planovalgus posture during gait.
  - Subtalar motion. This can be checked by inverting and everting the foot while the hindfoot is held steady. Alternatively, patients are asked to walk on the medial then lateral borders of their feet.
  - Arch at rest (non-weight bearing) and with toe raise. A flexible flatfoot has a normal arch while sitting, as well as with toe raise. During toe raise, the heel should

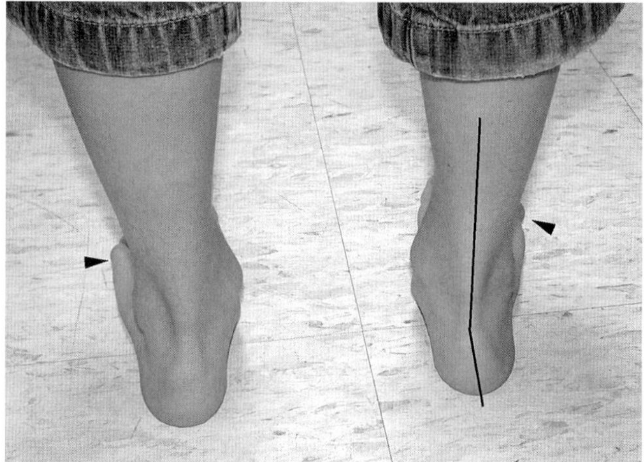

Figure 12–3: Flexible flatfeet. The heel is in valgus, with the weight-bearing stress transferred to the medial column of the foot. The compensatory forefoot abduction that results from a break in the midfoot leads to the "too many toes" sign (arrowheads). Normally, the lateral toes are not visible when the foot is viewed from behind.

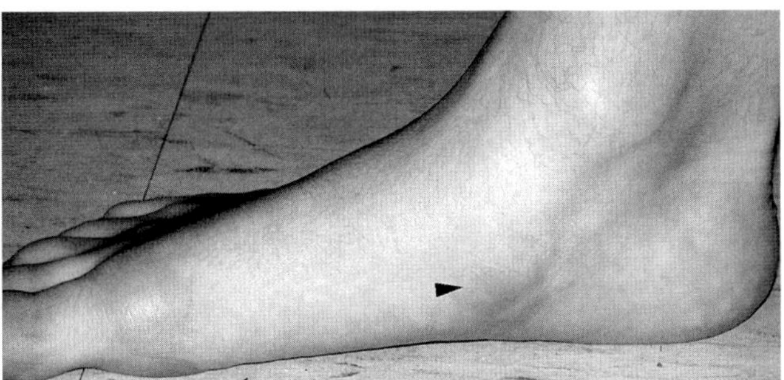

Figure 12–4: **Flatfoot associated with an accessory navicular. The arch is flat, and there is erythema, callus formation, and tenderness over the navicular (arrowhead).**

be seen to move into varus as well. This is not the case with a rigid foot seen with a tarsal coalition. The Jack test consists of dorsiflexing the great toe, which should cause the arch to form in a seated patient.

- Specific areas of pain. These may point to other diagnoses, such as accessory navicular or osteochondritis (Fig. 12–4).

Radiographs

- Radiographic examination should begin with weight-bearing anteroposterior, lateral, and oblique plain films (Fig. 12–5).
- If an accessory navicular is suspected, an oblique taken with the beam angled medially 45° may be obtained (Fig. 12–6).
- Computed tomography (CT) scanning is helpful to rule out the presence of a tarsal coalition.
- Unilateral foot deformities should prompt a thorough neurologic examination, and MRI may be indicated to rule out a tethered cord, lipomeningocele, etc.

Treatment

- Treatment options include reassurance, Achilles stretching, arch supports, and surgery.
- For the majority of patients with flexible flatfeet, no treatment is needed. For those with a tight Achilles tendon, daily stretching may offer some benefit.
- If the feet are painful from collapse of the arch and medial skin irritation, a cushioned arch support may be

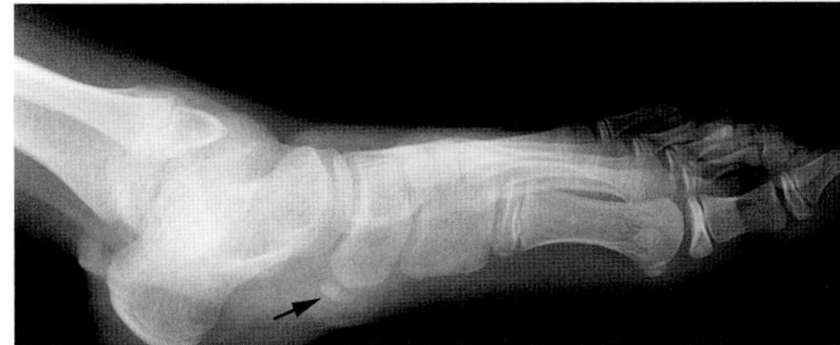

Figure 12–6: **Medial oblique radiograph demonstrating an accessory navicular (arrow).**

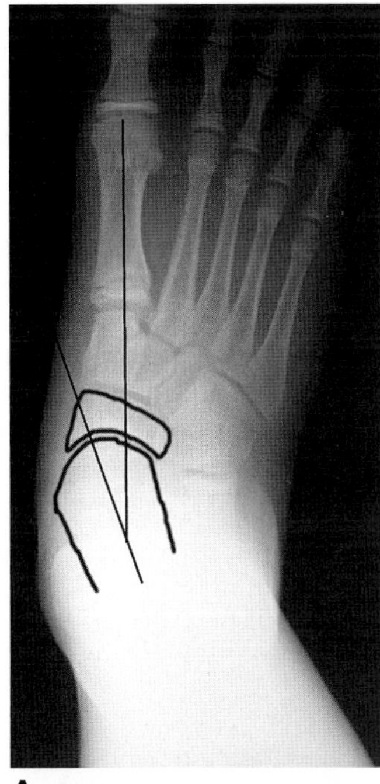

A

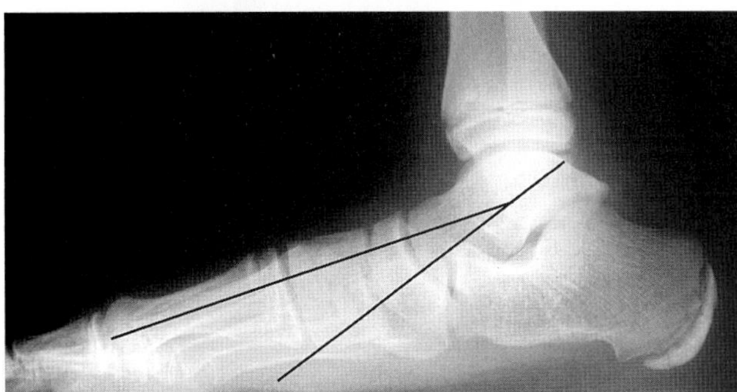

B

Figure 12–5: **Anteroposterior and lateral (standing) views of a flexible flatfoot. A, The talus is significantly uncovered by the navicular due to abduction of the forefoot, and becomes a weight-bearing structure, leading to pain. Note the divergence of the talus-first metatarsal angle (TFMTA). B, Lateral view of the same foot. There is a significant "sag" of the midfoot, measured by an increased TFMTA, as well as decreased calcaneal pitch. Note the loss of the normal arch.**

helpful. A more rigid University of California Biomechanics Laboratory insert is occasionally helpful for more severe feet, but many children do not tolerate a rigid orthosis.

- Treatment with shoe inserts will not alter the eventual shape of the feet.
- Patients with intractable symptoms despite maximized non-operative treatment may benefit from surgery.
- Arthrodesis, using silicone or Silastic implants placed through small incisions laterally, has received much attention, as it is an extraarticular, minimally invasive procedure. Although the podiatric literature cites the

successful use of this technique, in our experience the technique is not particularly effective, and a reactive synovitis from the implant is not uncommon. One surgeon at our facility has combined this technique with a calcaneal osteotomy with some success.

- Our current procedure of choice is a lateral column lengthening, often combined with a percutaneous Achilles lengthening if required. The technique has been well described by Mosca and others (Davitt et al. 2001) (Fig. 12–7). In general, the calcaneus is cut posterior to the calcaneocuboid joint, and a wedge-shaped graft from the iliac crest is inserted. Medial imbrication of the talonavicular capsule has also been described as an adjunctive procedure. Other authors choose to perform a sliding calcaneal tuberosity osteotomy.
- Triple arthrodesis may be helpful as a salvage procedure but should not be performed on an adolescent with a flexible flatfoot.

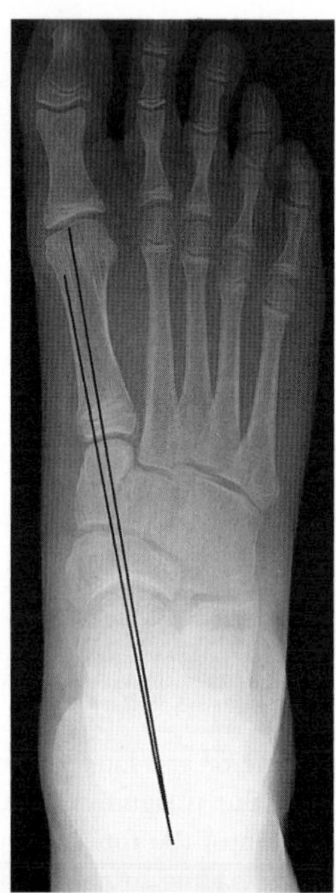

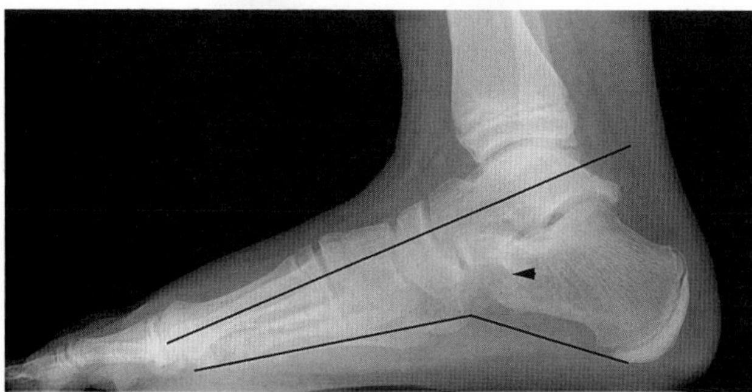

Figure 12–7: Radiographs of the patient seen in Figure 12–6 after undergoing percutaneous Achilles lengthening and lateral column lengthening with iliac crest bone graft. On both views, the talus-first metatarsal angle is restored. The talus is well covered by the navicular and is no longer prominent. The calcaneal pitch and arch are restored. The arrowhead is pointing to the healed osteotomy.

Tarsal Coalitions

Introduction

- Tarsal coalitions occur in at least 1% of the population, but many are not symptomatic.
- Commonly arise between the calcaneus and navicular, or between the talus and calcaneus, particularly the middle facet of the subtalar joint.
- Other variations have been described (i.e. talonavicular).
- Coalitions can also be seen in congenital limb anomalies, such as fibular hemimelia, leading to a "ball and socket" ankle joint.
- Tarsal coalitions commonly present with painful flatfoot deformities, referred to as the "peroneal spastic flatfoot."
- In some cases, the arch is of normal height.
- They are thought to arise as a variation of normal development.
- Between 50 and 60% are bilateral.
- While many may be treated non-operatively, some will eventually require surgery.

Clinical Presentation

- Symptoms usually begin in early adolescence, possibly as the coalition ossifies and becomes more rigid. The cause of these symptoms is debated but is most likely from abnormal movement from the remainder of the foot.
- Pain is usually described as being from the area of the sinus tarsi laterally. It is usually increased with activity, particularly that which stresses the subtalar joint, such as walking over uneven ground.
- Physical examination reveals limited mobility of the hindfoot.
  - The foot is in an everted position.
  - Peroneal "spasm" resists inversion.
  - The heel does not move into varus during single-leg toe raise.
  - The patient often will be unable to walk on the lateral border of the foot.
- Initial radiographs should consist of anteroposterior, lateral, oblique, and axial heel (Harris) views.
  - A calcaneonavicular coalition is best seen on the oblique view, while a talocalcaneal coalition may be best seen on the lateral or Harris view. Other coalitions are less commonly seen and may also be visible on plain films (Fig. 12–8).
  - Secondary findings include "beaking" of the talus, narrowing of the posterior talocalcaneal facet, and broad-

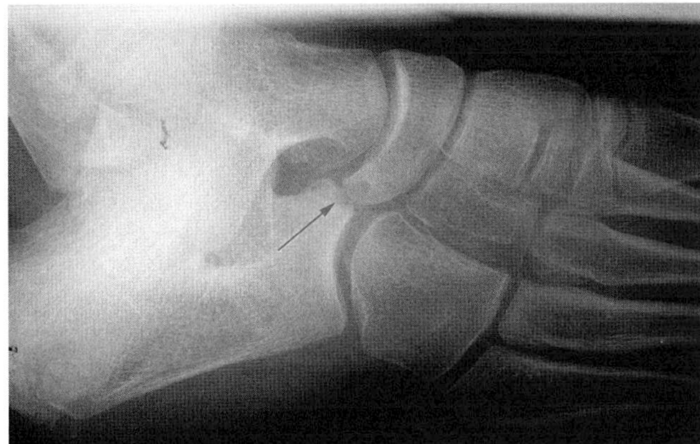

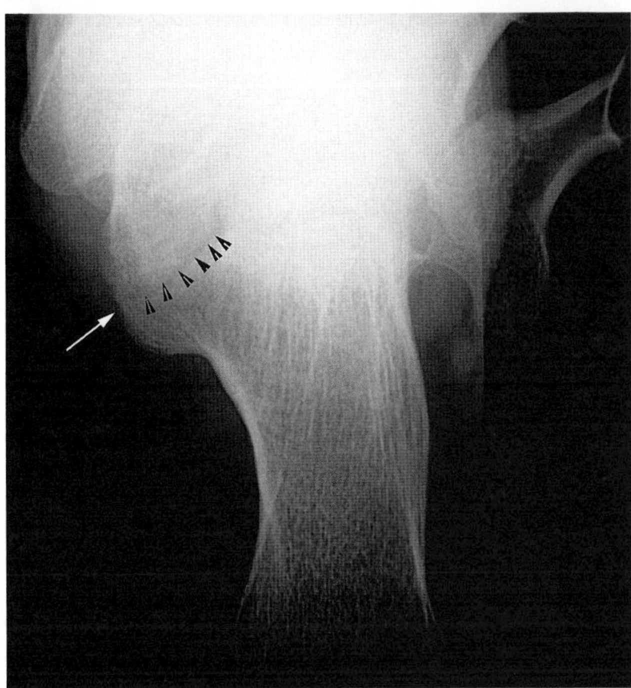

Figure 12–8: Radiographic appearance of tarsal coalitions. A, A calcaneonavicular coalition; B, a talocalcaneal coalition. The coalitions are noted by arrows. Note oblique slope of the medial facet seen in the talocalcaneal coalition (arrowheads).

ening of the lateral process of the talus. Talar beaking was once felt to represent arthrosis but is probably just an adaptive change resulting from abnormal movement and traction from the joint capsule (Fig. 12–9).

- CT remains the "gold standard" for tarsal coalitions. Even if a calcaneonavicular coalition is clearly seen on plain radiographs, a CT scan should be obtained to rule out the presence of an additional coalition (Fig. 12–10). CT is helpful both as a means to establish the diagnosis and as a guide to treatment (see below).
- MRI has been used recently to aid in the diagnosis of fibrous coalitions, but its full utility and role in this condition have not yet been defined.

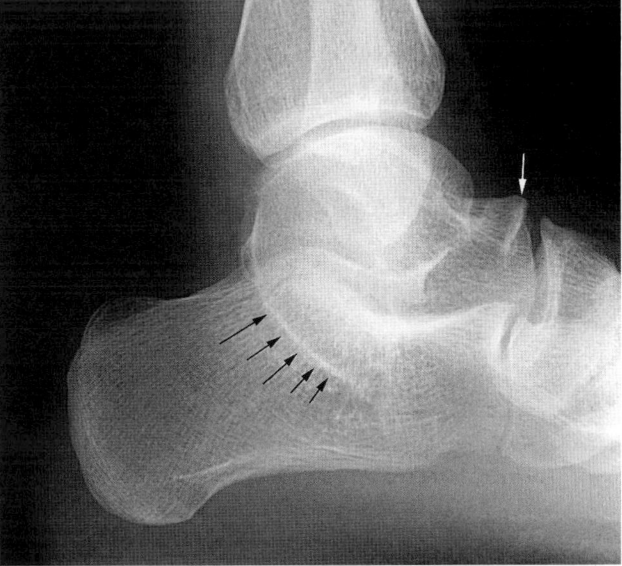

Figure 12–9: Lateral radiograph of a talocalcaneal coalition. Talar "beaking" (white arrow) and the "C sign," which represents the fused middle facet (black arrows).

Treatment

- Patients presenting with coalitions should be initially treated conservatively.
- Activity modification, anti-inflammatory medications, and arch supports designed to reduce hindfoot motion (i.e. University of California Biomechanics Laboratory orthosis [UCBL]) can be helpful.
- Occasionally, a trial period in a short leg walking cast may be successful for recalcitrant cases.
- For patients failing these regimens, surgery can often be helpful. Surgical treatment varies by the type of coalition and the extent of involvement.

Calcaneonavicular Coalitions

- Because these do not involve a normal articulation in the foot, wide excision is usually successful. The foot is approached through an Ollier-type incision over the sinus tarsi. The coalition is excised completely. The excision should extend from the lateral border of the talonavicular joint to the medial border of the calcaneocuboid joint. In particular, care should be taken not to narrow the excision plantarly; the coalition will often extend down several centimeters toward the sole of the foot. Failure to excise the entire coalition will probably result in an unsatisfactory result.
- After resection, the space between the bones should be filled to prevent recurrence. Traditionally, the extensor digitorum brevis muscle is sutured down into the defect. This leaves a contour defect in the foot, however, and in some patients the muscle will not reach to the bottom of the foot. Our preference is to use fat harvested from the

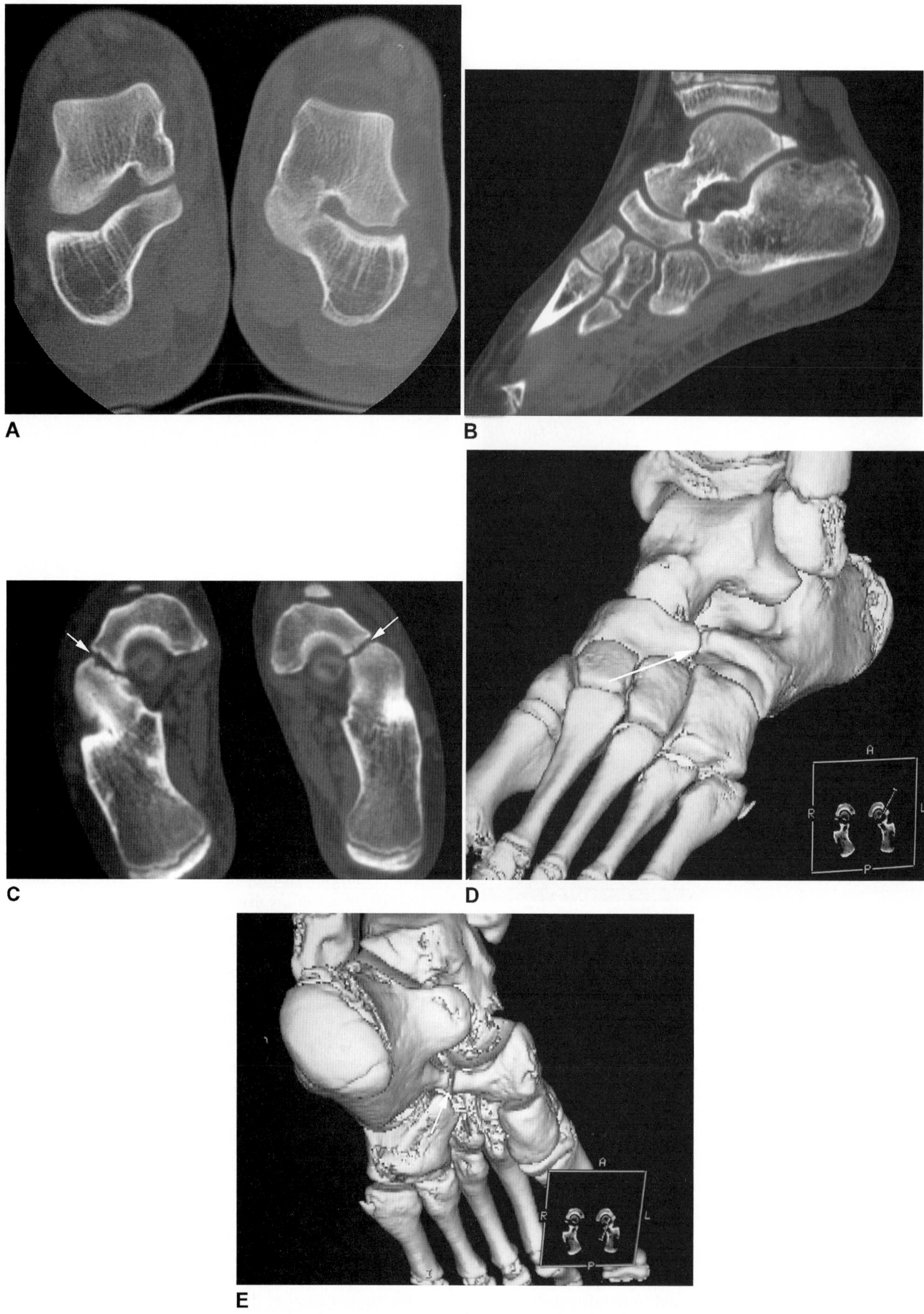

Figure 12–10: Computed tomography views of tarsal coalitions. **A**, A talocalcaneal coalition on the left foot, compared with a normal foot on the right. **B** and **C**, Bilateral fibrocartilagenous calcaneonavicular coalitions. **D** and **E**, Three-dimensional reconstructed tomography demonstrating the large extent of the coalition (white arrows).

ipsilateral natal crease. The fat of the buttock is copious and globular, and nicely fills the space. We have not seen any recurrences using this technique (Fig. 12–11).

Talocalcaneal Coalitions

- Results of surgery are not as predictable as calcaneonavicular coalitions, which are extraarticular.
- These occur through a joint, and therefore disturb the normal function of the foot if a large coalition exists.
- Non-operative treatment should be attempted prior to considering surgery.
- A preoperative CT scan is mandatory to assess the coalition. The amount of the subtalar joint involved can be estimated.
- Several authors have attempted to quantitate a resectable coalition. Wilde et al. (1994) suggested avoiding resection for patients in whom the coalition was greater than 50% of the area of the posterior facet, in whom the amount of

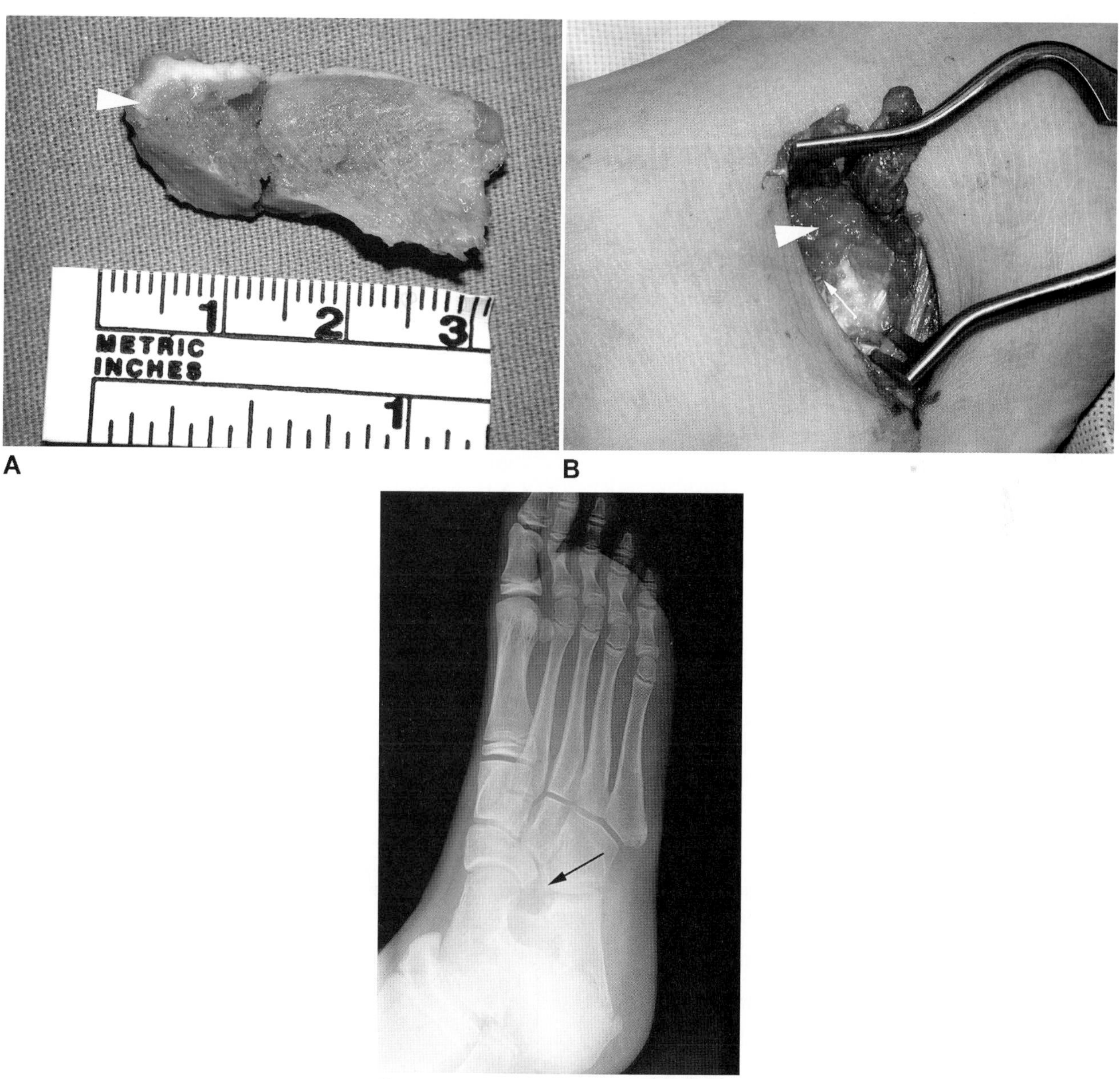

Figure 12–11: Surgical excision of a calcaneonavicular coalition. **A**, The excised fragment (arrowhead marks the dorsum). The depth of the coalition is often surprising. **B**, Fat harvested from the buttock is placed in the gap after resection (arrowhead). The edge of the calcaneus can be seen (small arrow). In this figure, the toes are to the left, heel to the right. **C**, Radiograph of the foot seen in (A) after resection. Note the wide gap that extends from the calcaneocuboid joint laterally to the talonavicular joint medially.

preoperative valgus noted on the CT was greater than 16°, and in those patients with significant narrowing of the posterior subtalar joint. Comfort et al. (1998) suggested that if the area of the coalition is less than one-third of the area of the entire subtalar joint, the likelihood of a successful resection was 80%. Degenerative changes in the foot also portend a worse prognosis. Talar beaking is currently viewed as an adaptive change, and as such does not preclude resection.
- In practice, the measurements described in these studies may be difficult, and parents and patients should be warned preoperatively about the possibility of persistent symptoms requiring further treatment.
- Resection is performed through the medial portion of the Cincinnati incision. Normal subtalar joint is identified anterior and posterior to the coalition, which is then resected. Care is taken to protect the neurovascular and tendonous structures. The flexor hallucis longus tendon, which usually is running directly beneath the sustentaculum tali (i.e. the medial facet coalition) must be carefully identified as well. After resection, fat harvested from the retrocalcaneal area may be inserted in the newly formed space. Other authors have recommended excision of the sustentaculum tali as the mainstay of this procedure, but we have no experience with this technique (Westbury et al. 2003).
- For large coalitions, or in patients who fail to respond to excision, subtalar fusion is indicated.

Congenital Vertical Talus

Introduction

- CVT is a common cause of a rigid rocker bottom foot deformity commonly seen in children from birth to 2 years.
- The etiology remains unknown, although muscle imbalance or intrauterine positioning has been implicated. An autosomal dominant inheritance pattern and a HOX gene mutation have also been shown (Shrimpton et al. 2004).
- Rarely appearing independently, CVT is associated with neural tube defects, neuromuscular disorders, and chromosomal abnormalities (Box 12–2).

History and Physical Examination

- A patient with a CVT deformity will have a rigid, rocker bottom foot. The deformity is bilateral approximately 50% of the time. Classically, there is an irreducible dorsal dislocation of the navicular on the talus and a calcaneocuboid joint dislocation.
- The forefoot is abducted and dorsiflexed due to tight peroneal and anterior tibial tendons. A prominent talar head is palpable at the medial convex sole of the foot, and the hindfoot is in equinovalgus.

Box 12–2 Associated Conditions of Congenital Vertical Talus

Chromosomal
- Trisomy 13
- Trisomy 14
- Trisomy 15
- Trisomy 18

Developmental
- Developmental dysplasia of the hip
- Arthrogryposis
- Prune belly syndrome
- Rasmussen syndrome
- Costello syndrome

Neurologic
- Myelomeningocele
- Tethered cord
- Neurofibromatosis
- Spinal muscular atrophy

- Patients may demonstrate a peg leg gait due to limited forefoot push-off. The foot may demonstrate some flexibility; however, it is not passively correctable, unlike a calcaneovalgus foot, an oblique talus, or a flatfoot with a tight heel cord. These are not rigid deformities and will usually correct with plantar flexion.
- A thorough birth history and neurologic examination should be assessed to determine any other associated conditions. The Coleman (Coleman et al. 1970) and the Lichtblau (1978) classifications separate CVT into anatomical and etiologic descriptions (Box 12–3).

Radiographs

- Bilateral three-view foot radiographs should be ordered to evaluate CVT; however, the diagnosis is confirmed by a lateral x-ray in maximum plantar flexion.
- In a normal foot, a longitudinal line through the axis of the talus to the first metatarsal falls dorsal to the

Box 12–3 Congenital Vertical Talus Classification

Coleman
- Talonavicular dislocation.
- Talonavicular dislocation with calcaneal-cuboid dislocation.

Lichtblau
- Teratogenic: Bilateral, rigid, positive family history, tight extensors and heel cords, associated with developmental dysplasia of the hip and mental retardation.
- Neurogenic: Muscle imbalance, varying deformity and rigidity, associated with myelomeningocele and neurofibromatosis.
- Acquired: Unilateral, partially correctable, due to intrauterine compression.

navicular. In a foot with CVT, there is fixed dorsal dislocation of the navicular on the talar neck, and a line through the talus is plantar to the navicular (Fig. 12–12).

- A child younger than 3 may not have a visible navicular because it has not ossified, therefore position is identified by position of the metatarsals that align with the talar neck.
- A screening spine MRI should be considered in a child with a unilateral vertical talus.

Treatment

- A CVT is usually not amenable to conservative treatment. Long leg casting with the foot in maximum plantar flexion and inversion facilitates the operation by stretching the skin, soft tissues, and extensor tendons over the dorsum of the foot.
- Surgery is the gold standard for treatment of CVT; however, the type of procedure depends on the severity of the deformity, patient age, and associated diagnoses. Surgery is usually delayed until about 12-18 months old and can be done as a single- or two-stage procedure.
- The authors prefer a single-stage procedure through a Cincinnati incision in order to reduce the talonavicular joint and to lengthen the toe extensors and peroneals in order to reduce the forefoot. Failure to reduce the navicular will lead to a poor result. Reduction of the talonavicular joint is maintained with the use of K wires (Fig. 12–13). Release of the bifurcate ligament and calcaneocuboid joint capsule reduces the cuboid on the calcaneus, and Achilles lengthening with posteromedial and posterolateral releases reduces the equinus contracture, talonavicular, and subtalar joints. Finally, in older children the correction may be stabilized with transfer of the anterior tibialis muscle under the neck of the talus.
- A postoperative splint or bivalve cast for 6-12 weeks protects the correction and leads to excellent or good results (Zorer et al. 2002).
- In older children with severe or recalcitrant deformity, excision of the talus or navicular with medial column shortening, or a subtalar or triple arthrodesis, can be utilized to correct the deformity. Often, these lead to good results, although they can result in overcorrection and represent an extreme treatment.

Accessory Navicular

Introduction

- An accessory navicular is an ossicle located on the medial side of the foot, proximal to the navicular and in continuity with the tibialis posterior tendon that is often bilateral, and is seen in 2-15% of people.
- Three types have been demonstrated (Ray and Goldberg 1983). In a type 1, the ossicle is contained in the tendon, whereas in the type 2 the ossicle is connected to the

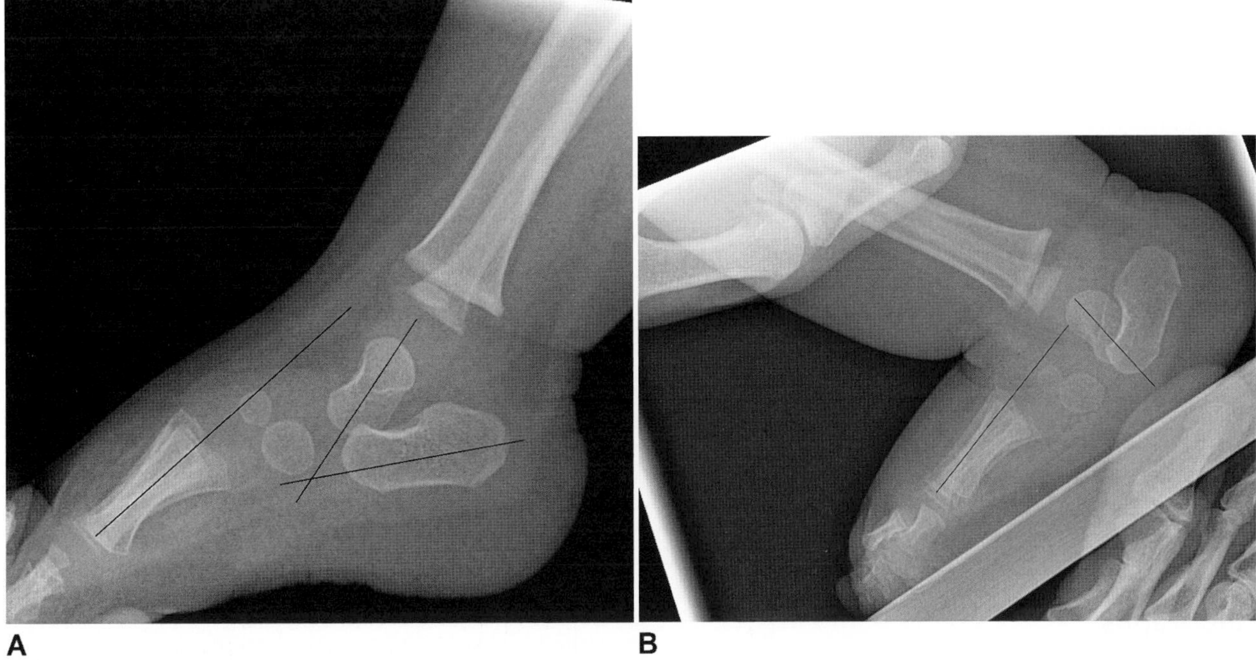

Figure 12–12: Lateral radiographs of a patient with a congenital vertical talus. **A**, Forced plantar flexion view of foot. The axis of the first metatarsal passes dorsal to the talus. The long axis of the calcaneus passes plantar to cuboid. **B**, Forced dorsiflexion demonstrates plantar flexion of talus and calcaneus, with the forefoot lying dorsally in the subluxed position. As opposed to the calcaneovalgus foot, where the calcaneus is dorsiflexed, here the calcaneus is plantar flexed.

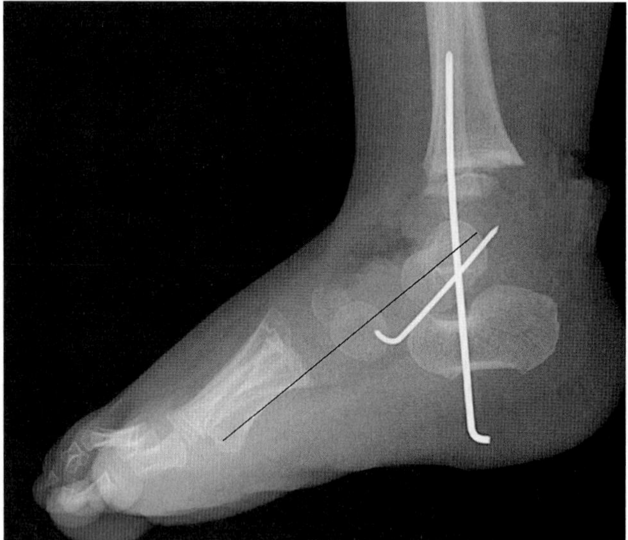

Figure 12–13: Lateral radiograph of postoperative congenital vertical talus. K-wire fixation of talus and calcaneus with axis of talus no longer passing plantar to the first metatarsal.

navicular by a cartilaginous bridge. A type 3 is an accessory navicular that has fused with the native navicular.

- Generally, the accessory navicular does not ossify until the age of 9, and in about 50% of cases will fuse to the navicular. Normally, an accessory navicular is not painful. A valgus stress injury may fracture the attachment of the ossicle to the navicular, resulting in abnormal motion.
- Insertion of the posterior tibialis tendon into the accessory bone displaces the tendon and allows the foot to deviate into a valgus position, resulting in a flatfoot with a prominent accessory bone and navicular (see Fig. 12-4).

History and Physical Examination

- The patient with an accessory navicular typically is an active adolescent who may report minor trauma and presents with a flexible flatfoot, although an accessory navicular does not itself cause a flatfoot (Kanatli et al. 2003).
- The foot should be evaluated for pain or a prominence on the medial side of the foot.
- Tenderness, swelling, and erythema directly over the prominence of the navicular can be observed, and even callus formation may occur. Pain is often worse with tight-fitting shoes. Pain over the prominence with resisted inversion also supports the diagnosis of an accessory navicular.

Radiographs

- A lateral oblique view of the foot is the radiograph of choice to evaluate an accessory navicular, because the standard medial internal oblique view will not show the accessory ossicle in profile (see Fig. 12–6).
- Radiographs may not be helpful if the accessory navicular is not ossified. Although it is actually attached by fibrous tissue or cartilage, the accessory navicular may appear distinct from the navicular on x-rays.
- CT scan may be beneficial to define the native navicular from the accessory navicular.

Treatment

- An asymptomatic flatfoot with an accessory navicular may not require treatment.
- In cases of local skin irritation, a doughnut-shaped piece of moleskin placed on the skin and around the prominence will relieve pain and tenderness.
- For deep pain, cast immobilization for 6 weeks or a UCBL that relieves pressure over the medial foot and decreases pronation may be helpful. Surgery is indicated for persistent symptoms after conservative measures have failed.
- The Kidner procedure removes the accessory navicular through excision of the accessory navicular and reinsertion of the posterior tibialis tendon, usually with much success (Kopp and Marcus 2004). Correction of the flatfoot is not expected to improve, and may require lateral column lengthening or a similar procedure if indicated.
- The incision is placed on the medial side of the foot, dorsal to the navicular prominence extending from the first cuneiform to the sustentaculum tali. A painful scar may result if the incision is placed directly over the prominence.
- The posterior tibialis tendon is identified at its insertion site on the navicular, and is teased away from the accessory navicular, leaving a wafer of bone attached to the tendon. The entire accessory navicular and the prominent portion of the navicular are excised, and the posterior tibialis tendon is advanced to the plantar surface of the navicular.
- The authors prefer simple excision of the accessory navicular with removal of the medial prominence of the navicular. The Kidner procedure has been shown to be no better than simple excision (Kopp and Marcus 2004). Both repairs require postoperative cast or splint immobilization.

Miscellaneous Forefoot Deformities

Metatarsus Adductus

Introduction

- Metatarsus adductus describes a foot with medial displacement of the metatarsals on the cuneiform, leaving the forefoot adducted at the tarsometatarsal joint. The foot has a bean-shaped appearance, with a curved lateral border. Normally, a line bisecting the heel on the plantar surface of the foot will pass through the second toe. In metatarsus adductus, this line moves laterally. Anatomical studies demonstrated medial deviation of the articular surface on the medial cuneiform, and adduction of the second through fifth metatarsal metaphyses (Morcuende and Ponseti 1996).

- Typically seen in the first year, although capable of presenting at any age, it is the most common congenital foot deformity, with an incidence of 1 in 1000, and the risk of an affected second child is nearly 1 in 20. Bilateral deformity will be present in 50% of patients. Torticollis is common, and developmental dysplasia of the hip is associated 10-15% of the time.
- The etiology remains unknown, although intrauterine positioning has been shown to cause medial subluxation of the tarsometatarsal joint when the foot is dorsiflexed (Reimann and Werener 1975).

History and Physical Examination

- Kite (1967) characterized metatarsus adductus by six distinct features: a high arch, concave medial border of the foot, separation of the first and second toes, fixed adductus of the forefoot when the hindfoot is in neutral, and a bean-shaped sole.
- The hindfoot is usually normal or in slight valgus, and the fifth metatarsal base is prominent with forefoot deviation. There is usually full range of motion in the ankle and subtalar joints. Internal tibial torsion may contribute to the intoed appearance, as well as other abnormalities included in the differential diagnosis (Box 12–4).
- Initially, determine whether the forefoot deformity is passively correctable past neutral by holding the heel static, and applying a lateral force to the medial border of first metatarsal. An actively correctable foot will correct with medial border stimulation.
- The foot may be rigid and associated with significant hindfoot valgus, a tarsometatarsal medial soft tissue crease and soft tissue contracture preventing passive correction. A tight abductor hallucis can be palpated medially when abduction of the forefoot causes big toe abduction.

Radiographs

- Radiographs are usually unnecessary if the forefoot is passively correctable and the hindfoot is normal.

Box 12–4 Differential Diagnosis of Metatarsus Adductus

- Skew foot
- Tibial torsion
- Femoral anteversion
- Metatarsus varus
- Clubfoot deformity
- Calcaneovalgus foot
- Oblique talus

However, severe cases will demonstrate medial deviation of the metatarsals at the tarsometatarsal joint, hindfoot valgus, and possible medial deformation of the metatarsal shaft.

Treatment

- Approximately 85-90% of affected feet will resolve spontaneously without treatment. A foot passively correctable past neutral requires no treatment, although some patients may benefit from passive stretching, stimulation, or straight last shoes.
- Serial above-knee casting and manipulation, most effective before 1 year old, is indicated for a rigid or persistent adductus.
- Severe uncorrectable deformities require operative treatment with release of the abductor hallucis, capsulotomy, and metatarsal osteotomy followed by cast correction.

Polydactyly and Syndactyly

Introduction

- Polydactyly, a very common foot deformity, is a duplication of a toe that occurs bilaterally in 40-50% of patients. Nearly 80% of these patients have postaxial polydactyly (duplication of the fifth toe), which often is not symmetric. Preaxial polydactyly affects the big toe and occurs in 15% of patients, while central duplication comprises the remaining 5% of patients, often duplicating a hypoplastic metatarsal ray.
- Often autosomal dominant with incomplete penetrance, polydactyly occurs in 2 out of 1000 live births, with a slight predisposition in boys. Polydactyly of the hand occurs in one-third of patients. Syndactyly of the toes occurs in about 20% of patients.
- Polydactyly is associated with Down syndrome, trisomy 13, Ellis-Van Creveld syndrome, Apert syndrome, and tibial hemimelia. Two types of polydactyly exist: type A, which exhibits a well-formed articulated digit, or type B, characterized by a rudimentary digit.
- In older patients, the main complaint is difficult shoe wear. The work-up of a child with polydactyly must include weight-bearing anteroposterior and lateral foot radiographs to define the anatomy.
- Syndactyly, or congenital webbing of toes, is a common deformity usually between the second and third toes, although it can affect any toe. It may have a family history. Syndactyly is classified as either simple, when only the skin is involved, or complex, when adjacent toes have not separated. The deformity is further defined as complete, when the webbing extends to the distal end of the toe, or incomplete. The toenails may be united in severe cases.
- Syndactyly is a cosmetic issue and usually does not lead to functional problems. Therefore it does not require treatment, except when present with polydactyly or for cosmesis.

Treatment

- Surgical excision, at 1 year of age, of the most medial or lateral toe will improve cosmesis and shoe wear, and allows the greatest potential for remodeling.
- Preaxial excision requires careful soft tissue balancing to prevent hallux varus, a complication of preaxial surgery. Central polydactyly is best treated with amputation of the duplicated central digit and reapproximation of the intermetatarsal ligament, followed by casting to prevent forefoot splaying.
- Postaxial polydactyly responds very well to simple excision of the duplicated digit, with nearly 90% of patients with excellent results (Nogami 1986). Attention should be taken to completely remove a prominent metatarsal in order to prevent a painful postoperative prominence.

Curly Toes and Overlapping Toes

Introduction

- Curly toes are an autosomal dominant deformity in which there is flexion and medial deviation of the proximal interphalangeal joint of the affected toe. Most commonly seen in bilateral third and fourth toes, lateral rotation at the distal interphalangeal joint leads to underlapping of the adjacent normal toe (Fig. 12–14).

Figure 12–14: Curly toes of the lateral two digits.

- Congenital contracture of the flexor digitorum longus and brevis tendons has been shown to cause the malrotation and flexion deformity of the toes.
- Symptoms of pain and corn formation are a result of abnormal pressure on the tips of the toes.
- Overlapping toes are characterized by dorsal adduction and external rotation of the fifth toe (Fig. 12–15). Contracture of the extensor digitorum longus tendon may occur, and in some cases dislocation of the metatarsophalangeal joint. Often, the deformity is familial and bilateral, and it is usually asymptomatic. Similar to

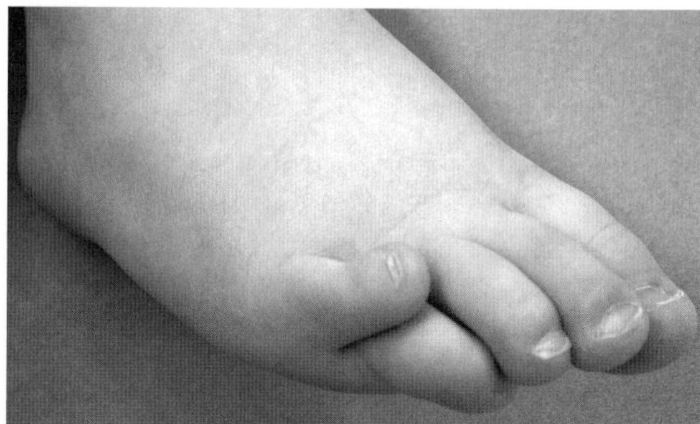

Figure 12–15: Overlapping toes. **A**, Overlapping fifth toe that caused difficulty with shoe wear. The fourth toe is a curly toe and was symptomatic from dorsal pressure from the third toe. **B**, Postoperative foot with straightened fourth and fifth digits. The fourth toe was treated with a simple tenotomy of the toe flexors, and the fifth with a modified Butler procedure, where the extensor tendon is sectioned, the metatarsophalangeal joint is released, and the toe is reduced using a Y to V advancement of the skin. In older patients, temporary pin fixation is advisable.

curly toes, shoe wear may be difficult and pain may be present over the dorsum of the toe with callus formation.

Treatment

- Curly toe deformity in the infant and young child should initially be observed. Percutaneous tenotomy of the long and short toe flexors is recommended at age 3-6 years (Ross and Menelaus 1984).
- A Girdlestone-Taylor procedure, which involves flexor to extensor transfers, can be utilized for more severe deformity; however, results are similar to those of open flexor tenotomy (Hamer et al. 1993).
- Overlapping toes can be corrected with a DuVries or Butler correction, which involves release of the extensor digitorum longus tendon, dorsal joint capsule, and medial collateral ligament (see Fig. 12–15). The toe should passively remain in the corrected position to prevent tension on the digital vessels.
- It is unclear whether treatment is beneficial in all patients. Redness, irritation, and pain are reasonable indications.

Fractures

Introduction

- Ankle growth plate fractures are extremely common injuries in children between 10 and 15 years of age, coinciding with physeal closure, which occurs over a 1- to 2-year period, starting with the tibial growth plate centrally, then medially, and finally laterally. These account for 15% of physeal injuries (Table 12–1). The most common ankle epiphyseal injury is Salter-Harris (SH) type 2 of the distal tibia caused by supination and external rotation (Fig. 12–16).
- The deltoid and lateral ligaments of the ankle joint insert into the epiphysis of the distal tibia and fibula, and because ligaments are stronger than the physis, twisting injuries of the ankle will often cause growth plate fractures as opposed to sprains. A child presenting with pain over the lateral malleolus with radiographs showing only soft tissue swelling can be assumed to have an SH type 1 fracture of the distal fibula.

Table 12–1: Common Pediatric Growth Plate Fracture

FRACTURE	PRESENTATION	TREATMENT
Salter 1 fibula	Lateral ankle pain and swelling	Short leg cast for 3 weeks
Salter 2 distal tibia	Rotational injury—may look "dislocated"	Closed reduction to within 3 mm of displacement May require open reduction
Salter 3 or 4 medial malleolus	Similar to adult ankle fracture	Open reduction Avoid crossing the physis with threaded fixation, if possible
Triplane or Tillaux fracture	Rotational injury	Closed treatment if minimally displaced, otherwise open or percutaneous reduction and fixation

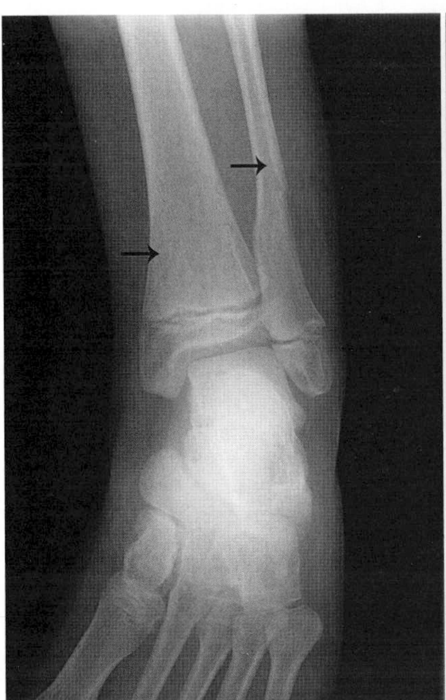

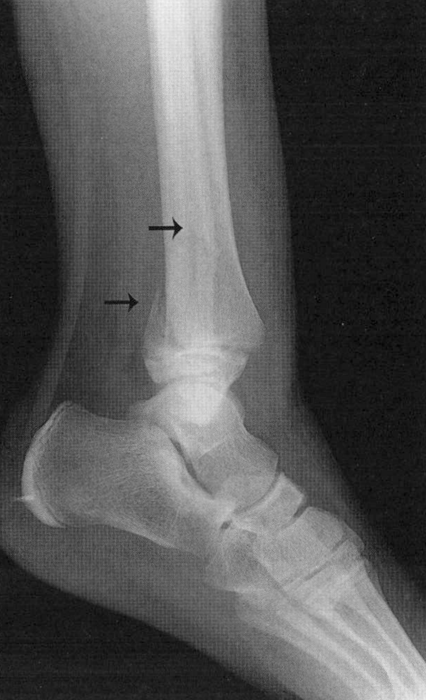

Figure 12–16: Radiograph of Salter-Harris type 2 fracture of distal tibia. **A**, Anteroposterior radiograph with arrow demonstrating fracture line of distal tibia and distal third fibula fracture. **B**, Lateral radiograph with tibia and fibula fracture lines marked. As is commonly seen, there is a large Thurston-Holland fragment, and the epiphysis is displaced posteriorly.

- Typically, patients will present with complaints of pain, swelling, ecchymosis, and an inability to ambulate. Goals of treatment are to restore joint congruity and mechanical alignment, and to minimize the potential for growth arrest, limb length discrepancy, and angular deformity.
- Three-view radiographs of the ankle are the gold standard to diagnose physeal fractures, with oblique radiographs distinguishing SH type 3 from type 4 fractures. CT scan of the ankle can be extremely beneficial for preoperative assessment and treatment.
- Transitional fractures are those that result from the particular sequence of distal tibial physeal closure. The plate closes centromedially, then medially, and finally laterally. Thus the anterolateral fragment may be avulsed.
- A Tillaux fracture is an SH type 3 fracture involving avulsion of the anterolateral tibial epiphysis (Fig. 12–17). It occurs in older adolescents, usually 12-15 years of age, after the middle and medial parts of the epiphyseal plate have closed, but prior to lateral closure.
- This fracture occurs in adolescents with nearly mature growth plates, thus there is minimal potential for deformity due to growth plate injury. The injury results from an external rotation force with stress placed on the anterior tibiofibular ligament, causing the anterolateral distal tibial epiphyseal plate to avulse and displace with lateral rotation.
- Three views of the ankle are needed to distinguish a Tillaux fracture from a triplane fracture. The common triplane fracture will contain an SH type 3 fracture similar to a Tillaux fracture on the anteroposterior view, in addition to the tibial physeal fracture, which appears to be an SH type 2 on the lateral view. A CT scan of the reduced and casted ankle is beneficial to delineate fracture fragments and direct potential operative treatment (Horn et al. 2001).
- Triplane fractures occur in older children, approximately 1 year prior to epiphyseal closure, rarely resulting in physeal arrest and angular deformity. The typical mechanism of injury is forced external rotation.
- Two-part and three-part triplane fractures exist. A two-part fracture is an SH type 4 fracture that occurs when the medial portion of the distal tibial epiphysis is closed and the posterior fracture extends across the epiphyseal plate into the metaphysis. This may be comminuted, with complete separation of the posterior half from lateral

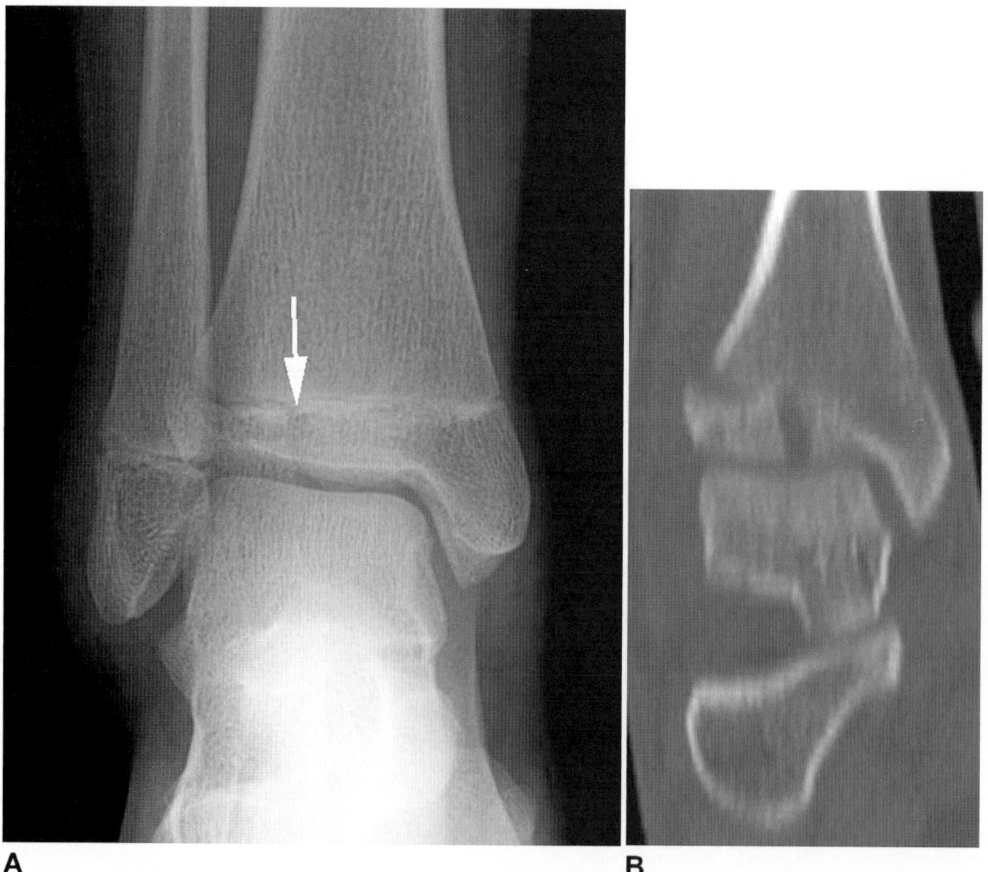

Figure 12–17: Radiograph and computed tomography (CT) scan of a Tillaux fracture. **A,** Anteroposterior radiograph demonstrates the fracture (arrow). Transitional fractures are best visualized with CT. **B,** The coronal reconstruction shows the lateral displacement.

Continued

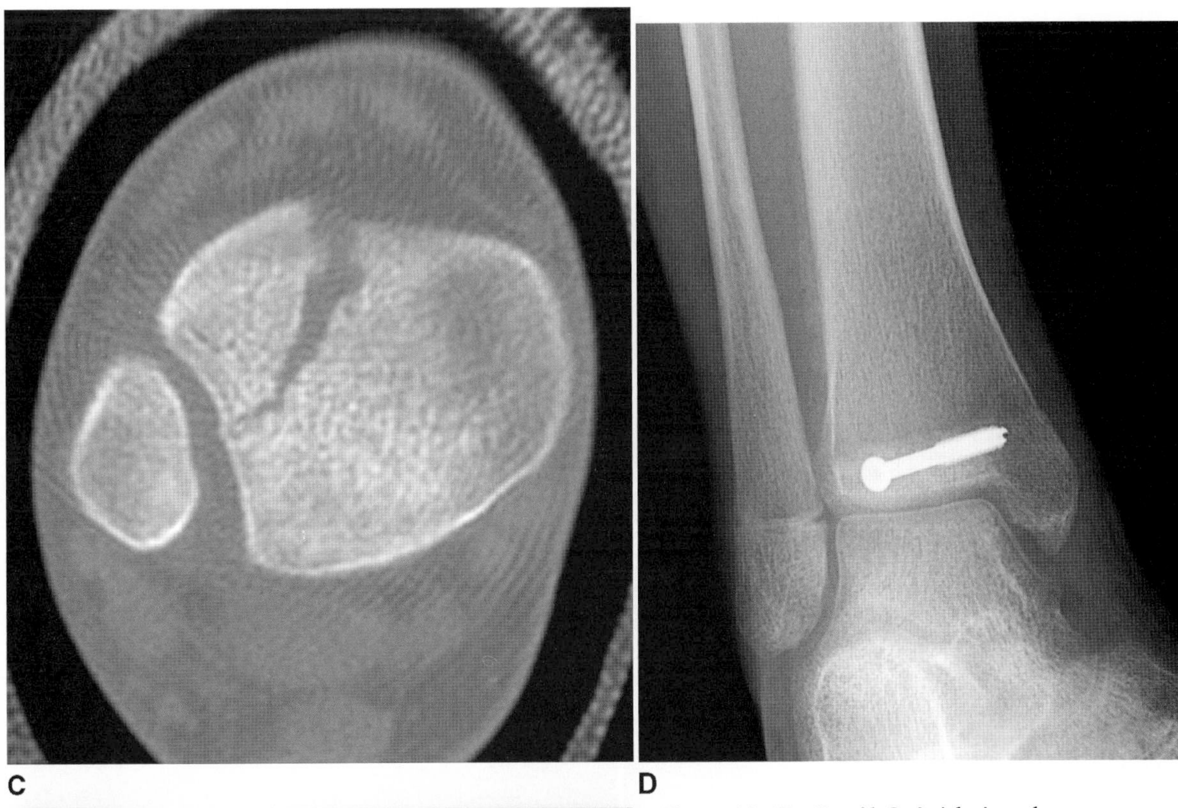

E

Figure 12–17: Cont'd **C,** Axial views best demonstrate the displacement as that of lateral rotation. **D** and **E,** Postoperative films show reduction of the fracture using a percutaneously placed cannulated screw. Note that the direction of screw placement is from anterolateral to posteromedial, perpendicular to the fracture line.

three-fourths. Three-part fractures occur when the middle portion of the distal tibial epiphysis is closed. A portion of the anterolateral, medial, and posterior distal tibia epiphysis is fractured, with an accompanying metaphyseal fragment (Fig. 12–18). The medial malleolus is intact; however, the fibula may be fractured.

- Evaluation of the fracture begins with obtaining three views of the ankle. Three-part fractures appear as an SH type 3 on the anteroposterior view and an SH type 2 on the lateral. There may be an associated fibular fracture as well. A CT scan demonstrates displacement of the articular surface and will potentially guide operative fixation.

Treatment

- Non-displaced SH type 1 and 2 fractures of the tibia can be treated effectively in a non-weight-bearing long leg cast for a minimum of 4-6 weeks, with minimal chance for growth disturbance. Displaced fractures should undergo gentle reduction to avoid growth plate damage and may require conscious sedation. Failure to obtain

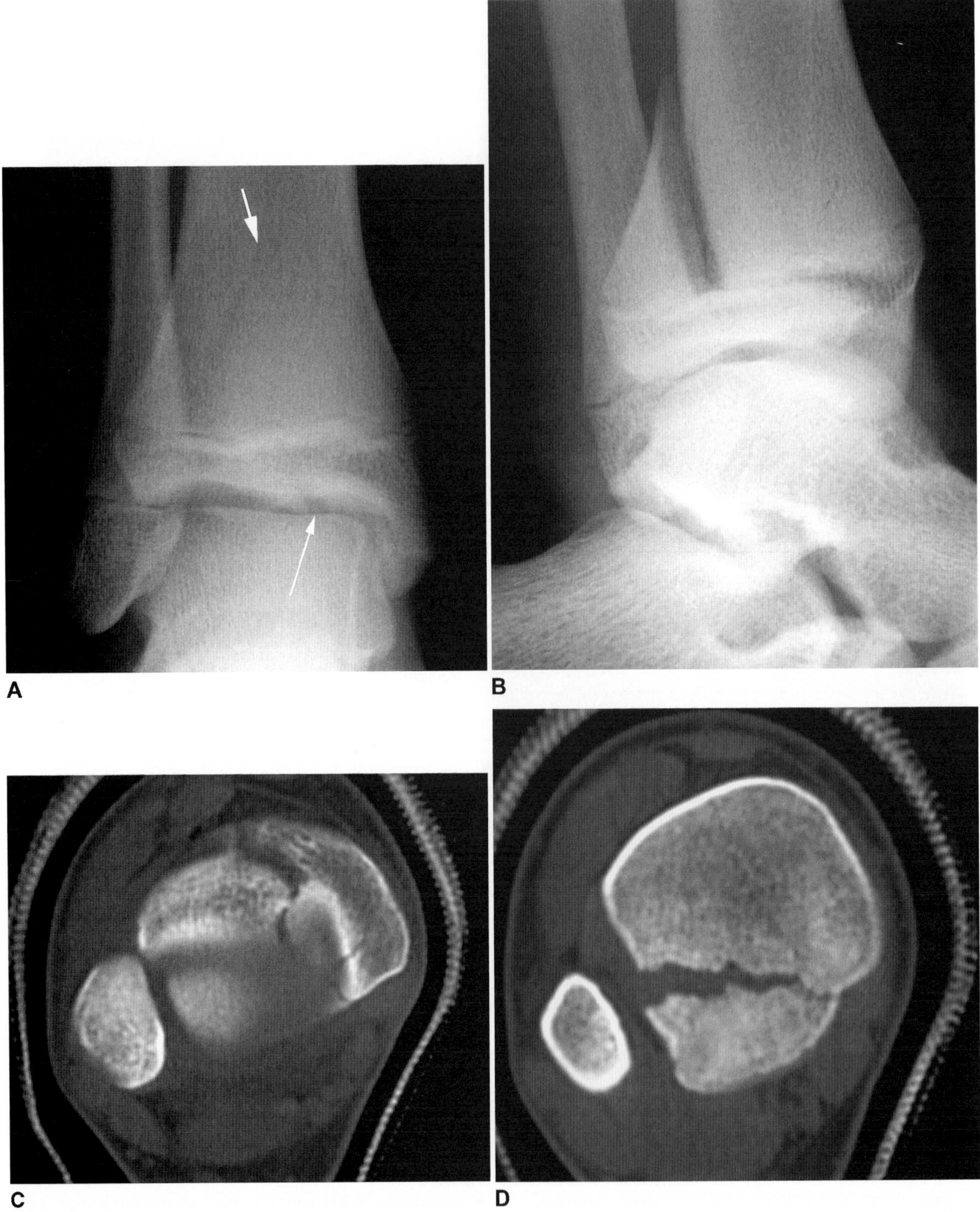

Figure 12–18: Triplane fracture. **A**, Anteroposterior radiograph of ankle, arrow marking fracture extension into the articular surface. This portion resembles a Salter-Harris (SH) type 3 component. The posterior fracture of the metaphysis is also visible (thicker arrow). **B**, The lateral view demonstrates the SH type 2 component. **C**, Computed tomography views demonstrate these fractures as a sagittal plane fracture extending into the articular surface, and **D**, a coronal plane fracture proximal to the physis. The fracture plane through the physis, which connects the other two fractures, is the third plane of the triplane.

Continued

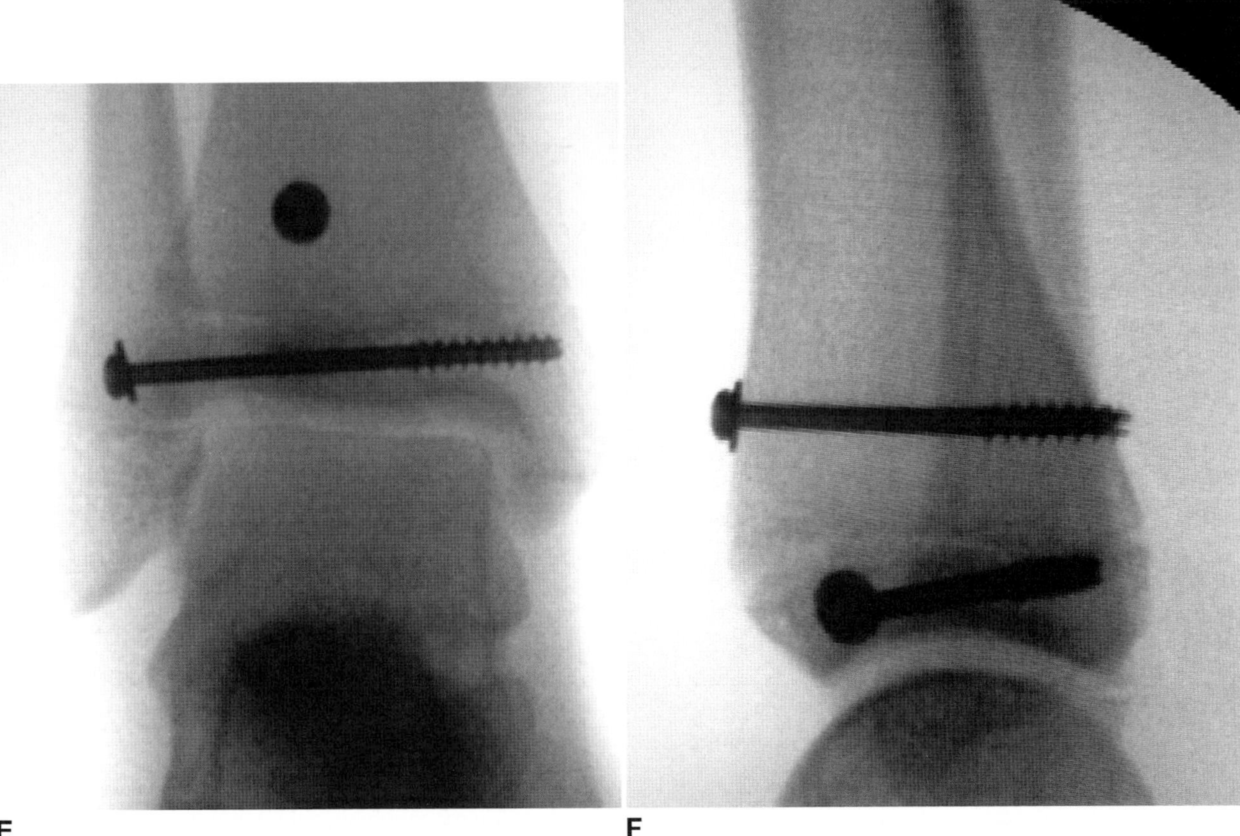

Figure 12–18: Cont'd E and F, Fluoroscopic intraoperative radiographs demonstrate anatomical reduction achieved with percutaneously placed clamps and placed parallel to the physis.

satisfactory reduction is often due to interposed periosteum, which may need to be extracted surgically. Often, stabilization of the fracture with K wires is helpful to prevent redisplacement.

- Supination external rotation, and pronation external rotation injuries with SH type 1 or 2 components of the distal tibial and fibular epiphysis are adequately treated by a non-weight-bearing long leg cast for a minimum of 6 weeks, which may be exchanged for a short leg cast until healing is complete.
- Patients less than 10 years old with SH 1 and 2 fractures may accept some displacement, because remodeling will occur with further growth. Inadequate reduction may be due to interposed periosteum, which then requires open reduction. Unlike SH type 4 fractures, there is no indication that anatomical open reduction will decrease the incidence of growth arrest in SH type 2 ankle fractures.
- SH type 3 and 4 fractures require anatomical reduction, which may be accomplished with closed or open reduction. Care must be taken to avoid damage to the perichondrium around the physis, and to avoid encroaching into the joint with wires or screw fixation. Intraoperative lateral radiographs help avoid this complication. A long leg cast is used postoperatively, which may require a change after a week due to swelling.
- Closed reduction of a Tillaux fracture, which involves internal rotation of the ankle and supination of the foot, may be attempted. Displacement greater than 2 mm should not be tolerated, and can be treated with single, cannulated screw fixation (see Fig. 12–17D,E). After reduction, patients should be placed in a non-weight-bearing long leg cast. Satisfactory reduction yields good ankle motion and articular congruity.
- Two-part triplane fractures displaced less than 2 mm and a congruous joint surface can be treated with closed reduction. Reduction is achieved by internal rotation of the foot and long leg cast immobilization for a minimum of 4 weeks. Significant soft tissue swelling prior to and after reduction make it difficult to maintain reduction in a cast, and occasionally lead to malreduction after the swelling has subsided.
- Open reduction and internal fixation is indicated for greater than 3 mm of displacement. The fracture pattern is often complex, making reduction difficult. Care should be taken to avoid placing screws into the growth plate, unless the patient is at the end of growth (Fig. 12–18E,F).

Complications

- Growth arrest may occur in SH type 1 and 2 fractures, because significant compression may occur at the time of injury. Visible signs may be delayed for 6 months or longer, thus ankle fractures should be followed for approximately 2 years.
- In SH type 1 and 2 fractures, growth plate arrest is usually central, whereas SH type 3 and 4 fractures undergo peripheral and more significant growth plate arrest (Barmada et al. 2003). Avascular necrosis, malunion, and non-union can occur with triplane fractures; however, due to skeletal maturity at the time of these fractures, growth deformities are uncommon.
- Angular deformities occur due to asymmetric arrest of distal tibial and fibular growth plate (Fig. 12–19). A varus deformity with or without an osseous bridge in the medial part of the physeal plate is common, especially after a supination inversion injury.
- Immediate growth arrest should be considered once a varus deformity is observed. A valgus deformity can be demonstrated with asymmetric arrest of the distal fibular physis.
- Other complications can include malunion or non-union, avascular necrosis, and a leg length discrepancy. A leg length discrepancy is seen in about 10-30% of cases, although the average discrepancy is only 1 cm.
- Because the distal tibial physis grows 2-3 mm/year, if the expected discrepancy is greater than 2 cm an epiphysiodesis of the contralateral proximal tibia and fibula at the appropriate age is indicated.

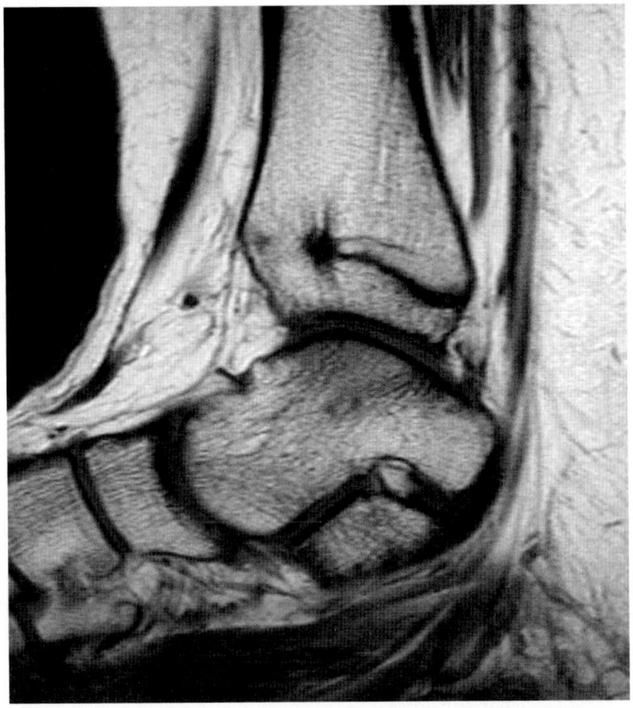

Figure 12–19: Angular deformities due to growth arrest. Magnetic resonance imaging scan of a 14-year-old girl who had a Salter-Harris type 2 fracture of the distal tibia 1 year prior. She had a clinical increase in dorsiflexion compared with the contralateral side. The growth arrest can be seen anteriorly. Note the sloping of the physis that resulted from the anterior tether.

Overuse Injuries of the Foot and Ankle in Children

Introduction

- Sports participation among children continues to increase, with many athletes participating year-round.
- In the immature skeleton, the growth plates are subjected to significant stress, and overuse injuries subsequently develop. Stress fractures can also be seen in the hindfoot and forefoot.
- Understanding the role of conditioning and activity modification in the prevention and treatment of these conditions is paramount.

Calcaneal Apophysitis (Sever Disease)

- Heel pain is a common complaint among pediatric athletes (Box 12–5).
- Sever described this phenomenon as an inflammation of the calcaneal apophysis, although others have thought it to be caused by microtrabecular injury in the apophysis due to overuse.

Box 12–5 Causes of Heel Pain in Children

Overuse
- Sever apophysitis
- Achilles tendonitis

Trauma
- Calcaneal stress fracture
- Acute hindfoot fracture

Inflammatory
- Juvenile arthritis (especially subtalar joint)
- Reiter syndrome (calcaneal enthesopathy, conjunctivitis, urethritis)

Neoplastic
- Benign (i.e. aneurysmal bone cyst, osteoid osteoma)
- Malignant (less common, i.e. leukemia, osteosarcoma)

Infection
- Osteomyelitis
- Soft tissue abscess

Other
- Tarsal coalition
- Contusion

- Patients present with complaints of heel pain, usually bilaterally, which occurs after running sports.
- Limping is less common, although it may occur in longstanding disease.
- Often, the patient may have symptoms on rising in the morning, until the feet "loosen up," analogous to plantar fasciitis.
- A thorough history should be obtained, focusing on duration and nature of pain, associated symptoms, fever, appetite changes, and joint swelling. Although this is most commonly a benign condition, the differential diagnosis can encompass a wide range of conditions.
- Physical examination begins with a general assessment. The heel cords are examined for flexibility, and are often found to be tight. There is usually pain to palpation over the heel, over the medial portion of the distal calcaneus.
- Gait examination may be normal or may reveal an absence of the normal heel-toe pattern. Patients may avoid pressure on the calcaneus, and may even toe walk.
- In bilateral disease with a reasonable history, radiographs are unnecessary. In unilateral disease, radiographs may rule out the presence of fracture, tumor, or infection (Fig. 12–20) The apophysis may appear fragmented as a normal developmental variant, and thus is usually not diagnostic for Sever disease in the absence of a suspicious history and examination. MRI may be helpful if stress fracture or tumor is suspected.
- Treatment is divided into several stages.
  - Eliminate the inflammation. Non-steroidal antiinflammatory drugs (NSAIDs) and ice are helpful for patients with significant pain.
  - Protect the area. We prefer an over the counter cushioned heel cup to be worn during sports.
  - Improve flexibility. Often, the most important factor in eliminating symptoms is to improve heel cord flexibility.
  - Remove stressor. In patients with significant, unrelenting pain, cessation of sports activity may be necessary until symptoms abate. We have not found this to be necessary for mild symptoms, but if the child limps or complains of discomfort for more than 12 h after a sporting event, some modification of activities is usually necessary.
- The vast majority of patients treated in this manner are able to resume sports without significant discomfort within 4-8 weeks. Prolonged symptoms may require further activity modification and evaluation. In extreme cases, casting is occasionally recommended by some authors, although this is rarely our practice.

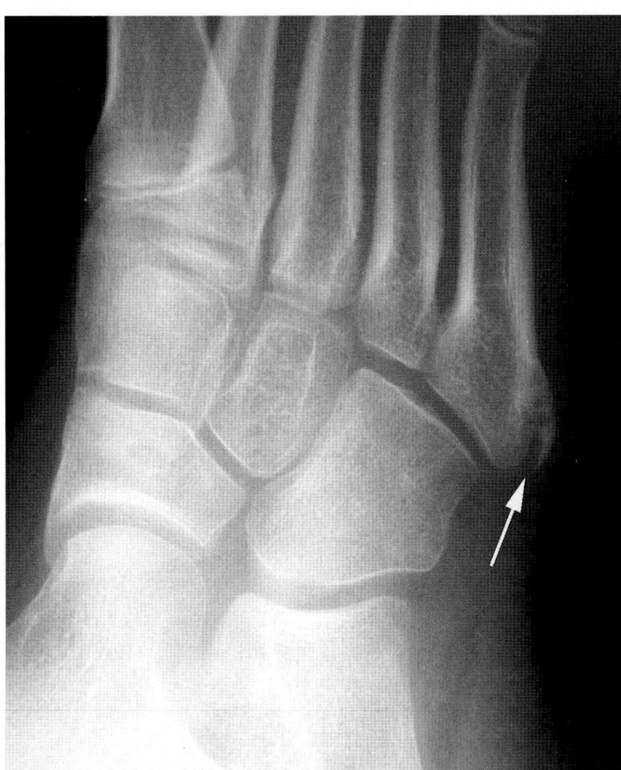

Figure 12–20: Iselin disease. The apophysis of the fifth metatarsal is sclerotic, with new bone formation.

Fifth Metatarsal Apophysitis (Iselin Disease)

- Seen in children and adolescents who participate in running and cutting sports that place an inversion stress on the foot.
- A history of an inversion injury may be present.
- Physical examination shows swelling and tenderness over the apophysis of the fifth metatarsal.
- Hindfoot posture that promotes inversion stress may be present (i.e. cavovarus foot).
- Pain is present with resisted eversion.
- Radiographs should be obtained to rule out fracture. They may be normal in Iselin disease, or may show widening or fragmentation of the apophysis (see Fig. 12–20).
- Treatment usually consists of physical therapy, orthotics, NSAIDs, and activity modification. Most athletes do well with conservative measures, although Canale and Williams (1992) noted a persistently painful non-union in one patient in their series.

Stress Fractures

- Children who participate in aggressive running sports are vulnerable to stress fractures of the foot and ankle (Box 12–6).
- Metabolic disease should be looked for, such as hyperthyroidism or parathyroid disease. Female endurance athletes, in particular, may suffer from amenorrhea and osteoporosis, increasing their risk.
- Often, there has been inadequate conditioning in the off-season, followed by an aggressive preseason activity regimen.

Box 12–6 Stress Fractures of the Foot in Children

Metatarsals
- Running, long marches, dancing, tennis

Sesamoid Bones
- Ballet, running sports

Calcaneus
- Jumping sports, long-distance marching, running sports

Navicular
- Sprinting, hurdling

Cuboid
- Running, jumping sports

Talus
- Pole vaulting, jumping sports

Medial Malleolus
- Basketball, running

Proximal Phalanx of Great Toe
- Sprinting, jumping

- Patients present with localized pain, usually activity-related. While it may initially occur only with sports, eventually the pain lasts throughout the day.
- Pain at rest is an ominous sign. Infection and tumor must be ruled out.
- Initial evaluation consists of physical examination to determine area of maximal tenderness, with radiographs of the offending area obtained.
- If films are negative despite persistent pain, bone scan or MRI may be helpful to identify occult fractures.
- Treatment consists of immobilization, activity modification, and analgesics until symptoms resolve, followed by a gradual return to activities. A rule of thumb is to increase mileage run by no more than 10% per week until the goal is achieved. Aggressive cross-training (swimming, biking, etc.) is helpful to avoid deconditioning. Proper shoe wear and orthotic use is helpful to avoid reinjury.
- Recalcitrant cases may benefit from adjuvant measures such as ultrasound or pulsed electromagnetic fields, although the efficacy of these treatments in children is unknown, and the cost is probably not justified for the uncomplicated case. In rare cases, surgery is required to achieve bony union.

References

Clubfoot

Cummings RJ, Davidson RS, Armstrong PF et al. (2002) Congenital clubfoot. J Bone Joint Surg 51: 385-400.

This is an excellent review of the subject, including background, history, examination, and operative and non-operative treatment. Primary and revision treatments are discussed. There is also an extensive bibliography.

Davidson RS. (2003) Clubfoot salvage: A review of the past decade's contribution. J Pediatr Orthop 23: 410-418.

This review article nicely summarizes the difficulties that arise in treating patients with a recurrent deformity after clubfoot surgery. The various deformities seen, radiographic evaluation, and treatment strategies are reviewed in detail. It is sobering to note the difficulties experienced even by seasoned clubfoot surgeons.

Dobbs MB, Rudzki JR, Purcell DB et al. (2004) Factors predictive of outcome after the use of the Ponseti method for the treatment of idiopathic clubfeet. J Bone Joint Surg 86: 22-27.

Despite its popularity, the Ponseti method of treatment often can fail if proper compliance with postmanipulation splinting is not achieved. Non-compliance with splinting was the most common reason for failure. This study pointed out the relationship between the educational level of the parents and compliance. The necessity for the bracing regimen must be explained clearly to parents in a manner that is easily understood by parents of all educational backgrounds.

Noonan KJ, Richards BS. (2003) Nonsurgical management of idiopathic clubfoot. J Am Acad Orthop Surg 11: 392-402.

This review discusses the non-operative management of clubfoot deformity. The Ponseti method is reviewed, as is the French physiotherapy method of manipulation, strapping, and continuous passive motion.

Ponseti IV. (1996) Congenital Clubfoot—Fundamentals of Treatment. New York: Oxford University Press, 1996.

This book describes in detail the pathophysiology, anatomy, presentation, and treatment of congenital clubfoot. Dr. Ponseti's method is explained in detail, and subsequent surgical procedures, such as anterior tibial tendon transfer, are described as well. As this technique has rapidly come into favor recently in the USA, this book is an important reference for anyone who treats patients with clubfeet.

Flatfoot

Comfort TK, Johnson LA. (1998) Resection for symptomatic talocalcaneal coalition. J Pediatr Orthop 18: 283-288.

The authors report good and excellent clinical results for excision of coalitions involving less then one-third of the total subtalar joint surface, measured with CT. Increasing age was not a contraindication.

Davitt JS, MacWilliams BA, Armstrong P. (2001) Plantar pressure and radiographic changes after distal calcaneal lengthening in children. J Pediatr Orthop 21: 70-75.

This study reviews the outcomes of patients undergoing calcaneal-lengthening osteotomy for flatfoot. They noted excellent improvement in terms of both radiographic measurement and redistribution of plantar pressure measurements toward normal. The surgical technique is also reviewed.

Sullivan JA. (1999) Pediatric flatfoot: Evaluation and management. J Am Acad Orthop Surg 7(1): 44-53.

An excellent review of the topic, reviewing the differential diagnosis and management of common disorders associated with a flatfoot in the pediatric population.

Vincent KA. (1998) Tarsal coalition and painful flatfoot. J Am Acad Orthop Surg 6: 274-281.
An excellent review of the topic, including operative and non-operative treatments.

Westbury DE, Davids JR, Oros W. (2003) Surgical management of symptomatic talocalcaneal coalitions by resection of the sustentaculum tali. J Pediatr Orthop 23: 493-497.
The authors reviewed 10 patients who had undergone a resection of the sustentaculum tali as treatment of a talocalcaneal coalition. They report a majority of good and excellent results with this procedure, without progressive malalignment. This may be an alternative to traditional resection where the sustentaculum is left intact.

Wilde PH, Torode IP, Dickens DR et al. (1994) Resection for symptomatic talocalcaneal coalition. J Bone Joint Surg Br 76(5): 797-801.
This paper initially described the criteria for a successful resection of a talocalcaneal coalition. Patients whose coalition involved more than 50% of the area of the posterior facet (based on the preoperative CT), and who had heel valgus greater than 16° with degenerative changes seen in the posterior facet, did poorly with resection. Talar beaking, previously thought to be a sign of arthrosis, had no effect on outcome.

Congenital Vertical Talus

Coleman SS, Stelling FH III, Jarrett J. (1970) Pathomechanics and treatment of congenital vertical talus. Clin Orthop 70: 62-72.
A historical article classifying the CVT based on anatomy. The first is a simple talonavicular dislocation, and the second type is a talonavicular dislocation with concomitant calcaneal-cuboid dislocation.

Herring JA. (2002) Disorders of the foot. In: Tachdjian's Pediatric Orthopaedics, from the Texas Scottish Rite Hospital for Children, 3rd edn. Philadelphia: Saunders. pp. 891-1038.
This book chapter is devoted to discussing every aspect of pediatric foot disorders. Specific attention is placed on prevalence, clinical presentation, diagnosis, evaluation, and treatment.

Lichtblau S. (1978) Congenital vertical talus. Bull Hosp Joint Dis 39(2): 165-179.
A classification scheme for CVT was designed to separate three different etiologies—neurogenic, teratogenic, and acquired—to aid in clinical decision making.

Napiontek M. (1995) Congenital vertical talus: A retrospective and critical review of 32 feet operated on by peritalar reduction. J Pediatr Orthop Br 4(2): 179-187.
The Grice-Green procedure combined with peritalar reduction led to overcorrection in 7 of 16 feet in children with CVT.

Shrimpton AE, Levinsohn EM, Yozawitz JM et al. (2004) A HOX gene mutation in a family with isolated congenital vertical talus and Charcot-Marie-Tooth disease. Am J Hum Genet 75(1): 92-96.
DNA was isolated from 36 family members with both CVT and Charcot-Marie-Tooth disease present. A single missense mutation was sequenced from six HOX genes. This mutation evidenced linkage to family members with both CVT and Charcot-Marie-Tooth disease.

Zorer G, Bagatur AE, Dogan A. (2002) Single stage surgical correction of congenital vertical talus by complete subtalar release and peritalar reduction by using the Cincinnati incision. J Pediatr Orthop Br 11(1): 60-67.
Seventeen feet in 12 patients with CVT were treated with a single-stage procedure using a Cincinnati incision. Follow-up averaged 42 months, with outcomes measured clinically and radiographically. Good outcomes can be achieved using a single-stage procedure.

Accessory Navicular

Kanatli U, Yetkin H, Yalcin N. (2003) The relationship between accessory navicular and medial longitudinal arch: Evaluation with a plantar pressure distribution measurement system. Foot Ankle Int 24(6): 486-489.
Ninety-two patients with accessory navicular were analyzed in the authors' gait laboratory. The medial longitudinal arch was calculated using a pressure picture. The presence of an accessory navicular did not correlate with the height of the medial longitudinal arch, and is not associated with a flatfoot.

Kopp FJ, Marcus RE. (2004) Clinical outcome of surgical treatment of the symptomatic accessory navicular. Foot Ankle Int 25(1): 27-30.
Fourteen feet with symptomatic accessory navicular were reviewed after surgical treatment. All patients had a type 2 accessory navicular and were observed for an average of 103 months. Simple excision and anatomical repair of the posterior tibialis tendon proved to be a successful intervention with respect to pain and patient satisfaction.

Ray S, Goldberg VM. (1983) Surgical treatment of the accessory navicular. Clin Orthop Relat Res 177: 61-66.
Twenty-nine feet with an accessory navicular were surgically corrected using the Kidner procedure. Follow-up ranged from 2 to 10 years. The Kidner procedure effectively treated 26 patients.

Ugolini PA, Raikin SM. (2004) The accessory navicular. Foot Ankle Clin 9(1): 165-180.
This article is an excellent review of accessory navicular. Prevalence, clinical presentation, diagnosis, evaluation, and treatment of this common foot disorder are presented in this review.

Metatarsus Adductus

Gordon JE, Luhmann SJ, Dobbs MB et al. (2003) Combined midfoot osteotomy for severe forefoot adductus. J Pediatr Orthop 23(1): 74-78.
Fifty feet were reviewed after undergoing a one-stage combined midfoot osteotomy for severe forefoot adductus for nearly 2 years. Clinical and radiographic improvement was seen in 90% of cases. The mean talo-first metatarsal angle decreased from 15 to 3° at final follow-up.

Kite JH. (1967) Congenital metatarsus varus. J Bone Joint Surg Am 49(2): 388-397.

A historical article describing the clinical presentation of a foot with metatarsus varus. The Kite features of metatarsus adductus have continued to remain the standard of clinical diagnosis.

Morcuende JA, Ponseti IV. (1996) Congenital metatarsus adductus in early human fetal development: A histologic study. Clin Orthop Relat Res 333: 261-266.

The medial cuneiform demonstrated a trapezoid shape, and the first cuneometatarsal joint angled medially and dorsally.

Reimann I, Werener HH. (1975) Congenital metatarsus varus: A suggestion for a possible mechanism and relation to other foot deformities. Clin Orthop Relat Res 110: 223-226.

Fourteen stillborn normal feet were dissected, and a metatarsus varus deformity was created after extensive capsulotomies in the tarsometatarsal joints distal to the joint of Chopart. This suggests that metatarsus varus results from a maximally dorsiflexed foot, with subsequent development of contractures of the soft tissues.

Toe Deformities

Hamer AJ, Stanley D, Smith TW. (1993) Surgery for curly toe deformity: A double-blind, randomised, prospective trial. J Bone Joint Surg Br 75(4): 662-663.

A randomized, prospective clinical trial compared results of flexor to extensor tendon transfer with those of open flexor tenotomy. Similar results were demonstrated with either procedure.

Kawabata H, Ariga K, Shibata T et al. (2003) Open treatment of syndactyly of the foot. Scand J Plast Reconstr Surg Hand Surg 37(3): 150-154.

Fifteen patients with simple syndactyly were treated by an open technique utilizing a dorsal rectangular flap to cover the bottom of the web. This method of reconstruction was cosmetically satisfactory in all patients after a mean follow-up of 5 years.

Nogami H. (1986) Polydactyly and polysyndactyly of the fifth toe. Clin Orthop Relat Res 204: 261-265.

Thirty-seven patients with 46 affected feet with polydactyly were classified and treated. Thirty-three patients with 42 toes were surgically treated. Children achieved good results when treated early or before they could walk.

Ross ER, Menelaus MB. (1984) Open flexor tenotomy for hammer toes and curly toes in childhood. J Bone Joint Surg Br 66(5): 770-771.

Sixty-two children with curly toes were observed for an average of 9 years after flexor tenotomy. No loss of flexion strength was demonstrated. The authors concluded that open flexor tenotomy is an effective method for correcting curly toes.

Thompson GH. (1996) Bunions and deformities of the toes in children and adolescents. Instr Course Lect 45: 355-367.

An excellent review of children's toe and foot deformities, including clinical evaluation and treatment.

Trauma

Barmada A, Gaynor T, Mubarak SJ. (2003) Premature physeal closure following distal tibia physeal fractures: A new radiographic predictor. J Pediatr Orthop 23(6): 733-739.

Premature physeal closure was investigated in 92 fractures of the distal tibia, with at least 1 year follow-up or until physiologic closure of the growth plates. Closed reduced SH type 1 and 2 fractures that required open reduction had entrapped periosteum at the fracture site. This led to residual gaps and can lead to an increased incidence of premature physeal closure.

Cass JR, Peterson HA. (1983) Salter-Harris type-IV injuries of the distal tibial epiphyseal growth plate, with emphasis on those involving the medial malleolus. J Bone Joint Surg 65(8): 1059-1070.

Thirty-two patients with an SH type 4 fracture of the distal tibial epiphysis were evaluated over a 5-year period. Eighteen patients had fractures of the medial malleolus, 13 had triplane fractures, and 1 involved the tibial plafond. Nine of the 18 patients demonstrated premature physeal closure, resulting in angular deformity or limb length discrepancy. The triplane and tibial plafond fracture did not heal with angular deformity or result in growth arrest, because the patients were nearly skeletally mature at the time of injury.

Dailiana ZH, Malizos KN, Zacharis K et al. (1999) Distal tibial epiphyseal fractures in adolescents. Am J Orthop 28(5): 309-312.

Three Tillaux fractures and five triplane fractures were followed from 1 to 11 years. All were treated with open reduction and internal fixation using either malleolar screws or K wires. No patients complained of pain or joint stiffness, and none healed with a congruous joint.

Horn BD, Crisci K, Krug M et al. (2001) Radiologic evaluation of juvenile Tillaux fractures of the distal tibia. J Pediatr Orthop 21(2): 162-164.

The accuracy of radiographs and CT scan to assess Tillaux fractures with varying amounts of displacement was evaluated using four cadaveric specimens. CT scans were more sensitive in detecting displacement greater than 2 mm, and are therefore the preferred imaging modality to assess Tillaux fractures.

Nenopoulos SP, Papavasiliou VA, Papavasiliou VA. (2003) Rotational injuries of the distal tibial growth plate. J Orthop Sci 8(6): 784-788.

Nine rotational injuries of the distal tibial growth plate were treated with closed reduction and long leg casting for 6-8 weeks. Final results yielded good to excellent results in all nine patients, with a follow-up of at least 1 year.

Spiegel PG, Mast JW, Cooperman DR et al. (1984) Triplane fractures of the distal tibial epiphysis. Clin Orthop Relat Res 188: 74-89.

Triplane fractures of the distal tibia can occur with a distal fibula fracture. Displacement greater than 2 mm on any view of a radiograph or CT scan is an indication for open reduction with screw fixation for the metaphyseal and epiphyseal fragment. Results are good if satisfactory reduction has been achieved.

Overuse Injuries

Canale TS, Williams KD. (1992) Iselin's disease. J Pediatr Orthop 12: 90-93.

This study reviews several cases of this ailment. Interestingly, the authors report a case of symptomatic delayed healing of the apophysis.

Nerve Disorders

Anthony Hinz*

*M.D., Orthopedic and Neurosurgical Care and Research Center, Bend, OR

- Nerve disorders and entrapment syndromes in the foot and ankle generally are caused by abnormal pressure on nerves, generated by anatomical structures such as bone, ligaments, fascia, and/or muscle.
- Many different conditions can lead to abnormal pressure, such as trauma, soft tissue masses, or other scar-generating processes. One must always consider other primary nerve disorders, such as peripheral neuropathy or neurilemmomas, as an etiology for any given nerve-mediated problem.
- When evaluating a patient for an entrapment syndrome in the foot, it is possible to access any of the peripheral nerves in question with injection, which may provide both diagnostic and potentially therapeutic blockade. Agents such as bupivacaine or lidocaine may be used to inject proximal to the site in question. Patient response may confirm or exclude a specific diagnosis. The addition of antiinflammatory agents such as prednisolone or triamcinolone may provide long-lasting relief as well as potentially reverse the etiology.
- Recovery from nerve surgery is highly variable due to the high variability of nerve injury, ranging from *neurapraxia* with a simple conduction block to *axonotmesis* or *neurotmesis*. Therefore surgery for nerve disorders must be well planned, and patients must be properly informed that recovery may be delayed or possibly never achieved.

Interdigital (Morton) Neuroma

Description

- Morton neuroma is a compression neuropathy of the plantar digital nerve with associated perineural fibrosis.
- It presents with a burning and tingling sensation in the forefoot/toes, radiating sometimes into the leg. Occasionally, there may be numbness in the affected toes.
- Patients may describe worse pain in the evening, improved with massage and removal of shoe wear.

Etiology

- Nerve irritation is produced by compression of the interdigital nerve near the distal edge of the transverse intermetatarsal ligament, more recently and more accurately described as *interdigital neuritis*.
- It may also be caused by ischemic changes to the perineural tissue or from repetitive neurovascular trauma.
- There is a strong predilection for the middle-aged woman (Wu 1996), but it can occur in a wide-ranging population.
- Any process that diminishes space available for the nerve may cause interdigital neuritis (such as metatarsophalangeal synovitis, ganglion cysts, or trauma with swelling).
- Excessive pressure from poorly fitted shoe wear (i.e. pointed, high-heeled shoes) has been linked to development of interdigital neuritis.
- Activities that require repetitive hyperextension at the metatarsophalangeal joint (walking, running, or squatting) may contribute to the problem.
- Atrophy of the forefoot fat pad can lead to increased trauma to the nerves from decreased shock absorption.
- The highest predilection is in the **third intermetatarsal space**, which may be due to dual contribution of the digital nerve from both *medial* and *lateral plantar nerves*, leading to more tethering and increased traction on that nerve (Mann and Reynolds 1983).

- The second interspace is the second most common location. It is very unusual to have concomitant lesions, so one must suspect more of a neuralgia as opposed to a true interdigital neuritis when the patient presents with more than one symptomatic interspace.

Clinical

- There will be tenderness and paresthesias with plantar pressure directed between the metatarsal heads and just proximal to the heads. This should reproduce the patient's pain (compression test).
- An audible, painful click when performing concomitant lateral, dorsal, and plantar compression of the metatarsal heads in the affected region is called the Mulder click, and is considered to be supportive of the diagnosis (Mulder 1951).
- Imaging for Morton neuroma has limited utility and specificity (i.e. enlarged nerve on ultrasound or magnetic resonance imaging, MRI, helps support the diagnosis but by itself is not diagnostic).
- X-ray helps rule out other bony disorders that may be in the differential diagnosis.
- Relief of the pain with local anesthetic agents supports the diagnosis.
- Nerve conduction studies may show significant latency in the foot and help support the diagnosis.

Associated Conditions and Differential Diagnosis

- Patients with interdigital neuritis may have elevated forefoot pressures due to a tight gastrocnemius.
- There may be hypermobility of the first metatarsal, leading to overload of the second and third metatarsal heads, with neuritis a direct result.
- Pain in the second or third interspace may arise from conditions other than neuritis, such as metatarsophalangeal synovitis.
- The Morton neuroma is probably over-diagnosed. It is important to remember that there are many causes of metatarsalgia, and to restrict the diagnosis of interdigital neuritis to patients with tenderness at a single interspace not having any of the other diagnoses (Box 13–1).

Non-operative Treatment

- Perhaps the first treatment should include shoe wear modifications, especially lower heels and wider toe boxes.
- The addition of an orthotic with metatarsal relief or a metatarsal bar on the sole of the shoe will take pressure away from the interspace and transfer it more proximally.
- Thicker, more cushioned soles decrease impact and pressure on the interspace.
- Plantar pads applied to the insole proximal to the neuroma elevate the metatarsal head, decrease pressure, and possibly open the space between the metatarsal shafts/heads.

Box 13–1 Differential Diagnosis of Metatarsalgia

- Plantar fat pad atrophy
- Tight gastrocnemius
- Hypermobile first metatarsal with transfer metatarsalgia
- Interdigital neuritis (Morton neuroma)
- Metatarsophalangeal synovitis
- Metatarsophalangeal arthritis
- Cavus foot

- Non-steroidal antiinflammatory drugs (NSAIDs).
- Tricyclics or antiseizure medications (such as amitriptyline [Elavil], gabapentin [Neurontin], and topiramate [Topamax]) are off-label by the US Food and Drug Administration for the treatment of this disorder, but may significantly lessen symptoms.
- *Corticosteroid injection* may have long-lasting relief. A single injection has a 14% chance of completely relieving symptoms. By repeating injections several times, the overall cure rate rises to 30%.
- Caution should be taken when repeating injection to the site multiple times, due to potential for local tissue atrophy and skin pigmentation changes.
- Even though a single injection is not commonly curative, such an injection can be useful as a diagnostic test for interdigital neuritis.
- There may be some utility to radiofrequency ablation.

Operative Treatment

- The nerve can be approached from either a dorsal or plantar approach. Most surgeons prefer the dorsal approach for primary operation, and the plantar for revision surgery.
- Some advocate decompression of the nerve (with a transverse ligament release and possible neurolysis), but most orthopaedists rely on excision (neurectomy with or without intermuscular transposition of the proximal stump).
- Transverse ligament release has been reported to relieve symptoms in 80% of patients. Endoscopic transverse ligament release may have less morbidity and quicker recovery.
- The success rate of traditional neuroma resection (neurectomy) is generally considered to be 80%. This reflects the multifactorial nature of metatarsalgia. If the interdigital neuritis is a result of forefoot overload (rather than the primary problem), then resection of the nerve will relieve only a portion of the symptoms (forefoot overload will continue).
- Persistent pain from a recurrent stump neuroma can be a problem. This is why some surgeons bury the proximal stump in the interosseus muscle.
- Other complications include a synovial sinus, hypertrophic scar, wound infection, and chronic regional pain syndrome (Coughlin and Pinsonneault 2001).

Tarsal Tunnel Syndrome

Description

- Tarsal tunnel syndrome is a nerve entrapment produced by pressure on the posterior tibial nerve or any of its three major distal branches (the medial plantar nerve, lateral plantar nerve, and medial calcaneal nerve), as they pass under the flexor retinaculum behind the medial malleolus.
- Variability in anatomical location of these branches may affect the propensity for acquiring the disorder.
- Tarsal tunnel syndrome is characterized by pain and paresthesias radiating from the medial side of the ankle distally into the foot and sometimes proximally into the leg.

Etiology

- True tarsal tunnel syndrome probably is quite rare. Many cases have a space-occupying lesion in the tarsal tunnel, such as a hypertrophic non-union of the sustentaculum tali, a neurilemmoma, synovial sarcoma, or epineural ganglion cyst.
- Hypermobile flatfoot deformity has also been associated with increased pressure/tension on the tibial nerve (Daniels et al. 1998).
- Because tarsal tunnel syndrome is relatively rare, it is important to rule out other disorders, such as peripheral neuropathy and plantar fasciitis.

Clinical

- There will be complaints of vague pain at the medial ankle. Some may have more dramatic findings of paresthesias and numbness in the posterior tibial nerve distribution.
- A positive **Tinel sign** is considered by many to be a requisite finding when making the diagnosis. Percussion is most properly performed not only at the fibroosseous tunnel behind the medial malleolus, but also into the foot along the leading edge of the abductor digiti quinti, or any location of suspected compression.
- Activity may worsen symptoms, and rest typically will decrease the intensity of the symptoms.
- Imaging studies (x-ray, MRI, or ultrasound) may help isolate extrinsic compressive/space-occupying lesions.
- Electromyography and/or nerve conduction studies can be helpful. Latency in nerve conduction velocities across the ankle or motor latency of the abductor digiti quinti or abductor hallucis help support the diagnosis, but inconclusive findings do not rule out the possibility of tarsal tunnel syndrome.

Non-operative Treatment

- Decreasing nerve tension from planovalgus foot deformity with a suitable orthotic is appropriate.
- NSAIDs and corticosteroid injections may prove useful for alleviation of symptoms.
- Physical therapy may help reduce local soft tissue swelling around the ankle and improve biomechanics (stretching of the calf/gastrocnemius to minimize the deforming effects on the foot).
- Night splints may help alleviate pressure/tension on the tibial nerve generated by foot deformity.

Operative Treatment

- When there is a space-occupying lesion, resection of the lesion should lead to a good result.
- Neurolysis of any tethering scar or adhesions is recommended, and occasionally release of the epineurium is indicated for severe scar formation around the nerve.
- Knowledge of the nerve anatomy and its variability will improve outcomes by ensuring adequate visualization and release of all the appropriate branches, as well as decrease iatrogenic injury.
- Outcomes tend to be good when the proper diagnosis has been made and the compressive lesion adequately removed (Gondring et al. 2003; Sammarco and Chang 2003).

Anterior Tarsal Tunnel Syndrome

Description

- *Anterior tarsal tunnel syndrome* is a compression syndrome affecting the deep peroneal nerve as it passes beneath the inferior extensor retinaculum.
- The superficial peroneal nerve may also be a site for compression as it pierces the fascia in the lower third of the leg. While much less common than other nerve compression disorders, it must be considered in the differential.

Etiology

- Compression of the deep peroneal nerve probably arises from repetitive trauma from tight shoe straps.
- Internal structures also put pressure on the nerve, including osteophyte from the dorsum of the first or second metatarsal base joints, and ganglion cysts.

Clinical

- The most common findings are pain, hyperesthesia, and occasionally decreased sensation, particularly in the first dorsal web space.
- A positive Tinel sign is often present.
- Weakness or atrophy of the extensor digitorum brevis muscle belly may also be present, so electrodiagnostic studies may have positive findings corresponding to sensory latencies as well as denervation potentials.

Treatment

- Attempts should be made to relieve pressure on the nerve. Shoe modifications or pads may help.

- Injection therapy may be both diagnostic and therapeutic.
- Surgical decompression is reserved for failed conservative measures, and involves simple decompression of the nerve by releasing the inferior extensor retinaculum and removing any intrinsic compressive structures.

Incisional or Traumatic Neuromas

Description

- Neuromas are generated by injury to sensory branches in the foot.
- Because the foot has very little soft tissue cushioning, and shoe wear is frequently snug over the majority of its surfaces, incisional or traumatic neuromas can be very problematic.
- Careful attention to placement of incisions and protection of sensory branches can help prevent the majority of these neuromas.
- Trauma/crush mechanisms often cause significant injury to the relatively subcutaneous nerves of the foot and ankle.

Clinical

- Pain, sensory disturbances, burning, and positive Tinel sign are the most common findings.
- Patients with pain, allodynia, and paresthesias/dysesthesias need to be properly identified and distinguished from patients with complex regional pain syndrome (CRPS) by making sure that the anatomical location of the symptoms can be explained with specific nerve injury.
- Electrodiagnostic studies may help elucidate the level or location of nerve injury by identifying specific sensory/motor latencies along the course of the nerve.

Treatment

- Modifications of shoe wear may alleviate pressure on affected nerves.
- Local injection therapy can be both a diagnostic and a therapeutic agent.
- Medications include NSAIDs, antidepressants, and anticonvulsant agents.
- Manual therapy to work on release of adhesions between skin and underlying nerve tissue may help reduce neuropraxia associated with a specific site of injury.
- Surgery is reserved for failed cases, and is aimed at neurolysis and releasing the nerve from scar. Occasionally, resection of the nerve at a more proximal level may be indicated, but can lead to more problems with further painful neuroma formation.
- There is limited experience with techniques such as wrapping the nerve with a vein graft.

Complex Regional Pain Syndrome/Reflex Sympathetic Dystrophy

Description

- These chronic pain conditions are believed to be the result of dysfunction of the central or peripheral nervous system.
- **CRPS type 1**, otherwise known as *reflex sympathetic dystrophy* (*RSD*), is a pain disorder characterized by a clinical picture of burning pain, sensory abnormalities, edema, autonomic dysfunction, functional impairment, and trophic changes of the skin and underlying bony structures. It can be incited by simple trauma, surgery, or other factors.
- **CRPS type 2**, or *causalgia*, has the same clinical presentation but has an identifiable nerve injury.
- Extensive research supports involvement of the sympathetic nervous system (sympathetically maintained pain) as well as other pathophysiologic pathways (sympathetically independent pain).
- These disorders are most common in adults but can also occur in children, for whom the prognosis is believed to be better.
- May have a genetic and/or phenotypic propensity.

Clinical

- There is a history of soft tissue, bone, or nervous system trauma resulting from a sprain, fracture, surgery, or crush injury.
- Typically, a triad of findings on examination with a combination of sensory abnormalities and autonomic and motor disturbances.
  - Ongoing pain, allodynia, or hyperalgesia that usually exceeds the distribution of a single nerve (hence the regional nature of the disease).
  - Evidence of edema, blood flow abnormalities (such as splotchy or mottled skin).
  - Abnormal sudomotor activity in the region of pain.
  - Trophic changes to the skin, such as abnormal hair/nail growth.
  - X-rays may show patchy osteoporosis.
  - May have dystonia in the affected extremity that can lead to progressive muscle atrophy and loss of range of motion/stiffness of joints involved.
- There are reports of the pain syndrome spreading, and even skipping over contiguous regions and manifesting in a different limb (Maleki et al. 2000).

Differential Diagnosis and Diagnostic Procedures

- Sympathetically maintained pain can also accompany diabetic peripheral neuropathy, stroke, postherpetic neuralgia, and herniated disk lesions.

- Although still controversial, there may be separate stages:
  - Stage 1: 1-3 months, characterized by severe burning pain along with muscle spasms, joint stiffness, rapid hair growth, and alterations in blood vessels that lead to skin discoloration and thermal changes.
  - Stage 2: 3-6 months, characterized by intensifying pain; swelling; decreased hair growth; cracked, grooved, brittle, or spotty nails; softened bones; muscle weakness/atrophy; and stiff joints.
  - Stage 3: There are irreversible skin and bone changes, pain tends to be unyielding, and there are marked limb changes ranging from simple loss of function to contractures and deformity.
- *Thermography* has been shown to have some utility in making the diagnosis (Gulevich et al. 1997).
- *Triple-phase bone scan* may be helpful but has limited sensitivity, as low as 50% in some studies. Increased diffuse uptake on the delayed images (phase 3) is considered the most suggestive and sensitive finding (Werner et al. 1989).
- *Sudomotor function testing*: Sweat test (sympathetic skin response), quantitative sudomotor axon reflex test, and chemical sweat test are all tools available at some centers to help establish a diagnosis.
- *Quantitative sensory testing* measures painful response to mechanical and thermal stimuli. There is a profoundly lower threshold for pain in patients with CRPS.
- Sympathetic blockade remains one of the most important diagnostic and treatment modalities available. While typically only effective for sympathetically maintained pain syndromes, the duration of its efficacy generally outlasts the duration of the local anesthetic.

Treatment

- The treatment is highly dependent on the condition of the patient at time of diagnosis, and modalities available to the individual practitioner.
- Response and long-term results are highly dependent on early recognition and aggressive treatment. Even early appropriate treatment does not prevent long-term sequelae and relapse.
- Modalities include physical therapy, occupational therapy, recreational therapy, and medication/pharmacologic, surgical, and psychologic therapy.
  - Physical therapy/occupational therapy: Steady progression of gentle weight-bearing exercise individually designed to restore function of the affected extremity. May incorporate a desensitization program (Stanton-Hicks et al. 1998).
  - Recreational therapy: Helps to reengage the patient in previously enjoyable activity.
  - Psychologic therapy: A multidisciplinary approach including treatment of psychiatric illness, such as underlying depression as a result of chronic pain and disability.
  - Medications: opioid analgesics (morphine, tramadol), non-opioid analgesics (NSAIDs, acetaminophen), antidepressants (tricyclics [e.g. amitriptyline, doxepin], serotonin reuptake inhibitors [e.g. paroxetine, fluoxetine], and others [e.g. venlafaxine, bupropion]), anticonvulsants (carbamazepine, phenytoin, gabapentin), corticosteroids, topical anesthetic agents (5% Lidoderm patches).
- Sympathetic blockade helps arrest the cycle of sympathetic hypersensitivity and relieves pain. Controversy exists over surgical sympathectomy; it should probably be considered only in severe recalcitrant cases with documented sympathetic involvement.
- Spinal cord stimulation has shown promise in refractory cases (Kemler et al. 2004).
- Intrathecal drug pumps that provide continuous infusion of epidural opioids and local anesthetics at much lower, safer doses than those required for oral administration.
- Peripheral stimulation has shown promise in several studies but is probably most effective when there is prominent involvement of one major nerve.
- For patients in whom surgery is to be undertaken in the involved extremity, great caution should be exercised, as there is frequently exacerbation of CRPS with any new injury. This should be anticipated and treated with a sympathetic block preoperatively, and possibly with epidural blockade postoperatively.
- Amputation of an extremity is frequently complicated with persistent pain and even recurrent CRPS in the stump, and therefore should be avoided (Dielissen et al. 1995).

References

Interdigital Neuroma

Coughlin MJ, Pinsonneault T. (2001) Operative treatment of interdigital neuroma: A long-term follow-up study. J Bone Joint Surg 83A: 1321-1328.

In a clinical series of surgically treated patients, 85% were found to have good results, but one-third had incomplete relief of pain.

Mann R, Reynolds C. (1983) Interdigital neuroma—a critical clinical analysis. Foot Ankle 3: 238-243.

In a series of patients treated surgically, 85% were improved after surgery. About two-thirds had persistent tenderness following resection, and two-thirds noted interspace numbness.

Mulder J. (1951) The causative mechanism in Morton's metatarsalgia. J Bone Joint Surg 33(B): 94-95.

A description of the classic test for a neuroma.

Wu K. (1996) Morton's interdigital neuroma: A clinical review of its etiology, treatment, and results. J Foot Ankle Surg 35: 112-119.

A review of interdigital neuroma.

Tarsal Tunnel Syndrome

Daniels T, Lau J, Hearn T. (1998) The effects of foot position and load on tibial nerve tension. Foot Ankle Intl 19: 73-78.

Hindfoot eversion that accompanies flatfoot deformity increases tension on the tibial nerve. Flatfoot deformity may explain some causes of tarsal tunnel symptoms in patients with no space-occupying lesion.

Gondring W, Shields B, Wenger S. (2003) An outcomes analysis of surgical treatment of tarsal tunnel syndrome. Foot Ankle Int 24: 545-550.
In a series of 60 patients treated surgically, 85% were seen to improve objectively, but only half of all patients thought they were better.

Nagaoka M, Satou K. (1999) Tarsal tunnel syndrome caused by ganglia. J Bone Joint Surg Br 81: 607-610.
Although rare, space-occupying lesions can cause tarsal tunnel syndrome. In these cases, surgical removal led to complete relief of symptoms.

Sammarco G, Chang L. (2003) Outcome of surgical treatment of tarsal tunnel syndrome. Foot Ankle Int 24: 125-131.
In a large clinical series, tibial nerve compression was due to vascular leashes, varicosities, and some space-occupying lesions.

Complex Regional Pain Syndrome

Dielissen P, Claasen A, Veldman P. (1995) Amputation for reflex sympathetic dystrophy. J Bone Joint Surg Br 77: 836.
In a small series of patients with RSD who underwent amputation, the majority had recurrence of symptoms in the stump.

Gulevich S, Conwell TD, Lane J, et al. (1997) Stress infrared telethermography is useful in the diagnosis of complex regional pain syndrome, type I (formerly reflex sympathetic dystrophy). Clin J Pain 13: 50-59.
Telethermography was seen to be a good test for RSD, with high specificity and sensitivity.

Kemler MA et al. (2004) The effect of spinal cord stimulation in patients with chronic reflex sympathetic dystrophy: Two years' follow-up of the randomized controlled trial. Ann Neurol 55: 13-18.
A randomized trial comparing spinal cord stimulation with therapy to physical therapy alone found significant improvements in outcome measures with stimulation.

Maleki J, LeBel A, Bennett G. (2000) Patterns of spread in complex regional pain syndrome. Pain 88: 259-266.
In a small retrospective series, most patients were seen to have spread of RSD symptoms to adjacent areas in the same limb, as well as sites in other extremities. A small minority had symptoms develop in the same part of the contralateral extremity.

Stanton-Hicks M, Baron R, Boas R, et al. (1998) Complex regional pain syndromes: Guidelines for therapy. Clin J Pain 14: 155-166.
A multidisciplinary approach to treating pain syndromes, with a central theme of functional restoration.

Werner R, Davidoff G, Jackson MD et al. (1989) Factors affecting the sensitivity and specificity of the three-phase technetium bone scan in the diagnosis of reflex sympathetic dystrophy syndrome in the upper extremity. J Hand Surg Am 14: 520-523.
This retrospective series found the sensitivity to be only 50%.

CHAPTER 14

Ankle Arthritis

Michael Brage[*] and Catherine M. Robertson[§]

[*]M.D., Associate Clinical Professor, Department of Orthopaedics, University of California, Irvine, CA
[§]M.D., Department of Orthopaedics, University of California, San Diego, CA

- Posttraumatic arthritis is the most common cause of ankle degenerative disease. Ankle arthritis may also arise from instability (recurrent sprains), from inflammatory disease, after infection, or from a handful of rarer causes. Idiopathic arthritis of the ankle is uncommon compared with that of other large joints such as the hip and knee, with rates 9 times lower in the ankle.

Posttraumatic

- Posttraumatic causes account for approximately 50% of ankle arthritis cases. Arthritis correlates with fracture type, degree of cartilage injury, and incongruity of the articular surface.
- Radiographic evidence of arthritis is usually apparent within 2 years of injury in high-energy injuries. However, in many cases it may be decades before pain becomes severe.
- Arthritis occurs after approximately 14% of ankle (malleolar) fractures. Weber C (proximal) fractures have a higher rate of arthritis (33%), as do trimalleolar fractures. Maintaining fibular length and reduction of the posterior malleolar fragment improve outcome. Larger posterior malleolar fragments involve a greater proportion of the articular surface and accordingly result in a higher rate of arthritis.
- Unreduced syndesmotic injuries are a common cause of posttraumatic arthritis. Because most Weber C injuries include syndesmotic disruption, failure to adequately reduce the syndesmosis may have accounted for the higher rate of arthritis with these injuries in the past.
- Widening of the syndesmosis by 1 mm increases peak contact pressures in the ankle by 50%.
- Pilon fractures are a higher energy injury and often result in increased rates of cartilage injury. Consequently, there is a higher rate of arthritis and avascular necrosis (AVN) as well as a higher complication rate. Soft tissue injury may also be extensive and compromise both healing in the acute setting and future surgical procedures. Early range of motion may decrease the risk of arthritis.
- Talus fractures are less common but result in rates of posttraumatic arthritis as high as 50-97%. The risk of AVN is also high; AVN is the cause of much of the reported arthritis after talar fractures. The talus is particularly prone to AVN because of its tenuous blood supply and predominately cartilaginous surface.
- Osteochondral lesions of the talus typically do not lead to severe arthritis. Although they can cause pain, they typically involve a small surface area. The natural history of osteochondral lesions, whether small or large, is not well documented.
- Other causes of ankle arthritis are shown in Table 14–1.

Biology of Ankle Cartilage

- The ankle bears the highest load per surface area of any joint in the body, yet has a small surface contact area of only 350 mm^2. The ankle bears up to 5 times the body weight with normal walking.
- Ankle cartilage is thinner than in the knee and hip (thickness: 1-1.7 mm).

Table 14–1: Causes of Ankle Arthritis

ETIOLOGY	FEATURES
Posttraumatic	Most common cause Result of intraarticular ankle fractures Can also be late result of tibial shaft or calcaneal malunion
Chronic ligamentous instability	Recurrent ankle sprains may lead to chronic instability of the ankle Instability can result in joint incongruence and cartilage damage Often see anterior subluxation of talus
Postinfectious	Cartilage destruction occurs secondary to inflammatory cascade Antibiotics and surgical irrigation and debridement may limit cartilage damage
Inflammatory arthritis	Characterized by thickened synovium or pannus, bony erosions, and osteopenia Generally symmetric Forefoot and midfoot more common than ankle Ankylosing spondylitis, Reiter syndrome, and psoriatic arthritis most common in ankle
Crystalline arthropathy	Gout and calcium pyrophosphate deposition disease cause episodic pain and inflammation Best treated with gout-specific medications Less common in the ankle than in other foot joints such as the first metatarsophalangeal
Neuropathic arthropathy	Diabetes most common cause, but paralysis, peripheral nerve injury, Charcot-Marie-Tooth also rare causes Characterized by bone loss and deformity
Hemochromatosis	Recurrent hemarthroses are painful and over time lead to cartilage destruction
Tumor	Osteoid osteoma in young patients, pigmented villonodular synovitis, synovial chondromatosis
Idiopathic	Rare

- Biomechanically, the ankle joint is highly congruent, and its cartilage is uniform and stiff, allowing it to withstand high forces.
- In the normal situation, this congruency keeps the contact pressures at an acceptable level. But if the surface area of the joint is decreased or the congruency is lost, then the pressures rise quickly, leading to arthritis.
  - This is in contrast to the knee, where slight incongruencies can be compensated for by the menisci.

Evaluation of the Arthritic Ankle

History and Physical Examination

- Pain is the most common presenting symptom and is characteristically deep in the anterior ankle or dorsal foot.
- History should include any previous trauma or infection, history of systemic disease such as diabetes or inflammatory arthritis, previous treatments, shoe wear, use of orthotics, and tobacco use.
- Physical examination should include areas of tenderness, alignment, and range of motion. Assessment of alignment of the ankle and hindfoot is particularly important, as the presence of severe deformity changes treatment options. The presence and location of calluses may point to underlying deformity or malalignment, while scars are evidence of previous trauma or surgery.
- Observation of the appearance of the soft tissues, palpation of pulses, and monofilament sensory testing provide additional information about healing potential. If pulses are not palpable, vascular assessment is needed. If any signs of neuropathy are found, the source of the neuropathy must be identified.
- Examination of the foot as well as the ankle can yield additional useful information.
  - Hindfoot flexibility, stability, and alignment should be noted.
  - Arthritis at adjacent joints may require concurrent treatment to obtain relief of symptoms.
- Gait analysis in patients with ankle arthritis typically shows decreased velocity, stride length, and cadence, and more time in double-limb stance. However, a formal gait analysis is generally not required in the work-up of ankle arthritis.

Imaging

- Radiographs should include weight-bearing anteroposterior, lateral, and mortise views of the ankle as well as anteroposterior, lateral, and medial oblique views of the foot. Radiographs should be assessed for joint space narrowing, alignment, and bone quality. The location and size of osteophytes should also be noted, especially when impingement is suspected. Obtaining a weight-bearing film is critical to assess true deformity and joint space narrowing. Congruity of the mortise and fibular length should also be assessed if there is concern for instability.
- Alignment should be evaluated on both sagittal and coronal views. A procurvatum or recurvatum deformity may be noted by examining the relationship of the tibia to the talus, which should be centrally located with its lateral process under the midline of the tibia.

In the coronal plane, varus-valgus alignment should be at approximately 0°, measured by the intersection of the midtibial line and the talar dome.

- Radiographs and a gross photo of ankle arthritis are shown in Figure 14–1.
- Additional specialized views may be useful in certain patients. The weight-bearing hindfoot alignment view shows coronal alignment of the hindfoot. The Harris view shows axial alignment of calcaneus, and the Broden view shows the subtalar joint.
- Other imaging modalities are generally not needed for diagnosis and surgical planning unless diagnosis is in doubt. Bone scans may identify occult arthritis, stress fracture, infection, or reflex sympathetic dystrophy. Computed tomography (CT) can be used to identify a subtle syndesmosis injury and for complex fractures. Magnetic resonance imaging is most useful for investigating the soft tissues, such as in cases of infection and tumor.

Other Diagnostic Modalities

- Selective diagnostic injections of local anesthetic, such as lidocaine, may be injected in the ankle and adjacent joints to determine relative contributions to symptomatology. For example, pain from subtalar arthritis may be confused with ankle-related pain, and may be clarified with selective injections to aid surgical planning and improve outcome.
- Laboratory data are generally not helpful in diagnosing ankle arthritis. However, if there is concern for infection, complete blood count, erythrocyte sedimentation rate, and C-reactive protein are sensitive indicators.

Non-surgical Treatment

Activity Modification and Bracing

- A number of non-surgical treatments may relieve the symptoms of ankle arthritis. Non-surgical, non-pharmaceutical modalities may alleviate pain and carry a low risk of complication, although effectiveness may be less in severe arthritis.
- Activity modification may minimize the pain of ankle arthritis. Steps include recommending low-impact activities such as swimming and stationary bicycle over high-impact exercise, for example jogging, and sedentary work over occupations that require prolonged standing.
- Weight loss may also alleviate symptoms by decreasing force across the joint, and may improve results of future surgical procedures.
- A cane carried in the contralateral hand may partially off-load the joint.
- Shoe modifications, orthotics, and braces can also be used to temper the pain of an arthritic ankle.
  - A shoe with a rocker sole may allow more comfortable gait by decreasing the amount of ankle motion needed.
  - A high-top shoe, boot, or lace-up ankle brace can provide some support and immobilization of the ankle.

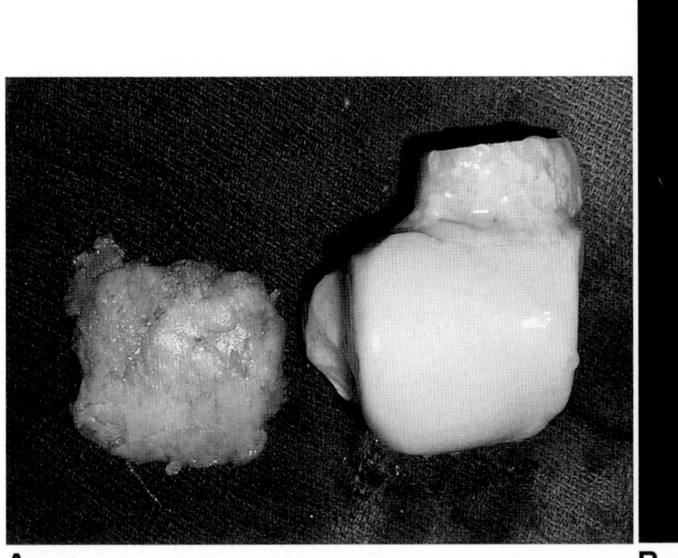

A

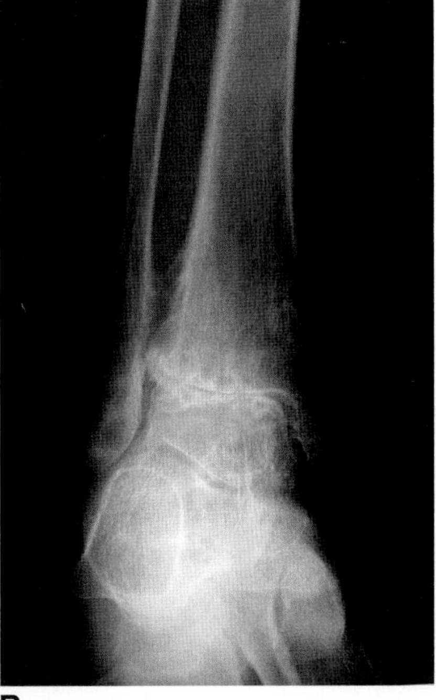

B

Figure 14–1: A, Gross photo and B, C, radiographs of the arthritic ankle. A, On the right is a normal talar dome, and the left shows an arthritic one, with loss of cartilage and subchrondal slerosis.

Continued

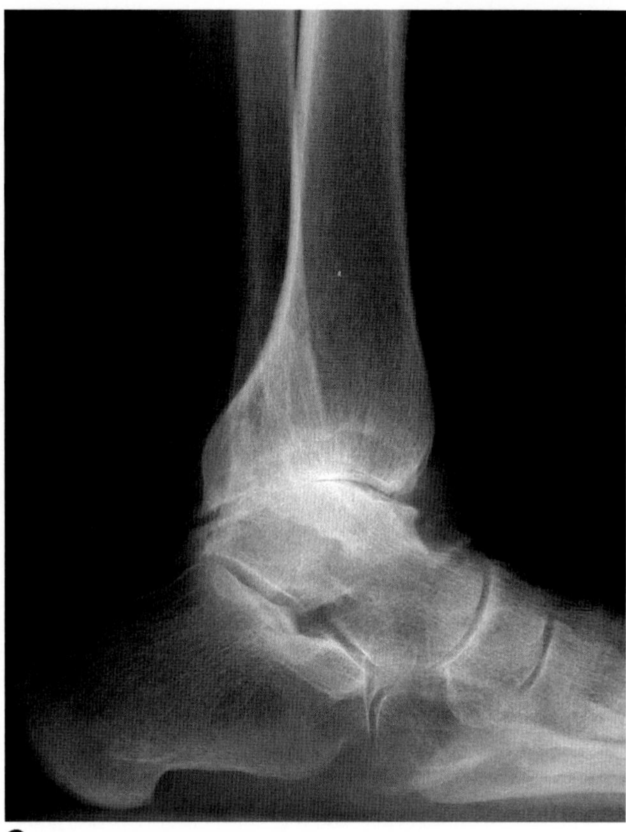

Figure 14–1: Cont'd

- An ankle-foot orthosis also immobilizes the ankle joint, improves axial alignment, and can improve gait.
- An off-loading brace that transfers load away from the ankle and to the patellar tendon and proximal tibia can be used in extreme situations. However, these braces are bulky and cumbersome.

- Casting may be viewed as the ultimate brace for the ankle, and offers pain relief by immobilizing the ankle joint. A short leg walking cast can be used for 6 weeks to reduce inflammation and pain, although post-immobilization stiffness should be expected.

Medications

- Medications may also be used to relieve the pain and inflammation of ankle arthritis. Non-steroidal anti-inflammatory drugs (NSAIDs) act by blocking cyclooxygenase (COX) to limit prostaglandin production and thus inflammation. They also have a central effect, which is responsible for their analgesic action. The most common complication of NSAID use is gastrointestinal upset and bleeding, and renal and hepatic screening is recommended in some patient groups. Newer COX-2 inhibitors offer similar pain relief with fewer gastro-intestinal consequences, but newer studies have identified cardiovascular side effects for some.
- Glucosamine is a building block of proteoglycans, the primary component of cartilage matrix. Although data are limited and primarily addresses osteoarthritis of the knee, it has been shown to offer some pain relief to patients and result in decreased inflammation in arthritic joints. Glucosamine is commonly coupled with chondroitin, another cartilage matrix protein, and sold as an over the counter supplement in a largely unregulated fashion. Quantity and bioavailability of the active agents in these preparations is largely unknown.
- Steroid injections may be used in the ankle and adjacent joints to decrease inflammation and alleviate pain. The ankle joint is injected via the medial or lateral gutter with the needle directed posteriorly. Steroid injections have been shown to be beneficial for short-term pain reduction but are no different from placebo in the long term. Repeated injections separated by several months continue to be effective in some patients but often show diminishing returns. Complications include a low risk of infection and skin depigmentation.
- Only anecdotal evidence exists for injectable hyaluronans in the ankle.

Surgical Treatment

Debridement

- Debridement of the ankle, either open or arthroscopically, has been advocated for treatment of ankle arthritis in certain cases. The ideal patient for this procedure has a specific indication, such as hypertrophic synovium, loose body, or impinging osteophytes, with relatively preserved joint space. Small chondral lesions, less than 1 cm, may also be treated effectively with debridement and drilling. Results of debridement in generalized arthritis with joint space narrowing or deformity are poor (Fig. 14–2) (Cheng and Ferkel 1998).
- For arthroscopic debridement, the anteromedial and anterolateral portals are used as the working portals. Care must be taken to avoid injuring neurovascular structures near the portal sites, particularly branches of the superficial peroneal nerve.
- Arthroscopy allows removal of loose bodies, debridement of hypertrophic synovium, drilling of osteochondral defects, and removal of impinging osteophytes. However, treatment of extensive osteophyte complexes may not be possible through an arthroscopic approach, and may require an anterior approach to the ankle joint. Impinging bone should be removed to provide an anterior tibia to talar neck angle of greater than 60°.
- In one series, 70% good or excellent results were achieved in a series of 57 patients with arthroscopic treatment of synovitis, loose bodies, or osteophytes, compared with only 12% in patients with generalized arthritis. Furthermore, 75% of these arthritic patients went on to fusion or other further surgical treatment after debridement (Martin et al. 1989).

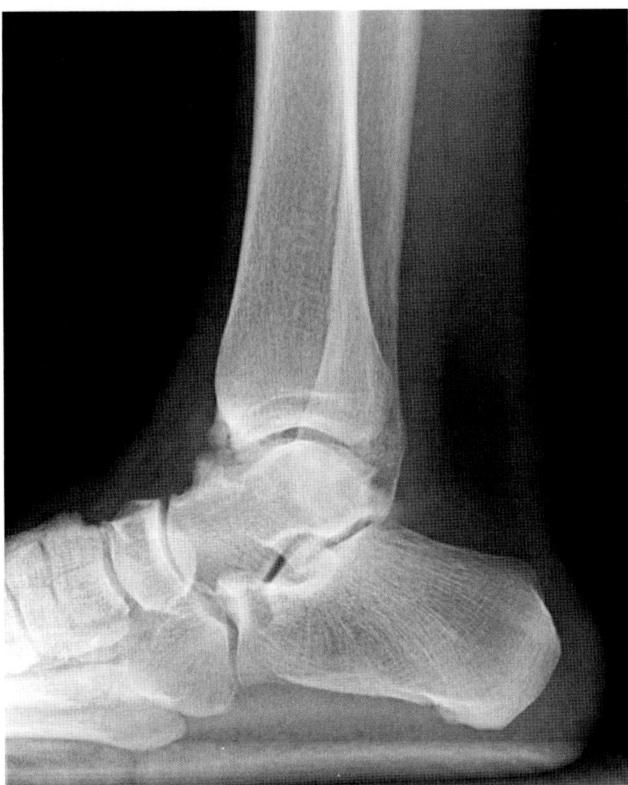

Figure 14–2: **Early ankle arthritis. Anterior osteophyte with joint space preservation: a good candidate for anterior debridement.**

Osteotomy

- After fibular fracture, if the distal fibula is not anatomically reduced, instability and resultant arthritis can occur. The fibula is most often shortened and externally rotated, allowing abnormal subluxation of the talus. These patients may present late, after fracture healing, with persistent pain.
- Radiographs may show decreased overlap of the distal fibula and anterior tibia on the anteroposterior view, or widening of the tibiofibular clear space on the mortise view. Comparing radiographs with the contralateral ankle or obtaining a CT scan of both ankles may identify subtle injuries.
- Fibular osteotomy may be indicated in these patients with fibular malunion and pain to restore fibular length and ankle stability. The goal of fibular osteotomy is seating of the distal fibula into the incisura fibularis and restoration of a symmetric joint space. Osteotomy as an isolated procedure, however, is contraindicated when there is joint space narrowing of the ankle, indicating that extensive cartilage damage has already taken place.
- Distal tibial osteotomy may be useful in certain circumstances.
- The tibia osteotomy is usually a medial or lateral closing wedge with internal fixation. It is most useful for angular deformities with loss of joint space on the medial or lateral side of the joint. By realigning the joint, weight-bearing forces are transferred from the affected to the unaffected side of the joint.
- Short-term results of distal tibial osteotomy are generally good for the rare patient with the correct indication. However, as in the knee, the surgeon should expect arthritis to slowly worsen with time.

Distraction

- Distraction arthroplasty is a possibility for a minority of patients with ankle arthritis. The theory is that, by distracting and off-loading the joint for 3 months, symptoms will reduce and the cartilage may actually repair itself.
- A thin wire (Ilizarov) external fixator is placed across the ankle in distraction.
- The technique is based on data from animal studies in which immobilization and distraction reduce mechanical forces across the joint while maintaining intraarticular flow and pressure. Because chondrocytes depend on diffusion for nutrition, maintenance of intraarticular flow without mechanical stress may promote enhanced repair of cartilage. There are, however, no human data showing cartilaginous repair, and animal data show only suggestive evidence. Alternatively, the technique may enhance joint space and relieve symptoms by increasing fibrosis of the joint (Marijnissen et al. 2003).
- Published data include solely patients with severe degenerative joint disease of the ankle with joint space narrowing. The technique is generally used in younger patients who prefer an alternative or temporizing measure prior to fusion or arthroplasty. Perhaps the best candidate is a young person with severe arthritis but preserved ankle motion (for whom fusion would not be ideal).
- The technique has thus far been limited to patients with posttraumatic or primary arthritis, as previous reports in patients with inflammatory arthritis of the hip showed poor results.
- Relative contraindications include an infected or a neuropathic joint and, as noted above, inflammatory arthritis. Although deformity may be addressed by Ilizarov technique, simple distraction does not affect alignment and should not be used as an isolated treatment in a severely deformed joint. Most importantly, the Ilizarov technique requires a committed and compliant patient and a watchful surgeon.
- The Ilizarov external fixator is placed with proximal and distal tibial rings, a half-ring around the heel with calcaneal wires, a half-ring over the forefoot with metatarsal pins, and a final wire through the talus and attached to the foot frame to prevent subtalar distraction. Distraction may be accomplished acutely in the operating room or by distracting 0.5 mm twice daily until 5 mm total of distraction is achieved. The frame is then worn for up to 3 months, with weight bearing generally allowed

after the first 1-2 weeks. The frame may be adjusted to concurrently correct equinus deformity. Angular deformity correction with an Ilizarov frame generally requires osteotomies.

- Patients require a special shoe secondary to rigidity of the foot and ankle, and must perform careful pin care and skin checks.
- Common complications include pin site infections requiring oral antibiotics, and pin breakage.
- The goals of ankle joint distraction are relief of pain through widening of the joint space. A report by van Valburg et al. (1999) did show increased joint space after distraction, but this finding has not been consistent. However, even if joint space and range of motion are not improved, a handful of case series show patient satisfaction in two-thirds to three-quarters of patients, with better functional scores over time. This implies a progressive improvement of symptoms after completion of the distraction. Approximately one-quarter of patients require fusion within 1-2 years.
- One study of 17 patients randomized to arthroscopy or distraction showed improved symptom relief in the distraction group. This study was limited by a small sample size, lack of blinding, and poor control treatment (as arthroscopy has limited benefit in generalized arthritis) (Marijnissen et al. 2002).
- In summary, distraction arthroplasty shows promising preliminary results in young patients with severe degenerative joint disease. Although it is unclear whether joint space expansion is maintained or whether cartilage repair is actually taking place, patients report improvement in the majority of cases and continue to see improvement with time, at least in 2- to 5-year follow-up. Additionally, distraction does not preclude future arthrodesis or arthroplasty. However, this technique does require a relatively sophisticated patient and committed surgeon to carefully monitor the somewhat difficult and complex Ilizarov frame.
- Distraction arthroplasty remains a viable option because of the lack of good surgical options for the younger patient with arthritis.
- Radiographs of an ankle distraction case are shown in Figure 14–3.

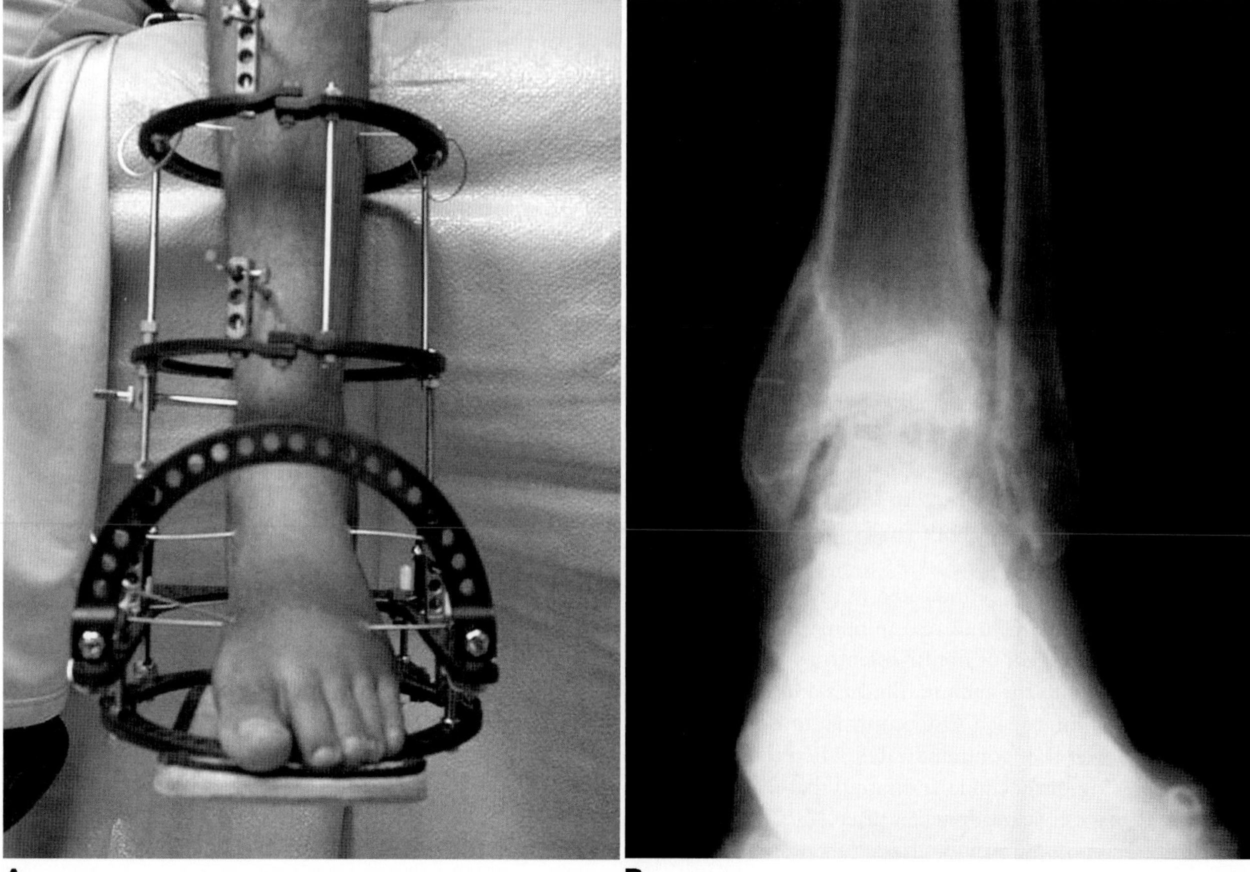

Figure 14–3: Distraction arthroplasty. **A,** The leg in the frame. **B,** Preoperative x-ray showing loss of joint space.

Continued

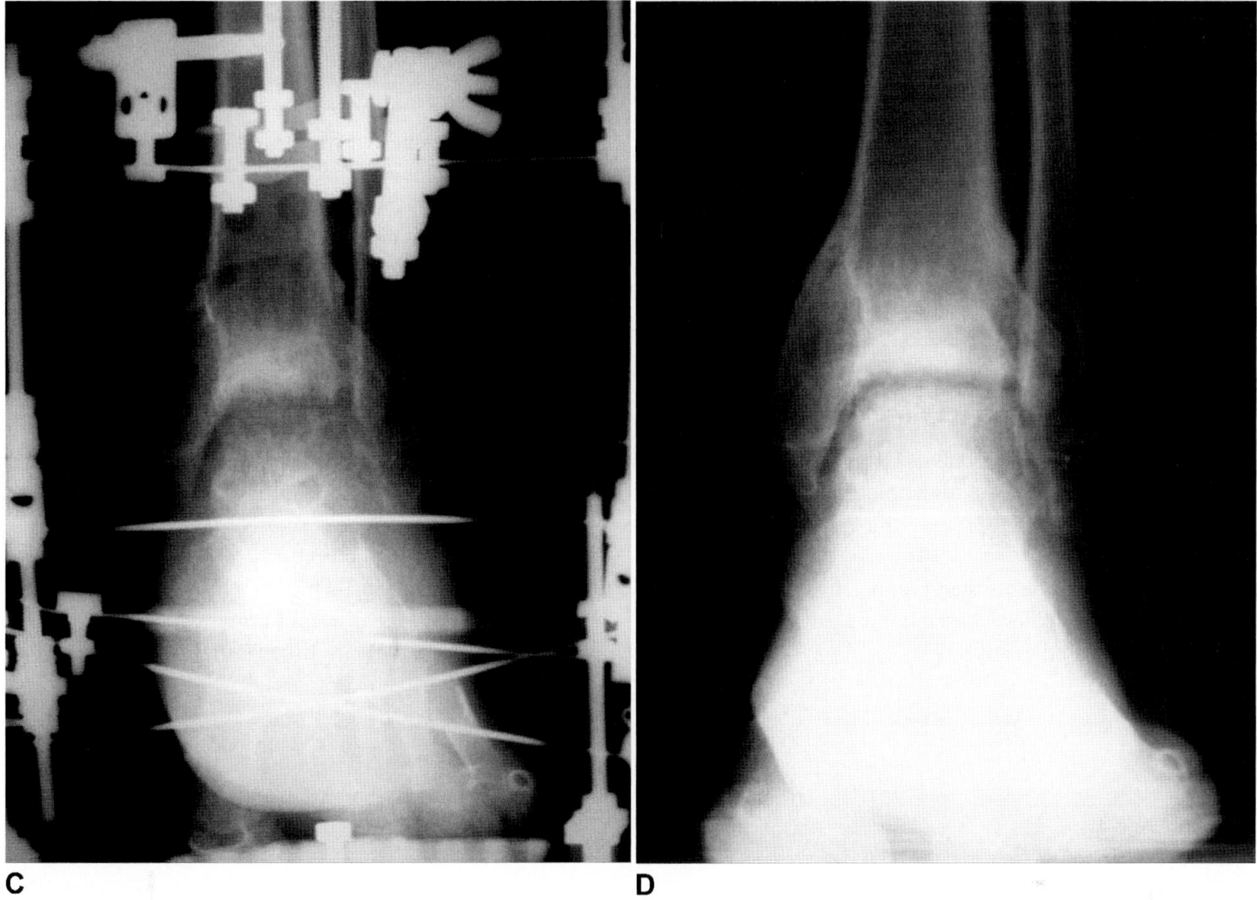

Figure 14–3: Cont'd **C**, **Radiograph during distraction. D, One-year follow-up, with suggestion of improved joint space.**

Allograft

- Fresh osteochondral allografting is another technique that offers promise to younger patients with severe ankle arthritis who wish to delay or avoid the functional limitations of arthrodesis. The technique uses a fresh cadaveric specimen to resurface the tibial plafond and talar dome with full-thickness cartilage and a thin layer of underlying bone that reliably integrates into the host bone.
- Fresh allografts offer a distinct advantage over frozen grafts used in tumor reconstructions, in that the damaged articular surface is resurfaced with viable chondrocytes. Limited second-look arthroscopy and retrieved specimen data have shown viable chondrocytes several years after implantation.
- Allografting of the arthritic ankle generally includes resurfacing the entire joint, but smaller allografts may be used for osteochondral lesions or focal AVN.
- Fresh allografts are harvested based on standard tissue procurement guidelines. Tissue is procured within 24-48 h and stored in enhanced media. Tissue is then matched to a recipient based on size, and transplanted within 2-5 weeks. Previously, tissue was transplanted within 7 days, but recent safety concerns have led to a 14-day holding period for microbiologic testing. No tissue matching or postoperative immunosuppressive therapy is currently employed.
- As with distraction, fresh allografts offer promise as a temporizing measure or potential alternative to fusion or implant arthroplasty in young, active patients with severe ankle arthritis. Published studies have limited recipients to those under 55 years of age. Obesity is also a relative contraindication, as allografts may be unable to tolerate the increased mechanical stress, particularly during early incorporation. Osteochondral allografts, like other bone graft materials, should not be placed in the setting of infection. Severe bone loss and malalignment are also relative contraindications to allografting (Box 14–1).
- The technique of fresh osteochondral allografting of the ankle borrows concepts from total ankle arthroplasty and tumor surgery. A temporary external fixator is first placed to allow joint distraction during allograft placement. An anterior approach to the ankle is then used to give wide exposure of the tibiotalar joint, as in total ankle arthroplasty. The surgeon then resects the distal tibia and

Box 14–1 Relative Contraindications to Allograft Arthroplasty

Patient Factors

- Age > 55
- Obesity
- Active infection

Local Factors

- Severe bone loss
- Severe deformity

talus, adjusting as indicated to correct mild angular deformity. Total ankle allograft cutting jigs may be used to improve precision of the resection. A size-matched allograft is then cut appropriately and fixed into the defect (Fig. 14–4).

- The patient should be assessed preoperatively to determine if an Achilles lengthening or gastrocnemius recession is required as well.
- Patients are generally kept non-weight bearing for 3 months during recovery to allow incorporation of the graft.
- A number of complications of fresh osteochondral allografting have been reported, including graft collapse, fracture, and tissue rejection. Collapse of the subchondral bone may occur, especially with heavier patients or thin grafts. Graft thickness must be balanced between the risk of collapse and a potential infectious or immunogenic risk from thicker grafts.
- No incidence of infection or disease transmission from an osteochondral allograft has been reported, although risk is probably equivalent to that of blood transfusion.
- The majority of allograft recipients show humoral cytotoxic antibodies indicative of an immune response to the foreign tissue, but no immune reaction has been noted in histologic examination of retrieved specimens.
- There is a risk of intraoperative or late fracture of the medial malleolus, which must be carefully preserved when making the tibial cut.
- Gross et al. reported a series of nine patients with focal grafts for osteochondritis dissecans lesions of the talus.

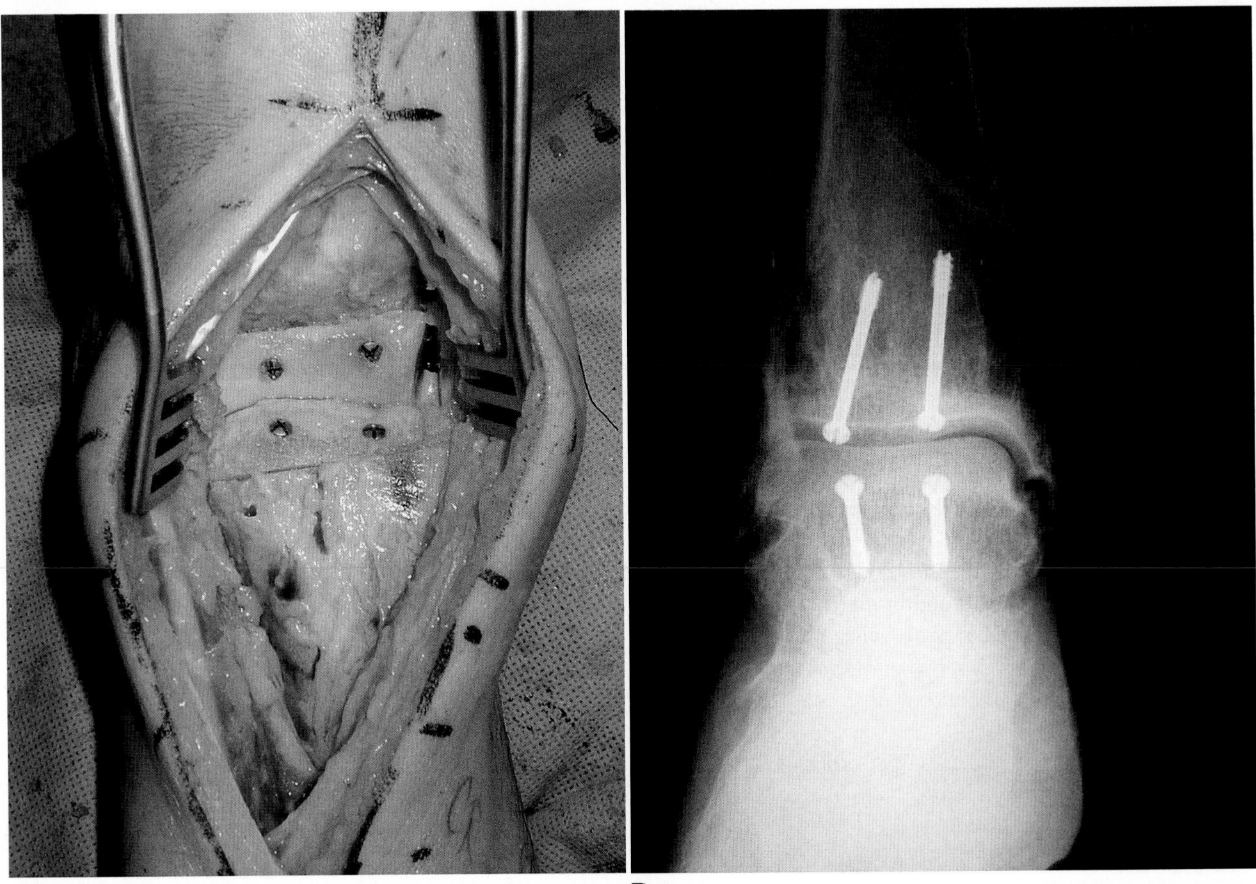

Figure 14–4: Allograft arthroplasty. **A,** Intraoperative photo showing allografts in place. **B,** Postoperative x-rays showing good incorporation of the graft.

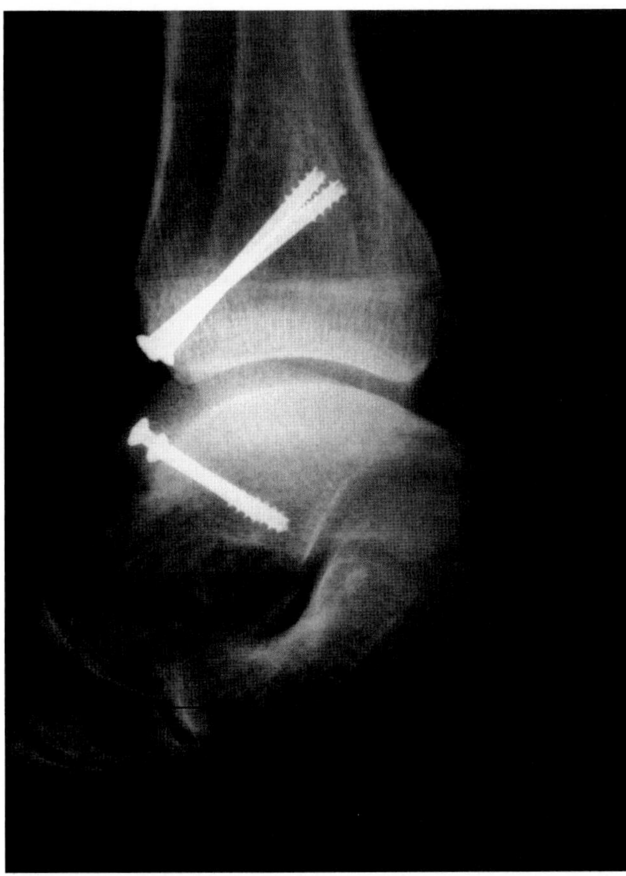

C

Figure 14–4: Cont'd C, Postoperative x-rays showing good incorporation of the graft.

Six of nine had good results with functional range of motion at 12 years' follow-up, while three suffered from graft fragmentation and underwent arthrodesis.

- Brage et al. reported a series of 11 patients with complete allograft arthroplasty (not focal), with follow-up of at least 2 years. Eight of 11 patients were satisfied (72%), with improvements in pain, gait, and walking. Two patients had regrafting for early failure secondary to collapse, and one had conversion to a total ankle arthroplasty. Risk factors identified as leading to poor outcome included graft-host mismatch (graft too small) and graft thickness less than 7 mm (graft too thin).
- In summary, fresh osteochondral allografting of the ankle represents a promising technique for young, active patients with severe ankle arthritis who are unwilling to accept the functional limitations of arthrodesis. Good results have been reported in long-term follow-up of allografts in the knee, but limited data are available for total resurfacing of the ankle.
- When compared with implant arthroplasty, allograft replacement of the ankle better preserves bone stock.
- Use of this technique is currently limited due to tissue availability and the necessity of size matching.

Arthrodesis

- Arthrodesis or fusion of the ankle is the "gold standard" of treatment for severe ankle arthritis.
- The goal of fusion is to provide a stable, painless, plantigrade ankle.
- General surgical principles of arthrodesis include:
  - a large bed of cancellous bone for healing
  - stable fixation, usually internal
  - interfragmentary compression to obtain a solid fusion mass.
- In contrast to other major joint fusions, ankle arthrodesis can result in a patient with little or no functional limitations. Good results are seen in patients with healthy subtalar and transverse tarsal joints, because these hindfoot joints provide motion to compensate for the ankle stiffness.
- Patients with arthritis in the hindfoot joints are less good candidates for ankle arthrodesis, because the final motion and comfort will not be as good.
- There are other situations in which ankle arthrodesis is not ideal. Smoking carries a 4 times greater risk of non-union. Patients with medical comorbidities also show compromised healing potential. Older literature cites poor outcomes in neuropathic joints, although fusion rates have improved with current techniques.
- The ideal ankle position is neutral dorsiflexion, 5° valgus, and 5° external rotation. Alternatively, the external rotation of the contralateral foot may be matched. Some authors advocate translating the talus posteriorly to shorten the lever arm of the foot and provide a biomechanical advantage, although this may decrease the surface area available for fusion (Box 14–2).

Approaches

- Arthrodesis is most commonly approached with an open incision, although some ankles with limited deformity are amenable to an arthroscopic or a mini-open approach. Fixation is not dependent on approach.
- With an arthroscopic approach, a joint distractor is first placed to open the joint, and then anteromedial and anterolateral portals are used to remove the distal tibial and talar cartilage with a burr and curette. Although this technique is limited to ankles with negligible deformity, the minimal bone resection potentially improves cosmesis and shoe wear. The arthroscopic approach may also yield a faster fusion due to limited soft tissue dissection (8.7 versus 14.5 weeks to fusion), with a similar fusion

Box 14–2 Ankle Position for Arthrodesis

- Dorsiflexion: Neutral
- Valgus: 5°
- External rotation: Matched to contralateral or 5°

rate. Other potential advantages are less intraoperative blood loss and a shorter hospital stay.

- The miniopen approach uses a similar technique but with enlarged portals for improved exposure.
- The open approach is the standard approach for ankle fusion, and maximizes exposure of joint surfaces and ability to correct deformity. The transfibular or lateral approach uses an incision centered over the fibula, with an oblique fibular osteotomy just above the joint line.
- There are several options for handling the fibula in a transfibular approach.
  - The fibula can be removed and mulched into bone graft. This option destroys normal ankle morphology after fusion, which might be a problem if the patient was to consider converting to a total ankle arthroplasty in the future.
  - The fibula can be removed but preserved. At the end of the procedure, the medial cortex of fibula is removed, and it is lagged back into place alongside the talus.
  - The distal fibula may be left attached to posterior soft tissues and rotated posteriorly on the soft tissue hinge. At the end of the procedure, the medial cortex is removed with a saw, and it is replaced into its normal position. In theory, the fibula acts as a vascularized fibular graft.
- With a transfibular approach, an additional smaller incision at the anterior third of the medial malleolus may improve access to the medial side of the joint. Complete removal of cartilage from the medial gutter may be difficult using a single lateral incision and is aided by this additional medial approach. However, the medial malleolus should be preserved in order to maintain blood supply to the talus through the deep deltoid ligament.
- An anterior approach to the joint in the interval of the extensor hallucis longus and tibialis anterior tendons, or extensor hallucis longus and extensor digitorum longus tendons, may also be used for arthrodesis, as for arthroplasty. Care must be taken to preserve the anterior compartment neurovascular bundle with this approach. Disadvantages of this approach include potential damage to the extensor retinaculum, and neuroma formation in small cutaneous nerves or branches of the peroneal nerve.
- Regardless of approach, the joint space should be distracted with a laminar spreader or other instrument, and all cartilage carefully removed to expose bleeding bone. Articular cartilage should be removed with an osteotome, curette, or burr to maintain the ankle contour. Some surgeons use a large saw, making a transverse or chevron cut across the tibia and talus; these techniques result in more limb shortening. Sclerotic subchondral bone should be drilled to improve healing potential.

Fixation

- Ankle fusion was originally performed with cast immobilization. Charnley in 1951 introduced external fixation as an innovation that greatly improved fusion rates. This was followed by the use of internal fixation, the current standard.
- Internal fixation provides the greatest stability to the fusion construct. Numerous techniques for internal fixation have been described and yield reliable fusion rates.
- Overall, screws offer greater compression than plates, and probably higher fusion rates. Screw placement requires less soft tissue stripping than plating.
- It is possible to provide fixation with a plate, but a lateral plate is limited by the small area for purchase in the talus, therefore requiring a blade or locking plate. An anterior T-shaped plate will have good purchase and is cited by some surgeons to work as a tension band, but there are no proven benefits to this technique.
- When screws are used, three yield greater compression than two screws, and crossing screws greater than parallel.
  - Screws are placed from the tibia and directed laterally, medially, or anteriorly into the talar body or neck.
  - Alternately, some surgeons place two screws from the lateral process of the talus back up into the tibia.
- Regardless of location, screws should be placed with all threads past the fusion site, and not violate the subtalar joint. Fluoroscopic imaging may be used to ensure screw placement and bony alignment (Figs 14–5 and 14–6).
- For combined ankle and subtalar fusions, a blade plate or retrograde intramedullary nail may be used. A retrograde nail should not be normally used if the subtalar joint is healthy.
- External fixation may also be used to support the fusion, and historically was the first type of fixation used in ankle arthrodesis. External fixation is indicated in active infections, open wounds, and severely osteopenic bone that may not support internal fixation. A thin wire ring fixator (Ilizarov) may be particularly helpful in osteoporosis. Patients may begin to bear weight on an Ilizarov frame shortly after placement.
- The major disadvantage of external fixators is that they offer less interfragmentary compression than internal fixation, with perhaps a higher chance for non-union. Uniplanar external fixators provide less rotational and sagittal stability in biomechanical studies. External fixators also require careful pin care, excellent patient compliance, and frequent physician monitoring.
- Bone graft may be used to fill bony defects or as an aid when correcting deformity. Autograft has generally been shown to be superior to allograft bone in enhancing healing. A number of sources may provide bone graft during ankle arthrodesis. When a fibular osteotomy is used to gain access to the ankle joint, the fibula may be fully or partially morselized and used as bone graft. Local bone may be taken from the calcaneus or proximal tibia. Iliac crest graft may be useful if a large bony defect exists, for example with osteonecrosis of the talus, with Charcot

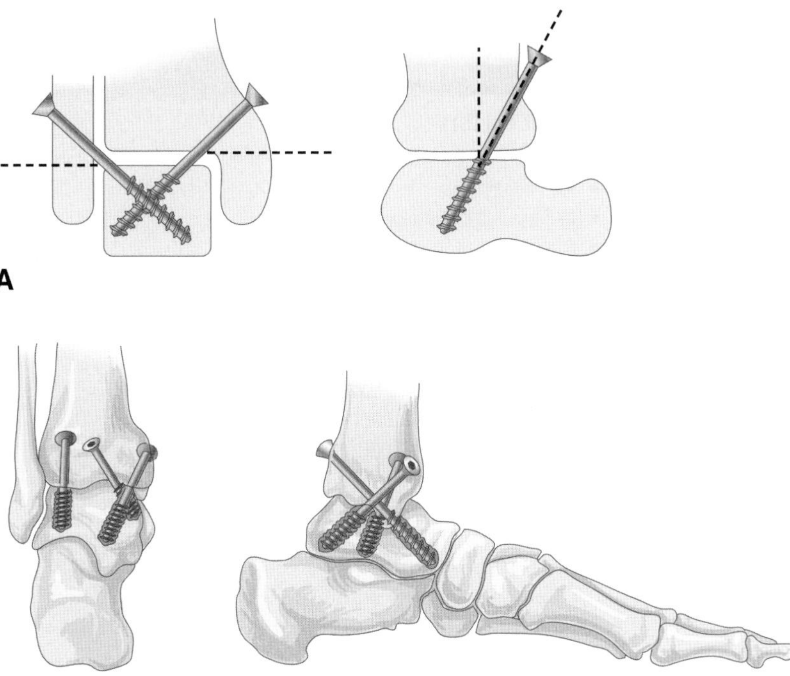

Figure 14–5: Screw placement in ankle arthrodesis. Screws can be placed in many different locations. These are two common patterns.

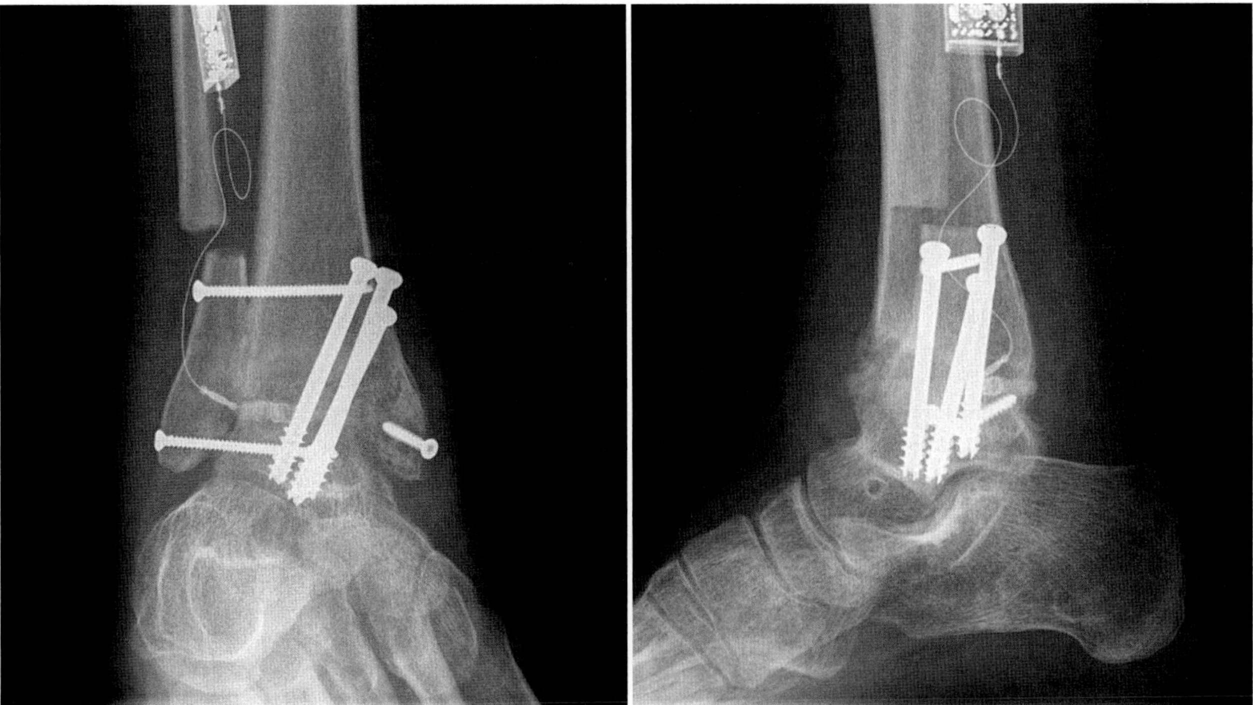

Figure 14–6: Radiograph showing ankle fusion. Ankle arthrodesis: postoperative films showing three screws across the joint and two screws bridging from the fibula. It is normally best to get screws that are crossing, not parallel, but parallel screws will work if rigid compression is achieved.

arthropathy, or after total ankle arthroplasty failure. In these cases, the graft is structural.

- Allograft bone is generally considered an inferior alternative, although a recent series reported the successful use of bulk frozen allograft during revision arthrodesis of ankles with large bony defects (Myerson et al. 2005).
- Postoperatively, patients are splinted until wound healing is evident. The patient is then placed in a short leg cast to maintain alignment, and kept non-weight bearing until radiographic signs of fusion are noted.
- Reports of time to healing after arthrodesis are extremely variable but average 3-4 months in most series. There is similar variability in terms of when a non-union is diagnosed. In the setting of delayed healing, patients should be observed with serial examination and radiographs. There is anecdotal evidence in some cases of healing after 6 months, and even 1 year with conservative treatment.

Complications

- The most common serious complications of arthrodesis include non-union, malunion, and infection.
- Infection rates of 0-28% have been reported after ankle arthrodesis. The risk may be reduced with perioperative antibiotics and prevention of wound hematomas. Certain patient groups are at higher risk for infection, including diabetics and those with renal and hepatic disease.
- Non-union is defined as a failure of bony healing or union. The rate of non-union using current techniques for ankle arthrodesis is generally less than 10%, but reported rates vary from 0 to 40%. Certain patient groups are particularly high risk, including smokers and those with impaired vascularity. Other risk factors for impaired healing are previous open fracture, pilon or talus fracture, AVN of the talus, local infection, and patient non-compliance.
- Age is not associated with non-union.
- Some surgeons feel that it is more difficult to obtain ankle fusion in the patient with previous subtalar fusion, but a few studies have failed to find this to be a significant risk factor.
- Non-union of an ankle arthrodesis generally presents with persistent pain. Radiographs may show a clear lucency at the bony interface, or more subtle signs. Lucency around the screws or shifting of the screws indicates motion at the fusion site. If radiographs are unclear, a CT scan offers a more detailed view of the fusion and may aid detection of a non-union. Once a non-union is diagnosed, identification of its cause is critical to treatment.
- Some non-unions are asymptomatic and require no further treatment (Box 14–3).
- Malunion may occur as a result of errors in intraoperative positioning, poor bone quality, or deformity at adjacent joints. Pain and increasing deformity may follow, at times leading to revision arthrodesis (Table 14–2).

Box 14–3 Risk Factors for Non-Union after Ankle Arthrodesis

Patient Factors

- Smoking
- Non-compliance
- Impaired vascular supply
- Diabetes
- Neuropathic joint

Local Factors

- Previous open fracture
- Previous pilon or talus fracture
- Avascular necrosis of the talus
- Prior or current infection

- Tibial stress fracture can occur months to years after fusion and presents with acute onset of pain. These fractures predictably occur in the distal half of tibia at a stress riser caused by the internal fixation. Treatment of tibial stress fractures is generally non-operative, consisting of casting and non-weight bearing.
- Soft tissue breakdown and skin slough may also occur after ankle arthrodesis. The ankle has a relatively thin soft tissue envelope that may be further compromised by previous injury, impaired vascularity, or systemic disease. Recognition and careful observation of patients with risk factors for wound-healing problems, as well as careful surgical technique, may reduce soft tissue problems. Wound breakdown may be treated conservatively with local wound care and dressing changes, or may require operative debridement. Rarely, a severe skin slough may require treatment with a vascularized free muscle flap.

Results

- Arthrodesis predictably alleviates pain, improves function, and allows acceptable gait. Several large series in patients with posttraumatic arthritis, rheumatoid arthritis, and osteoarthritis have shown good or excellent results in 90% of patients at long-term follow-up.
- Gait can be normal after ankle arthrodesis. If the contralateral limb is normal and there is uncompromised motion of the hindfoot joints, gait efficiency is decreased only 10% and energy requirement increases 3%. However, activities requiring more motion and energy than normal walking will be compromised after arthrodesis, such as walking on uneven ground or stairs.
- Many patients undergoing ankle arthrodesis have poor preoperative motion. Successful arthrodesis converts a stiff, painful, and sometimes deformed ankle into a stiff, straight, comfortable one.
- Although some studies have shown no change in hindfoot motion after ankle fusion, others have shown increased motion at the transverse tarsal joints. This

Table 14–2: Malunion after Ankle Arthrodesis

MALUNION TYPE	CONSEQUENCE	BRACING OPTION
Varus	Lateral foot pain Subtalar instability Pressure over base of fifth metatarsal	Neutralizing shoe modification or orthotic
Valgus	Medial knee strain Secondary foot deformity	Accommodative orthotic
Dorsiflexion	Heel pad pain and/or breakdown	Rocker bottom shoe
Plantar flexion/equinus	Metatarsalgia Back and knee pain	Solid ankle cushion heel shoe

hindfoot hypermobility partially compensates for the stiff ankle.

- The late development of adjacent joint arthritis remains a problem. Long-term follow-up of ankle arthrodesis shows a high rate of progressive subtalar and talonavicular arthritis (Coester et al. 2001). Eight years after fusion, approximately one-half of patients have adjacent joint arthritis, and after 22 years nearly all patients have arthritis in the subtalar or talonavicular joint.
- These adjacent hindfoot joints are subject to increased stress after ankle fusion. It is assumed that the increased stress leads to joint degeneration. However, it is possible that these increased stresses were present prior to fusion, when the ankle was arthritic and stiff. Adjacent joint arthritis may be a result of ankle arthritis, not just ankle arthrodesis.
- The complex issue of secondary adjacent arthritis after fusion has been a major impetus for the development of motion-preserving techniques for treating ankle arthritis.

Revision Arthrodesis

- Symptomatic malunion of an ankle fusion may require osteotomy through the fusion site. In some cases, wedge osteotomy in the distal tibia may be the simplest solution.
- In the case of a non-union, healing is the primary issue. The soft tissues, bone, hardware, and general medical condition of the patient must be carefully assessed to identify the contributors to the failure of healing. Patient non-compliance may also be a factor. Soft tissue healing and vascular sufficiency should be carefully assessed. If there is concern for an infected non-union, laboratory data such as complete blood count, C-reactive protein, and sedimentation rate may be helpful indicators, and cultures should be taken at revision. If avascular bone is present, it should be resected and grafted. If there is a failure of hardware, it must be removed and a stable construct devised. With osteoporosis or bone loss, lag screws may not be feasible. Fixed angle (blade or locking) plate or an external fixator may be a better option.
- The ankle may be fused concurrently with other hindfoot joints. Consideration of adjacent joints as an additional source of pain will result in improved selection of procedure and outcome.
- In summary, arthrodesis remains the gold standard for treatment of severe, painful arthritis of the ankle. Careful removal of cartilage, restoration of alignment, and use of compression fixation yield reliably high rates of fusion and good results. Although patients with an ankle fusion can have excellent pain relief and a relatively normal gait initially, painful adjacent joint arthritis eventually occurs.

Arthroplasty

- The success of arthroplasty in the hip and knee, coupled with the limitations of ankle arthrodesis, has generated interest in the development and implementation of a total ankle arthroplasty. However, more than 30 years after the first ankle replacement, and after more than 20 implant designs, it has proved difficult to recreate normal ankle kinematics, and long-term clinical results have been inferior to those of the hip or knee.
- The theoretical advantage of arthroplasty over arthrodesis is conservation of motion at the ankle, with improved gait and function. The preservation of motion might decrease the incidence of adjacent joint arthritis.

History of Total Ankle Replacement and Implant Design

- A number of first-generation designs were trialed in the 1970s. Most were composed of metallic tibial and talar implants that were cemented into place and separated by a polyethylene insert. These implants showed encouraging short-term results but high rates of loosening and component subsidence in the midterm, leading to high rates of conversion to arthrodesis. Problems cited with these initial designs were a large amount of bone resection, which compromised initial fixation and later salvage procedures, and a failure to reestablish normal joint kinetics.
- Early attempts at arthroplasty also suffered from technical errors. Deformities in the foot, which often coexist with ankle arthritis, must be corrected prior to ankle replacement.
- After this initial round of failures, total ankle arthroplasty has slowly regained ground with the use of two newer designs, the Agility total ankle replacement (TAR) and the Scandinavian total ankle replacement (STAR)

prostheses. A number of other TAR designs are in development or have limited use outside the USA (Easley et al. 2002).

- A number of factors intrinsic to the ankle joint make development of a prosthesis difficult.
  - The ankle bears a very high load over a small surface area, resulting in high mechanical stresses on the arthroplasty components.
  - There are high stresses at the implant/bone interface, with the potential for implant loosening and subsidence.
  - The metaphyseal bone of the distal tibia is spongiform and not ideal for stable, secure fixation.
  - The talus has a precarious blood supply that is centered in the talar body, the usual location for a keel in the component. Compromise of talus vascularity can impair bone ingrowth into the component.
  - The soft tissues around the ankle are thin and prone to scarring. Wound-healing problems can lead to devastating infection. Also, the propensity for scarring leads to ankle stiffness.
  - The joint cannot be dislocated during surgery, making implant placement during surgery more difficult.
- Two biomechanical factors that have guided implant design are congruence and constraint. Congruence or conformity is a geometric measure of the closeness of fit of the articulation of the prosthesis to the joint. Constraint is the resistance of an implant to a degree of freedom in a plane of motion. Conformity increases articular contact and generally leads to low polyethylene wear rates. However, high conformity can also result in elevated constraint and shear forces that can lead to loosening. The ideal implant optimizes conformity for low wear while minimizing constraint for decreased loosening.
- An additional design factor is the bearing type: fixed or mobile. A fixed bearing implant has a single interface of motion, generally between the polyethylene fixed in the tibial component and the talar component. Alternatively, a mobile bearing sits between the tibial and talar components with motion at each interface. A fixed bearing implant such as the Agility TAR is highly congruent but also shows high constraint. A mobile bearing implant, for example the STAR, potentially decreases constraint while maintaining congruence at each articulation. However, use of a mobile bearing increases design complexity and has a potential for dislocation.

Indications

- Generalized arthritis is the most common indication for ankle arthroplasty. A recent metaanalysis of the literature by Stengel et al. showed rheumatoid arthritis (38%), posttraumatic arthritis (28%), and osteoarthritis (26%) as the most common presenting diagnoses.
- The ideal candidate for TAR is elderly with low physical demands and normal bone, vascularity, and alignment. The patient should be underweight and thin, with relatively large bones and no osteoporosis. It is difficult to find the ideal candidate.
- The appropriate age restrictions for patients undergoing ankle replacement are somewhat controversial, but younger patients generally have a higher complication rate, leading some authors to advocate limiting use of TAR to patients 60 years of age and older. Ankle arthroplasty in young patients is a problem both because of a longer life required of the components and an expectation of higher activity level. Accordingly, some authors support limiting TAR even in high-demand elderly patients. Other patient characteristics associated with poor outcome after TAR include obesity, diabetes, and other medical comorbidities.
- Although mild deformity may be corrected with TAR, malalignment of greater than 15° of varus or valgus cannot be easily corrected with arthroplasty and may require treatment with arthrodesis or concurrent osteotomy.
- A contraindication to TAR is avascularity in the tibia or talus, which compromises ingrowth of components.
- Neuropathy is also a contraindication to implant arthroplasty, because of the potential for rapid failure (neuropathic joint degeneration).
- Absence of the medial malleolus or deltoid ligament incompetence are both problems, because the ankle replacement requires medial stability to prevent valgus collapse.
- Lack of the fibula is not an absolute contraindication but probably leads to poorer results (early failure).
- Indications do not vary considerably among implant designs.
- Relative contraindications to TAR are shown in Box 14–4.

Approach and Technique

- Surgical approach and placement of components are similar regardless of implant used. A temporary external fixator is first placed to allow joint distraction during component placement.

Box 14–4 Relative Contraindications to Total Ankle Replacement

- Age < 60
- High activity level
- Infection, past or present
- Severe deformity
- Charcot joint
- Poor soft tissue envelope
- Talar avascular necrosis

- The surgeon then uses the anterior approach to the ankle to expose the tibiotalar joint.
- The distal tibia and talar dome are resected using cutting jigs or, with experience, a freehand technique. Because the joint is not dislocatable, exposure of the joint surfaces can be difficult.
- The components are press fit into place after the bone is prepared. TAR implants may be cemented, but early experience has shown an unacceptably high rate of loosening with cemented components. Most current implants are hydroxyapatite or porous coated to enhance ingrowth.
- Appropriate soft tissue balance in surrounding muscles and ligaments is essential to success.

Complications

- Complications of TAR include wound problems, infection, aseptic loosening, subsidence of components, and osteolysis. There also are problems related to the surgical approach and joint preparation, including nerve injury and malleolar fracture.
- Wound problems and infection are related to the thin soft tissue envelope. Small wound irritations may need only close follow-up and oral antibiotics. Larger wound problems require surgical debridement, with possible component removal and antibiotics similar to with other joint replacements. Uncontrollable infection may occasionally require amputation.
- Patients with aseptic loosening may present with pain and radiographic lucency around components. Loosening is more common after TAR than in hip and knee replacement. It is often the talar component that fails to osseointegrate.
- Subsidence of either component can occur, and is more likely with obesity and osteoporosis. Settling of the joint from component subsidence leads to pain from malleolar impingement on the talus (Fig. 14–7).
- Tilting of the talus in the mortise is a difficult problem stemming from imperfect tissue balance. Tilting remains a problem even for the most experienced surgeon (Fig. 14–8).
- Osteolysis is loss of bone around the implant, usually due to polyethylene particulate debris in the joint. Osteolysis at the distal tibiofibular joint after TAR has also been observed in the setting of syndesmotic non-union. Severe osteolysis may result in loss of fixation and lead to

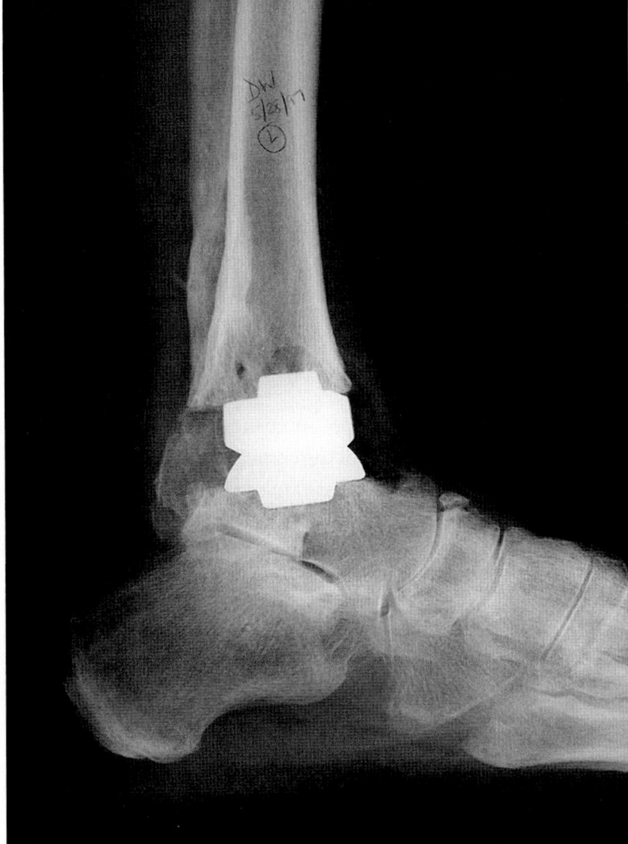

A

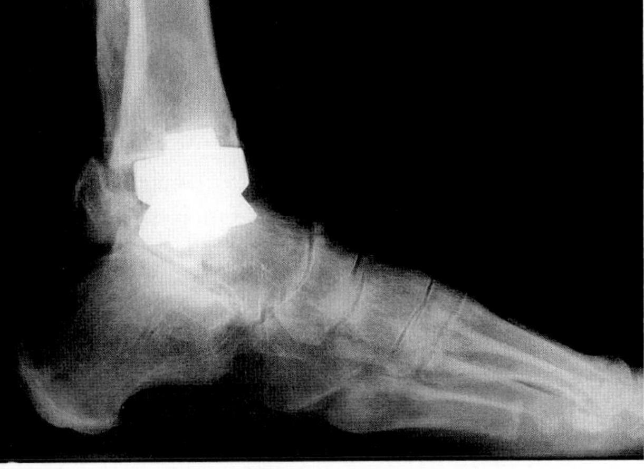

B

Figure 14–7: Total ankle arthroplasty. **A,** Total ankle arthroplasty at early postoperative stage. **B,** One year later, the talar component has subsided into bone. Revision ankle arthroplasty was carried out because of pain with a wider talar component.

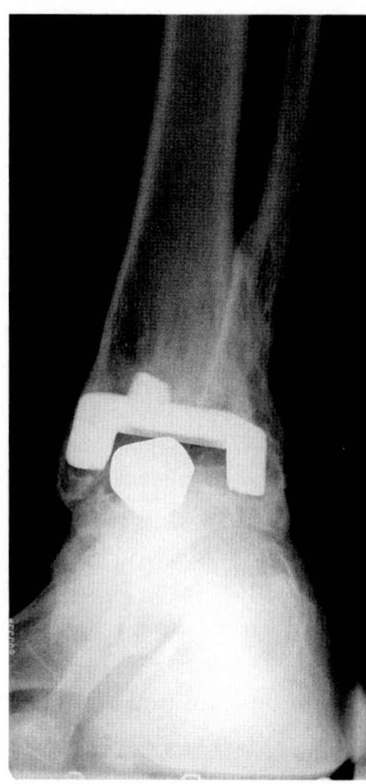

Figure 14–8: A total ankle arthroplasty tilting into valgus due to tissue imbalance. This patient had mild pain from lateral bone impingement, but the potential for catastrophic polyethylene fracture exists (because of edge loading of the talus into the polyethylene).

a difficult revision procedure, with extensive bone loss (Knecht et al. 2004).

Two-component Design

- The two-component Agility design is the only implant with US Food and Drug Administration approval currently.
- The Agility Ankle is a second-generation design that resurfaces the superior, medial, and lateral surfaces of the tibial plafond as well as the talus. A polyethylene insert is fitted to the larger tibial implant, which then articulates with the talar component (fixed bearing).
- Lack of congruency between the larger tibial and smaller talar components allows for some sliding and rotational motion.
- Because its solid tibial component incorporates the medial and lateral malleolar surfaces, fusion of the syndesmosis is required. Either through the same anterior incision, or a separate lateral approach, the syndesmosis is debrided and stabilized with screws.
- Failure of syndesmosis fusion leads to a higher rate of reoperation, with valgus tilting of the talus in severe cases. Motion at the unfused syndesmosis leads to "ballooning" osteolysis in the distal fibula.
- There is some evidence that use of a plate with the two syndesmotic screws may increase the rate of syndesmosis fusion.
- Advantages of the two-component design include complete resurfacing of the ankle and greater surface area to support the tibial component. This larger surface area distributes forces well across, and subsidence of the tibial component is not a common complication.
- Transformation of the ankle from a three-to a two-bone joint is controversial but does allow this total resurfacing, and after fusion avoids a painful distal tibiofibular joint. However, the larger component does require more extensive bone resection, and consequently a potentially more difficult salvage. Additionally, the syndesmosis fusion often requires a second incision, increasing the risk of soft tissue problems, and failure of syndesmotic fusion is problematic.
- The two large series of two-component TARs were published recently.
- In one study of 126 patients with mean follow-up of 9 years, the revision rate was 15%. Greater than 90% of patients reported satisfaction and pain relief. Average arc of range of motion was 18°. Complications included syndesmotic non-union in 8%, subsidence in 14%, and periimplant lucency in 76%. Importantly, a significant number of patients developed adjacent joint arthritis in the subtalar and talonavicular joints (Knecht et al. 2004).
  - The patients in this series were selected by the inventor of the Agility Ankle, and so were probably all ideal candidates.
- Spirt et al. (2004) reported a series of 306 consecutive ankle arthroplasties with an average 33-month follow-up. Overall, they observed less favorable results. Five-year survivorship was 80% using the end point of failed TAR, and 54% with reoperation as the end point. Younger patients (< 55 years) did significantly worse than older patients. Failure of syndesmosis fusion, loosening, and subsidence were cited as common complications. A few patients required below-knee amputation (BKA) as a salvage procedure.
  - This series had less strict inclusion criteria, including many younger patients, and most patients were not at all ideal candidates.
- Although data regarding outcomes of the Agility TAR are mixed, several points of agreement exist.
  - The majority of patients are satisfied in the short term, but long-term results are as yet unknown.
  - Younger patients tend to have worse implant survival and increased complications.
  - Range of motion is not fully restored after TAR, with an average of about 30°.
  - Syndesmosis fusion is important to successful Agility TAR.
  - Adjacent joint arthritis may occur after TAR, but it is unclear whether the rate of arthritis is lower than after ankle arthrodesis.

Scandinavian Total Ankle Replacement

- The STAR design is a second-generation, three-component implant that is undergoing US Food and Drug Administration trials in the USA but that has been used extensively in Europe. The components include coated, metal alloy tibial and talar implants with a mobile polyethylene bearing, termed a *meniscus*.

- Based on biomechanical examination of failed first-generation implants, a cylindric design, like that used in the STAR, appeared to have the lowest failure rate and least rotational stress at the bone-implant interface, minimizing loosening.
- The STAR prosthesis is *congruent*, in that the tibial and talar components are similarly sized, but *unconstrained* in that the polyethylene bearing is mobile and the entire joint is not resurfaced. The medial and lateral gutters remain to some degree.
- The meniscus is constructed of ultrahigh molecular weight polyethylene and is designed to rotate freely between the fixed components. In practice, the meniscus rotates minimally and serves to absorb compressive forces across the joint. Use of a mobile meniscus adds freedom to the construct but increases risk of polyethylene displacement or dislocation.
- The tibial component is a plate that does not resurface the malleoli. The syndesmosis is not fused. This avoids the problem of syndesmotic non-union but leaves the distal tibiofibular joint, a potential source of pain, unaddressed.
- In 2004, Kofoed reported a series of 55 patients who had undergone cemented or uncemented STAR arthroplasty. At 5 years, the cemented implants showed a 90% survivorship. The majority of failures were due to aseptic loosening. Careful patient selection was emphasized as a requisite for success.
- Other implants with similar design features are currently in use around the world.
- All modern TAR designs share the potential for tilting of the talus. Alignment of the TAR and balance in the foot are essential.
- Modern surgeons continue to work to minimize early failures from loosening, subsidence, and tilting. Once these problems are resolved, the longer term problems of polyethylene wear and osteolysis can be addressed.

Unresolved Questions

- It is unclear whether current TAR accomplishes the goals of recreating ankle kinematics and addressing the shortcomings of ankle arthrodesis.
- Range of motion after TAR is limited to approximately 30°, and gait studies show protected weight bearing of the replaced ankle and altered kinematics even in asymptomatic TAR. Twenty or thirty degrees of motion may be functional in the low-demand patient but is certainly not normal.
- It is unproven whether TAR decreases the development of adjacent joint arthritis. Rates of subtalar and talonavicular arthritis after TAR and arthrodesis are similar at 5-year follow-up. It is unknown whether adjacent joint disease in TAR occurs secondary to reduced range of motion, increased stress caused by abnormal ankle joint kinetics, or underlying disease.

Summary

- Total ankle arthroplasty continues to be an evolving technique. Second-generation implants show clear improvements over earlier cemented designs, but long-term results are not yet available. Each implant design shows individual benefits and drawbacks.
- Regardless of design, TAR results appear to lag behind results for hip and knee arthroplasty.

Amputation

- BKA is a viable reconstructive option for many patients.
- A well-functioning prosthesis will provide better function than ankle arthrodesis or arthroplasty in a healthy, young person.
- Patients with a BKA can have excellent function and quality of life. Unlike above-knee amputation, BKA requires only moderate increases in energy consumption. Most patients can be fitted with a prosthesis and ambulate successfully, particularly when comparing gait with a stiff and painful ankle.
- Disadvantages of amputation include cosmesis, psychologic distress, and stump difficulties that can result in more proximal amputation.
- Amputation also may be a salvage for patients who have no reasonable reconstructive option:
  - posttraumatic patients with impaired vascularity and soft tissue envelope, leading to failure of healing
  - patients with impaired blood supply secondary to primary vascular disease or diabetes not amenable to revascularization
  - patients with uncontrolled infection unresponsive to local measures and antibiotic treatment.
- Although isolated ankle or hindfoot fusions are well tolerated, the young patient with pantalar disease may be better served by BKA.

References

Abidi NA, Gruen GS, Conti SF. (2000) Ankle arthrodesis: Indications and techniques. J Am Acad Orthop Surg 8(3): 200-209.
Review of arthrodesis for ankle arthritis, with a discussion of indications, surgical technique, and complications including non-union.

Amendola A, Beaman DN, Brage ME et al. (2005) Emerging Methods for Treating Ankle Arthritis. AAOS Instructional Course Lecture. Washington: American Academy of Orthopaedic Surgeons.
Instructional course detailing reconstruction techniques for ankle arthritis, with expanded discussion of osteochondral allografts and joint distraction.

Anderson T, Montgomery F, Carlsson A. (2004) Uncemented STAR total ankle prostheses. J Bone Joint Surg Am 86-A(suppl 1): 103-111.

Reviews surgical technique for the STAR ankle prosthesis, using numerous surgical photographs, diagrams, and radiographs.

Cheng JC, Ferkel RD. (1998) The role of arthroscopy in ankle and subtalar degenerative joint disease. Clin Orthop 349: 65-72.

Review of ankle arthroscopy organized by specific lesion. Also includes brief discussion of subtalar arthrosis and arthroscopy.

Coester LM, Saltzman CL, Leupold J. (2001) Long-term results following ankle arthrodesis for post-traumatic arthritis. J Bone Joint Surg 83-A: 219-228.

At an average of 22 years' follow-up, the majority of patients developed arthritis in adjacent hindfoot joints on x-ray, and many were limited by the pain.

Demetriades L, Strauss E, Gallina J. (1998) Osteoarthritis of the ankle. Clin Orthop 349: 28-42.

Comprehensive review of ankle arthritis, with sections on etiology, treatment, and complications. Also included are brief summaries of clinical studies related to each of the common treatments (debridement, arthrodesis, arthroplasty).

Easley ME, Vertullo CJ, Nunley JA. (2002) Total ankle arthroplasty. J Am Acad Orthop Surg 10(3): 157-167.

Review of TAR, with interesting historical perspective and discussion of implant design. The article then discusses four implants, emphasizing design type, results, and common complications.

Katcherian DA. (1998) Treatment of ankle arthrosis. Clin Orthop 349: 48-57.

Review of ankle arthritis treatments, with emphasis on arthrodesis techniques, implants, and complications.

Knecht SI, Estin M, Callaghan JJ et al. (2004) The Agility total ankle arthroplasty: Seven to sixteen year follow-up. J Bone Joint Surg Am 86-A(6): 1161-1171.

Retrospective review of 126 patients undergoing total ankle arthroplasty with the Agility implant system. Mean follow-up of 9 years. Includes analysis of Ankle Arthritis Scale scores, range of motion, and radiographs. Survival curve is also calculated. Expanded discussion of non-union of the syndesmosis is also included.

Kofoed H. (2004) Scandinavian total ankle replacement (STAR). Clin Orthop 424: 73-79.

Discussion of STAR design and case series of 58 patients with average 9.4 years' follow-up. Includes cemented and uncemented prostheses. Patients with uncemented implants showed better survival, with 70% at 10 years having clinical improvement in symptoms and function.

Marijnissen ACA, van Roermund PM, van Melkebeek J et al. (2002) Clinical benefit of joint distraction in the treatment of severe osteoarthritis of the ankle: Proof of concept in open prospective study and in a randomized controlled study. Arthritis Rheum 46(11): 2893-2902.

Prospective case series that includes 46 patients undergoing joint distraction with mean follow-up of 2.8 years. Patients showed significantly decreased pain and increased function at 1 and 3 years. Radiographs showed increased joint space and decreased subchondral sclerosis. The progressive nature of the improvements is emphasized. Seventeen additional patients were included in a randomized trial of distraction versus arthroscopic debridement, with follow-up of 1 year. Patients in the joint distraction group had improved pain, function, and clinical status. The results are weakened by the choice of debridement as the comparison treatment for severe ankle arthritis instead of the gold standard, arthrodesis, or even arthroplasty.

Marijnissen ACA, van Roermund PM, van Melkebeek J et al. (2003) Clinical benefit of joint distraction in the treatment of ankle osteoarthritis. Foot Ankle Clin North Am 8: 335-346.

Review article detailing the biology and technique of joint distraction, with a limited summary of current clinical outcomes. The authors emphasize a worsening of symptoms in the first months following removal of the distractor, with improvement from baseline seen after the first year and progressive improvement with prolonged follow-up.

Martin DF, Baker CL, Curl WW et al. (1989) Operative ankle arthroscopy. Long-term followup. Am J Sports Med 17(1): 16-23.

Case series of 57 patients with arthritis of the ankle undergoing arthroscopy. Patients with generalized arthritis fared worse than those with specific conditions amenable to arthroscopic treatment, such as loose bodies and synovitis.

Mizel MS, Hecht PJ, Marymont JV et al. (2004) Evaluation and treatment of chronic ankle pain. J Bone Joint Surg Am 86-A(3): 622-632.

Review of chronic ankle pain, including several non-arthritic causes and helpful physical examination findings.

Myerson MS, Neufeld SK, Uribe J. (2005) Fresh-frozen structural allografts in the foot and ankle. J Bone Joint Surg Am 87(1): 113-120.

A series of structural allografts showing quite good results.

Spirt AA, Assal M, Hansen ST. (2004) Complications and failure after total ankle arthroplasty. J Bone Joint Surg Am 86-A(6): 1172-1178.

Retrospective review of 306 patients undergoing TAR with the Agility system, with a mean follow-up of 33 months. Reoperation rate of 54% and survival of 80% at 5 years. Younger patients, that is those less than 55 years, were found to have a higher complication rate with worse survival. Complications included infection, subsidence, non-union of the syndesmosis, and amputation.

Thomas SH, Daniels TR. (2003) Current concepts review: Ankle arthritis. J Bone Joint Surg Am 85-A(5): 923-934.

Current concepts review of ankle arthritis and treatment. Includes detailed discussion of etiology and cartilage biology of ankle arthritis. Limited review of emerging techniques is also included, with greater emphasis on arthrodesis and arthroplasty.

Tontz WL, Bugbee WD, Brage ME. (2003) Use of allografts in the management of ankle arthritis. Foot Ankle Clin North Am 8: 361-373.

Case series of 12 patients undergoing fresh osteochondral allografting of the ankle, with tibial and talar resurfacing in the majority. Average follow-up is 21 months. The majority of patients had improvement of pain and were satisfied with the procedure, although gains in mobility were modest. Complications included malleolar fracture, graft collapse, and pain at the talofibular joint requiring debridement.

van Valburg AA, van Roermund PM, Marijnnissen ACA et al. (1999) Joint distraction in treatment of osteoarthritis: A two-year follow-up of the ankle. Osteoarthr Cartil 7(5): 474-479.

Case series of 17 patients undergoing joint distraction of the ankle with a minimum 2-year follow-up. Patients had clinical improvement in pain and function but no radiographic change in joint space narrowing.

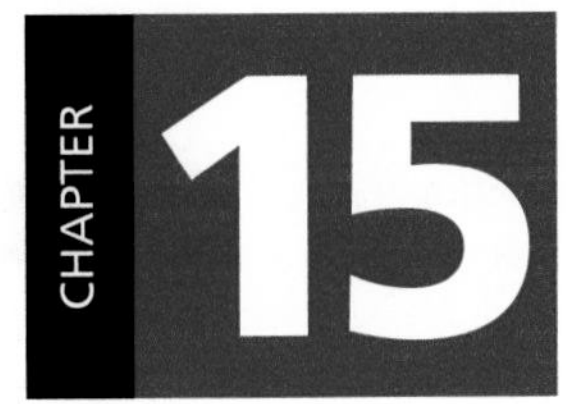

Heel Pain

Eric M. Berkson[*], Justin Greisberg[§], and George H. Theodore[†]

[*]M.D., Orthopaedic Sports Medicine, Massachusetts General Hospital, Boston, MA
[§]M.D., Assistant Professor of Orthopaedic Surgery, Columbia University College of Physicians and Surgeons, New York, NY
[†]M.D., Codirector, Foot and Ankle Service, Massachusetts General Hospital, and Clinical Instructor, Harvard Medical School, Boston, MA

- Heel pain is one of the most common complaints in the foot and ankle, second perhaps only to ankle sprains. Heel pain results in 1 million medical visits per year and comprises 1% of all visits to orthopaedic surgeons (Riddle and Schappert 2004).
- The majority of patients with heel pain will be treated successfully non-operatively.
- Heel pain can be plantar (subcalcaneal) or posterior. Posterior pain may be due to insertional Achilles tendinosis, retrocalcaneal bursitis, or Haglund deformity (also known as a pump bump). These are discussed further in Chapter 16.
- Plantar heel pain is most commonly caused by plantar fasciitis but has several possible causes (Box 15–1).

Box 15–1 Differential Diagnosis of Plantar Heel Pain

- Plantar fasciitis
- Fat pad atrophy
- Calcaneal stress fracture
- Plantar nerve impingement
- Cavus or calcaneus deformity
- Inflammatory enthesopathy

Normal Heel Anatomy

- The Achilles tendon inserts on the posterior calcaneus. Fibers continue plantarward to merge with the origin of the plantar fascia.
- The skin at the posterior heel is normally very supple and glides freely over the Achilles insertion.
- Between the Achilles tendon and the posterosuperior calcaneal tuberosity lies the retrocalcaneal bursa.
- The subcutaneous tissue under the calcaneus is the plantar fat pad. Fibrous septae enclose small "cells" of adipose, giving the entire structure the ability to absorb shock during gait.
- The plantar aponeurosis consists of three segments.
  - The medial and lateral segments cover the abductor hallucis and abductor digiti quinti.
  - The central portion of the plantar aponeurosis originates from the medial tuberosity of the calcaneus and is referred to as the plantar fascia.
  - The central portion inserts into the plantar plate of the proximal phalanges and through the sesamoids into the great toe.
- Hyperextension of the toes and metatarsophalangeal joints tenses the plantar fascia, raises the longitudinal arch of the foot, inverts the hindfoot, and externally rotates the leg. This apparatus, the windlass mechanism, provides a passive mechanism for increased foot stability.
- The tibial nerve branches just at or above the medial malleolus into the medial and lateral plantar nerves. The medial calcaneal nerve comes off the medial plantar nerve at this level to supply sensation to the medial, posterior,

and inferior heel. When making a posteromedial ankle incision, this nerve can be injured if the incision is carried too far distally.
- The first branch of the lateral plantar nerve runs under the inferomedial calcaneus and deep to the fascia of the abductor hallucis. It provides motor function to the abductor digiti minimi and the flexor digiti brevis, as well as innervation to some calcaneal periosteum.

Plantar Fasciitis

- Many people refer to this condition as a "heel spur," but only 50% of patients with the condition will have a plantar spur, and 15% of normal patients will also have a spur. The exact role of the plantar spur in the condition is not well defined, and treatment should not focus on the spur (Fig. 15–1 and Box 15–2).
- The condition is thought to be due to irritation of the proximal plantar fascia. There may or may not be a history of mild trauma. It is bilateral in 15-30% of patients.
- Patients will typically have pain under the plantar heel that is worse on initial weight bearing. The pain may improve as they "walk it off," but then returns with increased time on the feet during the day.
- Plantar fasciitis has been associated with a tight gastrocnemius and hamstrings. Some physicians credit the tight gastrocnemius with causing the problem.
- When sitting or resting for prolonged periods of time, the gastrocnemius and plantar fascia tighten up. If the patient rises without loosening up these structures, the forced dorsiflexion of normal standing will provide an acute stretch to the tight structures, with pain.
- On examination, there is usually tenderness at the proximal plantar fascia. Some patients may be tender only under the calcaneal tuberosity.
- Passive dorsiflexion of the toes tightens the fascia and may increase tenderness in the proximal fascia in patients with plantar fasciitis.
- Specialized imaging studies are not needed for the treatment of plantar fasciitis. In cases where the diagnosis is not clear, bone scans or magnetic resonance imaging (MRI) may help differentiate from other pathologies, such as stress fracture.
- Bone scans reveal increased uptake at the inferior aspect of the calcaneus. Patients with this finding may have a better response to local cortisone treatments.

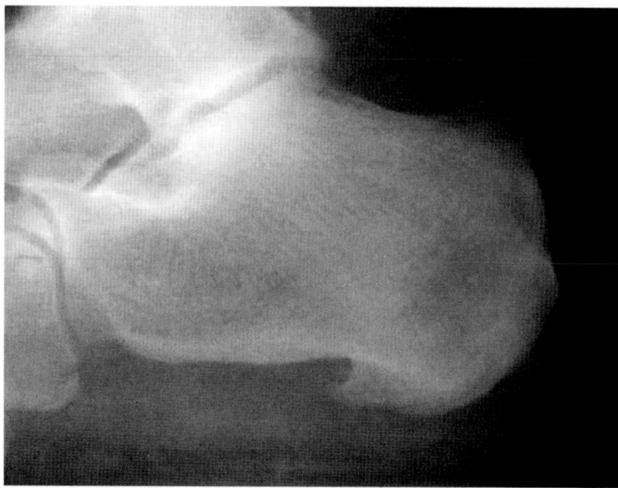

Figure 15–1: Lateral calcaneus with heel spur. Lateral radiograph of a heel spur. Heel spurs are caused by chronic inflammation and are not the primary etiology of heel pain. They are present in about 50% of those patients with subcalcaneal pain syndrome and about 15% of the general population.

Box 15–2 Heel Spurs

- Heel spurs were originally thought to be an etiology of heel pain (Fig. 15–1).
- Epidemiologic studies, however, have improved our understanding of their origin.
- Heel spurs are present in about 50% of patients with subcalcaneal pain syndrome, and in about 15% of the general population. Less than 5% of those with spurs have pain.
- Spurs were assumed to originate in the plantar aponeurosis but are actually located in the origin of the flexor hallucis brevis. This too casts doubt on the spur's role in the etiology of heel pain.
- Spurs are probably caused by chronic inflammation and are not the primary etiology of heel pain.

Treatment for Plantar Fasciitis

- There are many treatment options for plantar fasciitis. Similar to low back pain, many patients will improve spontaneously with time.
- Initial treatments include rest, antiinflammatories, heel cups, full orthotics, corticosteroid injections, stretching exercises, and immobilization (night splint or cast). There is probably some value to all these regimens.
- Because most patients with plantar fasciitis have a tight gastrocnemius, stretching is a logical treatment choice. A prospective study found that regular daily stretching of the plantar fascia and gastrocnemius, combined with an over the counter orthotic, was more effective than routine Achilles tendon stretching alone (DiGiovanni et al. 2003).
- Another study found a prefabricated orthotic to be as effective as a custom one for plantar fasciitis (Pfeffer et al. 1999). Correction of a planovalgus foot with orthotics will reduce strain on the origin of the plantar fascia.
- Tisdel and Harper (1996) found that 86% of patients improved after 4 weeks in a weight-bearing short leg cast.
- Although many physicians rely on corticosteroid injections, there is no evidence that injections are as good as, or better than, other options. Repeat injections can

lead to fat pad atrophy, a devastating complication. Plantar fascial rupture and calcaneal osteomyelitis are other rare complications of injection.
  - Miller et al. (1995) noted recurrence of symptoms in 13 of 24 feet at 5-8 months after injection.
- Botulinum toxin has been found to be effective in one randomized, placebo-controlled, double-blind study (Babcock et al. 2005). Additional study of this treatment method is required before widespread use is accepted.
- There has been recent interest in the use of extracorporeal shock wave therapy (Fig. 15–2). There are not uniform recommendations on the dose or energy level of the shock waves. Some studies show good improvements, while others do not find any benefit over placebo.
  - Extracorporeal shock wave therapy delivers shock waves that are thought to stimulate angiogenesis, promote new bone formation, disrupt calcific deposits, and increase cytokine diffusion.
  - A multicenter, randomized, placebo-controlled, prospective trial of shock wave therapy in 150 patients noted 56% improvement at 3 months and 94% at 12 months (Theodore et al. 2004).
  - A metaanalysis of six randomized controlled trials and 897 patients found a statistically significant result in favor of therapy, although the effect size was noted to be small.
- As a whole, 90% of patients will improve by 6 months. A recommended treatment plan is summarized in Box 15–3.

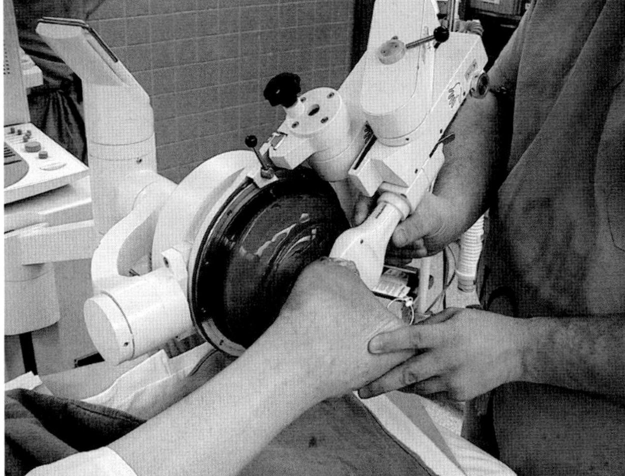

Figure 15–2: Extracorporeal shock wave therapy. Extracorporeal shock wave therapy delivers shock waves that are thought to stimulate angiogenesis, promote new bone formation, disrupt calcific deposits, and increase cytokine diffusion. As a second-line treatment for plantar fasciitis, several multicenter trials have found statistically significant success.

Box 15–3 A Treatment Plan for Plantar Fasciitis

- History and examination consistent with plantar fasciitis
  - Begin plantar fascia and gastrocnemius stretching multiple times daily.
  - Wear shoes with good support or use prefabricated orthotic.
  - Consider antiinflammatory medication.
  - If no improvement, confirm proper performance of exercises. Confirm appropriate frequency of exercises.
- If still no improvement:
  - consider alternative diagnoses
  - if still most consistent with plantar fasciitis, consider adding alternative treatment, such as night splint, casting, or corticosteroid injection.
- If symptoms persist more than 6 months:
  - can consider shock wave treatment
  - can consider surgery.

Surgery for Plantar Fasciitis

- If symptoms have persisted for more than 6 months despite appropriate treatment, surgery can be considered. There are several surgical options.
- Partial plantar fasciotomy can be done through a medial incision. The lateral bands of the fascia are left intact to prevent lateral column pain.
- Endoscopic partial plantar fasciotomy can be performed to minimize the skin incision. Although many assume that endoscopic surgery offers a faster recovery than traditional open technique, this has not been proven.
- In patients with a tight gastrocnemius, gastrocnemius recession may be the best choice. At least one surgeon has proposed plantar fascia release for the patient with a stable or high arch, and gastrocnemius lengthening for the patient with a low or collapsed arch.
- In case series, all the above techniques are effective, with 70-90% good results.
- The role of heel spur resection is unclear, and most orthopaedists do not include it in the surgical procedure.

Plantar Nerve Impingement

- Compression of the nerve to the abductor digiti minimi (first branch of the lateral plantar nerve) is a less common cause of heel pain. The nerve is impinged at the fascia of the abductor hallucis.
- Pain is generally felt more medial on the heel, rather than plantar. The area of maximal tenderness will be on the medial inferior border of the calcaneus, at the origin of the abductor hallucis.
- For the appropriate patient, surgical release of the medial plantar fascia and the fascia of the abductor hallucis may lead to improvement.

Fat Pad Atrophy

- The plantar fat pad provides essential shock absorption during gait. Loss of this function results in chronic heel pain.
- Direct trauma, as seen with a calcaneus fracture, may lead to fat pad atrophy. It can also result as a side effect of corticosteroid injections. Although a single injection rarely causes this complication, it can be seen with repeated injections.
- Treatment is focused on providing better padding and shock absorption with padded heel inserts and appropriate (well-padded) shoes.

Calcaneal Stress Fracture

- Stress fracture of the calcaneus will present with heel pain that is worse with activity and better with rest. In contrast to plantar fasciitis, stress fracture pain will usually be mild with the first step, and increase with further weight-bearing.
- Examination will show tenderness at the medial and lateral tuberosity, which is not seen with plantar fasciitis.
- After a few weeks, plain x-rays may show sclerosis. MRI or bone scan may be useful earlier.
- Treatment should focus on activity modification and rest. Some patients will need a cast, cast boot, and/or crutches.

Cavus Foot Pain

- The patient with a high-arched foot may have increased loads placed on the heel and metatarsal heads. This may lead to mechanical heel pain.
- Well-padded shoes or heel pads may provide good relief.
- A custom orthotic with good padding under the heel and a built-up instep to distribute weight-bearing forces away from the heel can also be helpful.
- For recalcitrant cases, osteotomies to lower the arch can be performed, but results may not be good. Pain in these difficult cases is multifactorial. A surgery that makes the foot and the x-ray look better to the surgeon may not improve the pain.

Enthesopathy

- Patients with inflammatory enthesopathies can develop plantar fasciitis as part of systemic disease. In cases of refractory or recurrent heel pain, referral to a rheumatologist should be considered, especially when other enthesopathies are involved.

References

Babcock MS, Foster L, Pasquina P et al. (2005) Treatment of pain attributed to plantar fasciitis with botulinum toxin A: A short-term, randomized, placebo-controlled, double-blind study. Am J Phys Med Rehabil 84(9): 649-654.

In a randomized, double-blind, placebo-controlled study of 27 patients (43 feet) with plantar fasciitis, feet were randomly injected with either saline or botulinum toxin A. At 8 weeks postoperatively, compared with placebo injections, the botulinum toxin A group improved in Pain Visual Analog Scale ($P < 0.005$), Maryland Foot Score ($P = 0.001$), and Pain Relief Visual Analog Scale ($P < 0.0005$). No side effects were noted.

Baxter DE, Pfeffer GB. (1992) Treatment of chronic heel pain by surgical release of the first branch of the lateral plantar nerve. Clin Orthop Relat Res 279: 229-236.

In a series of patients with entrapment of the first branch of the lateral plantar nerve, surgical release led to good results in more than 80% of patients.

Buchbinder R, Ptasznik R, Gordon J et al. (2002) Ultrasound-guided extracorporeal shock wave therapy for plantar fasciitis: A randomized controlled trial. JAMA 288(11): 1364-1372.

This prospective series found no benefit to shock wave therapy for plantar fasciitis.

DiGiovanni BF, Nawoczenski DA, Lintal ME et al. (2003) Tissue-specific plantar fascia-stretching exercise enhances outcomes in patients with chronic heel pain. A prospective, randomized study. J Bone Joint Surg Am 85-A(7): 1270-1277.

A prospective study found that exercises focusing on the plantar fascia were more effective than routine Achilles tendon stretches.

Miller RA, Torres J, McGuire M. (1995) Efficacy of first-time steroid injection for painful heel syndrome. Foot Ankle Int 16(10): 610-612.

In a prospective study, many patients receiving a single cortisone injection had short-term relief but recurrence of heel pain at final follow-up 5-8 months later.

Pfeffer G, Bacchetti P, Deland J et al. (1999) Comparison of custom and prefabricated orthoses in the initial treatment of proximal plantar fasciitis. Foot Ankle Int 20(4): 214-221.

In this study, prefabricated orthotics were seen to be as helpful as more expensive custom ones.

Riddle DL, Schappert SM. (2004) Volume of ambulatory care visits and patterns of care for patients diagnosed with plantar fasciitis: A national study of medical doctors. Foot Ankle Int 25(5): 303-310.

Data from the National Ambulatory Medical Care Survey and the National Hospital Ambulatory Medical Care Survey between 1995 and 2000 were retrospectively analyzed. One million patient visits per year were made to medical offices and hospital outpatient services for heel pain. Approximately 62% of all visits were made to primary care practitioners, and 31% were made to orthopaedic surgeons. One percent of all patient visits to orthopaedic surgeons were for plantar fasciitis.

Theodore GH, Buch M, Amendola A et al. (2004) Extracorporeal shock wave therapy for the treatment of plantar fasciitis. Foot Ankle Int 25(5): 290-297.

In a multicenter, randomized, placebo-controlled, prospective, double-blinded study, extracorporeal shock wave was compared with sham treatments. In the group receiving extracorporeal shock wave therapy, 56% success was noted at 3 months and

94% success at 12 months postoperatively. The control group reported 47% success at 3 months. The study was unblinded at 3 months and the control group offered treatment.

Thomson CE, Crawford F, Murray GD. (2005) The effectiveness of extracorporeal shock wave therapy for plantar heel pain: A systematic review and meta-analysis. BMC Musculoskelet Disord 6(1): 19.
A metaanalysis of six randomized, controlled trials, including 897 patients, supports shock wave therapy for the treatment of plantar heel pain, but the effect size was very small. A sensitivity analysis including only high-quality trials did not detect a statistically significant effect.

Tisdel CL, Harper MC. (1996) Chronic plantar heel pain: Treatment with a short leg walking cast. Foot Ankle Int 17(1): 41-42.
A trial of casting led to improvement in 86% of patients who failed routine initial interventions.

CHAPTER 16

Achilles Tendon Problems

Annette M. Smith[*] and Andrew K. Sands[§]

[*]M.D., M.S., Department of Orthopaedic Surgery, Kingsbrook Jewish Medical Center, Brooklyn, NY
[§]M.D., Chief, Foot and Ankle Surgery, and Director, Foot and Ankle Institute, Department of Orthopaedic Surgery, Saint Vincent's Medical Center, New York, NY

- The Achilles tendon is the conjoined tendon of the gastrocnemius, soleus, and plantaris. The gastrocnemius and plantaris take their origin from the posterior femoral condyles, while the soleus originates on the tibia and fibula. The tendon inserts into a 2 × 2 cm area on the posterosuperior aspect of the calcaneus.
- When the leg is extended, the gastrocnemius muscle has a stronger plantar flexion force because it originates proximal to the knee joint. When the knee is flexed, the soleus muscle has a stonger plantar flexion force because it originates below the knee (Fig. 16–1).
- The Achilles is the largest and strongest tendon in the human body. It crosses three joints: the knee, the ankle, and the subtalar joint.
- The forces that occur during running and jumping can be up to 10 times body weight.
- The blood supply to the proximal portion of the Achilles is from the muscle tissue. The distal tendon receives its blood supply from the calcaneal insertion. The peritenon that encases the tendon provides the remainder of the blood supply. In between the proximal and distal blood supplies, there is a watershed area from 2-6 cm above the insertion with relatively little blood supply.
- This watershed area can lead to a zone of hypovascularity with aging, which is thought to contribute to the development of many tendon problems.

Tendon Basic Science

- Tendons are composed primarily of type 1 collagen, which is organized into three α chains coiled into a right-handed helix with a left-handed supercoil. This structural organization gives tendons their strength and resiliency. The primary bundles are surrounded by the endotenon, containing mostly type 3 collagen. This tissue layer contains the vascular supply, lymphatics, and nerves.
- These secondary bundles are further grouped into tertiary bundles surrounded by a layer of connective tissue called the epitenon, which contains mostly type 1 collagen.
- Surrounding this is the paratenon. This double-layer sheath is composed of an inner, visceral layer and an outer, parietal layer. The visceral layer is connected to the parietal layer by bridges called mesotenon.
- When a paratenon is lined by synovium, it is called a *tenosynovium*. When there is no synovial lining, it is called a *tenovagium*.
- The Achilles tendon has a tenovagium, while the other tendons of the ankle have tenosynovium. The main blood supply to the middle of the Achilles tendon is via the blood vessels in the paratenon.

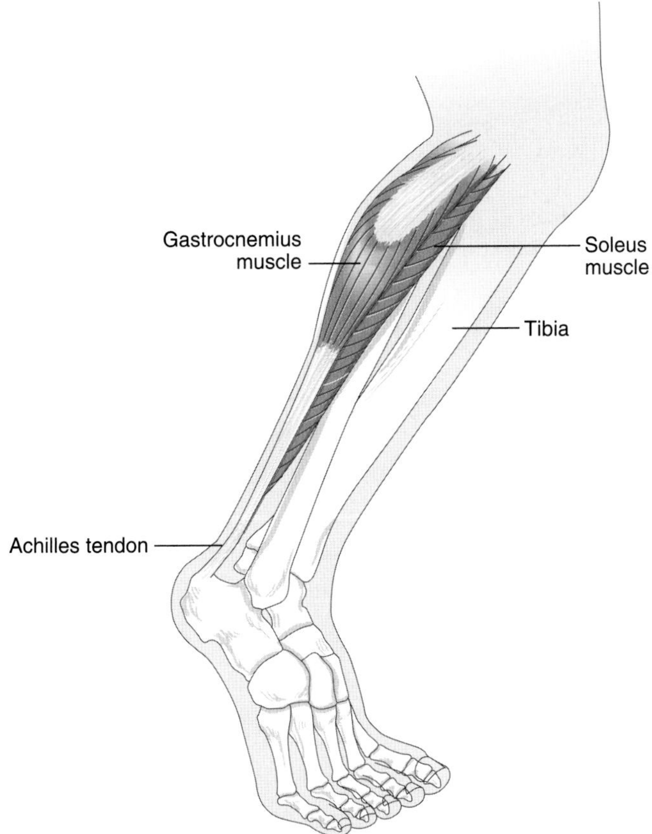

Figure 16–1: The Achilles tendon is the conjoined tendon of the gastrocnemius, soleus, and plantaris. Sometimes, the thin plantaris tendon will remain separate throughout its length.

Magnetic Resonance Imaging of Tendon Abnormalities of the Foot and Ankle

- Because most Achilles disorders are obvious clinically, MRI should be reserved for distinguishing between partial and complete Achilles tendon tears, or for clinically equivocal cases.
- Tendons have high collagen and low water content, which accounts for the low signal intensity (black) on MRI scans. Normal anatomy of tendons is best delineated with T_1-weighted images. Additional information like fluid, edema, hemorrhage, or scar around or within the tendons is more easily seen on T_2-weighted image.
- Asymptomatic patients will have fluid in the tendon sheath of the flexor hallucis longus (FHL), because of the occasional communication found between the FHL and the ankle joint. Fluid is almost never seen in the tendon sheaths of any of the anterior muscle groups. Tendons are best seen on axial images, which provide a cross-section of the tendons and are useful for detecting longitudinal splits and changes in girth.
- The anterior to posterior diameter of the Achilles tendon is equivalent throughout its length on sagittal images. The plantaris tendon is seen as a 2- to 3-mm black dot anterior and medial to the Achilles tendon.
- The myxoid degeneration found in tendinosis can lead to partial or complete rupture of the tendon. It is not surprising then, that advanced tendinosis may have the same MRI features as a partial tear.
- Tendinosis is best seen on the T_1 images, because it manifests itself as irregular or linear focal areas of increased signal intensity within the increased tendon's girth. Healed Achilles tendon tears can sometimes mimic the MRI appearance of tendinosis, because both conditions have an increased thickening in the tendon.
- The Achilles tendon is spared of the *magic angle* effect seen on MRI, because of its straight vertical course. All the other tendons of the ankle are susceptible to the magic angle effect as they curve down the ankle at or near 55° to the main magnetic field. The radiologist must look for additional pathologic features before misconstruing the artifactually increased signal as tendon disease.

Tendon Healing Following Acute Injury

- Tendons are dynamic structures that are capable of interacting with their environment by responding to stresses in a learned manner. Early protective rehabilitation has been shown to have many beneficial effects, suggesting that physiologic stresses not only can select for specific expression of proteins from the same population of cells, but may also select for specific cellular differentiation.
- A variation of the classic phases of wound healing occurs in the normal tendon repair process. The **inflammatory phase** occurs during the first 4-7 days after injury, followed by the **proliferative phase** from days 7-14. The final maturation phase occurs during the next 8-12 weeks while the tenocytes are maturing and collagen is remodeling in response to physiologic loading, parallel to the long axis of the tendon.
- The tendon must be protected from tensile forces during the healing process. Although tendons will generally look macroscopically healed at 8 weeks, it is not until roughly 12 weeks that the strength will approach normal.
- Non-steroidal antiinflammatory drugs protect the early soluble collagen from proteolytic enzymes, while cold therapy reduces the chemotactic factors and soft tissue swelling, spasm, and pain.

Overuse Achilles Tendon Disorders

- Overuse tendon disorders account for about 30-50% of all sports injuries and cost employers both time and money. A widely held assumption is that tendon overuse causes inflammation, and this causes pain, which is treated with anti-inflammatory medications. Recent research suggests that the pain of tendinopathy may be due to unidentified biochemical factors that activate peritendinous nociceptors, without any acute inflammation.

Tendon Histopathology in Athletes with Achilles Tendinopathy

- Symptomatic Achilles tendons reveal degeneration and a disordered arrangement of collagen fibers, as well as increased vascularity. Some argue that it is not the torn collagen that hurts, but rather the *intact* collagen that carries a greater load because adjacent collagen is injured. The persisting collagen is stressed beyond its normal capacity into a painful overload zone.
- Several studies of ultrasound in patellar tendon disorders have not found a correlation between the amount of abnormal collagen and pain.
- Inflammation may not play an important role in chronic tendon disorders. Tendinosis is probably a more accurate description of chronic Achilles problems than tendinitis. Pathologic studies have shown that Achilles tendinopathy is a degenerative process characterized by a curious *absence* of inflammatory cells and a poor healing response (Astrom and Rausing 1995).
- Research continues in Achilles tendon disorders. The neurotransmitter glutamate is a mediator of pain and has been found in higher concentrations in the Achilles tendons of subjects with tendinopathy than in control subjects. Several different research groups have been studying the mechanism where eccentric strengthening reduces tendon pain. The fat pad of Kager's triangle may be a specific form of the nociceptive peritendinous tissue that is sensitive to biochemical irritants.

Achilles Tendinopathy

- Achilles tendinosis frequently occurs in the midsubstance of the tendon, in the area of hypovascularity. Patients will complain of pain, initially when first getting up from bed or the seated position. They will also be bothered by athletic activity.
- Examination will usually find thickening of the midsubstance of the tendon, with local tenderness.
- Non-operative treatment includes antiinflammatory medications and avoiding offending activity. A heel lift can be used to decrease tension on the Achilles. Physical therapy, emphasizing Achilles stretching exercises, is an important part of the non-operative plan.
- If symptoms persist despite an adequate trial of non-operative therapy, surgery can be considered. The tendon is explored, and non-viable tissue is debrided. In cases where most of the tendon is diseased, or where there are risk factors for failure (perhaps smoking), the FHL can be transferred to the Achilles insertion.
- The FHL has a very low muscle belly, so an FHL transfer will bring the vascular muscle belly into direct contact with the diseased Achilles tendon. Some studies have shown improved outcomes with the use of the FHL transfer, although its exact role is not yet defined.

Insertional Tendinosis

- In some cases, patients develop the symptoms of Achilles tendinosis at the insertion. There will be focal tenderness, and a lateral radiograph may reveal ossification (calcification) of the insertion of the tendon (Fig. 16–2).
- Non-operative treatment is the same as for midsubstance tendinosis. In addition, shoes with a soft heel counter, or even open back shoes, should be worn to minimize local irritation.
- Surgery includes debridement of diseased tendon. In mild cases, the tendon insertion can remain on the calcaneus. With extensive disease or large areas of tendon ossification, the tendon should be removed from the calcaneus and then reattached. This will require a prolonged period of restricted weight bearing.

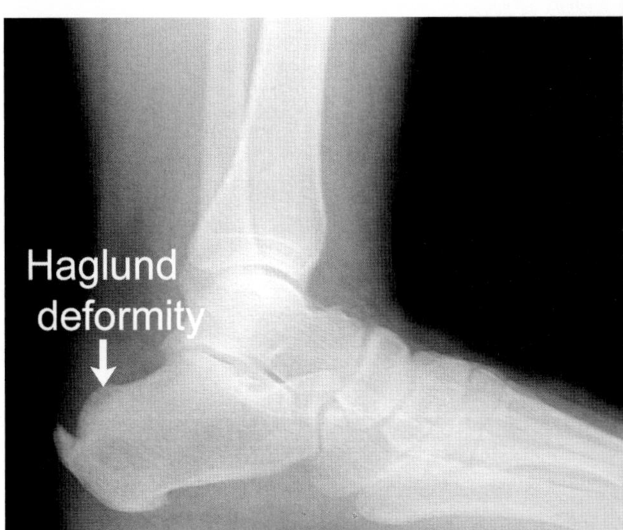

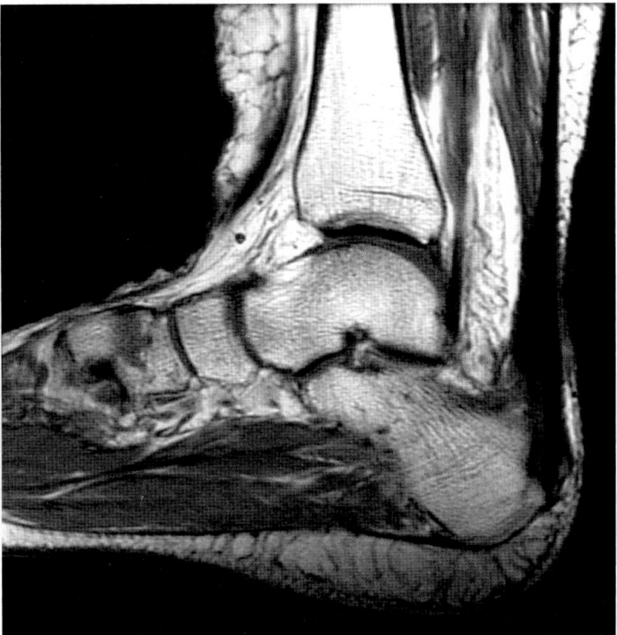

Figure 16–2: **A,** This woman had years of pain at the back of the heel. Plain radiographs reveal ossification (calcification) at the insertion of the Achilles tendon and a small Haglund deformity. **B,** This magnetic resonance imaging (MRI) scan shows increased signal in the distal tendon, suggestive of insertional Achilles tendinosis. **C,** This MRI scan of the same section shows retrocalcaneal bursitis and the Haglund deformity. The patient required distal tendon debridement, resection of the tendon ossification, and resection of the Haglund bump for pain relief.

- In many cases of insertional tendinosis, there will be a prominence on the calcaneal tuberosity, a Haglund deformity. This superolateral bony prominence may rub against the retrocalcaneal bursa and the distal Achilles tendon. Any Haglund deformity should be aggressively removed during surgery.
- In many of these cases, there will also be retrocalcaneal bursitis, or inflammation of the tissue between the calcaneus and the tendon just above the insertion. This tissue should be debrided during surgery.
- In cases of limited bursitis with a Haglund deformity, surgery may lead to a quick cure. But most cases of insertional tendinosis heal slowly, with improvement noted over many months. Incomplete pain relief may result in a significant minority of patients (one-third in one study).
- There is debate over whether cortisone injections should be given with tendinosis. It is agreed that intratendinous injections should be avoided.
- Animal models have shown that peritendinous injections can weaken the tendon, and many surgeons recommend

against any peritendinous injections around the ankle (Hugate et al. 2004).
- But at least one study has shown that injections adjacent to, but not in, the Achilles tendon are safe and help relieve symptoms.

The Role of Gastrocnemius Contracture

- Isolated tightness of the gastrocnemius is frequently seen in the adult population. It has been proposed that gastrocnemius contracture can place excess tension on the Achilles, leading to Achilles tendon disorders. There have not been any studies defining the role of the tight gastrocnemius in Achilles disorders, in part because of the difficulties in accurately measuring gastrocnemius tightness.
- Although the role of the tight gastrocnemius is somewhat controversial, most physicians would agree that Achilles- and gastrocnemius-stretching exercises are a fundamental part of the non-operative treatment of tendinopathy.
- If gastrocnemius contracture is identified in a patient undergoing surgical treatment of Achilles tendinopathy, serious consideration should be given to simultaneous gastrocnemius lengthening.

Box 16–1 Rehabilitation of Acute Injuries (such as Partial Tears) of Tendons of the Lower Extremity

Phase 1 (first 7-10 days after injury or surgery)

- Protection (bracing or protective weight bearing), rest (limitation of aggravating activities), ice (control of edema), compression, elevation.

Phase 2 (next 7-10 days after phase 1)

- Soft tissue cross-fiber friction massage to prevent tendinous adhesions and to promote subcutaneous and skin healing.
- Begin gentle passive range of motion and progress to arc-limited active range of motion as restricted by discomfort.
- Ultrasound and posttherapy ice massage.

Phase 3 (the following 2-3 weeks)

- Progressive strengthening of the myotendinous structures.
- Hydrotherapy, bicycling, and other closed chain activities may be performed.

Phase 4 (after the initial 6-8 weeks)

- Gradual resumption of activities of daily living.
- Start more progressive and aggressive weight training, whole body conditioning, and sport-specific exercises before resuming athletic activities.

Partial Tendon Tears

- Athletes may injure the Achilles tendon during sport. Examination will show a tender tendon, and MRI imaging will reveal a partial tear.
- It is possible that these partial tears are simply an acute presentation of Achilles tendinosis.
- Rehabilitation of these partial tears follows the general rehabilitation for any "sprain" or partial soft tissue injury around the ankle (Box 16–1).

Achilles Tendon Ruptures

- The incidence of Achilles tendon ruptures is higher in industrialized countries with sedentary lifestyles. Acute ruptures are becoming more prevalent as the "baby boomers" age and try to remain as active as possible. They seem to affect slightly overweight men (five males:one female) who have a more sedentary job and participate in recreational sports (such as basketball and softball) where there is a sudden explosive load to the Achilles tendon. These recreational athletes usually do not stretch or warm up properly before exercise.
- Achilles tendon ruptures are less common in developing countries where physical work and exercise are part of daily existence.
- The use of oral or injected steroids has been shown to cause collagen dysplasia and reduce the tensile strength of the Achilles tendon. Other risk factors for tendon rupture include past Achilles tendon injury, fluoroquinolone use, gout, hyperthyroidism, and renal insufficiency.
- While an Achilles laceration can be caused by direct penetrating trauma, acute ruptures are more often due to indirect trauma. There probably is preexisting tendon degeneration, and most acute ruptures occur in the watershed area.
- Typical scenarios for injury include:
  - an unexpected rapid dorsiflexion of the foot while contracting the gastrocnemius and soleus (e.g. stepping on a curb or into a hole)
  - forceful plantarflexion of the foot while the knee is extended
  - a strong dorsiflexion force on a plantarflexed foot (e.g. jumping or falling from a height).
- Tendon ruptures may occur at the musculotendinous junction or at the insertion on to the calcaneus.
- The diagnosis is made by history and physical examination. Patients will hear an audible pop or feel a snapping sensation in the posterior leg, followed by acute onset of pain and difficulty walking. They will be unable to rise on their toes.
- There will be a palpable gap within tendon itself, usually 2-6 cm from the calcaneal insertion at the most avascular region of the tendon.
- There will be a positive *Thompson test.* Have the patient kneel on a chair or lay in the prone position on the

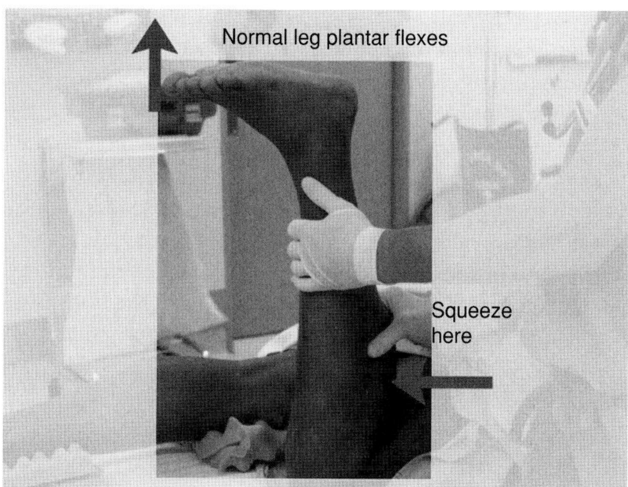

Figure 16–3: A Thompson test performed intraoperatively. The calf is squeezed with one hand. In the normal leg, the foot will plantar flex considerably. With an Achilles rupture, no plantar flexion will occur. It is best to compare the injured leg with the normal side.

examination table with the feet beyond the end of the chair or table. If squeezing of the calf muscle causes the foot to plantar flex, the Thompson test is negative. If the foot cannot move much or not at all, this is positive and diagnostic of an Achilles tendon rupture (Fig. 16–3).

- Some patients are able to actively plantar flex the foot with an intact plantaris, or with the peroneals or long toe flexors. Active ankle plantar flexion is not a good test for acute rupture, but ability to rise up on the toes is.
- A lateral ankle radiograph should be obtained to rule out an avulsion of the calcaneus with a small piece of the tuber.
- Plain x-rays may reveal a defect in the shadow of the Achilles tendon. The triangular lucency of the fat pad anterior to the Achilles tendon is generally obliterated. Kager's triangle can show increased density due to soft tissue swelling. This is the posterior triangular area of adipose tissue bordered by the anterior aspect of the Achilles, the superior surface of the calcaneus, and the posterior surface of the flexor tendons.
- Diagnosis is based on clinical examination, but an ultrasound is better than an MRI scan for obtaining a true picture of the gap between the tendon ends, especially if non-operative treatment is being considered.

Treatment of Achilles Ruptures

- There are persistent debates as to whether operative or non-operative treatment is best for the acute rupture. Several facts seem consistent.
- Operative treatment generally leads to a lower rate of rerupture in most studies (0-5% for operative, 5-20% for non-operative), although a few studies have shown very low rates of rerupture with non-operative treatment.
- Operative treatment gives predictably good return of strength, while non-operative treatment may not consistently restore maximum strength. This is one reason why many practitioners recommend surgery for athletes. There may not be a noticeable difference in non-athletes.
- Operative treatment will lead to a quicker return to normal life and work, and usually a quicker return to sport.
- Operative treatment carries a higher risk of complications, such as sural nerve injury, infection, and scar sensitivity. Some of these complications (especially infection) can have devastating consequences.
- Patients at higher risk for complications with surgery, such as those with diabetes, peripheral edema or venous stasis, morbid obesity, renal failure, and chronic corticosteroid use, should be considered for non-operative treatment.
- Patients with vascular insufficiency in the lower extremity are at risk for wound problems, so this is a relative contraindication to open surgical treatment.

Non-Operative Treatment

- In 1772, Louis-Jacques Goussier described the "Equipment used to reunite the Achilles tendon," which included a knee cap brace and a slipper, a winch for the slipper, and a key to crank the winch.
- Modern non-operative treatment includes an initial gravity equinus cast for 4 weeks with no weight bearing, and then a second cast in a more neutral position. A third neutral cast is worn for a final month with weight bearing.
- Concerns with prolonged cast immobilization include muscle atrophy, adhesion formation, joint stiffness, cartilage atrophy, degenerative arthritis, and deep venous thrombosis.
- One surgeon has described his experience with full weight-bearing casts from the beginning of treatment, and has achieved a 6.25% rerupture rate (Josey et al. 2003).
- Rerupture may be higher in athletes younger than 30 years when compared with less athletic adults in an older age group (31-50 years).

Operative Treatment

- In theory, delaying surgery by 1 week after rupture will allow consolidation of the tendon ends, thus making the repair technically easier.
- A longer delay is not a problem, because a primary repair can often be done even 6 weeks after injury. Delay beyond 6 weeks usually makes primary repair impossible, and alternative strategies must be used.
- There are three different surgical strategies: open, percutaneous, and miniopen. The goal of all is to restore integrity of the tendon at the appropriate length to allow earlier rehabilitation.

- In the percutaneous technique, the surgeon passes a suture through the skin and the tendon multiple times, making tiny incisions through which to bury the knots. In theory, the repair might not be as strong as with traditional open techniques, and in reality there is a much higher chance for sural nerve injury.
- In one study over a 14-year period comparing 70 patients who had an open procedure with 38 patients who underwent a percutaneous repair, there were less reruptures, more sural nerve lesions and palpable suture knots, and no wound infections in the percutaneous repair (Haji et al. 2004).
- An open repair can be done with the patient prone or supine. Many surgeons advocate preparing both legs, so that the tension in the repaired tendon can be compared with that of the normal side. General, spinal, or peripheral nerve block (popliteal) can be used.
- The incision should be made just medial to the midline to avoid injury to the sural nerve, which perforates the crural fascia at the myotendinous junction and passes subcutaneously distally on the lateral aspect of the Achilles tendon.
- Soft tissue technique is important to minimize wound complications. No flaps are made, but the dissection is carried sharply straight down to paratenon. The skin edges are not traumatized during the procedure (Fig. 16–4).
- If there is suspicion of a tendon avulsion from the calcaneal insertion, then the incision can be carried more plantarward to give better exposure.
- The paratenon is carefully opened, so that it can be closed after the repair. This minimizes adhesions between the tendon and the skin.
- An open repair is performed with a non-absorbable suture, such as a #5 Ethibond or #3 Dacron, in a Bunnell or Krachow pattern. Some surgeons use a smaller stitch running around the epitenon for support.
- The plantaris can be woven through the repair for extra strength (Fig. 16–5).
- For an avulsion off the insertion of calcaneus, curette the calcaneus to remove the overlying fibrous tissue down to the cancellous bone. Place two or three drill holes in the calcaneus where the tendon has been avulsed, and bring the ends of the suture through the drill holes within the substance of the bone. Tie these securely to the bone. If a plantaris tendon is present, it can be used to augment the repair.
- Meticulous wound closure in layers is performed. A bulky compressive dressing with a plaster splint in mild plantar flexion is applied (Fig. 16–6).

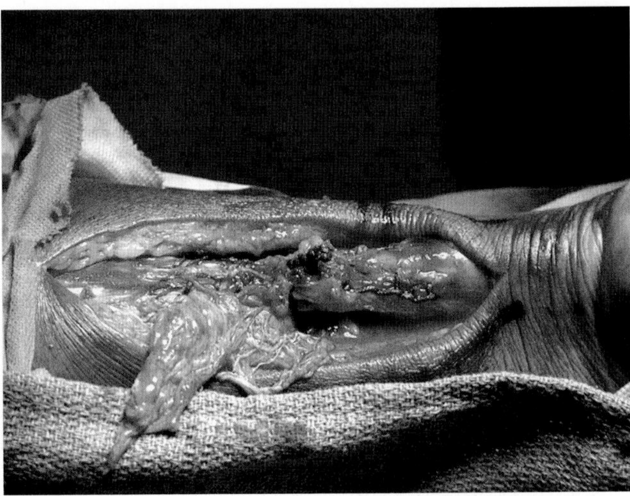

Figure 16–5: A running, locking stitch is the foundation for the tendon repair. It is nice to bury the knots below the tendon if possible, because prominent knots can irritate the patient and, rarely, rupture through the skin.

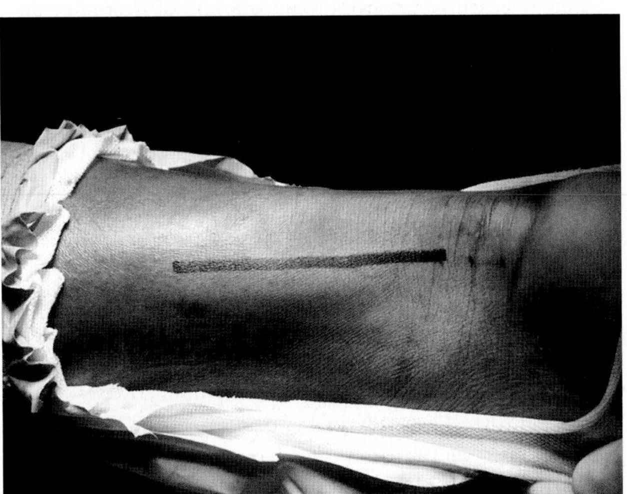

Figure 16–4: The typical incision for an open repair of the Achilles is made just medial to the midline, in order to protect the delicate skin directly posterior to the tendon.

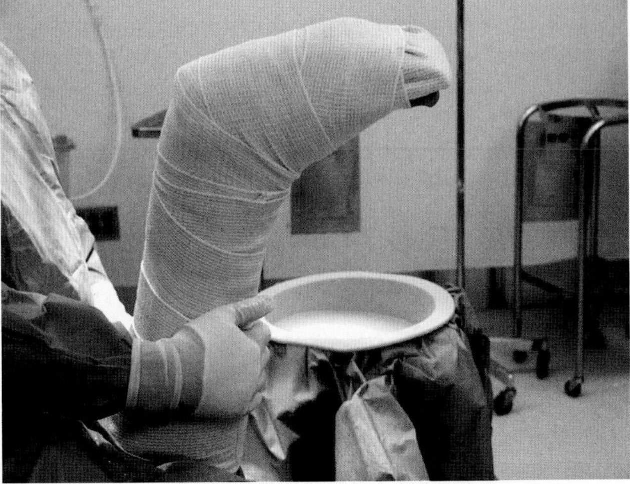

Figure 16–6: Following repair, the ankle is immobilized in mild plantar flexion to take tension off the repair and the skin.

- Open repair facilitates an earlier return to work than non-operative treatment, and ensures an accurate repair of the tendon. This gives the best chance for restoration of maximum strength. The cost of this advantage is higher risk of wound complications, especially infection.
- Superficial infections may simply require oral antibiotics. Deeper infections should be managed aggressively, with serial debridements. Unresolved infection can lead to loss of the entire tendon in severe cases.

Mini-incision Repair

- A new device has been created to facilitate a mini-incision repair. The goal was to achieve the benefits of traditional open repair without the wound complications, and also without the sural nerve injuries, of the percutaneous technique.
- The device is shaped like a fork, with four tines. After making a small incision at the level of the rupture, two of the tines are passed alongside the tendon inside the paratenon, and the other two tines remain outside the skin. Sutures are passed through a hole in each of the tines straight across, and then the fork is removed. The end result is a suture passed through the tendon, but then with both ends out of the open wound.
- It is possible to hit the sural nerve when passing the suture, but because it is then pulled out, the suture does not remain in or around the nerve.
- In two series of mini-incision repairs, the rerupture rate was similar to that with traditional open techniques, with most of the ruptures related to patient non-compliance. There were no deep infections.

Rehabilitation of Achilles Tendon Repair

- After a short course of immobilization for wound healing, the patient is placed in a removable cast boot. Active range of motion is begun.
- Weight bearing in the boot is begun between 2 and 8 weeks after surgery, depending on the surgeon's preference and the strength of the repair.
- Formal physical therapy is started at week 6 or 8, depending on the progress and age of the patient. A 1-inch heel lift can be placed in the shoe until 10° of dorsiflexion is obtained. Active strengthening begins at this time.
- Friction massage techniques can be directly applied to the tendon to help prevent the buildup of adhesions, to reduce swelling, and to aid circulation.
- Although a surgical repair has a lower incidence of rerupture than a non-operative repair, a continuous program of stretching should be maintained for up to 1 year after surgery.

Chronic Rupture

- When a rupture is identified more than 6 weeks out from injury, additional surgical techniques are needed to achieve a strong repair.
- Patients with chronic (old) untreated ruptures will complain of weakness in rising up on their toes, and altered gait patterns. Pain, if present, may be under the heel, because the foot assumes a relatively dorsiflexed position with chronic muscle imbalance (the dorsiflexors are stronger than the plantar flexors).
- Perhaps 20% of acute ruptures are initially missed for a variety of reasons. Patients with progressive degenerative tendinosis, such as occurs with rheumatoid arthritis and systemic connective tissue disorders, may develop a more gradual rupture. Initially, there may be Achilles tendinosis pain. With time, patients lose the ability to rise up on to the toes. A palpable defect may not be evident.
- Non-operative treatment for a chronic rupture includes a heel lift, molded ankle-foot orthosis, and/or laced-up high top shoes or boots that may decrease the demands to plantar flex the foot. However, none of these options restores the push-off strength of the tendon.
- For a subacute midsubstance tendon rupture, a V-Y lengthening of the gastrocnemius at the musculotendinous junction can be performed. Also, a tendon turndown will give more length.
- In recent years, an FHL transfer has gained popularity. The FHL is in phase to the Achilles in the gait cycle, and provides a strong muscle and a strong repair. The FHL can be attached to the distal tendon stump or secured directly to the calcaneus.

Partial Gastrocnemius Tear

- A partial gastrocnemius tear is a common injury. It used to be referred to as a plantaris rupture.
- The patient will complain of pain in the midcalf after a sudden movement. Although it may be confused with an acute Achilles rupture, the area of tenderness will be in the midcalf, well above the tendon. The Thompson squeeze test will be normal, and there will be no swelling or tenderness around the tendon itself.
- These injuries can be treated with a short course of immobilization and rest, and then mobilization and rehabilitation as tolerated.

Xanthomas

- Xanthomas of the Achilles tendon are found in patients with familial hyperlipidemia, and appear as an abnormal stippled appearance on the T_1 MRI image.
- It may be difficult to distinguish from Achilles tendinopathy, because both have heterogeneous and

morphologic changes in the tendon. Ultrasound is more effective in detecting discrete lipid deposits than MRI.

References

Achilles Tendinosis

Astrom M, Rausing A. (1995) Chronic Achilles tendinopathy. A survey of surgical and histopathologic findings. Clin Orthop Relat Res 316: 151-164.

An analysis of specimens retrieved at surgery found consistent degenerative tendinosis, with a noticeable lack of inflammatory cells and a poor healing response.

Hugate R, Pennypacker J, Saunders M et al. (2004) The effects of intratendinous and retrocalcaneal intrabursal injections of corticosteroid on the biomechanical properties of rabbit Achilles tendons. J Bone Joint Surg Am 86-A(4): 794-801.

Local injections of corticosteroid, both within the tendon substance and into the retrocalcaneal bursa, adversely affected the biomechanical properties of rabbit Achilles tendons. Additionally, tendons from rabbits that had received bilateral injections of corticosteroid demonstrated an additive adverse effect, with significantly worse biomechanical properties compared with tendons from rabbits that had received unilateral injections of corticosteroid.

Achilles Rupture

Assal M, Jung M et al. (2002) Limited open repair of Achilles tendon ruptures: A technique with a new instrument and findings of a prospective multicenter study. J Bone Joint Surg 84-A: 161-170.

Experience with a new device and a new technique of limited incision open repair of Achilles tendons found a low rerupture rate, with no deep infections and no sural nerve injuries.

Haji A, Sahai A, Symes A et al. (2004) Percutaneous versus open tendo Achilles repair. Foot Ankle Int 25(4): 215-218.

This small retrospective series of patients found a higher incidence of sural nerve injuries in the percutaneous group and a higher wound infection rate in the open group, but these differences were not significant. Both groups had good functional outcomes.

Josey RA, Marymont JV et al. (2003) Immediate, full weightbearing cast treatment of acute Achilles tendon ruptures: A long-term follow-up study. Foot Ankle Int 24(10): 775-779.

This series of 48 tendon ruptures treated non-operatively with early weight bearing found good functional outcomes, with only a 6% rerupture rate.

Moller M, Movin T et al. (2001) Acute rupture of tendon Achilles. A prospective randomised study of comparison between surgical and non-surgical treatment. J Bone Joint Surg Br 83: 843-848.

This study of 112 patients found a higher incidence of rerupture in patients treated non-operatively, but similar functional outcomes if no rerupture occurred.

CHAPTER 17

Other Tendon Problems

Eric M. Bluman*

*M.D., Ph.D., Chief, Orthopaedic Foot and Ankle Surgery, and Chief, Orthopaedic Traumatology, Department of Orthopaedic Surgery, Madigan Army Medical Center, Fort Lewis, WA

- Diagnosis of disorders of the "lesser tendons" of the foot and ankle in some ways may be more difficult than that of the Achilles and posterior tibial tendons. Their proximity to one another, as well as to other structures, makes the differential diagnosis more challenging to narrow down.
- Acute injuries as well as overuse syndromes are common in this group of tendons. These tendons are subjected to tensile, compressive, and shearing forces, all of which can contribute to tendon pathology.
- A complete history as well as a foot and ankle examination needs to be done on patients suspected of having one of these disorders to ensure that alternative diagnoses are not being missed.
- There have been a multitude of descriptors given to inflammatory and non-inflammatory conditions of tendons. In the past, the terms *tenosynovitis*, *peritendonitis* and *tenovaginitis* have all been used to describe the inflammation of the paratenon. These terms have been supplanted by more accurate descriptors.
- **Paratenonitis** is the correct term to describe the presence of acute inflammatory cells in the paratenon and adjacent non-tendinous connective tissue. Paratenonitis usually arises from mechanical irritation and is completely reversible. Rupture secondary to pure paratenonitis is a rare phenomenon. Isolated paratenonitis refractory to non-operative therapies may be treated by tenolysis.
- **Tendinosis.** Paratenonitis with tendinosis describes tendon thickening and intrasubstance degeneration. Tendon nodules may be present with this condition (Fig. 17–1 and Box 17–1).

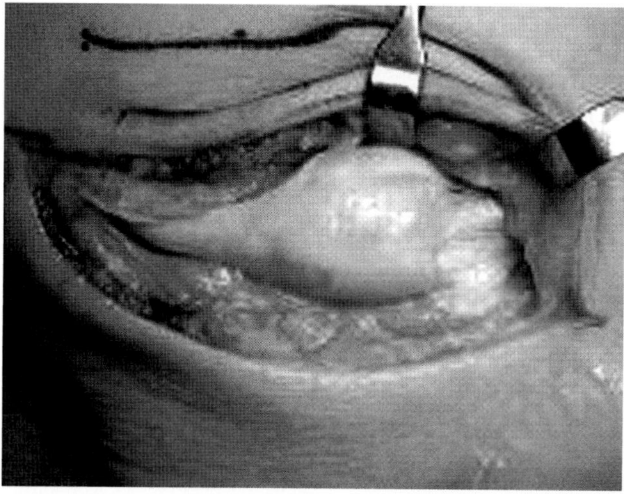

Figure 17–1: Tendon thickening from tendinosis.

Box 17–1 Tendinitis Versus Tendinosis

Most pathologies we call tendinitis are actually tendinosis, because there is no inflammation. There is intrasubstance degeneration consisting of collagen degeneration and angiofibroblastic ingrowth. Histologically, there is mucoid degeneration with chondroid metaplasia. The tenocytes, which are normally spindle-shaped, become more rounded and numerous. The normally highly ordered collagen fibers become disorganized, fragmented, and fibrillated. Occasionally, there may be calcium deposition within the tendon. These areas of tendon degeneration lead to tendon weakening and increase the risk for tendon rupture.

- Paratenosis with tendinosis occurs when both conditions are present simultaneously.
- Insertional tendonitis is an example of paratenonitis with tendonosis.
- Paratenonitis with tendonosis refractory to conservative therapies may be treated with therapies ranging from excision of the diseased portion of the tendon with primary repair to excision with tendon transfer.
- Perhaps 36% of all paratenonitis occurs in the foot and ankle.
- Selective injections into tendon sheaths or neighboring anatomical structures may be invaluable in helping discern among competing diagnoses. Diagnostic injections should consist of local anesthetic preparations alone.
- Corticosteroid injection into the tendon proper, the tendon sheath, or in the proximity of the tendon carries with it the risk of weakening the tendon. Corticosteroid injections in the vicinity of tendons should be done with extreme caution and in most cases should be avoided altogether.
- Rehabilitation of injured or surgically repaired tendons should follow four general phases. These four phases are outlined in Table 17–1.

Fluoroquinolones and Tendon Disease

- Fluoroquinolones have been shown to increase the risk of spontaneous rupture of tendons. Tendon rupture or drug-induced tendonopathy should be strongly considered in those who have a tendon injury and have recently taken these drugs.

Table 17–1: The Four Phases of Tendon Rehabilitation

PHASE	APPROXIMATE TIMES	REHABILITATIVE ACTIVITY
1	First week	Immobilization Cryotherapy Light compression Elevation
2	Second week	Continued immobilization Cross-fiber friction massage (prevents adhesions) Early gentle passive mobilization with progression to active assisted range of motion Cryotherapy Ultrasound therapies
3	Third through sixth week	Functional bracing Progressive strengthening Hydrotherapy Closed chain exercises
4	Seventh week onward	Gradual resumption of activities of daily living Weight training Sport-specific exercises

- Fluoroquinolones are bactericidal and function through disruption of bacterial DNA gyrase. Fluoroquinolone-induced tendonopathies have recently been reported in the literature. Many orthopaedists utilize these drugs in the perioperative setting for infections, because they do not increase the effect of warfarin in the same manner as other antimicrobials, such as trimethoprim-sulfamethoxazole.
- The relative risk of Achilles tendon disorders with use of these drugs is estimated at 3.2 times that of a control population. This increased risk may be limited to those patients who are over 60 years of age. Use of fluoroquinolones with corticosteroids in those over 60 further increases the risk of tendonopathy to 6.7 times that of a control population. Apparently, the risk of tendonopathy is increased in those currently using the drugs and not in those who have used them in the past.
- Shakibaei et al. (2000) demonstrated that even limited doses in a rat model of fluoroquinolone-induced Achilles tendonitis resulted in degenerative alterations of the tenocytes. Cells lost normal cell-matrix relations as well as interactions with the extracellular matrix. It is believed that these adverse effects are the result of altered fibroblast metabolism. Culture of tendon fibroblasts with ciprofloxacin resulted in 66% reduction in cell proliferation relative to control cultures. Collagen synthesis and proteoglycan synthesis were also decreased. Fluoroquinolones also stimulate tendon matrix degradation by proteases. It is likely that fluoroquinolones not only decrease the synthesis of tendon structural components but also accelerate their degradation.

Peroneal Tendons

Function

- Primary function of peroneus longus is plantar flexion of the first metatarsal, and its secondary function is eversion of the foot.
- Primary function of the peroneus brevis is eversion of the foot; its secondary function is plantar flexion of the foot.
- The peroneal tendons provide 63% total eversion power to the hindfoot; 35% is accounted for by the longus, 28% by the brevis.

Anatomy

- The peroneals are lateral compartment muscles. The peroneus longus originates from the lateral condyle of the tibia as well as the head and lateral aspect of the fibula. The peroneus brevis arises from the lower two-thirds of the lateral fibula and the anterior and posterior intermuscular septum.
- The peroneus longus muscle lies just lateral and posterior to the brevis in the lateral compartment of the leg.

The brevis tendon lies anterior to the longus tendon at the level of the lateral malleolus.

- Both muscles are innervated by the superficial peroneal nerve.
- The musculotendinous junction of both peroneals normally lies above the superior peroneal retinaculum. The junction of the peroneus brevis lies 2-3 cm above the lateral malleolus. Occasionally, the muscle belly of the brevis muscle may lie within the retinaculum.
- Microvascular studies have not identified a watershed area found in some other tendons (e.g. Achilles and posterior tibial), and there seems to be good blood supply to all areas of the tendons.
- The common peroneal synovial sheath starts approximately 4 cm proximal to the lateral malleolus, and then bifurcates at the inferior margin of the superior peroneal retinaculum.
- A fibroosseous tunnel helps to maintain the peroneals in the retrofibular groove. The borders for the tunnel are the superior peroneal retinaculum posterolaterally; the posterior talofibular ligament, the posterior inferior tibiofibular ligament, and the calacaneofibular ligament medially. The anterior border is the posterior groove (retromalleolar sulcus) of the fibula (Fig. 17–2).
- The retrofibular groove or sulcus is concave in 82% of individuals, flat in 11%, and convex in 7%.
- It is the superior peroneal retinaculum that is most important in keeping the tendons in the retrofibular groove. Inferior to the lateral malleolus, the tendons then pass the peroneal tubercle and below the inferior peroneal retinaculum (Fig. 17–3).
- The peroneus brevis then continues anteriorly and inserts into the proximal fifth metatarsal.
- The peroneus longus passes inferior to the cuboid in a tunnel formed by the cuboid groove superiorly and the long plantar ligament inferiorly. The tendon then continues anteromedially on the plantar aspect of the foot to insert on the base of the first metatarsal and medial cuneiform.
- The os peroneum is a sesamoid bone that lies within the peroneus longus tendon. It is located where the tendon passes around the cuboid to enter the plantar aspect of the foot (Fig. 17–4). As with other sesamoid bones, the os peroneum may be unipartite, bipartite, or multipartite. Approximately 5-15% of individuals have an ossified os peroneum. Probably all individuals have an os perineum, but most remain cartilaginous.
- The peroneus quartus is an accessory muscle that is present in 11-23% of individuals. When present, it arises from the muscle belly of the brevis, passes through the tendon sheath, and inserts into the peroneal tubercle on the lateral aspect of the calcaneus.

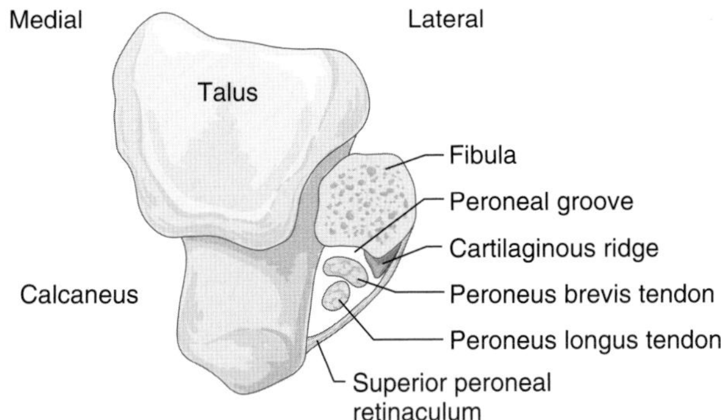

Figure 17–2: **Borders of the peroneal tunnel.**

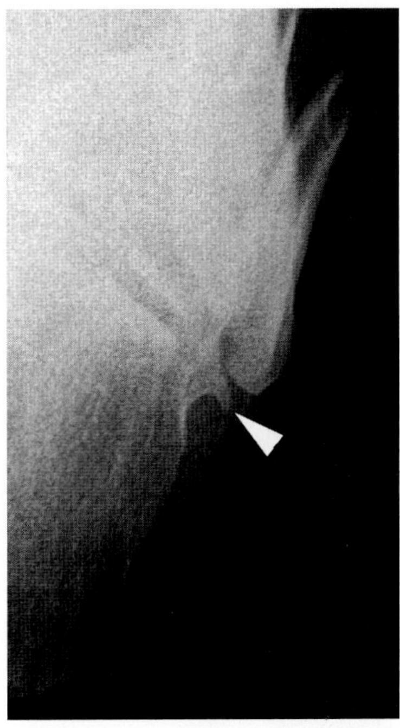

Figure 17–3: **Enlarged peroneal tubercle noted on the axial view of the calcaneus.**

Physical Findings

General

- Peroneal pathology can arise along the entire length of the tendon. Many non-peroneal disorders can also lead to lateral-sided ankle pain and/or instability. Lateral ankle pain must be explored completely to prevent a missed diagnosis or a misdiagnosis (Box 17–2).
- Individuals who are involved in sports with heavy cutting or twisting motions are predisposed to peroneal pathology. The position that is thought to put the peroneals at greatest risk of injury is foot eversion combined with ankle dorsiflexion. Skiers are the prototypical athletes who present with peroneal pathology.
- Radiographic evaluation should include anteroposterior, lateral, and oblique views of the foot and ankle. Magnetic resonance imaging (MRI) or sonography may demonstrate

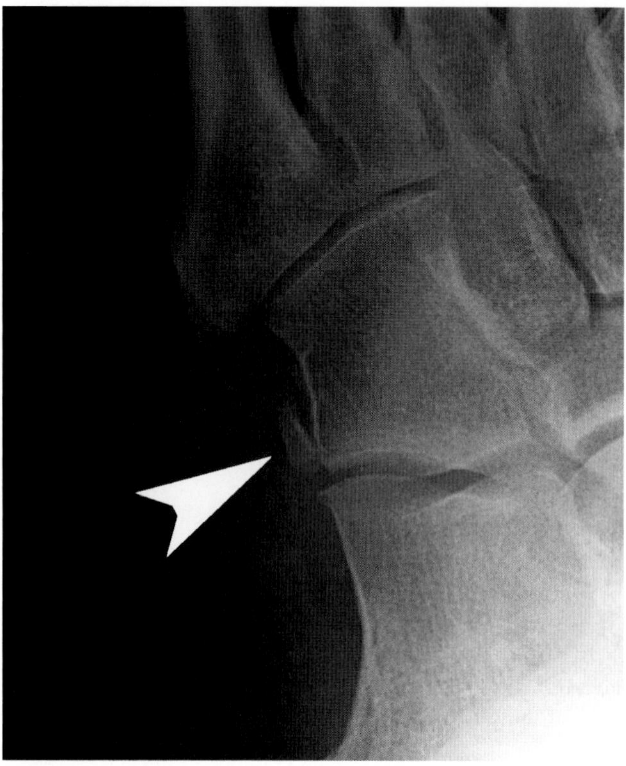

Figure 17–4: **The os peroneum lies in the peroneus longus tendon.**

peroneal strength may be found. Subtalar motion may also be painful because of peroneal muscle spasm.

- Patients with peroneal tendonitis may have a pronounced antalgic gait when walking over uneven surfaces.
- Common sites for stenosis: cuboid tunnel, peroneal tubercle, superior peroneal retinaculum.
- MRI usually not needed to make diagnosis.
- Options for conservative therapy include rest, non-steroidal antiinflammatory drugs (NSAIDs), cryotherapy, activity modification, and a lateral heel wedge to limit tendon excursion. Difficult cases may benefit from 6 weeks of immobilization in a cast or brace.
- Surgery is appropriate if symptoms persist despite adequate conservative treatment. Inflammatory tissue can be removed (tenolysis). If peroneus brevis tendinosis is seen, the damaged segment should be longitudinally excised, and the remaining healthy tendon repaired. If the amount of tendon needed to be removed is too large to allow repair of the tendon, then excision of the entire diseased portion and tenodesis to the peroneus longus should be performed (Fig. 17–5).
- If the peroneal tubercle is hypertrophied and contributing to the inflammation, it should be excised.
- A low-lying peroneus brevis muscle belly may result in paratenonitis by a mass effect. The increased girth of the

Box 17–2 Lateral Ankle Pathology That May Mimic Peroneal Tendon Disorders

- Fibular fracture
- Lateral ankle sprain
- Lateral process of the talus fracture
- Impingement lesions
- Syndesmosis injuries
- Osteochondral injury of talus
- Subtalar pathology
- Os trigonum
- Sural neuritis
- Anterior process of calcaneus fracture

the presence of tendinosis, paratenonitis, and even longitudinal tears or complete ruptures of the peroneals, but usually do not provide enough information to discern the extent of pathology.

Paratenonitis and Tendonosis

- Patients present with swelling and pain in the area of the peroneal tendons. There is point tenderness over the path of the tendons.
- Symptoms of peroneal tendonitis are exacerbated by passive plantar flexion with inversion, or active contraction of the peroneals against resistance. Decreased

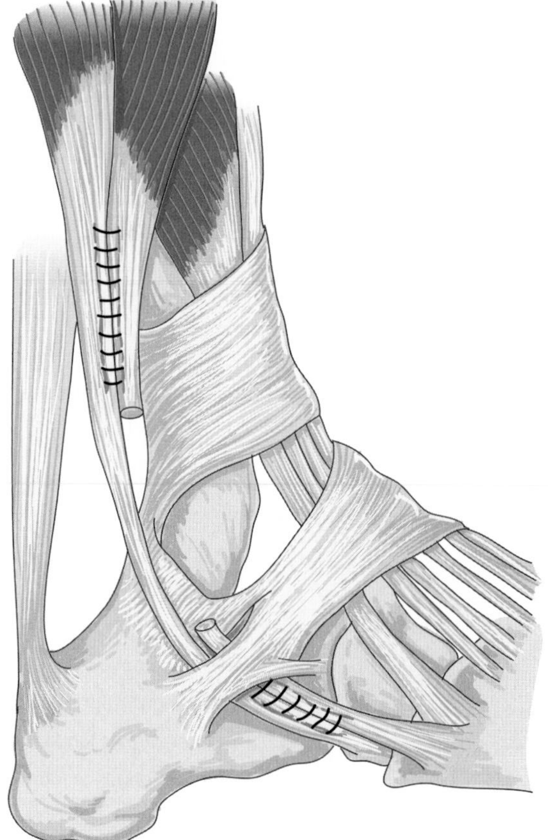

Figure 17–5: **Side to side repair of peroneus brevis to longus.**

low-lying muscle belly results in impingement and inflammation within the sheath. The low-lying fibers should be resected (Fig. 17–6).

- A peroneus quartus muscle can contribute to paratenonitis in two ways. First, irritation may arise because of the mass effect of the muscle belly passing through the peroneal sheath. Second, the pull of this muscle has also been implicated in hypertrophy of the peroneal tubercle and subsequent development of irritation as the tendons turn anteriorly at this point. The accessory muscle can be resected as needed.
- The most common location of involvement for paratenonitis caused by rheumatoid arthritis is the peroneal tendons. Treatment for those with rheumatoid arthritis should mirror that used for non-rhematoid-induced paratenonitis.

Painful Os Peroneum Syndrome (POPS)

- POPS is a set of pathologic conditions grouped together by their colocalization in the region from the peroneal tubercle to the cuboid groove.
- POPS has five described variants:
  - acute os peroneum fracture
  - chronic (healing) os fracture
  - attrition or partial rupture of peroneus longus tendon
  - frank rupture
  - large peroneal tubercle on lateral calcaneus that entraps the tendon or the os peroneum.
- Presentation of POPS can be acute or chronic.
  - Acute presentations result from a sudden traumatic episode, commonly involving ankle inversion and supination. This results in either an os peroneum fracture or a diastasis of a bipartite or multipartite os peroneum. There is loss of peroneal function with acute presentations.
  - Chronic presentations arise from repetitive inversion/supination injuries. Symptoms akin to a sprained ankle may fluctuate in intensity over an extended period of time. There is no loss of peroneal function.
- Symptoms may include tenderness and thickening of the peroneus longus tendon at the peroneal tubercle or at the cuboid tunnel. Some patients may have the sensation of "stepping on a pebble" if the pathology has resulted in malalignment of the os peroneum at the cuboid groove. There may be sensations consistent with a sural neuritis, because the distal branches of this nerve are located nearby.
- Initial evaluation of a suspected POPS should include plain radiographs of the foot. The oblique view may reveal os peroneum fracture, diastasis, or migration. Axial views of the calcaneus will allow evaluation of the size and shape of the peroneal tubercle. MRI can be used to evaluate for tendon tears or rupture.
- Acute, displaced os perineum injuries with loss of peroneal function should be treated with surgical repair.

Longitudinal Tears and Rupture

- These injuries probably lie along a continuum with paratenonitis. Inflammation of the tenosynovium over time may weaken the tendon and lead to longitudinal tears. The history and examination are similar to that in patients with tendonitis.
- Acute injury or chronic repetitive injury can both result in longitudinal tears of the peroneals, more commonly in the brevis (Fig. 17–7).
- These longitudinal tears can be seen in association with subluxation or dislocation of the tendons out of the peroneal groove.

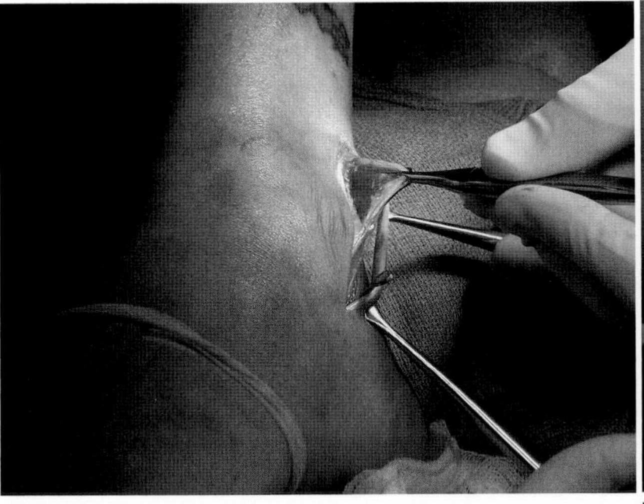

A

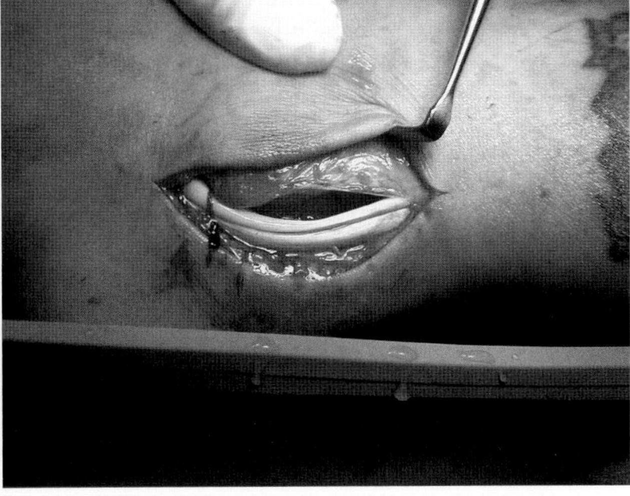

B

Figure 17–6: Low-lying peroneal brevis muscle belly. **A,** Muscle belly seen lying adjacent to the peroneus longus behind the lateral malleolus. **B,** The tendons with plenty of room after the low-lying muscle fibers are resected.

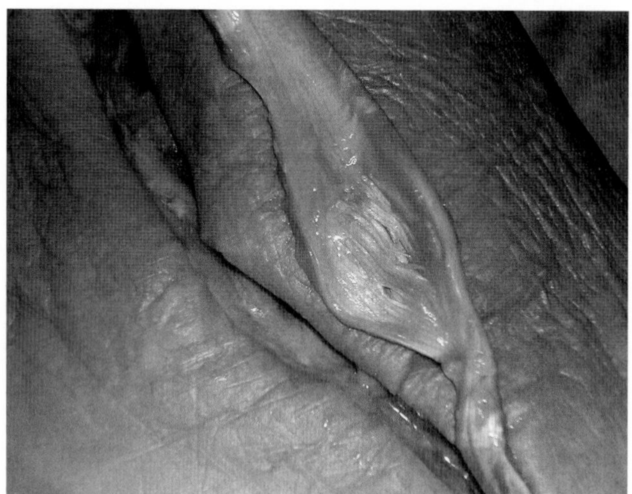

Figure 17–7: **A longitudinal tear of peroneus brevis.**

- The most frequent position for a longitudinal tear to be found is in the region of the peroneal groove of the fibula. This is thought to occur because the brevis becomes compressed and attenuated between the longus tendon and the fibula during activity. This attenuating effect may be aggravated by repetitive scraping of the tendon along the posterolateral lip of the peroneal groove.
- The prevalence of longitudinal tears is not exactly known. Cadaver studies have placed the prevalence between 10 and 20% of the population (Sobel et al. 1991). An observational study conducted in patients with lateral ankle instability who were undergoing lateral ankle reconstructions found that 23% of patients demonstrated longitudinal tears.
- Non-surgical treatment of longitudinal tears is unsuccessful in most cases, even after prolonged treatment courses.
- Surgical treatment of longitudinal tears.
  - Tendons that have longitudinal tears that affect less than 50% of their diameter may be debrided and repaired with an absorbable suture.
  - Those tears that involve grater than 50% of the diameter of the tendon should have the degenerated section excised to a level above and below the peroneal retinaculum, with tenodesis of the proximal and distal limbs to the remaining peroneal tendon in a side to side fashion (see Fig. 17–5).
- Frank acute rupture is rare. Non-acute ruptures usually result from attrition brought about by mechanical and inflammatory factors. Both chronic and acute ruptures need to be surgically repaired. Ruptures usually occur where paratenonitis with tendinosis is observed. Ruptures will result in weakening or complete loss of eversion. In those with little body fat, loss of the peroneal tendon outline on the lateral aspect of the calcaneus may be observed (Fig. 17–8).

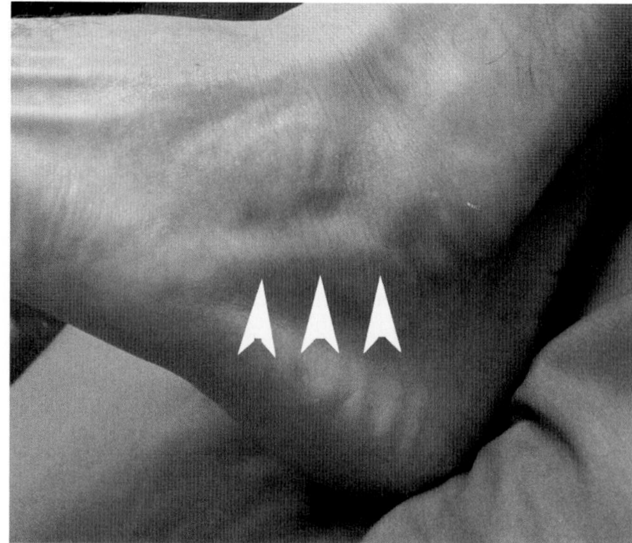

A

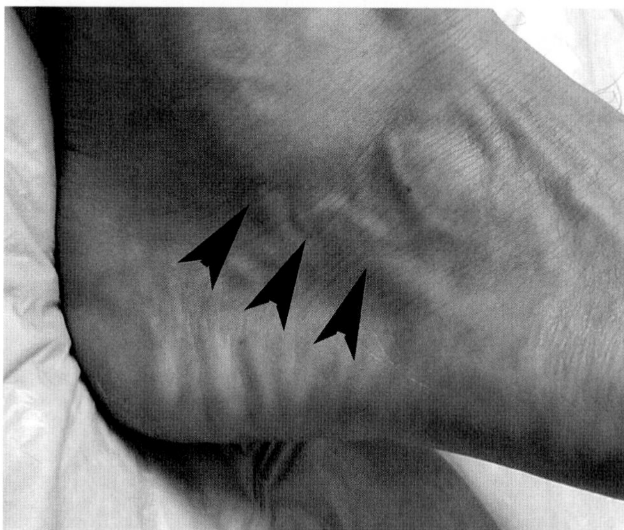

B

Figure 17–8: **Clinical appearance of peroneal tendon rupture. A, Normal peroneal tendons lateral to the heel. B, Absence of the peroneal prominence after rupture.**

- If peroneus brevis rupture is left unrepaired, the foot may drift into varus over time from the resulting tendon imbalance.
- An operative management scheme for peroneal tendon tears was recently proposed by Redfern and Myerson (2004) (Fig. 17–9).
- If a longitudinal tear is present but the tendons are grossly intact (type 1), a debridement is performed and the defect is repaired by tubularization of the remaining tendon.
- When a rupture is present with the remaining tendon being usable (type 2), excision of the diseased portion and a tenodesis are performed.

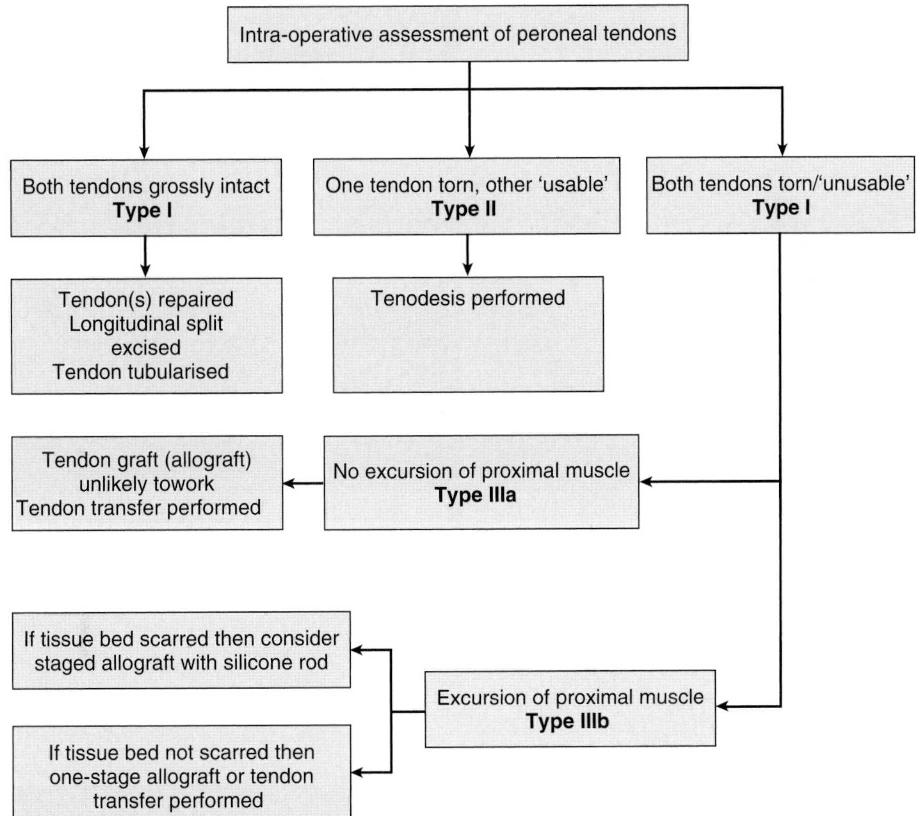

Figure 17–9: An operative management scheme for peroneal tendon tears, by Redfern and Myerson (2004).

- When both tendons are torn or are unusable, treatment decisions hinge on the excursion of the proximal musculature. If both tendons are torn and the muscle bellies are stiff or fibrotic (type 3a), another tendon must be used to recreate peroneal action. The flexor digitorum longus (FDL) or flexor hallucis longus (FHL) can be transferred behind the tibia to the lateral foot.
- If both peroneal tendons are lost but the muscle belly has good excursion (type 3b), an interposition tendon grafting can be done. In some cases, the tissues of the tendon sheath have no scarring, and a one-stage interposition grafting may be done. The presence of scarring requires a staged procedure in which a silicone rod is placed along the path of the peroneal tendons (Fig. 17–10). After 6-8 weeks to allow reestablishment of a sufficient sheath, the silicone rods are removed and interposition grafting is carried out.
- Calcaneal impingement of lateral ankle structures may result after calcaneal fracture with unreduced lateral wall "blowout," or with severe hindfoot valgus, as is seen in advanced posterior tibial tendon rupture. Chronic impingement may lead to peroneal erosion and eventual rupture. If detected before rupture occurs, the deformity should be corrected and tendons repaired (Fig. 17–11).

Subluxation and Dislocation

- Peroneal dislocation or subluxation may occur as an acute or a recurrent (chronic) event. Acute dislocations account for only 10% of reported cases.
- It has been proposed that a non-concave shape of the peroneal sulcus may predispose to dislocation (Fig. 17–12).

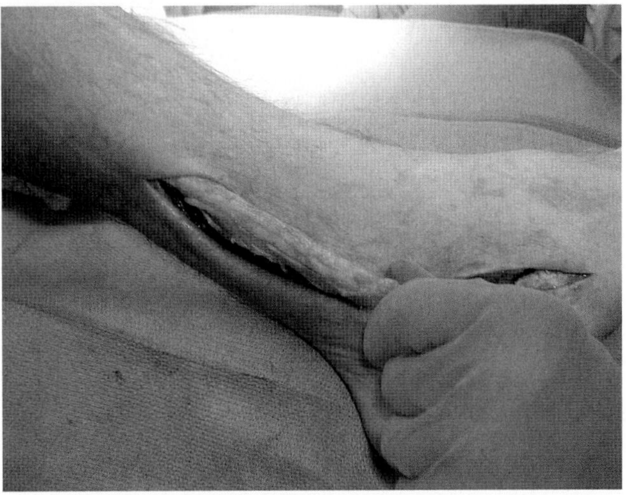

A

Figure 17–10: Reconstruction of chronic peroneal rupture. **A,** The peroneal muscle bellies are tested for normal excursion.

Continued

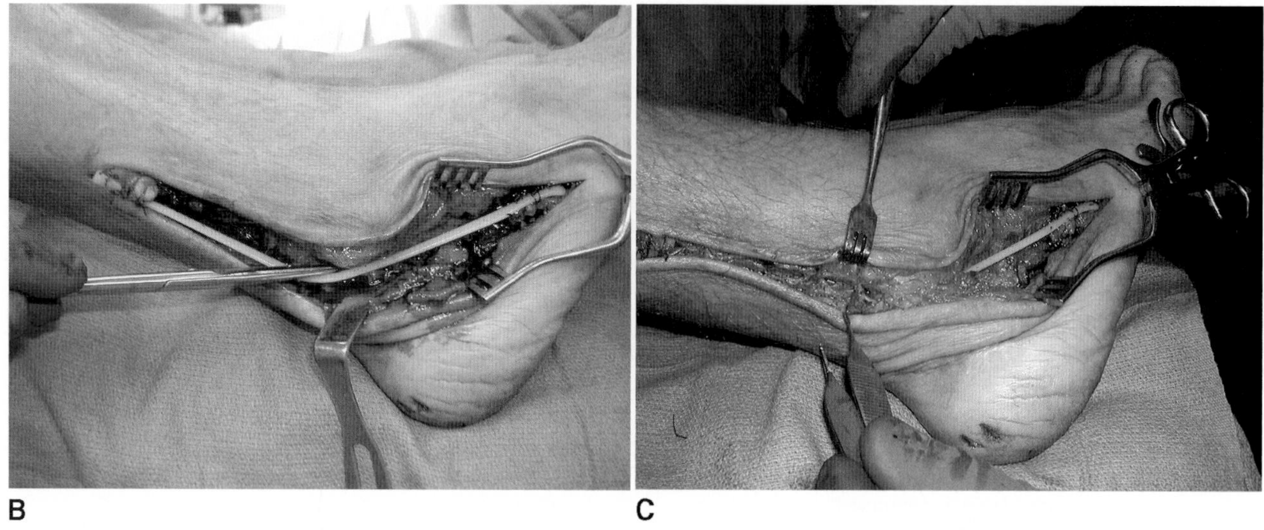

Figure 17–10: Cont'd **B**, The silicone rod is placed in the bed. **C**, The soft tissues are closed over the rod.

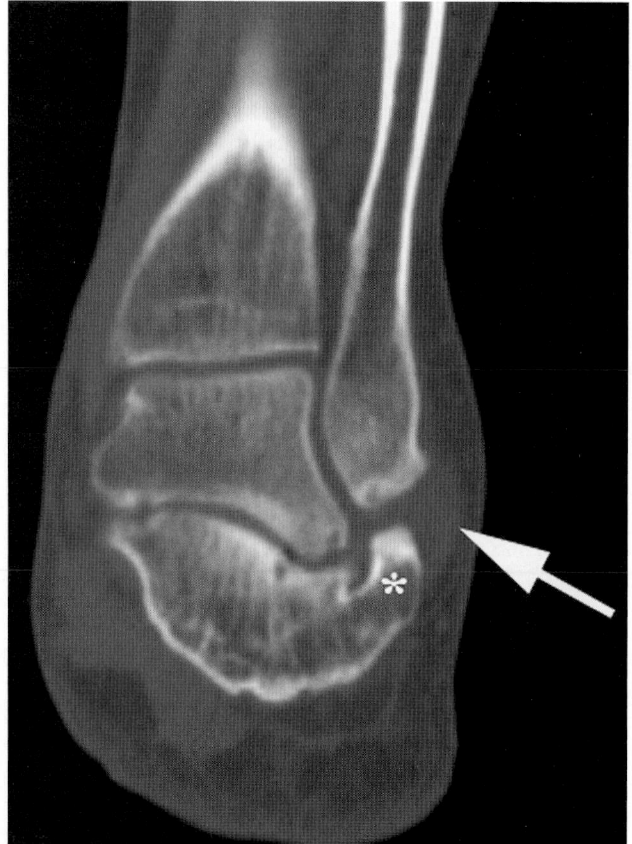

Figure 17–11: Coronal reconstruction from CT scan demonstrating peroneal impingement from a calcaneal fracture malunion. Note the limited space (arrow) between the fibula and the "blown-out" lateral wall of the calcaneus (asterisk). Figure courtesy of Richard deAsla, M.D.

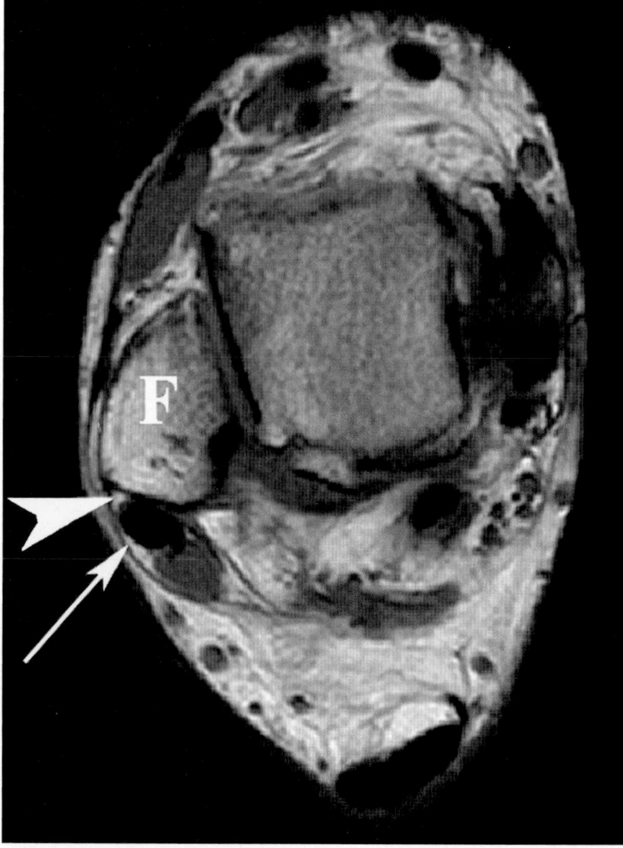

Figure 17–12: Axial T1-weighted image at the ankle demonstrating that the posterior surface of the fibula (F) is relatively convex (marked by arrowhead), facilitating subluxation of peroneal tendon (arrow). Peroneal tendons are not subluxed in this image.

- Acute dislocations usually result from a violent, forced dorsiflexion of the ankle with reflex contraction of the peroneals, causing a disruption of fibroosseous tunnel holding the tendons.
- There are four main types of acute peroneal tendon dislocation (Fig. 17–13):
  - elevation of fibular periosteum by the superior peroneal retinaculum, with anterior displacement of the tendons
  - complete tearing of the superior peroneal retinaculum, with anterior displacement of the tendons
  - avulsion fracture of the posterolateral aspect of the distal fibula by the superior peroneal retinaculum, with anterior dislocation of the tendons
  - avulsion of the superior peroneal retinaculum from its posterior insertion on the calcaneus, with anterior dislocation of the tendons over the retinaculum.
- Chronic dislocations are often seen in patients with a history of recurrent inversion ankle sprains and lateral ankle instability. These injuries lead to a failure of the superior peroneal retinaculum. Repetitive tendon subluxation leads to fraying and splitting of fibers as they become abraded over the posterolateral lip of the retrofibular sulcus (Fig. 17–14).
- Acute dislocations usually present with the tendons reduced within the retrofibular sulcus. The patient will probably have pain, swelling, and ecchymosis just posterior and lateral to the fibula.
- An anterior drawer test for ligament disruption is usually normal.
- Having the patient actively evert the foot while in a dorsiflexed position against resistance may cause redislocation of the tendons.
- A flake or avulsion fracture from the posterolateral fibula may be seen on routine radiographs, indicating the presence of a grade 3 injury. This is pathognomonic for peroneal tendon dislocation.

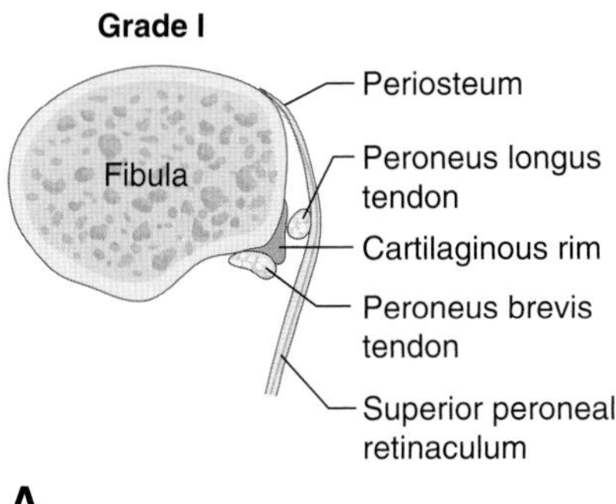

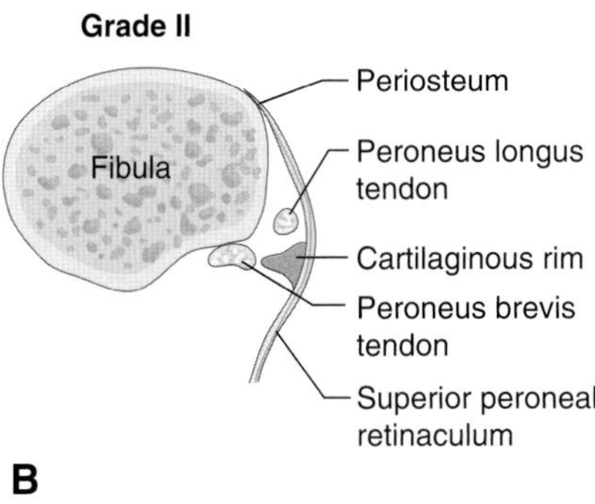

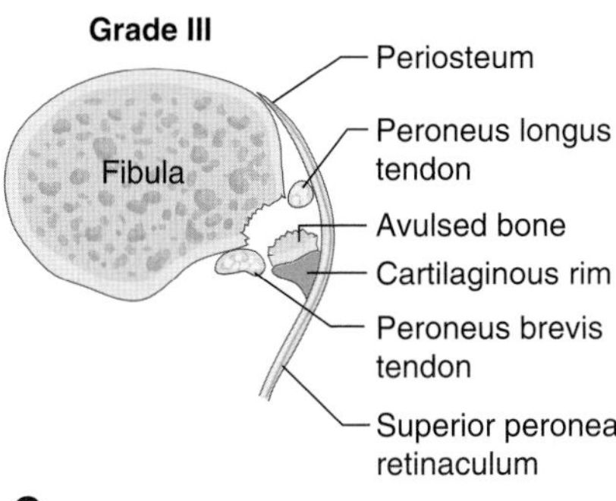

Figure 17–13: Eckert and Davis classification of acute peroneal tendon dislocation. This system comprises the first three parts of the four part grading system.

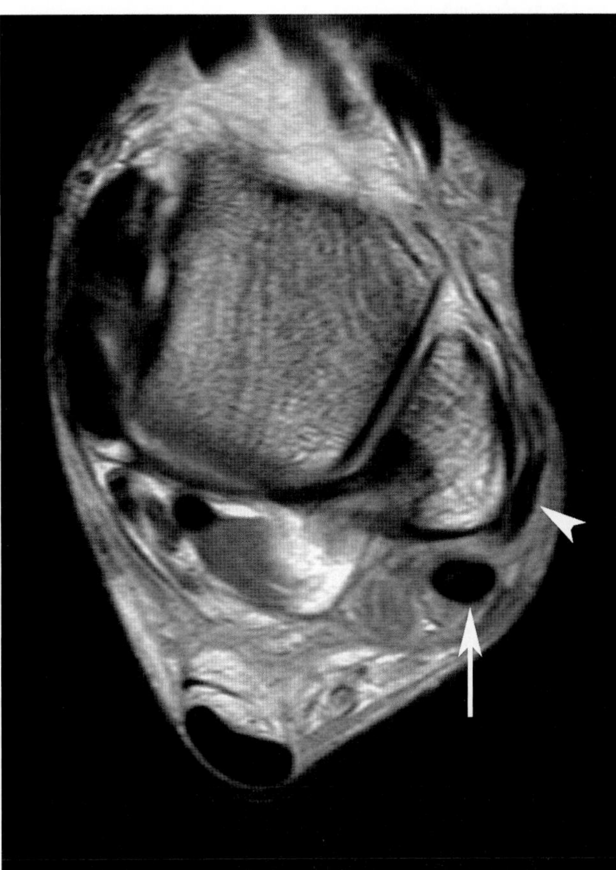

Figure 17–14: Chronically dislocated peroneal tendons. Axial MR imaging demonstrating chronically dislocated peroneus brevis (arrowhead) and peroneus longus remaining posterior to the fibula (arrow).

- With chronic dislocations, patients may describe snapping, popping, or crepitance, with repeated episodes of giving way or instability.
- Unreduced dislocations may be palpable at the subcutaneous border of the fibula.
- In contrast to acute dislocations, anterior drawer testing may be positive because of the association of this condition with lateral ankle instability.

Treatment of Subluxation

- Treatment is based on acuity, anatomical classification of injury, and activity level of the patient.
- All chronic subluxations/dislocations require treatment. Evaluation of any need for lateral ankle ligament reconstruction should be done in the office as well as intraoperatively. Reconstructive options for chronic peroneal subluxation/dislocation are:
    - direct repair
    - reconstruction of superior peroneal retinaculum using tendon graft
    - bone block procedures to create a barrier to dislocation
    - groove-deepening procedures (Fig. 17–15)
    - rerouting of the tendons deep to the calcaneo-fibular ligament
    - simultaneous lateral ankle ligament and tendon subluxation reconstructions.
- Non-operative therapy of acute dislocations/subluxations may be attempted if they fall into types 1 or 3 of the Oden-Eckert-Davis classification. In type 1 injuries, the tendons remain within the peroneal sheath. After reduction of the tendons within the peroneal groove, the avulsed fibular periosteum should be able to heal back down to the posterolateral aspect of the fibula with immobilization only. Type 3 injuries have a bony avulsion fragment off the posterolateral lip of the fibula, which may heal down into place with casting. Types 2 and 4 are less likely to do well with conservative treatment, because it is unlikely that the tendons will relocate into their sheath without operative reduction. Studies have shown a 30-40% rate of later redislocation of the tendons when types 2 and 4 are treated conservatively. Surgical treatment involves reducing the tendons and then repairing the retinaculum with sutures placed through drill holes in the posterolateral corner of the fibula.

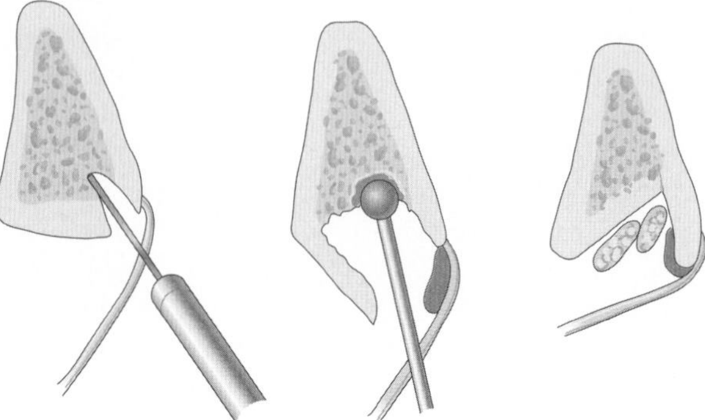

Figure 17–15: Groove-deepening procedures.

Tibialis Anterior

Function

- The tibialis anterior is the main dorsiflexor of the foot, and secondarily aids in inversion of the subtalar joint. It has minor functions in forefoot supination and adduction.
- It provides 80% of the dorsiflexion strength to the ankle, while extensor digitorum longus (EDL) and extensor hallucis longus (EHL) provide the rest.
- Eccentric firing of the tibialis anterior at heel strike modulates the approach to foot flat.
- Concentric firing during the swing phase of gait assists in clearance of the toes and foot.
- The tibialis anterior acts opposite the peroneus longus by providing dorsiflexion moment to first metatarsal-cuneiform joint.
- Earliest and most severely affected motor unit in Charcot-Marie-Tooth disease. This weakening leads to "peroneal overdrive," with resultant plantar flexion of the first metatarsal and cavus foot deformity with time.

Anatomy

- The tibialis anterior is the most medial of the muscles located in the anterior compartment of the leg (Fig. 17–16).
- Tendon makes up almost 50% of the length of the musculotendinous unit.
- Maximum excursion of the tendon is 2.9 cm.
- The tendon is easily palpated in most individuals just lateral to the anterior tibial crest.
- Originates from broad-based area stretching from Gerdy's tubercle to a point approximately halfway down the length of the lateral tibial surface. Additional fibers originate from the interosseous membrane, the overlying crural fascial, and the intermuscular septum.
- Inserts in a broad-based, fan-shaped fashion over the medial and inferior surfaces of the medial cuneiform and inferomedial base of the first metatarsal.
- Along its course, the tendon undergoes a 90° internal rotation. This is a result of the internal limb rotation that occurs during embryologic development.
- Innervated from branches off the superficial peroneal nerve.
- Microvascular studies demonstrate no hypovascular area along the length of the tendon. The tendon sheath contains a complete mesotenon and vinculae, which provide a good blood supply to the tendon in the area of the extensor retinacula.

Extensor Retinacula

- Superior and inferior extensor retinacula prevent bowstringing of tendons (Fig. 17–17).
- The retinacula contribute to the mechanical advantage of the musculotendinous unit.

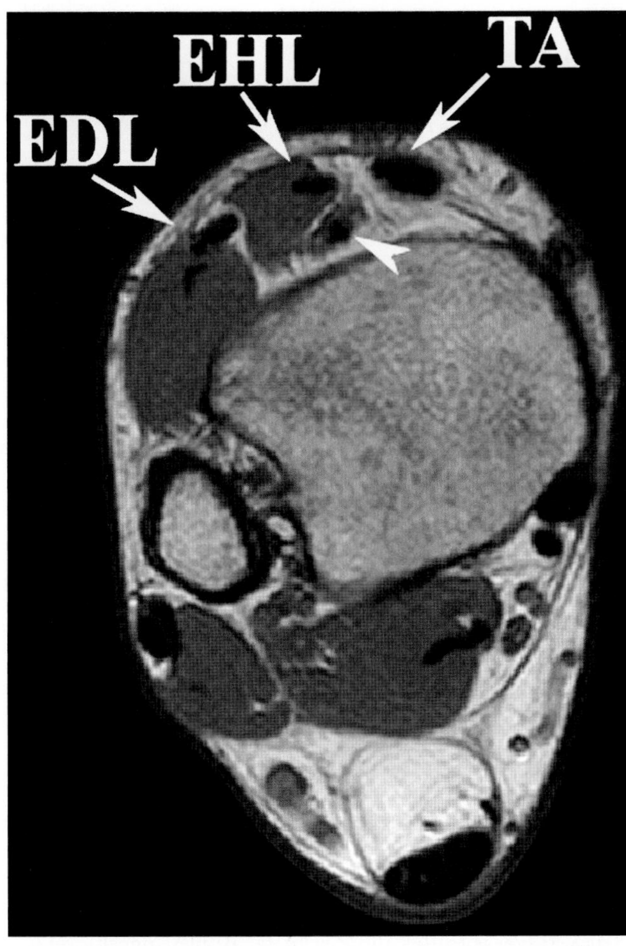

Figure 17–16: Axial magnetic resonance imaging scan of leg, showing tibialis anterior (TA), extensor hallucis longus (EHL), and extensor digitorum longus (EDL). Arrowhead points to anterior neurovascular bundle.

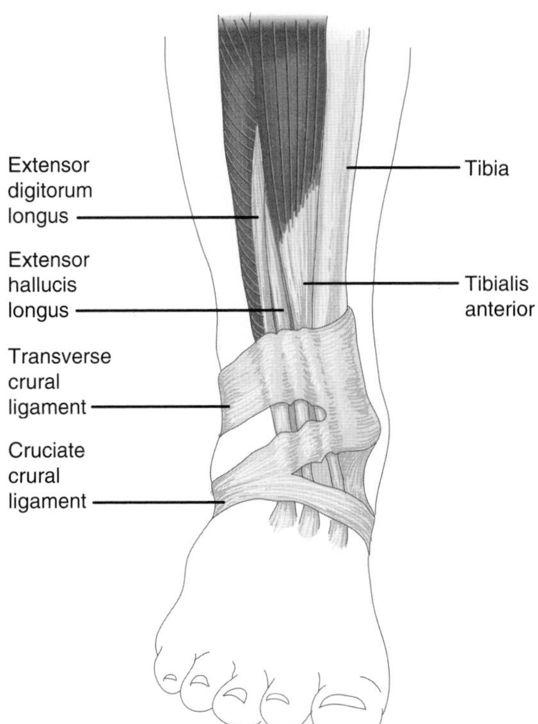

Figure 17–17: Line drawing of retinacula.

- Superior extensor retinaculum has attachments on anterolateral fibula just above distal metaphysis as well as medial distal tibial metaphysis.
- Inferior extensor retinaculum is a forked structure.
  - Lateral portion has a single limb that is contiguous with the inferior peroneal retinaculum and attaches to the lateral calcaneal wall.
  - Medial portion splits into two limbs, one that attaches just below the medial attachment of the superior extensor retinaculum, and one that spans the medial navicular cuneiform joint.

Scope of Injury and Diagnosis

- Paratenonitis is not common but may be seen in hikers and runners. May be caused or exacerbated by pressure from the tongue of boots over anterior ankle.
- Patients with tibialis anterior paratenonitis may have weakness or pain with resisted ankle dorsiflexion. Heel walking will be difficult.

Rupture

- Complete rupture can occur, typically in older patients, but may be shrugged off as a sprain.
- Elderly patients may not remember any acute injury.
- Sometimes, patients report pain over anterior ankle.
- Most common complaints relate to clumsiness when walking and a foot drop.
- In cases of chronic rupture, a bulbous nodule may be found in the area of the proximal tendon (Fig. 17–18).
- Complete rupture may be misdiagnosed as a peroneal nerve injury. With tibialis anterior rupture, the sensory distributions of the superficial and deep peroneal nerves remain intact. EHL, EDL, and peroneal motor function are also unaffected.
- Patients with complete rupture of the tibialis anterior may demonstrate eversion when asked to dorsiflex at the ankle. This occurs because the EHL and EDL functional substitution that occurs tends to pull the foot into eversion. These patients will not be able to effectively heel walk.
- With complete rupture, ankle dorsiflexion is difficult when the toes are plantar flexed. This occurs because of the loss of mechanical advantage of the EHL and EDL in this position.
- Most reliable sign of rupture is a lack of tibialis anterior bowstringing with resisted dorsiflexion of the foot. This is normally seen between the superior and inferior extensor retinacula over the anteromedial ankle.

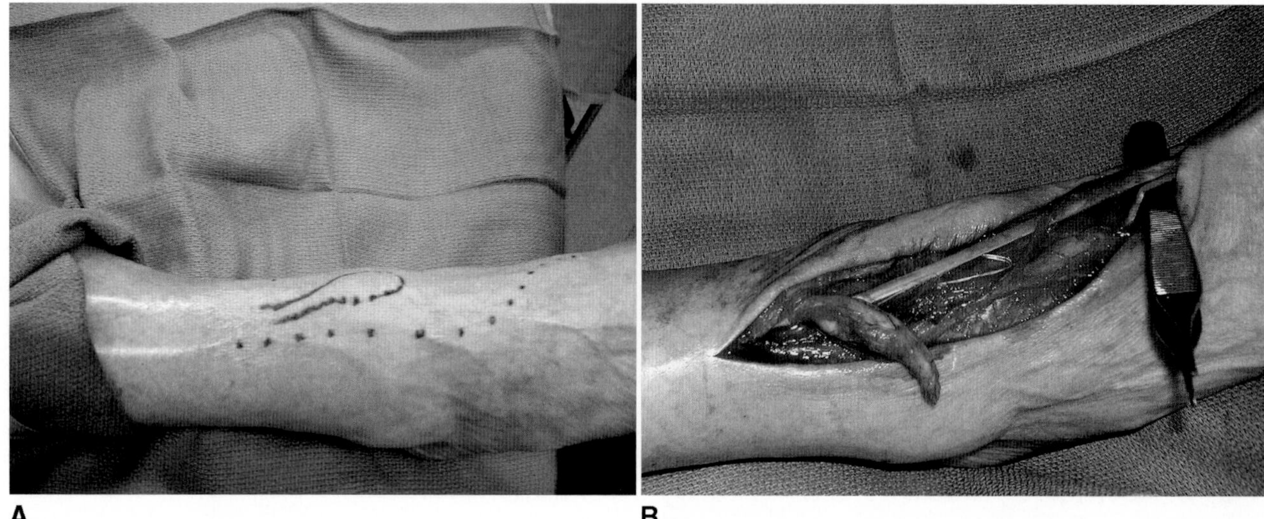

Figure 17–18: **A, Chronic ruptured tibialis anterior shows nodule of proximal stump in the lower calf. B, The proximal stump is exposed to the left. The intact extensor hallucis longus (EHL) and extensor hallucis brevis (EHB) are to the right. The EHL was used to bridge the gap in the tibialis anterior, and the distal EHL tendon was tenodesed to the EHB to prevent a flexion deformity at the first interphalangeal joint.**

- Most common site of rupture is 0.5-3.0 cm proximal to its insertion. Coincides with the location where the tendon passes under the distal band of the inferior extensor retinaculum.
- MRI is not usually required for diagnosis or treatment, because diagnosis is made on clinical grounds, and the location of the proximal tendon stump is frequently palpable over the anterior leg. Late presentations with extensive retractions of the proximal stump may need MRI to confirm the diagnosis.

Treatment Options

- Non-operative treatment of an anterior tibial tendon rupture will result in foot drop and difficulty clearing the toes on the swing-through phase of gait. For many less active patients, this is an acceptable option. If non-operative therapy is to be used, an ankle-foot orthosis may assist in ambulation.
- Generally, surgical repair is indicated in younger and more active individuals.
- Early diagnosis of an acute rupture can be treated with primary repair.
- When diagnosed late, delayed primary repair is difficult because of retraction of proximal tendon stump. For late cases, reconstruction with a tendon transfer is required. Tenodesis to the neighboring EHL is a useful strategy.
- Allograft tendon can be used to make up tendon length if the muscle belly is healthy.
- A non-anatomical reconstruction can be performed, with insertion of the tendon into the navicular or cuneiform.

Flexor Hallucis Longus

Function

- The FHL flexes the interphalangeal joint of the great toe.
- It also works to flex the first metatarsophalangeal joint, and is a secondary plantar flexor of the ankle.
- Electromyography studies have demonstrated that the FHL has its greatest activity during midstance, when it aids in stabilizing the midfoot. There is only minimal activity in heel-off with normal ambulation.

Anatomy

- The FHL is referred to as the "lighthouse of the posterior ankle," because it warns of proximity to the neurovascular bundle, which lies medial to the tendon (Fig. 17–19).
- The FHL originates from the distal posterior surface of the fibula, with a portion coming off the covering fascia and adjacent fascial septum.
- The tendon lies in the most posterolateral portion of the flexor retinaculum.
- Cradled between the medial and lateral talar tuberosities on the posterior aspect of the talus.
- The tendon runs through a fibroosseous tunnel as it passes inferior to the ankle. Its boundaries are: medially, medial tubercle of the talus; anteriorly, talar body; posteriorly, flexor retinaculum; and laterally, lateral tubercle of the talus.
- There is an interconnecting tendon slip between the FHL and FDL. This tether runs from the FHL to the more plantar FDL at the level of the master knot of Henry. The

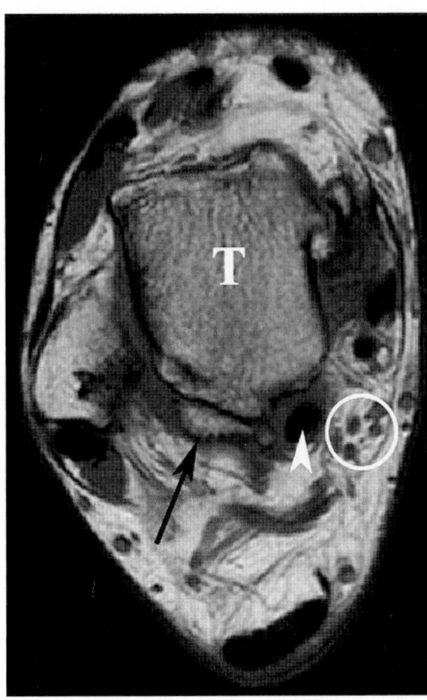

Figure 17–19: **A cross-section at the level of the talus (T) shows the neurovascular bundle (circled) just medial to the flexor hallucis longus (arrowhead). The arrow marks a normal os trigonum.**

interconnecting tendon couples flexion of the terminal interphalangeal joints of the hallux and lesser toes when either tendon fires. This coupling preserves flexion strength when a transfer of the FDL is performed, so long as the interconnection is not damaged in harvesting the tendon.
- Inserts in the proximal plantar aspect of the distal phalanx.
- The maximal excursion of the FHL is 1.7 cm.
- The FHL has two distinct synovial sheaths. The proximal sheath starts 2 cm proximal to the ankle joint, continues through the fibroosseous tunnel past the master knot of Henry, and terminates at the naviculocuneiform joint. This proximal sheath lacks a mesotenon but may have communications with the ankle joint, the FDL sheath, or the posterior tibial tendon. The distal sheath starts at the base of the first metatarsal, continues with the tendon as it passes through the intersesamoidal space, and terminates with the insertion of the tendon on the distal phalanx.

Epidemiology

- The FHL is uncommonly injured in the general population.
- Injury of the FHL is most frequently encountered in athletes and others involved in frequent, repetitive push-off movements. Ballet dancers and other jumping athletes are more prone to injury. Because of the high incidence of paratenonitis in the former population, it has been termed the "dancer's Achilles heel."

Clinical Findings

- Patients may complain of snapping or triggering exacerbated by toe flexion or pushing-off activities.
- Pain will be located posteromedially, and is frequently described as being within or just behind the ankle.
- Paratenonitis or partial ruptures need to be differentiated from os trigonum pathology, posteromedial talar osteochondritis dissecans lesions, FHL tendinosis, and posterior tibial tendon pathology (Table 17–2).
- FHL may be damaged by errant saw blade cuts during total ankle arthroplasty.
- Fibrosis of the tendon may limit excursion after low tibial fractures, ankle fractures with a posterior malleolar fragment, posterior talar fractures, or calcaneal fractures.

Treatment Options

- Conservative options include rest, ice, antiinflammatory medications, strapping or taping of the foot, and stiff-soled shoes or rigid inserts. A Morton extension added to an orthosis will limit the amount of dorsiflexion of the hallux at toe-off. If paratenontitis alone is present, the decreased excursion and pressure will diminish the pain experienced. In the case of paratenonitis with tendinosis, the limited excursion will prevent the thickened proximal portion of the tendon from being drawn into or against the fibroosseous tunnel.
- Conservative methods often fail if there is a critical stenosis of the fibroosseous tunnel conducting the tendon behind the talus.
- Operative treatment consists of release of the flexor retinaculum with resultant decompression of the tendon (Fig. 17–20).
- There is a risk of rupture of the central fibers of the tendon after fibroosseous tunnel release.
- The FHL is often "borrowed" as a tendon transfer for other pathologies. There is controversy as to whether this tendon should be sacrificed in high-level athletes needing Achilles tendon repairs or tendon transfers.

Table 17–2: Syndromes of Posterior Ankle Pain in Dancers

POSTEROMEDIAL CONDITIONS	POSTEROLATERAL CONDITIONS
Flexor hallucis longus tenosynovitis	Posterior bony impingement (os trigonum or Stieda's process)
Soleus syndrome	Fractured Stieda's process (Shepard fracture)
Posterior tibial tenosynovitis	Peroneal tenosynovitis
Posteromedial fibrous tarsal coalition	Soft tissue impingement (pseudomeniscus syndrome)

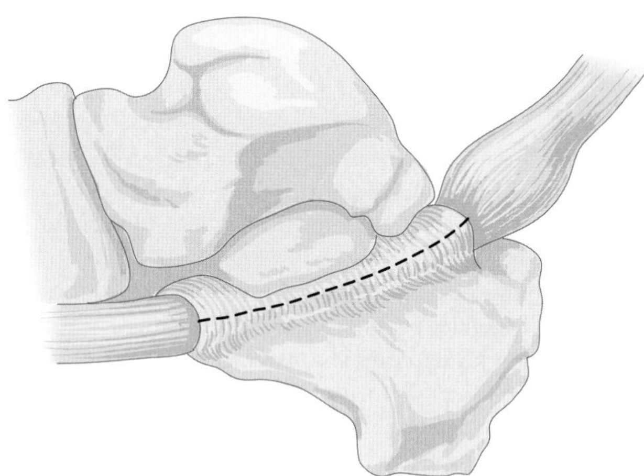

Figure 17–20: Posteromedial view of FHL tendon within fibroosseous sheath.

Os Trigonum and Stieda's Process

General

- Because of their intimate relationship with the FHL, the os trigonum and Steida's process present challenges in discerning between their pathologies and that of the FHL proper.
- The os trigonum, when present, is the ununited posterior portion of the lateral talar tubercle. It normally unites with the rest of the talus between 8 and 11 years of age.
- The Stieda's or trigonal process is an abnormally large lateral tubercle of the talus.
- Neither is a sesamoid bone, as they do not lie within the tendon but rather just lateral to it.

Anatomy

- The os trigonum may or may not have an articular process with the posterior talus. It is attached to the posterior process of the talus with a fibrous, fibrocartilaginous, or cartilaginous bridge. Inferiorly, it articulates with the calcaneus. The posterior talofibular and the talar component of the fibulotalocalcaneal ligament are attached to the posterior surface of the os trigonum.

Epidemiology

- The incidence of os trigonum had been reported to be between 2.7% and 7.7%.
- A symptomatic os trigonum or Stieda's process is most often seen in dancers and athletes, because of the frequency with which they are in extreme plantar flexion. Soccer players may also develop problems here.
- Symptoms with both of these conditions are unrelated to size of the bony prominence. Many dancers and athletes have either an os trigonum or a Stieda's process, but most are asymptomatic.

Conditions

- Both the os trigonum and Stieda's process may produce pathology by creating impingement on extreme plantar flexion of the ankle. The os or Stieda's process impinges against the posterior surface of the tibial plafond. This has been termed the *os trigonum syndrome*.
- Stieda's process may fracture and produce pain. This has been termed a *Shepard's fracture* from the author who first described it (Fig. 17–21).

Diagnosis

- Os trigonum and Steida's process pathology must be differentiated from FHL pathology, posterior soft tissue impingement, and posterior talar body fractures.
- Patients will usually present with complaints of pain in the posterior ankle.
- Pain may be of a sudden onset, as is seen with a fracture of Stieda's process, or develop gradually when chronic, repetitive impingement is the cause.
- Examination will reveal pain to palpation if it is a new fracture. Chronic conditions will have more vague findings.
- Forced ankle plantar flexion will reproduce the pain. This has been termed the *plantar flexion test*.

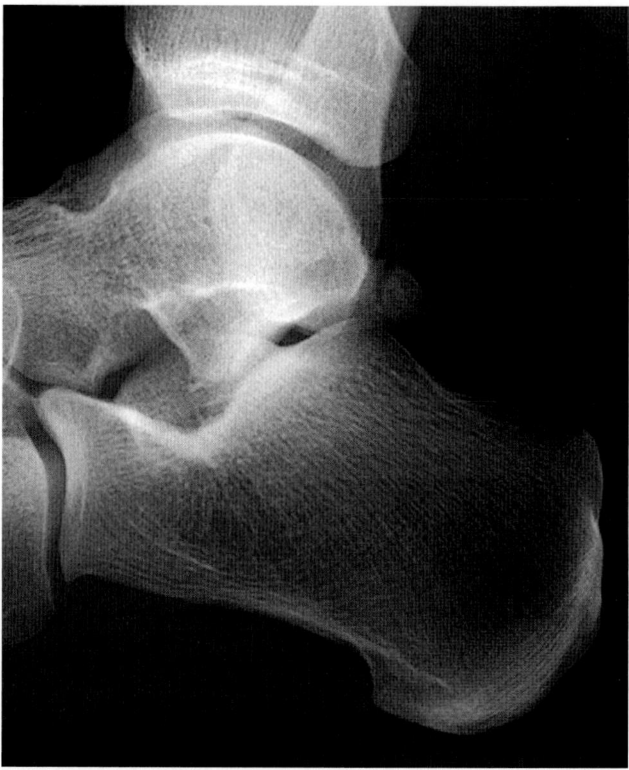

Figure 17–21: Radiograph of fractured Stieda's process.

- Some patients may experience pain with dorsiflexion and plantar flexion of the hallux, because the FHL movement at the area of the bony fragment irritates the inflamed tissues. This can complicate elimination of FHL pathology from the differential diagnosis.
- Radiographically, an os trigonum will show a smooth radiolucent line between the ossicle and the lateral tubercle of the posterior process of the talus. An acute fracture of Stieda's process will appear as an irregular rough line on plain radiographs (see Fig. 17–21).
- If there is inadequate resolution on the straight lateral view, a 30° subtalar oblique view may help differentiate between an os trigonum and a fractured posterior process.
- A lateral view of the ankle with the dancer en pointe, or with the athlete in full plantar flexion, may demonstrate impingement of the os on the posterior tibia.
- MRI is the study of choice in evaluation of os trigonum syndrome. T_2-weighted images will demonstrate high signal intensity at the posterior ankle, indicating inflammation in the area. Bone scans are generally not helpful in differentiating between pathologic entities of the posterior talus.

Treatment

- Initial treatment for each of these pathologic entities should be non-surgical. Immobilization in a short leg cast or boot, with or without weight bearing, has been reported in the literature.
- For a fracture of Stieda's process, repeat radiographs are utilized after 4-6 weeks of immobilization to evaluate bony union. Continued immobilization is warranted if bony union is not obtained.
- In addition to immobilization, NSAIDs can be helpful in the treatment of os trigonum syndrome. Local injection of corticosteroids has been suggested but puts the FHL at risk because of its proximity to the os trigonum. If utilized, it should be placed from the lateral side to avoid weakening of the FHL.
- Limited studies have shown that approximately 50% of patients will get better with conservative treatment of either fracture of Stieda's process or posterior bony impingement.
- Surgical excision of the ossicle or the fracture fragment is warranted if bony union or resolution of symptoms is not obtained within 3-6 months.
- Either a medial or a lateral approach may be used. A lateral approach endangers the sural nerve. A medial approach provides good visualization of the FHL and is generally safer. In the posteromedial approach, the FHL is swept medially to protect the tibial nerve and vessels.
- A recent study by Abramowitz et al. (2003) demonstrated that patients with symptomatic os trigonum for at least 3 months had substantial relief of their symptoms after excision through a lateral approach. Their findings also suggested that those who had surgery after reporting symptoms for 2 years or less had a better outcome than those with reported symptoms of greater duration. Their main complication was sural nerve sensory loss, which resolved spontaneously in only 50% of those affected.
- Arthroscopic excision of the os trigonum has been shown to be effective. Marumoto and Ferkel (1997) demonstrated substantially improved American Orthopaedic Foot and Ankle Society hindfoot and ankle scores, with attainment of maximal recovery within 3 months postoperatively. No complications were observed.

Tendon Lacerations

General

- Tendon lacerations of the foot and ankle are uncommon but potentially very debilitating injuries. Simple lacerations are not difficult to repair. The difficulty lies in diagnosis, which may be complicated by relatively small skin lacerations, partial lacerations that maintain some function, and substitution of function by other unaffected musculotendinous units.
- Careful neurovascular examination should be conducted with all cases of tendon laceration no matter how distal the level. Neurovascular damage can result in delayed tissue ulceration or ischemia if not recognized early.
- Lacerations without concomitant soft tissue defects can be repaired directly with any number of tendon-suturing techniques. Those associated with significant coverage defects may need to be tagged and buried under viable tissue until adequate coverage can be attained. This prevents tendon desiccation.
- Tendon lacerations associated with contaminated wounds present treatment dilemmas. It may be advantageous to perform an early repair to prevent tendon retraction. The surgeon may want to perform the repair with monofilament rather than braided sutures in these cases. The contaminated wound should be left open, and consideration should be given to placing a temporary non-absorbable drug delivery device (e.g. tobramycin-laden polymethyl methacrylate beads).
- Tendon salvage may have to be weighed against attaining prompt soft tissue coverage. Severe lacerating or mangling injuries may be better treated with early coverage, even if it means sacrificing a few non-essential tendons.
- Although negative pressure-assisted wound closure has become popular in wound management, the technique probably should not be applied directly over uncovered tendon.

Flexors

- Lacerations of the flexor tendons of the foot usually occur from an individual stepping on a sharp object.

- Children are more prone to this injury because of their propensity to run barefoot. Unfortunately, they are also those at risk for developing deformity from the resultant muscular imbalance if left untreated.
- The interconnecting ligaments between the FHL and FDL may prevent recognition, but also may obviate the need for flexor repair if the laceration is proximal to the master knot of Henry.
- Complete lacerations of the FHL distal to the master knot of Henry need to be repaired to prevent hallux cock-up deformity or painful interphalangeal hyperextension.
- For FHL lacerations in the area of the interphalangeal joint, a plantar approach provides the best access for repair. Lacerations proximal to the metatarsophalangeal joint should be approached medially.
- Functional rehabilitation permits plantar flexion but not dorsiflexion of the hallux.
- If a delayed diagnosis prevents a direct repair of the FHL, arthrodesis of the interphalangeal joint can be performed, depending on symptoms.
- FDL lacerations cause minimal functional deficit or cosmetic deformity, and therefore rarely warrant repair.

Tibialis Anterior and Toe Extensors

- Laceration of the tibialis anterior and toe extensors may occur from hockey skate injuries or from dropping sharp objects on the anterior ankle or dorsal foot (Fig. 17–22).
- Especially careful neurovascular examination should be conducted in these injuries, because of the relatively common concomitant laceration of the anterior neurovascular bundle.
- In the case of EHL laceration, toe extension may be absent or weak. Metatarsophalangeal extension may be present through substitution of extensor hallucis brevis action.
- Although there are many reports to the contrary, lacerations to the EHL should be repaired to avoid clawing of the hallux from imbalance between the FHL and the intrinsics. If the laceration is neglected and the patient presents with deformity, it is usually not possible to effectively repair the tendon. In this case, arthrodesis of the interphalangeal joint is necessary.
- Repair of distal lacerations of the EDL slips is not necessary, and spontaneous healing may occur in many cases. Lacerations within the common tendon should be repaired.
- Lacerations of the tibialis anterior tendon should be treated with direct repair. Late-presenting lacerations should be treated in the same manner as neglected ruptures, i.e. they should be repaired unless the surgical risks outweigh the gain in function that the patient will obtain.
- The skin incision should be slightly offset from the subcutaneous location of the tendon to avoid development of adhesions. Repair of the retinaculum helps prevent bowstringing of the tendon.

Peroneal Tendons

- Peroneus longus lacerations may occur behind the fibula, along the posterolateral aspect of the foot, or on the plantar aspect of the foot.
- Peroneus longus lacerations may be diagnosed by lack of plantar flexion strength of the first ray.
- Loss of function will result in metatarsus primus elevatus and possibly cavovarus of the foot. Peroneus longus lacerations should probably be repaired whenever possible.
- Peroneus brevis lacerations may occur along the lateral border of the calcaneus. Identification of isolated brevis

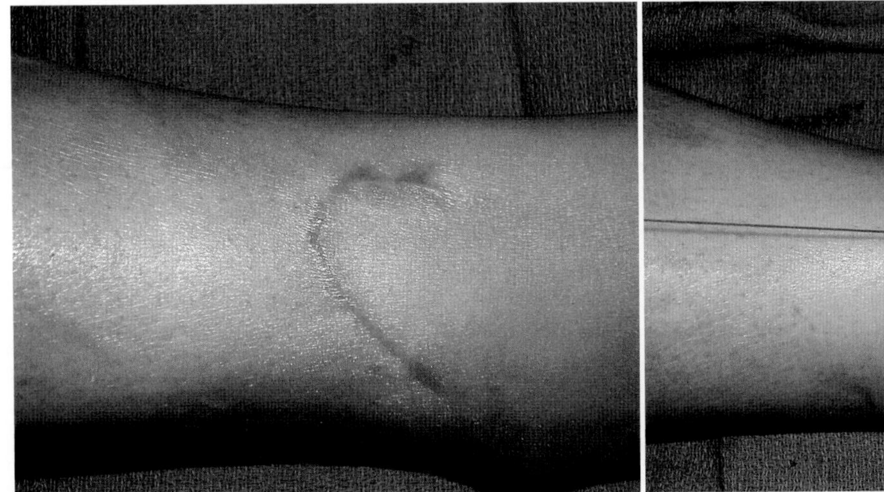

A

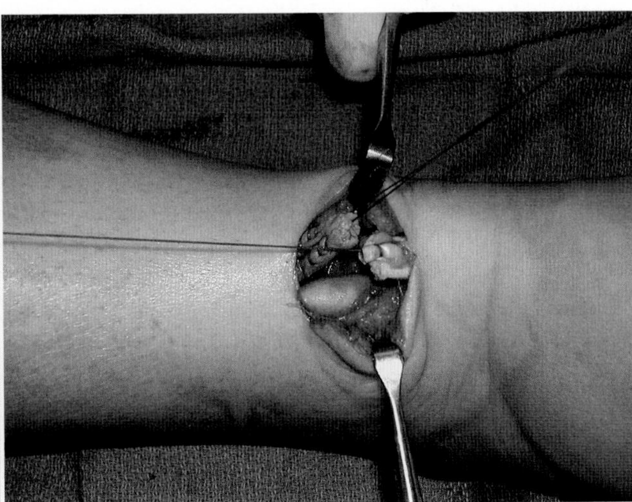

B

Figure 17–22: **Laceration of the tibialis anterior tendon. A, Healed laceration over distal leg at presentation. B, Direct repair of lacerated tibialis anterior.**

laceration may be difficult, because the longus tendon has substantial evertor function. Chronic varus deformity of the foot with or without ankle instability may occur if this injury is left untreated.

- If primary repair is not possible, a tenodesis with the peroneus longus may recreate brevis activity. If tenodesis is not possible, transfer of the FHL or FDL to restore eversion strength is recommended.

References

Abramowitz Y, Wollstein R et al. (2003) Outcome of resection of a symptomatic os trigonum. J Bone Joint Surg Am 85-A(6): 1051-1057.
Study showing good results in open treatment of symptomatic os trigonum. When the sural nerve was damaged in this study, only 50% of those recovered normal sensory function.

Armagan O, Shereff M. (2000) Tendon injury and repair. In: Disorders of the Foot and Ankle. Philadelphia: Saunders. pp. 942-971.
Another excellent chapter on the tendonopathies.

Chao W. (2004) Os trigonum. Foot Ankle Clin 9(4): vii, 787-796.
A good review on the pathologies of the posterior process of the talus and their treatment.

Clarke HD, Kitaoka HB et al. (1998) Peroneal tendon injuries. Foot Ankle Int 19(5): 280-288.
Good overall review of peroneal tendon pathology and treatment.

Eckert WR, Davis EA Jr. (1976) Acute rupture of the peroneal retinaculum. J Bone Joint Surg Am 58(5): 670-672.
Original description of grading system for acute dislocation of peroneal tendons.

Geppert MJ, Sobel M et al. (1993) Microvasculature of the tibialis anterior tendon. Foot Ankle 14(5): 261-264.
Microvascular study which demonstrates that there is no hypovascular area in the tibialis anterior tendon.

Kolettis GJ, Micheli LJ et al. (1996) Release of the flexor hallucis longus tendon in ballet dancers. J Bone Joint Surg Am 78(9): 1386-1390.
Retrospective study of 13 high-level ballet dancers who failed conservative therapy and required release of the FHL for relief. Releases were done through a posteromedial approach. Mean follow up was 6.5 months. All patients returned to dancing at a mean of 5 months postoperatively.

Krause JO, Brodsky JW. (1998) Peroneus brevis tendon tears: Pathophysiology, surgical reconstruction, and clinical results. Foot Ankle Int 19(5): 271-279.
Study demonstrating that non-operative treatment of longitudinal peroneal tendon tears is usually not effective, even when used for an extended period of time.

Major NM, Helms CA et al. (2000) The MR imaging appearance of longitudinal split tears of the peroneus brevis tendon. Foot Ankle Int 21(6): 514-519.
Study demonstrating that MRI was able to identify longitudinal tears of the peroneus brevis. Radiographically discernable statistically significant associated findings with the tears were increased signal within the tendon, bony changes, a flat peroneal groove, abnormal lateral ligaments, a lateral fibular spur, and a chevron-shaped tendon.

Markarian GG, Kelikian AS et al. (1998) Anterior tibialis tendon ruptures: An outcome analysis of operative versus nonoperative treatment. Foot Ankle Int 19(12): 792-802.
One of the largest studies done on tibialis anterior tendon ruptures. These investigators found no difference between operative and non-operative therapy of this problem. Despite this, they recommend that non-operative therapy be reserved for the low-demand elderly population.

Marumoto JM, Ferkel RD. (1997) Arthroscopic excision of the os trigonum: A new technique with preliminary clinical results. Foot Ankle Int 18(12): 777-784.
Report on the arthroscopic treatment of os trigonum pathology.

Myerson MS, Sammarco VJ. (1999) Penetrating and lacerating injuries of the foot. Foot Ankle Int 4(3): 647-674.
Review of penetrating trauma to the foot that has a particularly good section on tendon laceration.

Oden RR. (1987) Tendon injuries about the ankle resulting from skiing. Clin Orthop Relat Res 216: 63-69.
Modification of the Eckert and Davis classification of acute peroneal dislocations.

Puddu G, Ippolito E et al. (1976) A classification of Achilles tendon disease. Am J Sports Med 4(4): 145-50.
Provides the best nomenclature of tendonopathy in terms of pathophysiology and histologic findings in each stage of progression.

Redfern D, Myerson M. (2004) The management of concomitant tears of the peroneus longus and brevis tendons. Foot Ankle Int 25(10): 695-707.
Largest study on treatment and outcome of concomitant peroneus longus and brevis ruptures. A useful algorithm is presented that sets the standard for treating these injuries.

Sammarco GJ, DiRaimondo CV. (1988) Surgical treatment of lateral ankle instability syndrome. Am J Sports Med 16(5): 501-511.
This study looked at the prevalence of peroneal tendon tears in patients undergoing lateral ankle reconstruction for instability. The authors found that about one-quarter of patients demonstrated longitudinal tearing of their peroneal tendons. Although important in that it was conducted in living patients, it is probably biased, in that the population being studied already had lateral ankle pathology that may have resulted in, or from, the peroneal pathology.

Shakibaei M, Pfister K et al. (2000) Ultrastructure of Achilles tendons of rats treated with ofloxacin and fed a normal or magnesium-deficient diet. Antimicrob Agents Chemother 44(2): 261-266.
Electron microscopic studies of rat tendon after treatment with fluoroquinolones. Ultrastructural and cell-matrix relationships are shown to be altered after treatment. Provides histologic and cellular explanations for the increased rate of spontaneous rupture seen in those on these antimicrobial agents.

Sobel M, Bohne WH et al. (1991) Cadaver correlation of peroneal tendon changes with magnetic resonance imaging. Foot Ankle 11(6): 384-388.

Sobel M, Geppert MJ et al. (1992) The dynamics of peroneus brevis tendon splits: A proposed mechanism, technique of diagnosis, and classification of injury. Foot Ankle 13(7): 413-422.

Although both of these studies are important for defining the prevalence of peroneal tendon pathology in a study cohort not specifically afflicted with disorders of the foot and ankle, they probably suffer from an age bias. It is entirely possible that the prevalence of asymptomatic longitudinal tears of the peroneal tendons increases with age. This would predispose most of the cadaveric material under study to an inflated prevalence.

Sobel M, Pavlov H et al. (1994) Painful os peroneum syndrome: A spectrum of conditions responsible for plantar lateral foot pain. Foot Ankle Int 15(3): 112-124.

The definitive paper on POPS.

Stover CN, Bryan DR. (1962) Traumatic dislocation of the peroneal tendons. Am J Surg 103: 180-186.

Describes the redislocation rate of peroneal tendons after conservative treatment.

van der Linden PD, Sturkenboom MC et al. (2002) Fluoroquinolones and risk of Achilles tendon disorders: Case-control study. BMJ 324(7349): 1306-1307.

Large numbers of patients on fluoroquinolones were compared with those not taking these antibiotics as to the incidence of spontaneous tendon rupture. The relative risk of spontaneous rupture becomes even greater if these drugs are taken concomitantly.

Williams RJ III, Attia E et al. (2000) The effect of ciprofloxacin on tendon, paratenon, and capsular fibroblast metabolism. Am J Sports Med 28(3): 364-369.

Study demonstrating that fluoroquinolone antibiotics affect the biochemical processes of tendon, paratenon, and other connective tissue fibroblasts.

CHAPTER 18

Ankle Sprains and Ligament Injuries

Michael S. Aronow* **and Raymond J. Sullivan[§]**

*M.D., Associate Professor of Orthopaedic Surgery, University of Connecticut School of Medicine, Farmington, CT
[§]M.D., Assistant Clinical Professor of Orthopaedic Surgery, University of Connecticut School of Medicine, Hartford, CT

Anatomy and Biomechanics

- The fibula articulates with the incisura fibularis of the tibia to form a mortise that is held together by syndesmotic ligaments. The syndesmotic ligaments are the anterior inferior tibiofibular ligament, the interosseous ligament, the posterior inferior tibiofibular ligament, the transverse ligament, and the interosseous membrane (Fig. 18–1). While these ligaments prevent diastasis, they do allow slight motion of the distal fibula relative to the distal tibia with weight bearing.
- The talus articulates within this mortise and allows sagittal plane motion of the foot relative to the leg. The ankle joint is more stable in dorsiflexion due to the talar dome being wider anteriorly than posteriorly. It is also more stable with full weight-bearing load across the joint surfaces.
- The lateral ankle ligaments prevent excessive inversion, anterior translation, and posterior translation of the talus relative to the mortise. The lateral ankle ligaments are the anterior talofibular ligament, the calcaneofibular ligament, and the posterior talofibular ligament. The anterior talofibular ligament is the primary lateral restraint to anterior translation of the talus and varus tilt of the plantar flexed talus. The calcaneofibular ligament resists varus tilt of the talus, particularly in dorsiflexion, and is also one of the primary lateral stabilizers of the subtalar joint.
- The deltoid ligament prevents excessive eversion, anterior translation, and posterior translation of the talus relative to the mortise. The deltoid has a deep and superficial component, the latter of which has four components: the tibionavicular ligament, the anterior tibiotalar ligament, the posterior tibiotalar ligament, and the tibiocalcaneal ligament.
- The subtalar joint allows inversion and eversion of the calcaneus and more distal foot relative to the talus and leg. The lateral subtalar ligaments prevent excessive anterior translation, medial translation, and lateral varus gapping of the posterior facet of the calcaneus relative to the posterior facet of the talus.
- The lateral subtalar ligaments can be divided into three layers.
  - The superficial layer contains the calcaneofibular ligament, the lateral talocalcaneal ligament, and the lateral root of the inferior extensor retinaculum.
  - The intermediate layer contains the cervical ligament and the intermediate root of the inferior extensor retinaculum.
  - The deep layer consists of the interosseous talocalcaneal ligament and the medial root of the inferior extensor retinaculum.

Acute Lateral Ankle Ligament Sprains

General

- The vast majority of ankle sprains are lateral inversion injuries in which there is a fall down the stairs, a misstep

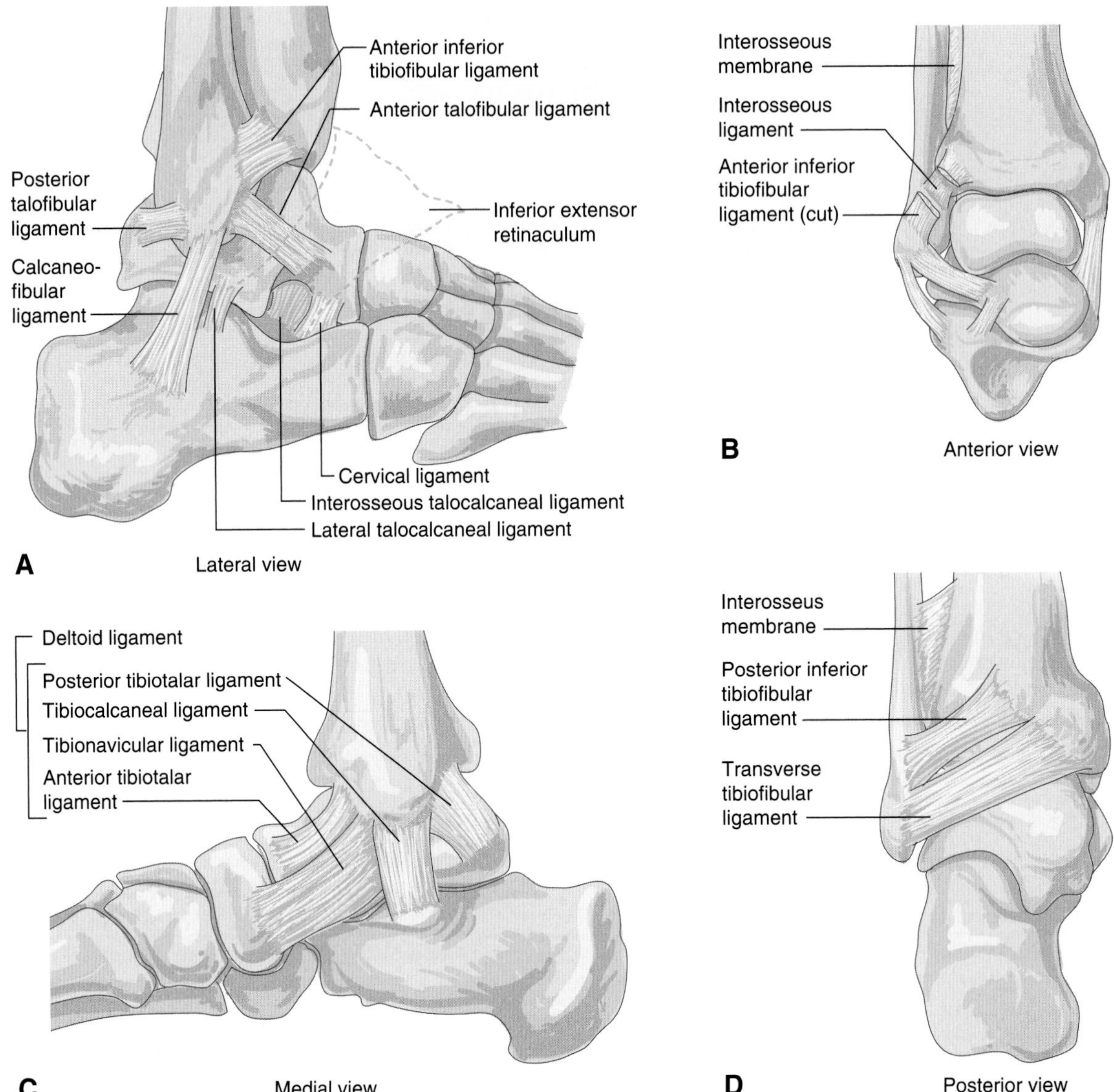

Figure 18–1: **Anatomy of the ligaments of the ankle and lateral subtalar joint. A, Lateral view. B, Posterior view. C, Medial view. D, Anterior view.**

off a curb, or landing on another person's foot, all situations in which the ankle is plantar flexed and not fully loaded.

- The anterior talofibular ligament is generally injured first.
- The calcaneofibular ligament may additionally be injured in more severe sprains. It may occasionally sustain an isolated injury with excessive inversion of the dorsiflexed ankle.
- The stronger posterior talofibular ligament is usually completely torn only in severe sprains and dislocations.
- There are multiple ankle sprain classification systems. The most commonly used is the American Medical Association classification system, in which grade 1 is a ligament stretch, grade 2 a partial ligament tear, and grade 3 a complete ligament rupture. Other classification systems take into account the number of ligaments torn and/or the clinical findings.

History and Physical Examination

- Clinical findings are proportional to the extent of ligament and surrounding soft tissue damage, and include ankle swelling and ecchymosis, tenderness over the affected ligaments, and difficulty weight bearing. With complete ligament tears, joint instability may be present.
- Associated pathology, as listed in Box 18–1, needs to be ruled out by physical examination and if necessary, radiographic studies.

Diagnostic Evaluation

- The modified Ottawa rules can be used as a guideline for whether or not to obtain plain x-rays after an ankle

Box 18–1 Differential Diagnosis of Acute Lateral Ankle Sprain

Tendon injuries

- Peroneal tendon tear or tenosynovitis
- Peroneal tendon subluxation
- Posterior tibial tendon tear or tenosynovitis
- Achilles tendon tear
- Anterior tibial tendon tear
- Flexor hallucis longus tear or tenosynovitis

Fractures and dislocations

- Proximal fibula (Maisonneuve fracture)
- Malleolar injuries
- Talar dome
- Posteromedial talar body fractures
- Os trigonum injuries
- Lateral process of talus (snowboarder's fracture)
- Anterior process of calcaneus
- Cuboid
- Navicular tuberosity
- Fifth metatarsal base
- Tarsometatarsal (Lisfranc) joints
- Medial subtalar dislocation

Neuropraxias

- Sural nerve
- Superficial peroneal nerve
- Deep peroneal nerve

Ligament instability

- Lateral ankle ligaments
- Syndesmotic ligaments
- Deltoid ligament
- Subtalar joint
- Lisfranc joints

sprain. Ankle x-rays should be obtained if there is pain in the malleolar region, and either bone tenderness at the tip or within the distal 6 cm of the posterior edge of either malleolus, or inability to bear weight both at the time of injury and for four steps in the emergency room. Foot x-rays should be obtained if there is pain in the midfoot, and either bone tenderness at the navicular or fifth metatarsal base, or inability to bear weight both at the time of injury and for four steps in the emergency room.

- X-rays should also be considered if there is clinical suspicion of other bone pathology, such as an anterior process of the calcaneus fracture, lateral process of the talus fracture, or Lisfranc injury, or if there is minimal clinical improvement after 4-6 weeks of appropriate treatment.
- Arthrography and stress x-ray may confirm complete ligament rupture. However, they are not commonly performed in the acute setting, as they are invasive and uncomfortable. Furthermore, whether or not there is a complete ligament rupture rarely affects clinical decision making for the initial treatment of an acute ankle sprain.
- Other studies, such as magnetic resonance imaging (MRI), computed tomography (CT), ultrasound, and bone scans, may be added if one clinically suspects other pathology, but physical examination and plain x-rays are not definitive.

Treatment

- Three types of treatment have been described for acute lateral ankle ligament injuries: cast immobilization, functional treatment, and acute operative repair.
- The literature is fairly clear that prolonged cast immobilization is inferior to functional treatment. However, in patients with significant discomfort after severe lateral ankle sprains, up to 2 weeks of immobilization with the ankle in dorsiflexion and the subtalar joint in slight eversion may be beneficial with respect to pain control.
- Functional treatment consists initially of rest, ice, compression, elevation, and if not contraindicated, anti-inflammatory and/or analgesic medication. Depending on the extent of injury, an elastic bandage, lace-up or stirrup brace, or controlled ankle motion walker can provide compression, limit hindfoot inversion, and allow protected ankle motion. Progressive weight bearing is allowed, using crutches if needed.
- Rehabilitation can be done as a home program or through formal physical therapy. Anti-inflammatory modalities are used to decrease swelling. Ankle range of motion exercises are performed, including in particular, gastrocnemius and soleus stretching to regain ankle dorsiflexion. Muscle strengthening is subsequently begun, particularly for the peroneus brevis and longus, the principal dynamic restraints to excessive hindfoot inversion. Finally, proprioception exercises are begun to retrain the injured proprioceptive nerve fibers in the ankle ligaments and decrease the peroneal reaction time to inversion stress.
- While one large randomized prospective study suggests that acute surgical repair leads to a lower incidence of residual pain, symptoms of giving way, and recurrent sprains than functional treatment (Pijnenburg et al. 2003), other studies suggest that there is no difference in clinical outcome between the two treatment methods (Kannus and Renstrom 1992). Furthermore, functional recovery has a faster recovery time, less morbidity, and is more cost-effective. Given these findings, the fact that the vast majority of ankle sprains do well with functional treatment, and that the results of delayed ligament repair for chronic instability are similar to those for acute repair (Cass et al. 1985), functional treatment is considered by most to be the treatment of choice for complete lateral ankle ligament ruptures.
- Accepted indications for acute surgical repair of lateral ankle ligament ruptures include recurrent sprains that

have previously failed appropriate conservative treatment and concurrent ankle pathology requiring surgical treatment, such as open ankle lacerations and displaced fractures. A more controversial possible indication would be injury in a high-performance athlete such as a professional ballet dancer.

Chronic Pain Status Post Ankle Sprain

General

- Approximately 10-30% of significant ankle sprains have chronic symptoms. These symptoms may be due to the torn ligament(s) not healing at the proper tension (chronic lateral ankle instability) and/or the disorders listed in Box 18–2.
- In patients with chronic lateral ankle instability, the previously torn lateral ankle ligament(s) have not healed, or more commonly have healed in a lax fashion.
- These patients have *mechanical instability*, which is defined as the presence of abnormal motion of the talus relative to the ankle mortise, usually anterior translation and/or varus tilt.
- There is also usually *functional instability*, which is defined as the symptomatic feeling of the ankle giving way, often associated with pain, recurrent ankle sprains, or difficulty with uneven terrain.
- Not all patients with mechanical instability have functional instability. In fact, the goal of non-operative treatment for chronic lateral ankle instability described below is not to restore the normal tension of the lateral ankle ligaments but to get rid of the symptomatic functional instability.
- Not all patients with functional instability have mechanical instability. Many of the disorders listed in Box 18–2 cause symptoms of pain, giving way, recurrent sprains, and difficulty with uneven terrain with intact lateral ankle ligaments and no talar subluxation or tilt. Impingement lesions, in which scar tissue, synovitis, chondral fragments, or ligament ends get intermittently pinched between the bones of the ankle or subtalar joint and cause symptoms similar to a torn knee meniscus are in particular very common.

Box 18–2 Chronic Ankle Pain Differential Diagnosis

- Lateral ankle ligament instability
- Deltoid ligament instability
- Syndesmotic instability
- Subtalar instability
- Ankle impingement lesion
- Osteochondral lesion of talus
- Occult fracture
- Peroneal tendon tear
- Peroneal tendon subluxation
- Posterior tibial tendon injury
- Flexor hallucis longus tenosynovitis
- Sinus tarsi syndrome (subtalar impingement lesion)
- Tarsal coalition
- Arthritis
- Neuritis
- Tumor

History and Physical Examination

- Patients with symptomatic chronic lateral ankle instability give a history of a previous sprain and complaints of functional instability.
- The physical findings usually include tenderness over the affected ligament(s) and instability and/or pain and guarding with stress testing. There may be associated peroneal weakness and a positive modified Rhomberg test, defined as the inability to balance solely on the affected extremity with eyes closed.
- Stress testing can be assessed on physical examination or radiographically. Guarding secondary to pain or apprehension can cause false negative results, as firing of the ankle musculature, particularly the peroneals, limits talar subluxation and tilt. For that reason, stress testing is more accurate if performed under anesthesia.
- The anterior drawer test measures anterior subluxation of the talus underneath the tibia, thereby assessing competency of the anterior talofibular ligament. The knee and ankle are flexed to relax the gastrocnemius-soleus complex. One hand stabilizes the anterior aspect of the distal tibia, while the other provides an anterior and internal rotation stress to the foot with the thumb palpating the anterolateral ankle. The test is positive if there is excessive anterior talar subluxation, lack of a firm end point, or dimpling of the skin over the anterolateral ankle.

Diagnostic Evaluation

- Weight-bearing ankle x-rays are obtained to rule out arthritis, occult fractures, displaced fibular ossicles, and other bone pathology.
- Ankle stress x-rays should be performed, either in the office or under anesthesia (Fig. 18–2). While performing an anterior drawer test, the distance between the posterior aspect of the tibial articular surface and the nearest point on the talar dome is measured on a lateral ankle. A jig such as a Telos device can be used to provide a predetermined anterior force but does not adequately provide the internal rotation component.
- The talar tilt test measures the angle between the articular surfaces of the distal tibia and talar dome on an ankle mortise x-ray. Either a Telos device is used or one hand stabilizes the distal tibia while the other cups the heel and provides a varus stress to the foot. While this test can also be done clinically, distinguishing abnormal varus talar tilt

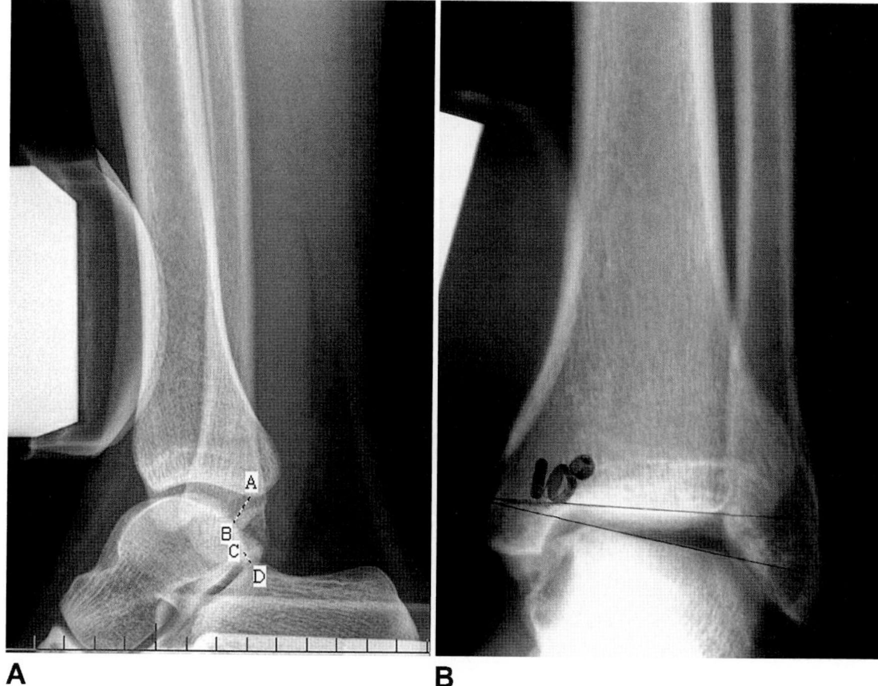

Figure 18–2: Ankle stress x-rays. **A,** Anterior drawer test performed on lateral ankle x-ray. The distance between markers A and B represents the tibiotalar distance. Significant anterior subluxation of marker D relative to C would be suggestive of lateral subtalar ligamentous instability. **B,** Talar tilt test performed on ankle mortise x-ray.

from normal subtalar inversion by palpating the superior anterolateral ankle is difficult.

- How much talar anterior subluxation or varus tilt is abnormal is controversial, with a wide range of values reported in the literature. Influencing variables include ankle size, film magnification, the amount of force applied, the amount of patient guarding, the value for the "normal" contralateral side, and whether the "normal" contralateral side is in fact normal or has been previously injured.
- A reasonable guideline for the anterior drawer test is to consider an absolute tibiotalar distance of ≥ 10 mm or 5 mm more than the contralateral side as positive, an absolute value of ≤ 5 mm as normal, and an absolute value between 5 and 10 mm as inconclusive.
- A reasonable guideline for the talar tilt test is to consider varus talar tilt of ≥ 10° or 5° more than the contralateral side as positive, an absolute value of ≤ 5° as normal, and an absolute value between 5 and 10° as inconclusive.
- MRI may show absence or evidence of previous injury to one or more of the lateral ankle ligaments. It may also show evidence of concurrent pathology to the other ligaments, tendons, bones, articular surfaces, and soft tissues of the foot and ankle.
- Ultrasound, CT, bone scans, laboratory blood work, and neurodiagnostic studies may be added as necessary.

Natural History

- The natural history of chronic ankle instability is unclear. There are studies describing patients with symptomatic ankle arthritis, often medial greater than lateral, and long standing ankle instability (Harrington 1979).
- Despite descriptions of these patients, other studies with appropriate control groups have not found an increased rate of arthritis in patients seen over 18 years previously for chronic ankle instability (Lofvenberg et al. 1994), or in patients treated 6-11 years previously, with functional treatment as compared with acute lateral ankle ligament repair (Pijnenburg et al. 2003).

Treatment

- Conservative treatment consists of ankle support to limit abnormal talar motion, increase proprioceptive nerve function, and prevent recurrent sprains. Options include lateral heel wedges, taping, ankle braces, high top shoes, or boots.
- Physical therapy involves ankle range of motion, strengthening, and proprioception exercises.
- Aggravating activities may be avoided and non-steroidal anti-inflammatory medication taken for associated pain and swelling.
- A local anesthetic and corticosteroid injection into the ankle or subtalar joint may address symptoms related to soft tissue impingement.
- Surgical repair or reconstruction of the ligaments is indicated if instability symptoms persist despite an adequate trial of conservative therapy and stress x-rays demonstrate mechanical instability.
- If adequate fluoroscopic stress x-rays of the ankle and, as described below, subtalar joint under anesthesia are normal, then lateral ankle instability is unlikely to be the cause of the patient's symptoms and a ligament reconstruction is not indicated. One possible exception is if ligament disruption is observed intra-operatively.

- If stress x-rays are inconclusive, then a lateral ankle ligament reconstruction should be considered if physical examination, diagnostic studies, and arthroscopy rule out other potential causes of the patient's symptoms.
- Another reasonable option is to defer preoperative stress x-rays on patients with recalcitrant functional instability, particularly those in whom an ankle anesthetic injection provides transient pain relief, and consent them for diagnostic ankle arthroscopy, more accurate fluoroscopic stress x-rays under anesthesia, and possible ankle ligament reconstruction.
- Concurrent pathology is common and should be addressed at the time of surgery. The anterolateral ankle joint should be assessed for intraarticular pathology. If there is tenderness overlying other parts of the ankle, particularly posteriorly or medially, or abnormal MRI findings, then strong consideration should be given toward also performing an ankle and, possibly subtalar joint, arthroscopy.
- The peroneal tendons must be visualized in order to access the calcaneofibular ligament, and any associated tendinopathy addressed. In cases where both the peroneus longus and brevis are non-functional, a flexor hallucis longus to peroneus brevis transfer may be considered to restore dynamic resistance to excessive inversion.
- Tarsal coalitions can be associated with recurrent ankle sprains and may need to be addressed by excision or fusion.
- In patients with varus hindfoot alignment, particularly those who have failed previous ankle ligament surgery, consideration could be made for a lateral displacement or Dwyer lateral closing wedge osteotomy to decrease the risk of recurrent ankle inversion injury.
- Stability may be restored by repairing or imbricating the previously torn ligaments and/or advancing local tissue, or by graft reconstruction of the ligament(s). While arthroscopic stapling and thermal capsular shrinkage of the anterior talofibular ligament has been described, the results have not been shown to be better than those with open procedures. Furthermore, the calcaneofibular ligament is an extracapsular structure deep to the peroneal tendons and is not readily amenable to these arthroscopic techniques.

Anatomical Repair

- The anterior talofibular and calcaneofibular ligaments are inspected and, if torn or avulsed from their insertions, repaired. The posterior talofibular ligament can also be inspected but is usually intact.
- More commonly, the ligaments are intact but lax. After confirming that the calcaneal and talar attachments are intact, the anterior talofibular ligament and, if lax or any question of subtalar instability is present, the calcaneofibular ligament are transected 1-5 mm from their fibular attachment along with the adjacent anterolateral ankle capsule (Fig. 18–3). The ligaments and capsule are then reefed at the proper tension into a bone trough at their normal fibular insertion sites using drill holes or suture anchors. The fibular cuff is then sewn over the repair in a "pants over vest" fashion. If avulsed distally, the ligaments can alternatively be advanced to their talar or calcaneal origins.
- The repair can be further augmented with a fibular periosteal flap or by advancing the inferior extensor retinaculum (Brostrom-Gould procedure) and/or lateral talocalcaneal ligament to the fibula.

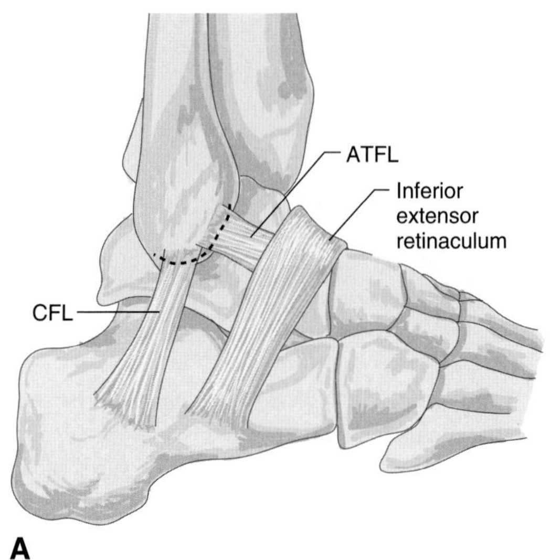

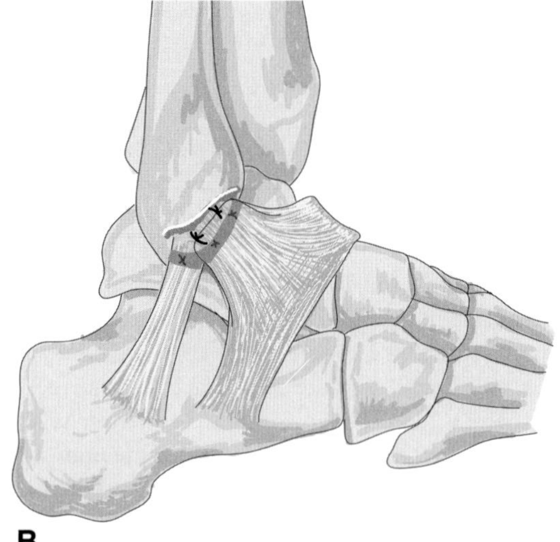

Figure 18–3: Brostrom-Gould lateral ankle ligament reconstruction. A, A continuous cut is made in the anterior talofibular ligament (ATFL), anterolateral ankle capsule, and calcaneofibular ligament (CFL) 1-5 mm from the fibular attachments (dashed line). B, The ligament/capsular flap is advanced at the proper tension into a trough made in the fibula, the other end that was left attached to the fibula is sewn over the ligament/capsular flap in a "pants over vest" fashion (shaded area), and the inferior extensor retinaculum is advanced to the fibula for additional reinforcement.

Ligament Reconstruction

- A graft is used to recreate or reinforce the lateral ankle ligaments. Among the tissues used are half of or the entire peroneus brevis or peroneus longus, the plantaris, slips of the extensor digitorum longus, hamstring tendons, fascia lata, allograft, and artificial ligaments. If present, the original ligaments should also be imbricated to add strength to the repair.
- Many of the historically popular reconstructions, such as the Evans, Watson-Jones, and original Chrisman-Snook procedures, did not place the grafts in the normal anatomical locations of the anterior talofibular ligament and calcaneofibular ligament (Fig. 18–4). While they

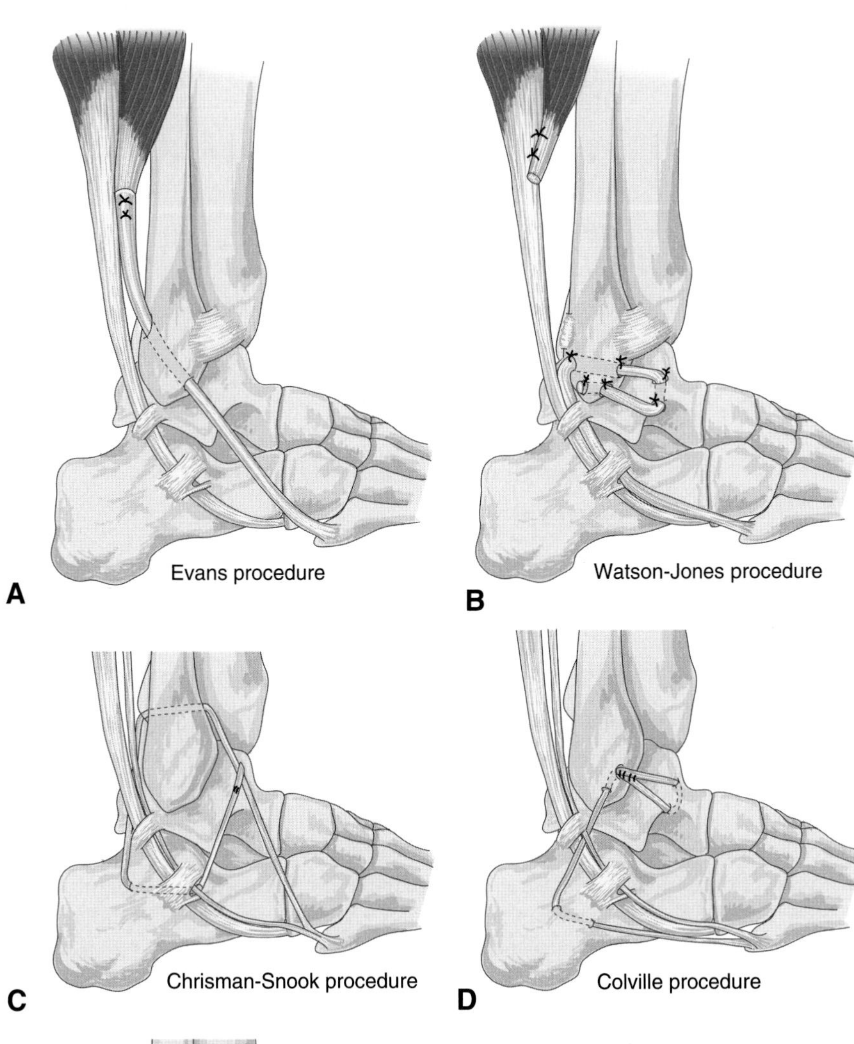

Figure 18–4: Lateral ankle ligament tenodeses. A, Evans procedure. B, Watson-Jones procedure. C, Chrisman-Snook procedure. D, Colville procedure. E, Burks and Morgan procedure.

provided initial ankle stability, these non-isometric repairs were often associated with subtalar stiffness and in long-term studies a high failure rate (Colville et al. 1992, Burks and Morgan 1994, Krips et al. 2002). They also often used the entire peroneus brevis, sacrificing the principal dynamic stabilizer of the lateral ankle.

- Alternative repairs, such as the original Elmslie procedure using fascia lata and more recent repairs described by Colville et al. (1992) and by Burks and Morgan (1994), attempt to recreate the original ligaments. Bone tunnels are made at the insertion sites of the anterior talofibular ligament and calcaneofibular ligament in the calcaneus, fibula, and talus, and fixation obtained with suture, suture anchors, or interference screws. Care is taken not to over-tension the graft, which may lead to excessive limitation of subtalar inversion. There is usually no significant loss of hindfoot eversion strength if only half of the peroneus brevis, distant autograft, or allograft is used.
- For most cases of recalcitrant ankle instability, an anatomical repair is sufficient and is preferable to a graft reconstruction (Hennrikus et al. 1996, Krips et al. 2002). The success rate is > 85%, there is no donor site morbidity or risk of allograft disease transmission, there is a lower risk of wound problems and nerve injuries, and there is decreased operative time.
- An isometric anatomical reconstruction with graft is indicated if there is insufficient ligamentous tissue to perform an adequate repair. Other relative indications include failure of a previous anatomical repair or reconstruction, generalized ligamentous laxity, large body mass, neuromuscular weakness, and possibly a greater than 10-year history of lateral ankle instability.

Postoperative Care

- Traditionally, patients were immobilized after ankle ligament repair or reconstruction for 6 weeks in a weight-bearing cast, followed by 7 weeks of functional bracing, and then 3-9 months of functional bracing or taping with athletic activity. With a good repair and a reliable patient, there has been a trend for early protected motion, limiting inversion and extreme plantar flexion in a functional brace instead of a cast. The potential benefits are decreased ankle and subtalar stiffness, decreased leg muscle atrophy, improved collagen organization and strength of the repaired tissue, and faster return to activity.

Acute Subtalar Sprain

General

- The mechanism of injury, clinical findings, differential diagnosis, and initial treatment of an acute lateral subtalar ligament sprain are similar to those of an acute lateral ankle sprain, and the two often occur together.
- The calcaneofibular and talocalcaneal ligaments are usually the first to tear with inversion stress, and sectioning them causes subtalar displacement. The cervical and interosseous talocalcaneal ligaments are also important stabilizers of the lateral subtalar joint and can be injured with further inversion stress.

History and Physical Examination

- There is a history of pain after a recent "ankle" sprain.
- On physical examination, there is usually lateral hindfoot swelling and ecchymosis, tenderness over the affected ligaments and sinus tarsi, and difficulty weight bearing.

Diagnostic Evaluation

- Radiographic studies are performed as needed to rule out fractures and other pathology.

Treatment

- Functional treatment is initiated, including rest, ice, compression, elevation, antiinflammatory and/or analgesic medication, bracing, progressive weight bearing with crutches as needed, and physical therapy.

Chronic Subtalar Instability

General

- Long-term symptoms are usually due to residual laxity of the injured ligament(s) or a soft tissue subtalar impingement lesion, also known as sinus tarsi syndrome.

History and Physical Examination

- The symptoms are similar to the functional instability seen in chronic lateral ankle instability, and include pain, giving way, recurrent sprains, and difficulty with uneven terrain. There is usually tenderness over the sinus tarsi, and guarding or instability with stress testing of the subtalar and often ankle joint. There may be physical examination findings related to concurrent pathology, such as peroneal tenderness or weakness.

Diagnostic Evaluation

- Stress Broden's x-rays are performed in addition to the previously described ankle mortise and lateral stress x-rays assessing talar tilt and anterior talar subluxation. The ankle is dorsiflexed 10°, the hindfoot inverted and internally rotated, and the forefoot adducted. The criteria for instability are loss of joint parallelism, more than 5° of talocalcaneal tilt, greater than 7 mm lateral talocalcaneal gap, or more than 5 mm medial calcaneal displacement (Thermann et al. 1997). However, a caveat is that there are studies which suggest that stress Broden's x-rays are similar for symptomatic and asymptomatic patients, and that abnormal stress Broden view may show normal subtalar alignment with the same stress on CT scan.

- Another criterion commonly used is excessive anterior translation of the posterior facet of the calcaneus relative to the posterior facet of the talus with anterior translation and internal rotation stress. This can be assessed on the same lateral view used to assess lateral ankle instability, or by direct visualization during subtalar arthroscopy.
- MRI can demonstrate ligament damage, osteochondral injuries to the subtalar joint, impingement lesions in the sinus tarsi and lateral gutter, tarsal coalitions, and other associated ankle and hindfoot pathology.

Treatment

- Conservative treatment is the same as for lateral ankle instability and includes bracing, high top shoe wear, physical therapy, non-steroidal anti-inflammatory medication, and if there are impingement symptoms, corticosteroid injections into the subtalar joint.
- Surgical intervention is considered for recalcitrant symptoms persisting for greater than 4 months despite adequate conservative treatment.
- Any associated impingement lesions in the sinus tarsi or lateral gutter deep to the calcaneofibular and talocalcaneal ligaments should be debrided arthroscopically or via an open arthrotomy.
- A modified Brostrom-Gould procedure with imbrication of the calcaneofibular ligament, along with advancement of the talocalcaneal ligament and inferior extensor retinaculum, will address mild to moderate subtalar instability along with any concurrent ankle instability.
- In the presence of poor-quality tissue or severe instability, a triligamentous reconstruction using a split peroneus brevis graft or allograft reconstructs the cervical, anterior talofibular, and calcaneofibular ligaments (Fig. 18–5).

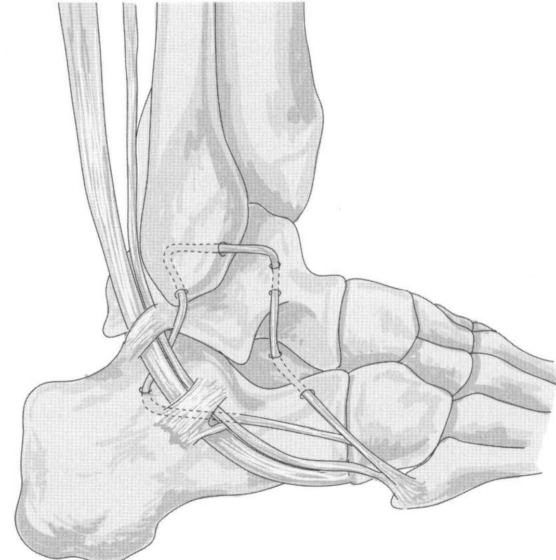

Figure 18–5: **Subtalar triligamentous reconstruction.**

Acute Syndesmotic Injuries

General

- The syndesmotic ligaments can be injured as part of ankle fracture patterns such as Maissonneuve or pronation external rotation fractures, which are discussed in chapter 19.
- In severe inversion injuries, the syndesmotic ligaments may be stretched or torn in addition to the lateral ligaments. These so-called "high ankle sprains" have been estimated to have an incidence of between 1 and 18% of all ankle sprains.
- Syndesmotic ligament(s) can also be injured in isolation or in conjunction with the deltoid ligament after external rotation stress to the dorsiflexed ankle.
- With isolated complete tears of the syndesmotic ligaments, there may be up to 2 mm of lateral subluxation of the talus and widening of the space between the distal tibia and fibula. There may also be posterior translation of the fibula relative to the incisura fibularis of the tibia. The amount of lateral talar subluxation and tibiofibular diastasis is often doubled if the deltoid ligament is also ruptured, and may be further increased with a concurrent fibular fracture.
- There may be frank diastasis, latent diastasis in which there is widening with external rotation stress, or no diastasis.

History and Physical Examination

- In addition to generalized ankle swelling and ecchymosis, there is usually tenderness over the anterior inferior tibiofibular ligament, and in more severe injuries, more proximally over the interosseous membrane.
- There is increased pain in the distal syndesmotic region with abduction and external rotation stress to the foot (Cotton test).
- There is also increased pain in the distal syndesmotic region with medial to lateral compression of the tibia and fibula in the midcalf (squeeze test).

Diagnostic Evaluation

- Weight-bearing anteroposterior, lateral, and mortise views of the ankle should be obtained to assess for fractures, widening of the medial "clear space" between the talus and medial malleolus, and widening of the tibiofibular clear space between the medial fibula and incisura fibularis.
- If widening is present, full-length tibia and fibular films are often necessary to rule out a proximal fibular fracture (Maisonneuve injury).
- Stress x-rays or fluoroscopy may be required to rule out latent instability, and are more accurate if performed under anesthesia or, less optimally, an ankle block. A Cotton test is performed and tibiofibular diastasis

assessed on a mortise view, and posterior translation of the fibula relative to the incisura fibularis evaluated on a true lateral view.

- Syndesmotic instability is suggested if the tibiofibular clear space 1 cm above the tibial plafond is greater than 6 mm on an anteroposterior or mortise ankle x-ray (Harper and Keller 1989), if the tibiofibular overlap 1 cm above the tibial plafond is less than 1 mm on a mortise view or less than 6 mm on an anteroposterior view, or if the medial clear space is greater than 4 mm or greater than the distance between the superior talar dome and tibial plafond (Fig. 18–6).
- Bilateral CT scanning (comparing with the normal side) is the best way to assess for lateral diastasis and posterior subluxation of the distal fibula, but may miss latent instability.
- MRI may also demonstrate displacement of the distal fibula along, signal changes within, or disruption of the individual syndesmotic ligaments.
- Although rarely used, bone scan may show increased activity in the distal syndesmotic region.

Treatment

- Acute syndesmotic sprains without instability are treated the same way as acute ankle sprains, but may take up to twice as long to recover.
- Frank instability is addressed with anatomical reduction and fixation of the distal fibula to the incisura fibularis with one or two syndesmotic screws or an endobutton-type device. If non-absorbable screws are used, consideration can be made for screw removal after 4 months to allow normal syndesmotic motion and avoid screw breakage. After screw removal, an intraoperative Cotton test should be performed under fluoroscopy to confirm adequate syndesmotic ligament healing. If an open reduction is performed, a suture may be placed in the torn ligaments.
- With latent instability, the options are to hold the syndesmosis reduced until the ligaments heal with syndesmotic screws, versus 6 weeks of cast immobilization followed by bracing to prevent external rotation stress on the ankle.

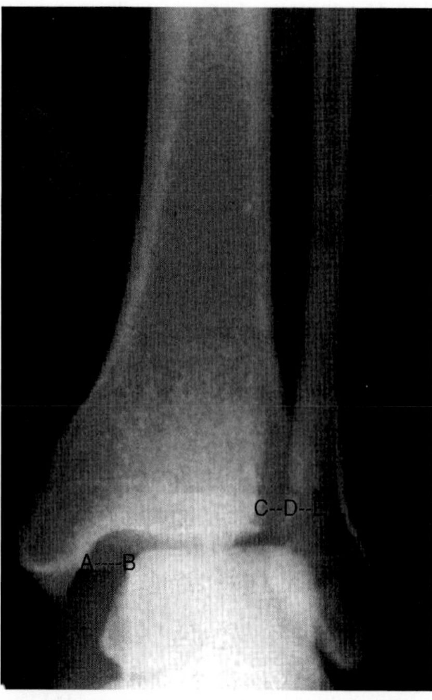

Figure 18–6: Anteroposterior ankle stress x-ray for syndesmotic ligament instability (Cotton test). A-B shows medial "clear space". C-D shows the tibiofibular clear space. D-E shows the tibiofibular overlap.

Chronic Syndesmotic Pathology

General

- Chronic symptoms may present related to persistent instability, residual lateral subluxation of the talus due to misdiagnosis or failure of acute treatment, ankle impingement lesions, or calcification of the syndesmotic ligaments.

History and Physical Examination

- There is history of previous injury, and there may be symptoms of functional instability.
- There may be tenderness over the syndesmotic ligaments, instability or pain with a Cotton test, and symptoms of ankle synovitis or arthritis such as joint line tenderness and decreased range of motion.

Diagnostic Evaluation

- Weight-bearing ankle x-rays or CT may show lateral talar subluxation, tibiofibular diastasis, arthritis, or calcification in the interosseous membrane.
- Stress x-rays may show persistent instability to a Cotton test.

Treatment

- Symptomatic talar subluxation and/or instability may be treated with bracing or surgical reconstruction. Scar tissue in the medial gutter is removed via ankle arthroscopy or arthrotomy. The lax syndesmotic ligaments may be imbricated and advanced to the fibula with drill holes or suture anchors, or reconstructed with the plantaris, toe extensors, or allograft. The repair is then protected with syndesmotic screw placement, avoiding over-compression of the syndesmosis. Alternatively, the distal incisura fibularis may be partially debrided arthroscopically followed by closed reduction of the fibula and percutaneous syndesmotic screw fixation.
- While there is biomechanical evidence that slight lateral talar subluxation dramatically alters tibiotalar contact

pressure, the long-term clinical studies supporting the suspicion that it will lead to long-term ankle arthritis do not yet exist. Therefore the reconstruction of asymptomatic lateral talar subluxation due to chronic syndesmotic laxity or fibular malunion to prevent future arthritis is controversial.

- However, one of the most common findings in patients with posttraumatic ankle arthritis is persistent widening of the syndesmosis. Because of this finding, many surgeons strongly advocate syndesmosis repair if degenerative changes are not yet present.
- The distal portion of the anterior inferior tibiofibular ligament is intraarticular, and partial tears followed by scar formation or synovitis can lead to painful impingement (Bassett lesion). Impingement lesions also can arise off the distal intraarticular portion of the interosseous and posterior inferior tibiofibular ligaments.
- Lesions that do not respond to antiinflammatory medication, bracing, or intraarticular cortisone injections may be arthroscopically debrided.
- Posttraumatic calcification of the syndesmotic ligaments is common. Symptomatic syndesmotic calcification is rare but can be treated with open excision.

Deltoid Instability

General

- Acute deltoid ligament injury may occur in conjunction with lateral ankle ligament injury in severe ankle inversion injuries, or alone or in conjunction with syndesmotic ligament injury or fibular fracture in ankle external rotation and eversion injuries.
- The deltoid ligament usually heals after functional treatment of the ankle sprain, syndesmotic screw placement, or fixation of the fibula fracture. Surgical repair of the deltoid is indicated only in the rare case of the torn ligament blocking reduction of the medial ankle joint.
- Chronic deltoid ligament insufficiency may rarely occur because of inadequate healing after an acute sprain. Chronic deltoid insufficiency may also arise from a longstanding hindfoot valgus deformity such as seen in posterior tibial tendon dysfunction.
- Chronic deltoid ligament insufficiency may be associated with chronic lateral ankle instability, and should be suspected as a potential cause of persistent instability after lateral ankle ligament repair or reconstruction.

History and Physical Examination

- In chronic deltoid instability, there is medial ankle pain and symptoms of functional instability. Unlike lateral ankle instability, the feeling of giving way is often medially based and a sense of going into valgus and eversion.
- There is tenderness over the anteromedial gutter of the ankle and the deltoid ligament.
- There may be pain, instability, and guarding with valgus stress to the ankle joint or an anterior drawer test with the foot held in external rotation.
- There may be an increased hindfoot valgus and flatfoot deformity, often asymmetric. There occasionally is associated tenderness over the posterior tibial tendon and spring ligament.
- In differentiation from posterior tibial tendon dysfunction, which it is sometimes associated with, in isolated chronic deltoid instability the hindfoot valgus and pes planus deformity correct with activation of the posterior tibialis, and there is ability to perform a complete single-leg heel raise.

Diagnostic Evaluation

- Weight-bearing ankle and foot x-rays are taken to assess for ankle arthritis, lateral subluxation or valgus tilt of the talus, longitudinal arch height, and lateral peritalar subluxation. Included is a Saltzman or Cobey view to assess for valgus tibiocalcaneal alignment.
- An ankle mortise x-ray with valgus stress applied to the foot may show valgus talar tilt, and a lateral x-ray with anterior-directed stress applied to the externally rotated foot may show anterior subluxation of the talus relative to the tibia.
- Concurrent lateral ankle instability may be demonstrated by the previously described stress x-rays assessing varus talar tilt and anterior drawer with internal rotation stress.
- MRI may show injury to the deltoid, spring, or other ankle and hindfoot ligaments; ankle arthritis or impingement lesions; tendinopathy; or other pathology.
- Diagnostic ankle arthroscopy may show partial avulsion of the deltoid ligament from the medial malleolus, impingement lesions in the medial gutter, evidence of lateral ankle instability, or other pathology.

Treatment

- Conservative therapy includes orthotic and brace management, physical therapy, and antiinflammatory medication.
- Surgical treatment consists of imbrication of the deltoid ligament versus reconstruction. Potential donor grafts include the flexor digitorum longus, the flexor hallucis longus, half of the posterior tibial tendon, the plantaris, and allograft.
- The anteromedial gutter is evaluated for an impingement lesion via arthroscopy or arthrotomy. Osteochondral lesions and lateral and posterior ankle pathology are evaluated and addressed arthroscopically.
- If present, concurrent lateral ankle ligament instability is addressed by an anatomical repair or reconstruction.
- The spring ligament is inspected, and if there is an associated tear, it is also repaired.

- In patients with hindfoot valgus and pronation deformity, and severe attenuation of the spring ligament, associated posterior tibial tendinopathy, or a similar asymptomatic deformity of the contralateral foot, strong consideration should be given for adding a calcaneal-lengthening and/or medial displacement calcaneal osteotomy to address the foot deformity, decrease subsequent strain on the deltoid ligament, and decrease the risk of recurrence.

References

Brostrom L. (1966) Sprained ankles. VI. Surgical treatment of "chronic" ligament ruptures. Acta Chir Scand 132(5): 551-565.

The author showed that in 57 of 60 cases of chronic lateral ankle instability, the previously torn or avulsed ends of the anterior talofibular ligament could be identified and repaired without a tendon graft, with good results. In a few cases with insufficient tissue for repair, a flap from the lateral talocalcaneal ligament was used instead. About one-fourth of the patients had evidence of a previous calcaneofibular ligament rupture, and there were two partial tears of the posterior talofibular ligament.

Burks RT, Morgan J. (1994) Anatomy of the lateral ankle ligaments. Am J Sports Med 22(1): 72-77.

The authors dissected cadaver ankles to determine the origin and insertion sites of the lateral ankle ligaments, which they used to describe an anatomical reconstruction using a free tendon graft. They demonstrated with radiographic markers that the Watson-Jones and original Chrisman-Snook procedures did not reconstruct normal ligament anatomy.

Cass JR, Morrey BF, Katoh Y et al. (1985) Ankle instability: Comparison of primary repair and delayed reconstruction after long-term follow-up study. Clin Orthop Relat Res 198: 110-117.

The authors reviewed 23 consecutive primary ligament repairs and 38 delayed Evans, Watson-Jones, or Chrisman-Snook reconstructions at a mean of 9.5 years after surgery. All patients filled out a subjective questionnaire, and a subset underwent clinical examination, stress radiography, and biomechanical gait analysis, with no significant measurable differences between the two groups.

Colville MR, Marder RA, Zarins B. (1992) Reconstruction of the lateral ankle ligaments. A biomechanical analysis. Am J Sports Med 20(5): 594-600.

The authors devised a split peroneus brevis lateral ankle reconstruction with bone tunnels that reproduce the anatomical orientation of both the anterior talofibular and the calcaneofibular ligaments. They compared this anatomical reconstruction in cadavers to the Evans, Watson-Jones, and Chrisman-Snook procedures, and found that it was overall better at resisting anterior displacement, internal rotation, and talar tilt, without restricting subtalar joint.

DiGiovanni BF, Fraga CJ, Cohen BE et al. (2000) Associated injuries found in chronic lateral ankle instability. Foot Ankle Int 21(10): 809-815.

Sixty-one patients undergoing surgery for chronic lateral ankle instability had intraoperative evaluation of their peroneal retinaculum, their peroneal tendons and, via arthrotomy, their ankle joint. All patients had associated injuries, including peroneal tenosynovitis (77%), anterolateral impingement lesion (67%), attenuated peroneal retinaculum (54%), ankle synovitis (49%), intraarticular loose body (26%), peroneus brevis tear (25%), talar osteochondral lesion (23%), and medial ankle tendon tenosynovitis (5%).

Hamilton WG, Thompson FM, Snow SW. (1993) The modified Brostrom procedure for lateral ankle instability. Foot Ankle 14(1): 1-7.

Twenty-eight Brostrom-Gould procedures were performed in 27 patients with symptomatic lateral ankle instability, with an average follow-up of 64.3 months. There were 26 excellent results, 1 good result, and 1 fair result with all 14 high-level professional ballet dancers, 5 of whose surgery was performed for acute grade 3 ruptures, having excellent results.

Harper MC, Keller TS. (1989) A radiographic evaluation of the tibiofibular syndesmosis. Foot Ankle 10(3): 156-160.

Based on a cadaver study radiographically evaluating normal as well as the progressively widened distal tibiofibular syndesmosis, the authors felt that a tibiofibular "clear space" on the anterior-posterior and mortise views of less than approximately 6 mm appeared to be the most reliable parameter for detecting early syndesmotic widening.

Harrington KD. (1979) Degenerative arthritis of the ankle secondary to long-standing lateral ligament instability. J Bone Joint Surg Am 61(3): 354-361.

The authors reported on 36 patients who had had lateral ankle instability for at least 10 years and complaints of increasing ankle pain. Thirty-one (86%) had at least mild degenerative changes in the medial ankle on weight-bearing x-rays, and five had severe degenerative arthritis. Twenty-two patients with mild to moderate arthritic changes underwent reconstruction of the lateral ankle ligaments, with 14 showing both symptomatic improvement and demonstrable widening of the medial joint space on weight-bearing roentgenograms.

Hennrikus WL, Mapes RC, Lyons PM et al. (1996) Outcomes of the Chrisman-Snook and modified-Brostrom procedures for chronic lateral ankle instability. A prospective, randomized comparison. Am J Sports Med 24(4):400-404.

Forty patients with chronic lateral ankle instability were randomized to either a Chrisman-Snook or a modified Brostrom procedure and evaluated at average 29-month follow-up. Both operations provided good or excellent stability in more than 80% of the patients. However, the modified Brostrom procedure resulted in higher Sefton scores and a statistically significant lower incidence of complications, particularly wound infection or dehiscence, sural nerve injury, and a feeling of the ankle being "too tight" as compared with the Chrisman-Snook procedure.

Hintermann B, Valderrabano V, Boss A et al. (2004) Medial ankle instability: An exploratory, prospective study of fifty-two cases. Am J Sports Med 32(1): 183-190.

The authors report on 51 patients (52 ankles) who underwent ankle arthroscopy and open surgical exploration and reconstruction for chronic medial ankle instability. Pain in the medial gutter was noted in all ankles, and arthroscopy verified clinically expected additional lateral instability in 77%. At average 4.4-year follow-up, there were 46 (90%) good/excellent, 4 (8%) fair, and 1 (2%) poor result(s). Three of the first five patients who had severe attenuation of or a defect in the superficial deltoid and/or spring ligament, and/or an asymptomatic valgus and pronation deformity on the contralateral foot, did poorly until revised with a lateral calcaneal-lengthening osteotomy and deltoid-shortening procedure. Therefore 11 subsequent patients with similar finding underwent primary calcaneal lengthening osteotomies with their initial deltoid ligament repairs.

Kannus P, Renstrom P. (1991) Treatment for acute tears of the lateral ligaments of the ankle. Operation, cast, or early controlled mobilization. J Bone Joint Surg Am 73(2): 305-312.

The authors reviewed 12 prospective randomized studies comparing functional treatment, cast immobilization, and/or acute surgical repair of grade 3 lateral ankle ligament ruptures. Their conclusion was that functional treatment was the treatment of choice, but that there were situations that were not adequately answered in which acute surgery might be appropriate, such as large avulsions of bone, severe medial and lateral ligament damage, and severe recurrent injuries.

Karlsson J, Bergsten T, Lansinger O et al. (1988) Reconstruction of the lateral ligaments of the ankle for chronic lateral instability. J Bone Joint Surg Am 70(4): 581-588.

One hundred and forty-eight patients (152 ankles) with chronic lateral instability of the ankle were treated with transection and imbrication of the anterior talofibular ligament, with 68 ankles also undergoing similar reconstruction of the calcaneofibular ligament. At average 6-year follow-up, there were 87% excellent or good results, all of which had radiographically improved mechanical stability. Sixteen of the 20 ankles that had an unsatisfactory result were in patients who had generalized hypermobility of the joints or longstanding local ligamentous insufficiency, or both, or who had had a previous operation. Reconstruction of both ligaments gave a better functional result than when only the anterior talofibular ligament was reconstructed.

Krips R, Brandsson S, Swensson C et al. (2002) Anatomical reconstruction and Evans tenodesis of the lateral ligaments of the ankle. Clinical and radiological findings after follow-up for 15 to 30 years. J Bone Joint Surg Br 84(2): 232-236.

The authors retrospectively compared the results of 54 patients who underwent anatomical imbrication of the lateral ligaments as described by Karlsson (1988) for chronic anterolateral instability, with 45 who had an Evans tenodesis. At average follow-up of 19.9 and 21.8 years, respectively, the patients undergoing the Evans procedure were more likely to have tenderness on palpation of the ankle, limited ankle dorsiflexion, a positive anterior drawer test, stress x-rays showing ligamentous laxity, degenerative changes on standard radiographs, a history of additional operations, and fair or poor outcomes according to the Good rating system.

Lofvenberg R, Karrholm J, Lund B. (1994) The outcome of nonoperated patients with chronic lateral instability of the ankle: A 20-year follow-up study. Foot Ankle Int 15(4): 165-169.

Thirty-seven patients conservatively treated 18-23 years previously for at least a 6-month history of chronic lateral instability ankle with no signs of arthritis per a radiologist's report were reevaluated. Thirty-four patients, 12 with previous bilateral instability and a control group of patients with recent acute ankle sprains, had non-weight-bearing ankle x-rays. Twenty-two patients, 12 with unilateral and 10 with bilateral symptoms, still had symptoms of instability, but only 3 considered further treatment. Degenerative changes were observed in 13% of the previously symptomatic ankles, 9.4% of the still symptomatic ankles, and 8.7% of the control group.

Pijnenburg AC, Bogaard K, Krips R et al. (2003) Operative and functional treatment of rupture of the lateral ligament of the ankle. A randomised, prospective trial. J Bone Joint Surg Br 85(4): 525-530.

Three hundred seventeen patients with a confirmed rupture of at least one of the lateral ligaments of the ankle were randomly assigned to receive either operative or functional treatment and evaluated at a median follow-up of 8 (6-11) years. Fewer patients allocated to operative treatment reported residual pain (16% versus 25%), symptoms of giving way (20% versus 32%), and recurrent sprains (22% versus 34%) compared with those who had been allocated to functional treatment. The anterior drawer test was less frequently positive in surgically treated patients (30% versus 54%), and the median Povacz score was significantly higher in the operative group (26 versus 22). There was no significant difference in the two groups with respect to percentage of good or excellent subjective outcome, return to sporting activities, or development of radiographic arthritis. Taking into account the high incidence of ankle ligament tears, the increased cost and morbidity of operative treatment, and the results of delayed ligament reconstruction, the authors believed that acute operative repair could be adopted in selected cases where higher functional demands are required.

Thermann H, Zwipp H, Tscherne H. (1997) Treatment algorithm of chronic ankle and subtalar instability. Foot Ankle Int 18(3): 163-169.

The authors reported at least 5-year follow-up results on 34 Chrisman-Snook procedures performed for isolated subtalar or combined ankle and subtalar instability, with the graft going through a talar tunnel only if ankle instability was present. Subtalar instability was determined by stress Broden's x-rays or intraoperative sinus tarsi exploration and evaluation of talocalcaneal interosseous ligament stability. There were 13 excellent, 18 good, and 3 satisfactory results. Twenty of the patients had a subtalar supination deficit averaging 7.2°.

CHAPTER 19

Malleolar Fractures

Stephen K. Benirschke* and Patricia Ann Kramer§

*M.D., Professor, Department of Orthopaedics and Sports Medicine, University of Washington, Seattle, WA
§Ph.D., Research Assistant Professor, Department of Anthropology, University of Washington, Seattle, WA

- Malleolar injuries generally result from a rotational or angular force on the foot relative to the leg.
- They are not usually the result of direct ankle trauma or axial load. Axial loading tends to lead to pilon (tibial weight-bearing surface), talus, and calcaneus fractures.
- The normal ankle joint distributes large forces over a large area, thus minimizing joint pressures. The articular surfaces are highly conforming. Any shifting of the talus relative to the tibia alters joint pressures dramatically, with late development of arthrosis.
- The goal of treatment of malleolar injuries is to preserve normal anatomy and keep joint pressures minimized. If these goals can be accomplished with early weight bearing and motion, then that is a bonus. If not, prolonged non-weight bearing and immobilization may be required.

Mortise Anatomy

- The ankle mortise is a tight socket for the foot. The medial and lateral malleoli connect the leg to the foot with strong ligaments.
  - The deltoid ligament connects the medial malleolus to the talus. The superficial fibers are broadly triangular, attaching superiorly from the malleolus and inferiorly to the navicular, calcaneus, and talus. Deep fibers connect superiorly from the tip of malleolus and inferiorly to the medial talus. Disruption of the ligament allows increased talar eversion and increased internal rotation (Michelson et al. 2002).
  - The distal tibia and fibula are connected by a syndesmosis. The anterior and posterior inferior tibiofibular ligaments maintain the alignment of these bones, with the aid of other smaller syndesmotic ligaments.
  - Laterally, the anterior and posterior talofibular ligaments bridge the ankle, while the calcaneofibular ligament connects the lateral malleolus to the calcaneus.
  - Malleolar injuries disrupt the medial and/or lateral sides of the ankle. In some cases, the malleoli fracture while the ligaments remain intact, and in other cases ligament disruption occurs with fracture.
  - The shape of distal fibula is complex, with a roughly triangular cross-section. The anterolateral face has a thick cortical layer, while the cortical thickness of lateral and posterolateral face is thinner.
  - The fibula is important for load bearing, carrying one-sixth of total load in the leg.
  - The tibial joint surface is concave, while that of the fibula is convex, forming the incisura. This articulation, not unlike that of the talar dome and tibia when viewed laterally, allows the fibula to seat with the tibia when both are anatomically reduced.
- Radiographs
  - The mortise view requires a neutral foot and approximately 15° of internal rotation of the leg, and allows visualization of the articular congruency of the ankle joint. In a good mortise view, the medial and lateral "clear spaces" will be visible around the talus.

- Normally, the superior, medial, and lateral clear space around the talus should all be the same thickness. Increase of medial clear space relative to superior suggests a deltoid disruption. Shifting of the talus just 1 mm laterally increases peak contact pressures considerably.
- There have been many studies looking at the absolute thickness of the medial clear space. More than 4 or 5 mm suggests deltoid ligament disruption, but of course the thickness will vary with the size of the individual. Perhaps the best test for medial clear space thickness is to compare it with the superior clear space, which should be comparable.
- When viewed on the mortise view, a continuous subchondral line can be seen in the tibia and fibula, analogous to Shenton's line in the hip. Discontinuity in this line suggests disruption of the mortise.
- The lateral view requires talar dome overlap, which is usually obtained with approximately 15° of internal rotation of the leg.
- It is important to obtain full tibia films in addition to ankle films, especially for "high risk" injuries. The classic injury is lateral translation of the talus without fibula fracture. There may be a proximal fibula spiral fracture, with syndesmotic instability.
- Most malleolar fractures do not involve the weight-bearing surface of the distal tibia, but some can, such as the trimalleolar or posterior pilon fracture pattern. Adduction and abduction injuries may have marginal impaction as well. Computed tomography scanning is valuable for evaluation of these injuries.

Classification of Injury

- The anatomical classification describes fractures based on the number of fractured malleoli. For example, all three malleoli are fractured in a trimalleolar injury. This classification has limited usefulness except for the most general of purposes.
- However, it can be said that most bi- or trimalleolar fractures are unstable. Isolated single-malleolus fractures can be either stable or unstable.
- The Lauge-Hansen scheme divides malleolar injuries by proposed mechanism of injury. Reduction must follow the injury mechanism in reverse order ("pathogenetic reduction"). The Lauge-Hansen classification emphasizes the position of foot, the direction of deforming force, and the severity of injury (grade) to describe malleolar fractures. For example, SER 4 is a grade 4 injury with a supinated-externally rotated foot. This system's usefulness derives from the attention it draws to the forces that caused the injury, forcing a deeper understanding of the relationship between the ligamentous and osseous injuries.
  - Supination-adduction 1-2
  - Supination-external rotation (eversion) (SER) 1-4
  - Pronation-external rotation (eversion) (PER) 1-4
  - Pronation-abduction 1-3
- The Lauge-Hansen classification is particularly useful for the orthopaedist, because the class of an injury will guide decision making, including need for surgery and surgical reduction techniques. For example, every PER 4 injury will be best treated by open reduction and internal fixation (ORIF) of the malleolar fracture(s) and stabilization of the syndesmosis.
- The (Danis-)Weber approach is based on the idea that the more proximal the fibular injury, the greater the potential for displacement of the lateral malleolus and for disruption of the syndesmosis, both of which are believed to be associated with the need for ORIF. The Weber classification is simple and uses the location of the fibular fracture to classify malleolar injuries.
  - Weber A injuries have a fibular fracture that is inferior to the plafond.
  - Weber B injuries are located approximately at the level of the plafond.
  - Weber C injuries have a fibular fracture that is superior to the plafond.
- However, not all injuries in a Weber class are treated the same. For example, Weber B injuries include both stable and unstable fractures.

General Treatment

- The goal is always "restoration of complete function with the least risk to the patient and the least anxiety for the surgeon."
- In many injuries, both the deep deltoid ligament and the medial malleolus remain intact. These injuries are stable, and the talus remains well reduced under the plafond. These injuries can usually be treated well non-operatively, with early weight bearing and mobilization.
- In other injuries, stability of the mortise will be lost. If an injury results in fracture or ligament disruption both medially and laterally, it is unstable. Unstable injuries are best treated with surgical reduction and fixation. Non-operative treatment of an unstable injury carries a higher risk of complications, especially posttraumatic arthrosis.
- When considering surgery, the following principles should be kept in mind.
  - The fibula must be restored to normal length and rotation. Anatomical reduction of the lateral malleolus is the key to proper functioning of the ankle joint.
  - It is generally helpful to check radiographs during surgery.
  - In most cases, patients are positioned supine on their ipsilateral side with a flank bump.
  - The key to closure is meticulous care for the soft tissue envelope.

Weber A/supination-adduction Injuries

- Weber A (infratectal) fibular fractures are generally caused by tension, resulting in a transverse fracture line. These may be inversion injuries, with avulsion of the tip of the malleolus by the lateral ankle ligaments.
- When the medial structures remain uninjured, Weber A injuries can be treated well non-operatively with a short leg cast, boot, or ankle brace, and early weight bearing.
- With more displacement, the medial malleolus will fracture, usually in a vertical pattern. There may be medial tibial plafond impaction. The medial fragment will have a proximal spike when viewed from the medial side.
- Unstable, bimalleolar adduction injuries should be treated with ORIF. Disimpaction of the marginal impaction fragments to form a congruous plafond is the first step. Bone graft may be needed to fill any defects. Then the malleolar fragment is reduced and stabilized with lag screws and possibly an antiglide medial plate.
- The fibula can be fixed using three methods.
  - Tension band wires are used for small fragments.
  - Lag screws in combination with K wires are used for medium-sized fragments. Two lag screws or one lag screw and a K wire are used, depending on the location and shape of the fragments.
  - A hook plate may be used for large fragments.

Supination-External Rotation Injuries

- SER (Weber B) injuries are caused by external rotation of the foot with tension on the medial side. The fibula is subjected to torsion. The fibular fracture pattern characteristically runs from posterosuperior to anteroinferior.
- When the injury is not severe, the fibula fractures but the medial malleolus and deltoid ligament remain intact (SER 2 pattern). The mortise is then stable. These SER 2 injuries can be treated with a short leg cast or brace, and early mobilization.
- If the injury is more severe, both malleoli fracture (SER 4). These injuries are best treated by ORIF.
- Although the typical SER 4 includes a medial malleolar fracture, in some cases (SER 4—deltoid variant), there may only be a disruption of the deep deltoid ligament. The mortise would then be unstable with only a lateral malleolar fracture. It is important to differentiate the SER 2 from the SER 4—deltoid variant patterns, because treatment and prognosis are quite different (Fig. 19–1).
- Usually, an SER 2 injury will have only lateral tenderness, while the SER 4—deltoid will have medial tenderness and ecchymosis. This is somewhat reliable but not diagnostic.
- An SER 2 injury should have less then 2 mm of fibular displacement, but this is also not diagnostic.

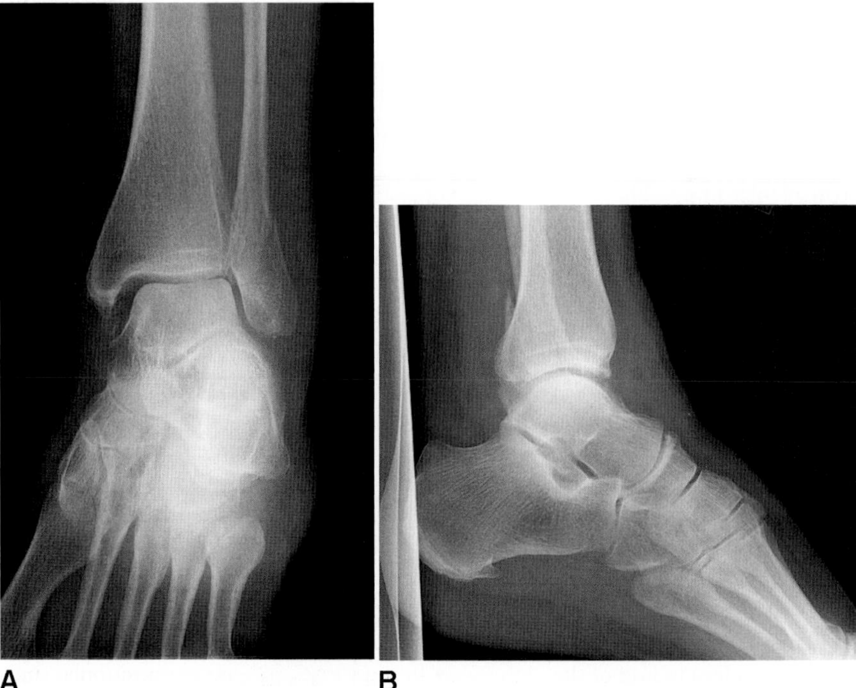

Figure 19–1: **Patient with a Weber B (SER) ankle fracture. A, Despite the relatively minimal displacement of the fibula, the medial "clear space" is widened. B, The lateral view shows the typical posterosuperior to anteroinferior fracture pattern.**

Continued

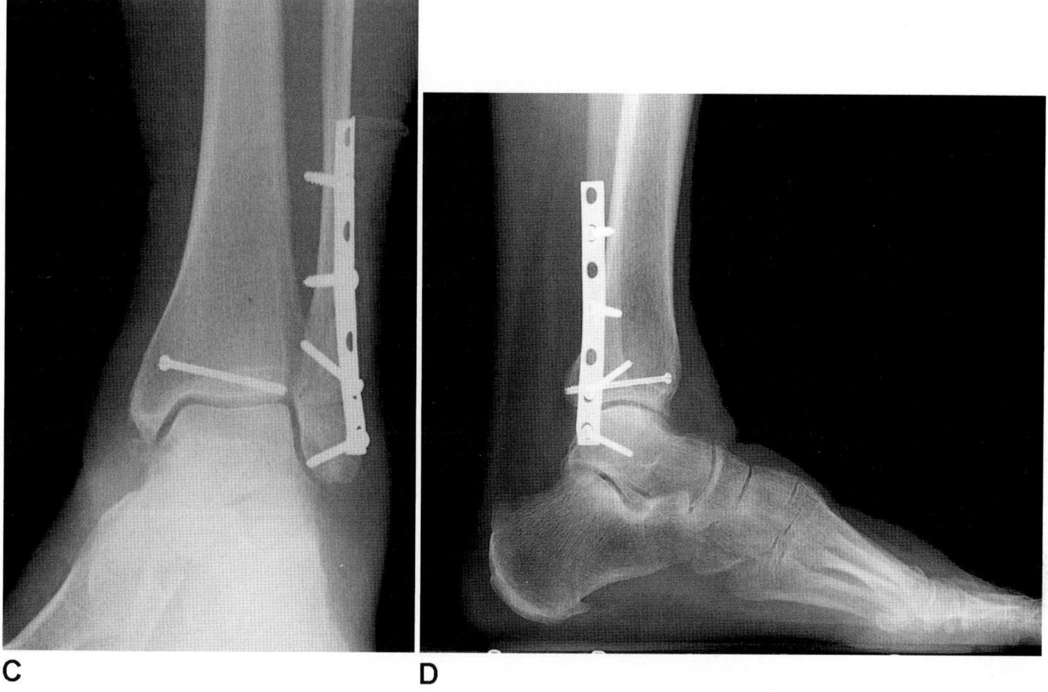

Figure 19–1: Cont'd **C,** A postoperative mortise view shows restoration of normal anatomy. **D,** On the lateral x-ray, a lag screw through the posterior plate is used.

- The best test to differentiate an SER 2 from an SER 4—deltoid variant is an external rotation stress x-ray. If the medial clear space widens on stressing, there is injury to the deep deltoid and the injury will best be treated surgically.
- When treating an SER 4 injury, the fibular fracture is reduced, restoring length and rotation, and held in place with K wires or a pointed reduction clamp. Simple oblique fractures can be fixed with a lag screw.
- Although direct lateral plating is commonly used, a posterolateral antiglide plate makes a biomechanically stronger construct. In the distal part of the fragment, longer screws can be used without impeding the fibulotalar joint. The posterolateral placement of the plate counteracts or neutralizes the joint forces more effectively than an anterolateral plate placement.
  - The anterolateral cortex provides more contact area for the lag screws than the posterolateral surface, dictating that the lag screws run from the posterolateral surface to the anterolateral surface. The antiglide plate can be used reinforce the thin posterolateral surface, i.e. the plate acts as a prosthetic cortex.
- Medial malleolar fractures are reduced and fixed with two screws. Small fragments are reduced and held in place with tension band wires.
- Deltoid ligament tears often allow the medial malleolus to remain intact, requiring no remedy unless deltoid interposition prevents mortise reduction. Some surgeons feel that individuals with deltoid tears should be kept immobile for at least 8 weeks (2 weeks longer than those with intact deltoids) to allow the ligament additional time to heal.
- Although SER injuries do not generally injure the syndesmosis, it should be stressed in the operating room to confirm stability, because an unrecognized syndesmotic injury can lead to posttraumatic arthritis.
- If rigid fixation is obtained and the syndesmosis is stable, the patient may be treated with early mobilization and early weight bearing.
- With less than ideal fixation or a syndesmotic injury, it will be necessary to restrict weight bearing for 6-8 weeks using use a short leg cast.

Pronation-External Rotation/Weber C Injuries (Fig. 19–2)

- Rotational injuries with a fibula fracture above the joint line usually disrupt the syndesmotic ligaments. External rotation stress x-rays can be taken if there is any doubt.
- Beware the isolated medial malleolar fracture! These may include a high fibula fracture with syndesmotic

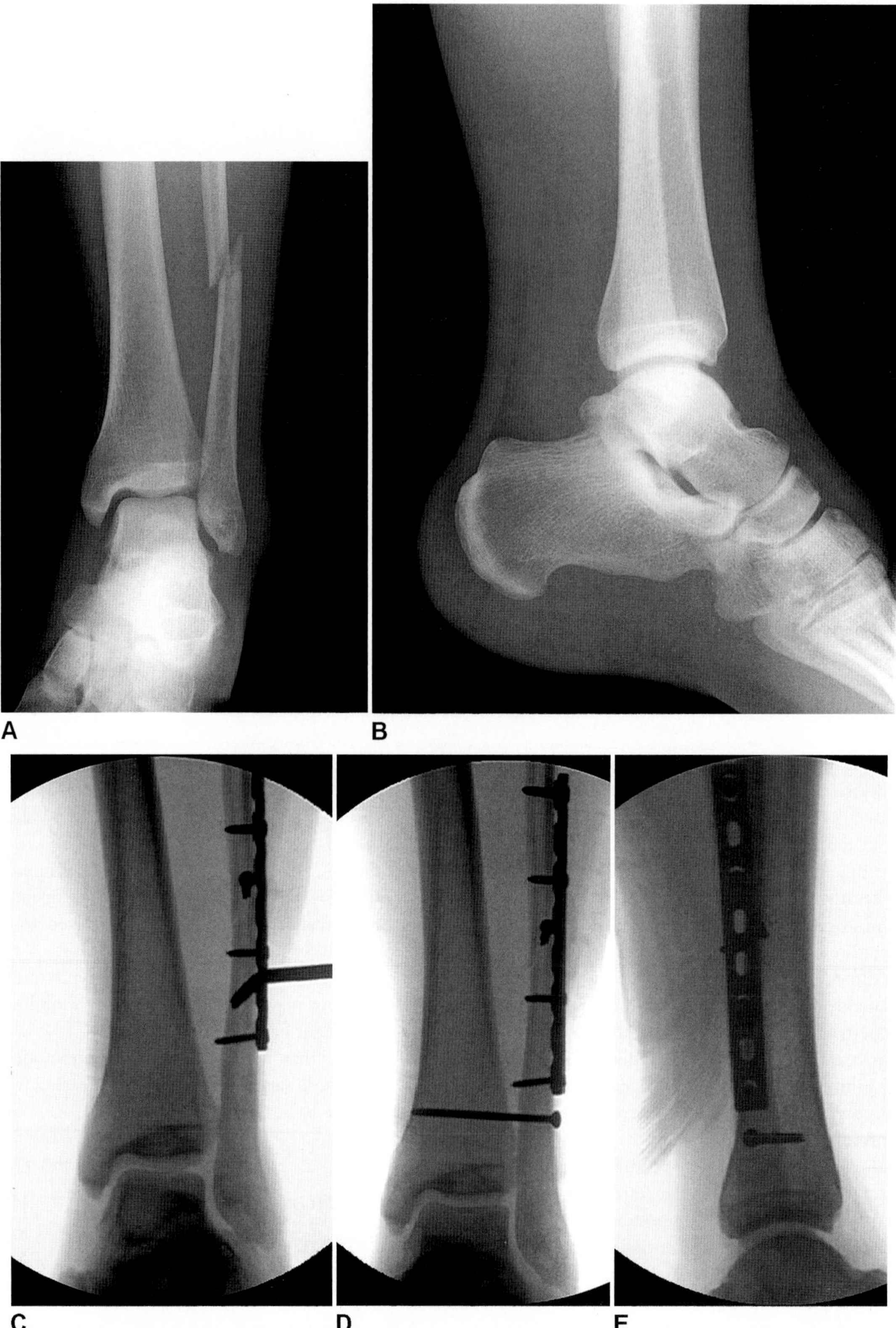

Figure 19–2: Weber C fracture pattern. **A**, Note the high fibula fracture and widening of the tibia-fibular space. **B**, The injury lateral shows that the fibular fracture is not the typical one for a supination-external rotation injury (as in Fig. 19–1), but is more typical of the irregular pattern seen with pronation-external rotation injuries. **C**, Intraoperatively, a small retractor applies a lateral stress to the repaired fibula. Instability (widening) at the syndesmosis is seen. **D**, After reduction of the syndesmosis, a four-cortex positioning screw holds the mortise. **E**, This lateral x-ray shows the long plate stabilizing the fibular fracture, and the syndesmotic screw passing from the fibula to the tibia.

Continued

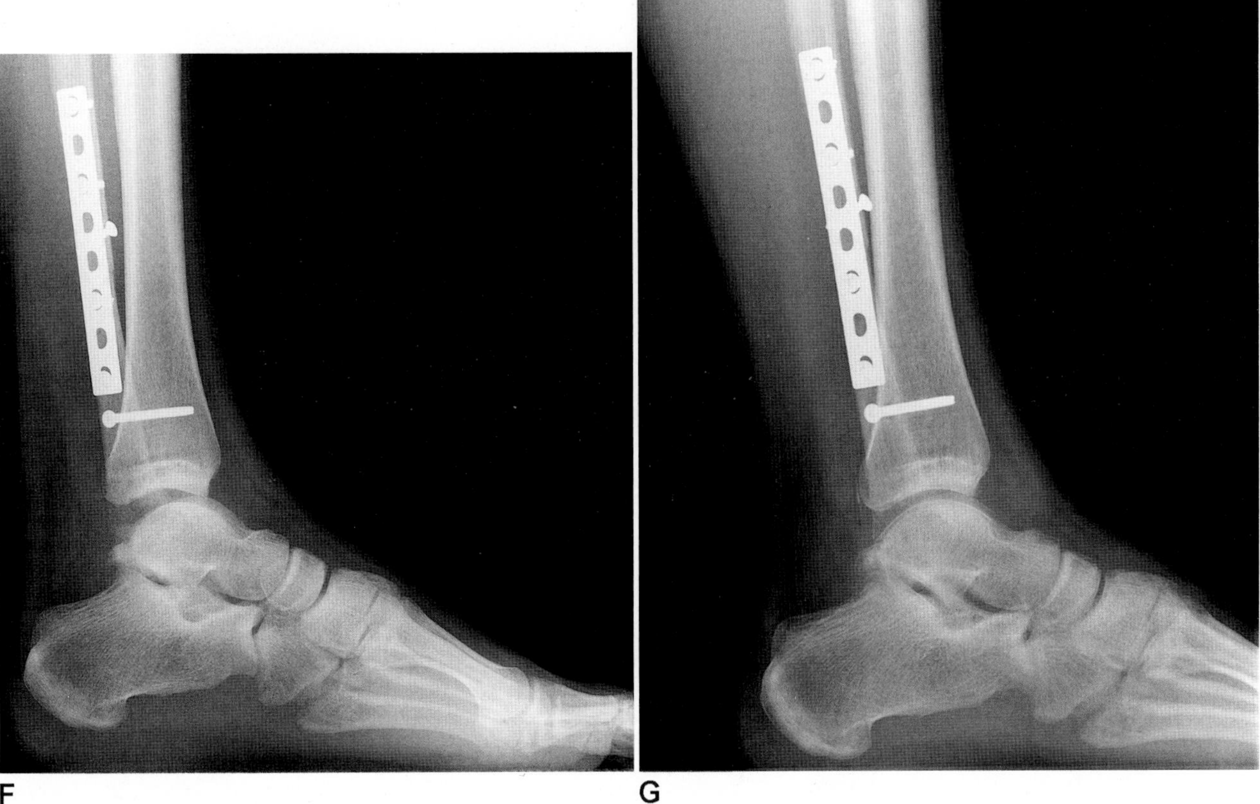

Figure 19–2: Cont'd F, At 3 months, a non-weight-bearing x-ray shows anterior subluxation of the talus from an associated injury to the anterior talofibular ligament and anterior capsule. Most Weber C injuries rupture the syndesmosis and deltoid ligaments, but less commonly the talofibular ligaments. G, At 1 year, a weight-bearing film shows restoration of alignment. Although many surgeons recommend routine removal of the syndesmotic screw, this patient had no symptoms from the retained screw.

disruption. Examine the entire calf and obtain tibia x-rays with isolated medial malleolar injuries.

- In these unstable injuries, the fibula must be restored to length and rotation without regard to the location of the fracture.
- If the fibular fracture is diaphyseal or metadiaphyseal, it is addressed with standard implants and techniques: one-third tubular plates, stacked one-third tubular plates, 2.7 or 3.5 DCP or periarticular plates. The key is to restore length, rotation, and alignment of the fibula, and to provide and maintain stable fixation.
- If the fibula fracture is at the fibular neck, it may be better to leave the fracture unexposed to prevent iatrogenic peroneal nerve injury. In this case, the syndesmosis should be exposed and reduced distally, correcting fibular shortening and external rotation.
- The syndesmosis is then stabilized. It may be helpful to use a large pointed reduction clamp to "squeeze" the syndesmosis closed while placing fixation.
- The syndesmotic injury is addressed with one or two screws implanted just above the tibiofibular joint. Either a 3.5-mm or a relatively new 4.0-mm screw, originally designed for Lisfranc injuries, is used, dependent on the size of the individual. Both have a higher pitch (number of threads per inch) than large fragment screws. Higher pitch allows for more contact between the screw and the cortical bone, allowing for a more persistent attachment. The core diameter of a 3.5 mm is 2.5 mm, while that of a 4.0 mm is 2.9 mm. The screw contacts all four cortices, and is left in for 6-12 months or until the screw loosens or breaks. With a broken screw, removal may require approaching the site both laterally and medially. Some surgeons no longer feel routine screw removal is necessary.
- The medial malleolus is addressed, depending on the size of the fragment, with lag screws or tension bands.
- All PER injuries involve the syndesmosis, so weight bearing is prevented for 8 weeks.

Pronation-Abduction Injuries (Fig. 19–3)

- Abduction forces can result in injuries with a transverse avulsion of the medial malleolus, and comminuted impaction of the lateral malleolus.

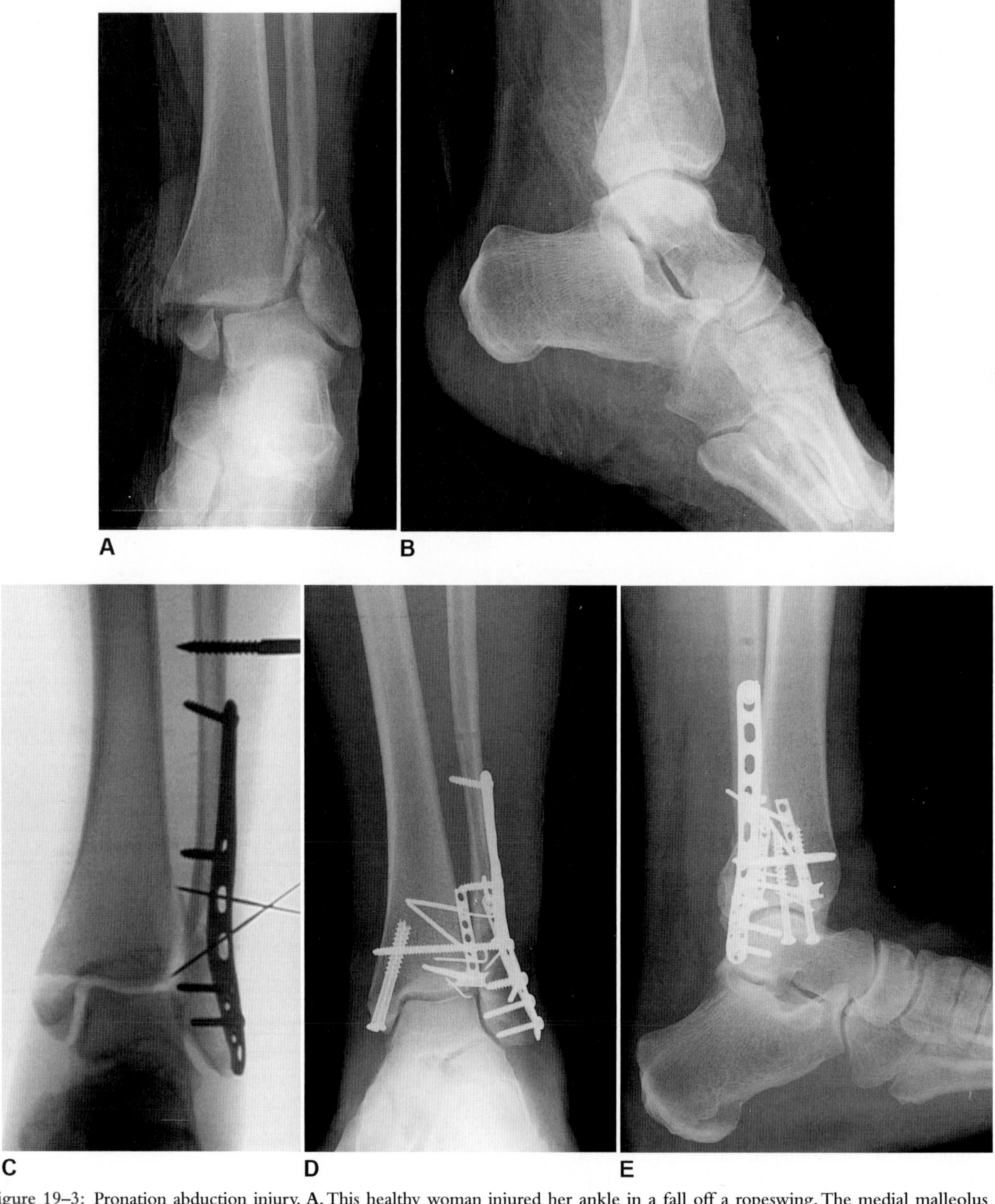

Figure 19–3: Pronation abduction injury. **A,** This healthy woman injured her ankle in a fall off a ropeswing. The medial malleolus shows the characteristic transverse avulsion, while the lateral malleolus is comminuted and impacted. The talus is tilted in valgus and subluxed laterally. **B,** The lateral view confirms lateral, but not posterior, displacement of the talus. **C,** Fibular length and rotation is restored using a distractor to facilitate reduction. **D,** Postoperative films show anatomical reduction of the mortise. All osseous elements are restored. **E,** Lateral view shows concentric reduction of the talus beneath the plafond.

- These injuries may have lateral plafond impaction. If present and not addressed, recurrent valgus tilting of the ankle may result.
- The unstable bimalleolar injuries should be treated surgically. It is usually easiest to reduce the medial side first, because there is no comminution. The fibular fracture often requires distraction to facilitate restoration of rotation and length of the metaphyseal comminution.
- Lateral plafond impaction can be reduced and fixed with mini or small fragment buttress plates and screws, possibly with bone graft.

Posterior Malleolus Injuries

- PER or SER injuries may include a posterior tibial plafond (posterior malleolus) fracture by avulsion of the posterior inferior tibial-fibular ligament.
- Very small fragments may be left unfixed. Alternatively, an anterior to posterior lag screw may stabilize the fragment without direct reduction.
- In rare cases, the posterior fragments will be large and often comminuted. This fracture pattern may be better described as a posterior pilon, because a large part of the plafond may be injured. Direct ORIF is needed for the posterior pilon injury.
- Exposure of the posterior pilon is difficult. An anterior incision is not adequate, because the intact anterior plafond blocks visualization and reduction attempts. A long medial incision with the dislocating approach of Shelton can be used. Alternatively, the patient can be positioned prone and the posterior plafond approached through posteromedial and posterolateral incisions.
- Reduction is best assessed with an externally rotated, lateral radiographic view.
- The posterior pilon is kept non-weight bearing for at least 8 weeks after surgery.

Syndesmotic Injuries (Fig. 19–4)

- Syndesmotic injuries can rarely present without osseous injury.
- They can be distinguished clinically from ankle sprains by instability of the joint in external rotation, and by pain and instability that do not resolve.
- A stress radiograph (external rotation) will show widened tibiofibular and talofibular joints.

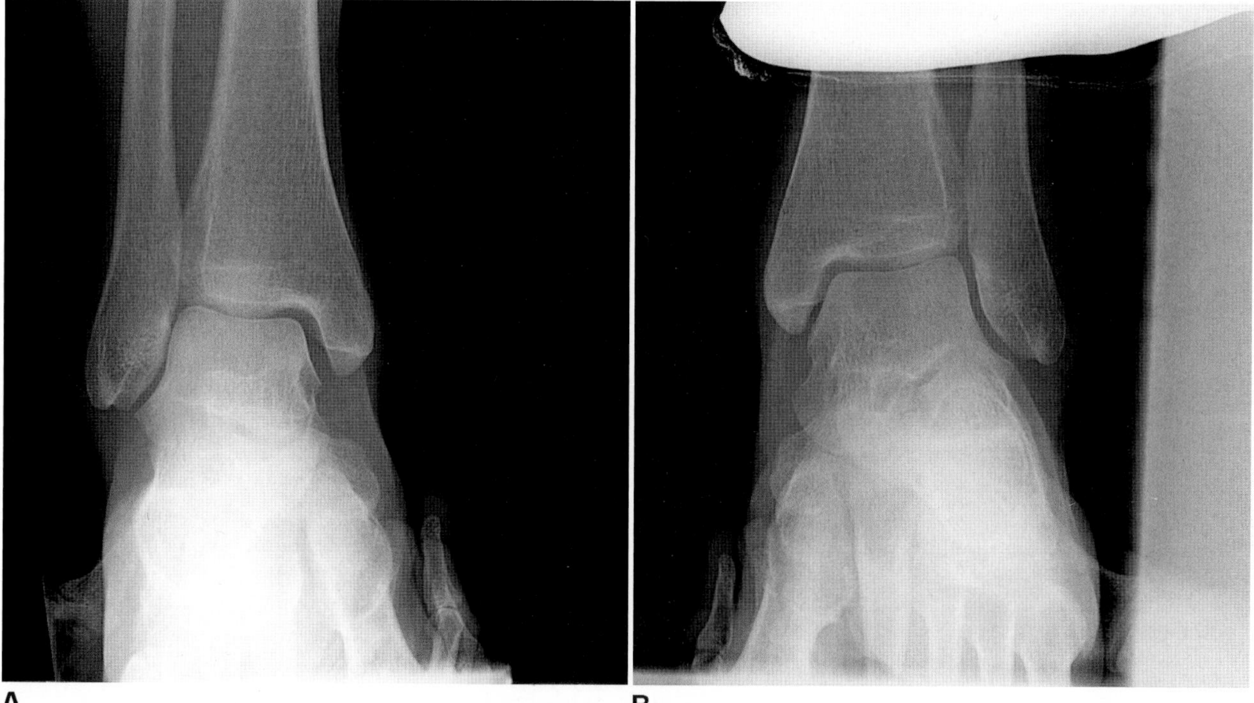

Figure 19–4: Syndesmotic rupture. **A**, The injured ankle under external rotation stress shows medial "clear space" widening. **B**, The uninjured contralateral ankle does not widen with stress.

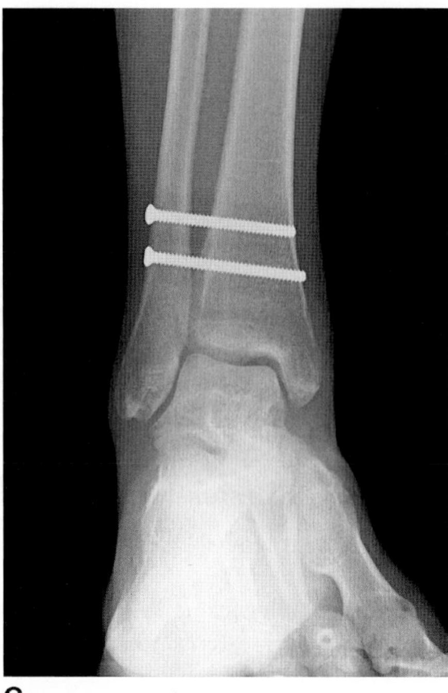

C

Figure 19–4: Cont'd C, The syndesmosis was reduced and then stabilized with two screws.

- These injuries should be treated with reduction and fixation with multiple screws.
- Rarely, syndesmotic injuries may extend through the proximal tibiofibular articulation. This disruption may be subtle, but any proximal migration of the fibula must be reduced.

Soft Tissue Technique for all Ankle Injuries

- All incisions are closed with appropriate care for the soft tissues.
- Periosteal closure over the implants is used if possible.
- Wound closure is obtained with symmetric tension.
- The skin is closed with standard mattress or Allgöwer sutures with knots tied on the posterior side. All skin sutures (3.0/4.0 monofilament) are placed before tying. Each suture is clipped with a snap to hold it in place.
- Steristrips may be used to reinforce the incisional closure.
- Avoid using staples, as the skin is friable, especially the anterior flap.
- No flap embarrassment should be tolerated!

Postoperative Care

- After the dressing is applied, the ankle is splinted in neutral position. Radiographs should be taken if indicated to demonstrate that the ankle is neutral and the tibiotalar joint is reduced, especially on the lateral view.
- Antiinflammatory medications may delay bone healing and probably should be avoided until bone healing is complete.
- Sutures are removed at 2-3 weeks, and radiographs taken if indicated. A cast or cast boot is applied with the ankle in neutral.
- At 6 weeks, radiographs are taken to confirm evidence of healing. More aggressive physical therapy is then begun.
- Syndesmotic injuries should remain strictly non-weight bearing for 8 weeks.
- At 10 weeks, the radiographs should demonstrate complete healing, and the patients should move on to functional recovery. Advanced balance and proprioception training is recommended.
- Syndesmotic screws should be removed when the screws break, which usually occurs between 6 and 9 months after surgery.
- There is a trend among many trauma surgeons not to routinely remove syndesmotic screws at all. Many patients are not bothered by the screws.
- Hardware removal from implants other than syndesmotic screws should wait until approximately 1 year after surgery.

Complications

- Wound complications rarely occur if proper technique is used to maintain the integrity of the soft tissues.
- Some surgeons will give prophylactic oral antibiotics to patients whose incisions do not seal by 3-4 days and do not heal within 2 weeks.
- Anterior subluxation of the talus is possible and should be treated with appropriate postoperative splinting or casting (see Fig. 19–2F,G).
- Delayed union, i.e. those fractures that do not demonstrate appropriate bone healing, should be treated with delayed weight bearing. Painful non-union is rare but should be treated aggressively with bone grafting and rigid fixation.
- When a non-union occurs, the surgeon should look for the reason:
  - smoking
  - patient non-compliance
  - unrecognized injury (plafond impaction or syndesmotic injury)
  - neuropathy.
- Displaced malleolar fractures treated non-surgically usually lead to a malunion. In the case of the external rotation injury, fibular osteotomy should be considered to minimize chances for late arthritis. The typical rotational malunion leaves the fibula short and externally rotated. Oblique fibular osteotomy with lengthening and internal rotation may help restore more normal kinematics.
- Unreduced syndesmoses should be reduced and stabilized, even if identified late, so long as adaptive degenerative changes have not yet developed.

- Posttraumatic ankle arthrosis develops in some patients by 1-2 years after surgery. It should be addressed as soon as it becomes evident.
- Appropriate accommodations include rocker bottom shoes, ankle lacers, and ankle-foot orthoses.
- Underlying conditions, such as gastrocnemius equinus, that compound the joint problems should be aggressively addressed.
- Salvage procedures include cheilectomy, debridement, and osteotomy. Ankle arthodesis or total ankle arthroplasty should be delayed as long as possible.

Osteoporosis

- When the bone is of poor quality, conventional methods may be less effective, especially on the fibula.
- The posterolateral plate may provide better purchase on the fibula. A locking plate can be used. K wires can augment the plate fixation. A 2.7 DCP plate will allow more screws into a small distal fragment. Precontoured distal fibular plates are available from some manufacturers, with more screw holes distally.
- Under-drilling through the metaphysis (1.5 mm for a 2.7-mm screw or 2.0 mm for a 3.5-mm screw) allows the screw to compact the adjacent bone as it engages the bone. This "radial prestress" produces a more persistent grip.
- Above the level of the plafond, the fibular screws can pass into the tibia for extra bone purchase. This is particularly useful for higher fibula fractures. Older patients are not bothered by screws spanning the syndesmosis, and routine screw removal is not needed (see Fig. 19–3C).

Stress Fractures

- Malleolar stress fractures are rare, and patients typically present with chronic pain with or without radiographic evidence of fracture (Fig. 19–5).

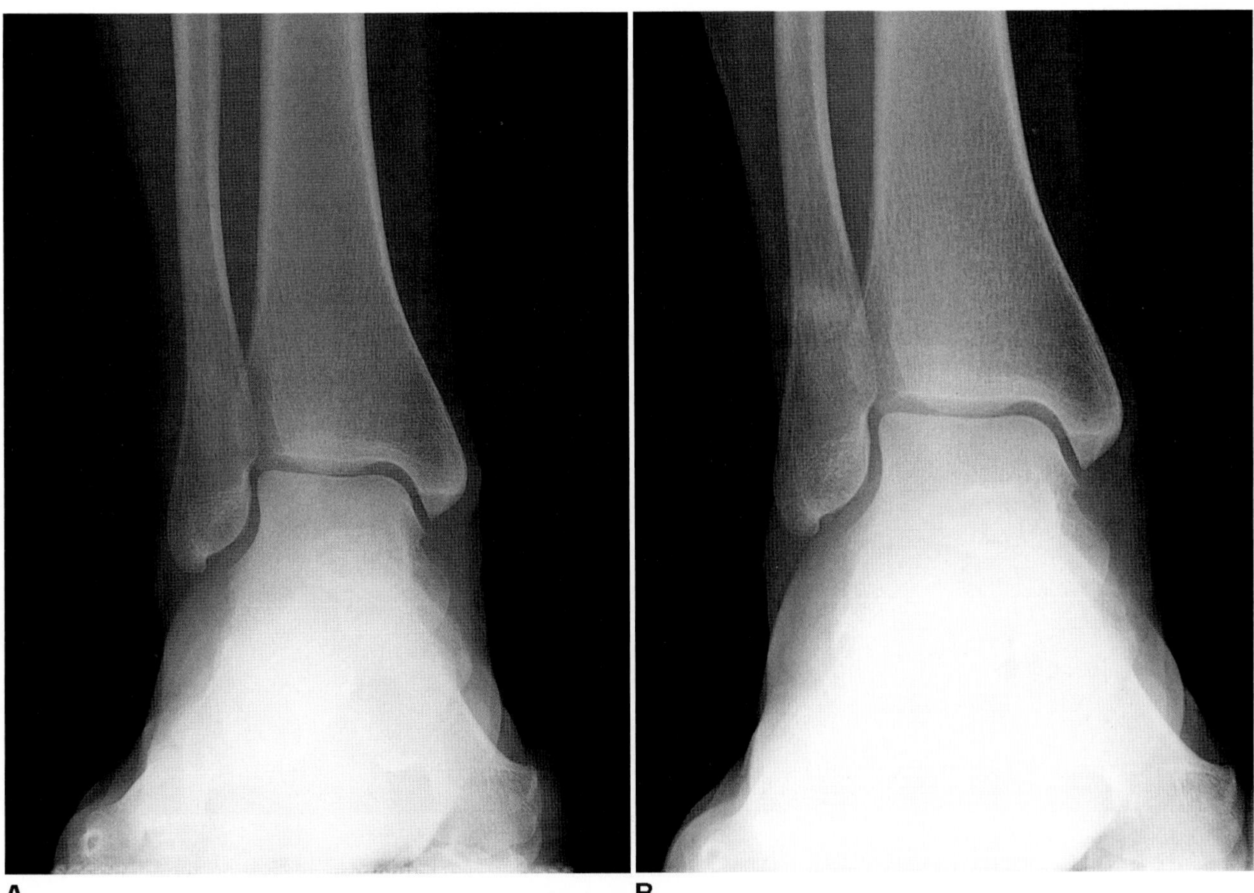

Figure 19–5: Lateral malleolar stress fracture. **A**, This patient with lateral ankle pain and swelling had no obvious findings on x-ray, although in retrospect there is slight sclerosis in the fibula just above the plafond. **B**, A follow-up x-ray 4 weeks later shows the characteristic periosteal reaction of a stress fracture.

- Medial malleolar stress fractures are usually associated with high-impact athletes such as runners and basketball players.
- When malleolar stress fractures do occur, aggressive treatment may be warranted, especially in those patients for whom conservative treatment has not been successful. Internal fixation and sometimes bone grafting are helpful.
- Rarely, postmenopausal women experience malleolar stress fractures.
- Patients with severe valgus hindfoot alignment may develop distal fibular stress fractures. These will generally heal with a short period of rest, but the misalignment should be addressed to prevent further complications (lateral ankle arthritis) (Fig. 19–6).

Outcome

- Short fibulae and wide ankle mortises are associated with the radiographic signs of osteoarthrosis, reduced mobility, and pain in long-term follow-up (Rukavina 1998).
- The fibular reduction is critical: 1 mm of displacement of the fibula equals a 42% decrease in joint contact area on average (Ramsey and Hamilton 1976).
- Outcome is correlated to reduction, but reduction does not completely explain outcome. For example, 87% of patients with an anatomical reduction had good or excellent outcome, yet 69% of patients with inadequate reduction also had good or excellent outcome (Lindsjo 1985).
- Although eventual ankle arthrosis correlates with initial reduction, some, perhaps 50%, of arthrosis cannot be explained by malreduction. This may be a manifestation of avascular necrosis of the periarticular fragments or of the talus.
- Lamontagne et al. (2002) did not demonstrate a difference in fixation failure, complications, or rate of hardware removal between Weber B patients treated with a posteriorly placed antiglide plate versus a laterally placed plate. Although both techniques produced equally good outcomes, the posterolateral plate does provide a stronger construct, less possibility of screw penetration into the joint, and less prominent hardware.
- Return to full function usually takes at least 1 year. Patients with Weber B fractures treated surgically continue to improve in physical function (36-Item Short-Form Health Survey) until 1 year post surgery, although pain may continue to decrease as long as 2 years after surgery (Bhandari et al. 2004).

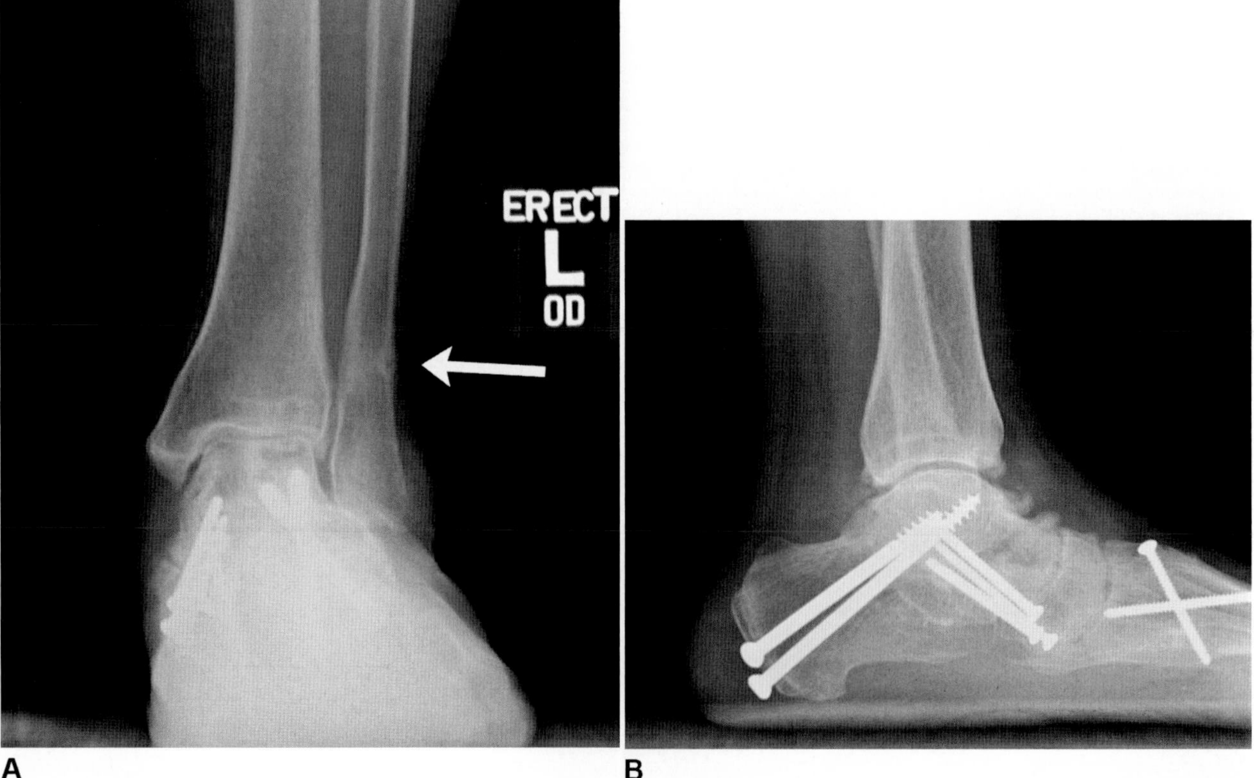

Figure 19–6: Lateral malleolar stress fracture. **A,** This woman with stage 4 posterior tibial tendonitis had previous hindfoot realignment and arthrodesis but remained in valgus alignment. Note the lateral ankle joint space narrowing. She developed pain over the lateral ankle. The mortise view shows the foot to be lateral to the weight-bearing axis of the leg. It also shows a stress fracture in the fibula (arrow). **B,** The lateral view reveals low calcaneal pitch due to under-correction of deformity at the previous surgery. She developed a fibular stress fracture because of persistent valgus forces due to misalignment.

Other Issues

- Open wounds should be managed with irrigation and debridement, acute fracture fixation, and wound closure.
- Patients who present with fibular malunions or nonunions should be aggressively treated using the techniques presented above. Fibular length and rotation are critically important to the long-term function of the ankle.
- Patients who present with persistent syndesmotic disruption should have syndesmotic reduction with screws and ligamentous reconstruction to reestablish stability. Occasionally, synostosis is necessary to maintain fibular position.

Tips

- Beware marginal (plafond) impaction!
- Use tension band wires for osteoporotic bone or small fragments.
- Pay close attention to the anterior capsule, and do not allow anterior extrusion of the talus to occur in the peri- and early postoperative period.
- Watch for gastrocnemius equinus and prevent it.
- Avoid devitalizing the skin flaps.

References

Bhandari M, Sprague S, Hanson B et al. (2004) Health-related quality of life following operative treatment of unstable ankle fractures: A prospective observational study. J Orthop Trauma 18: 338-345.

In this prospective study, outcome measures remained lower than normal over 2 years following an ankle fracture. Smoking and lower education level were associated with lower physical function.

Lamontagne J, Blachut PA, Broekhuyse HM. (2002) Surgical treatment of a displaced lateral malleolus fracture: The antiglide technique versus lateral plate fixation. J Orthop Trauma 16: 498-502.

Despite the biomechanical differences, no clinically relevant benefit was identified for the use of posterior fibular plating when compared with lateral plating in this retrospective review of 193 patients.

Lindsjo U. (1985) Operative treatment of ankle fracture-dislocations. A follow-up study of 306/321 consecutive cases. Clin Orthop Relat Res 199: 28-38.

Anatomical reduction of the mortise was important for a good outcome in this series of 300 patients.

Maynou C, Lesage P, Mestdagh H et al. (1997) [Is surgical treatment of deltoid ligament rupture necessary in ankle fractures?] Rev Chir Orthop Reparatrice Appar Mot 83: 652-657.

This retrospective review found no benefit to repair of the deltoid ligament in cases of unstable injuries with no medial fracture. The deltoid heals well, so long as the mortise is anatomically reduced with fixation of the fibula fracture and syndesmosis, as needed.

Michelson JD, Hamel AJ, Buczek FL et al. (2002) Kinematic behavior of the ankle following malleolar fracture repair in a high-fidelity cadaver model. J Bone Joint Surg Am 84-A: 2029-2038.

This biomechanical study examined in detail the kinematics of the injured ankle mortise. It is possible that disruption of ankle-stabilizing ligaments leads to altered motion during swing phase more than stance phase of gait.

Ramsey PL, Hamilton W. (1976) Changes in tibiotalar area of contact caused by lateral talar shift. J Bone Joint Surg Am 58: 356-357.

Key study showing that 1 mm of lateral talar shift decreases ankle contact area by 42%.

Rukavina A. (1998) The role of fibular length and the width of the ankle mortise in post-traumatic osteoarthrosis after malleolar fracture. Int Orthop 22: 357-360.

In this series, fibular shortening and widened mortises were more likely to be associated with posttraumatic arthritis.

Schaffer JJ, Manoli A. (1987) The antiglide plate for distal fibular fixation. A biomechanical comparison with fixation with a lateral plate. J Bone Joint Surg Am 69: 596-604.

Winkler B, Weber BG, Simpson LA. (1990) The dorsal antiglide plate in the treatment of Danis-Weber type-B fractures of the distal fibula. Clin Orthop Relat Res 259: 204-209.

Several studies have examined the mechanical in vitro strength of posterior versus lateral plating for fibular fractures. The posterior plating technique makes a stronger construct in the laboratory.

Yablon IG, Heller FG, Shouse L. (1977) The key role of the lateral malleolus in displaced fractures of the ankle. J Bone Joint Surg Am 59: 169-173.

A retrospective review found that inadequately reduced malleolar fractures were more likely to lead to arthritis. Unless the fibula is anatomically reduced, the talus will remain laterally subluxed.

Stress Fractures

Boden BP, Osbahr DC. (2000) High-risk stress fractures: Evaluation and treatment. J Am Acad Orthop Surg 8: 344-353.

This review article places medial malleolar stress injuries into a high-risk group and recommends aggressive treatment.

Iwamoto J, Takeda T. (2003) Stress fractures in athletes: Review of 196 cases. J Orthop Sci 8: 273-278.

A large series of patients with stress fractures is presented.

Kaye RA. (1998) Insufficiency stress fractures of the foot and ankle in postmenopausal women. Foot Ankle Int 19: 221-224.

In 12 patients presenting with stress fractures, 8 were metatarsal, 3 were in the fibula, and 1 was in the medial malleolus.

Shelbourne KD, Fisher DA, Rettig AC et al. (1988) Stress fractures of the medial malleolus. Am J Sports Med 16: 60-63.

A review of six patients with medial malleolar stress fractures. Half were treated surgically. All returned to activity within 8 weeks.

Tibial Pilon Fractures

Ivan S. Tarkin* and Peter A. Cole§

*M.D., Assistant Professor, Division of Orthopaedic Traumatology, University of Pittsburgh Medical Center, Pittsburgh, PA
§M.D., Professor and Chief of Orthopaedic Traumatology, University of Minnesota Physicians, Regions Hospital, St. Paul, MN

Terminology

- *Pilon* is a French term used to describe a fracture of the distal tibia usually characterized by high-energy traits including dissociation of the articular surface from the tibia shaft.
- Destot coined the term pilon, as he thought that the distal tibial metaphysis resembled a pharmacist's pestle.
- *Plafond* is also a French term, described by Bonin, referring to the distal tibial articular surface as the roof of the ankle joint.

Normal Anatomy

- At the level of the ankle, the distal tibia is intimately associated with the fibula through strong ligamentous attachments, including the anterior and posterior tibiofibular ligaments as well as the interosseous and inferior transverse ligaments.
- The articular surface of the distal tibia is concave in both the coronal as well as the sagittal plane.
- The talus has the opposite geometry of the tibial plafond, and therefore serves as a perfect template for assessing articular reduction of the distal tibia.
- The concave tibial plafond provides approximately 40% more posterior than anterior coverage.
- The talar dome is wider anteriorly than posteriorly, resulting in obligatory external rotation of the foot during ankle dorsiflexion in order to accommodate the wider anterior talus.

Fracture Anatomy

- The pilon fracture usually has an anterolateral (Chaput) fragment and a posterolateral (Volkmann) fragment, which usually remain attached to the distal fibula segment by the anterior and posterior tibiofibular ligaments.
- In the vast majority of pilon fractures, the fracture lines propagate from the fibular incisura laterally in the shape of a "Y" to exit anterior and posterior to the medial malleolus (Fig. 20–1A).
- Comminution, which frequently occurs with high-energy pilon fractures, is most typically located in the anterolateral and central regions of the plafond (Fig. 20–1B).

Surrounding Soft Tissue Anatomy

- The soft tissue envelope surrounding the distal tibia is vulnerable to injury, as it contains only retinacular tissue and tendons between skin and bone, rather than muscle tissue.
- The tendons of the anterior compartment, the dorsalis pedis artery, and the superficial and deep peroneal nerves can be encountered with anterior exposures at the level of the ankle joint.
- The tendinous and neurovascular structures are covered proximally by the investing fascia of the anterior compartment, and distally by the extensor retinaculum. The superficial peroneal and saphenous nerves are superficial to the fascia.

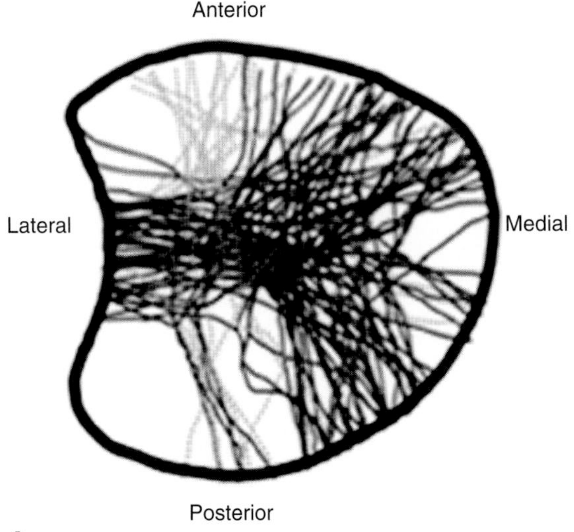

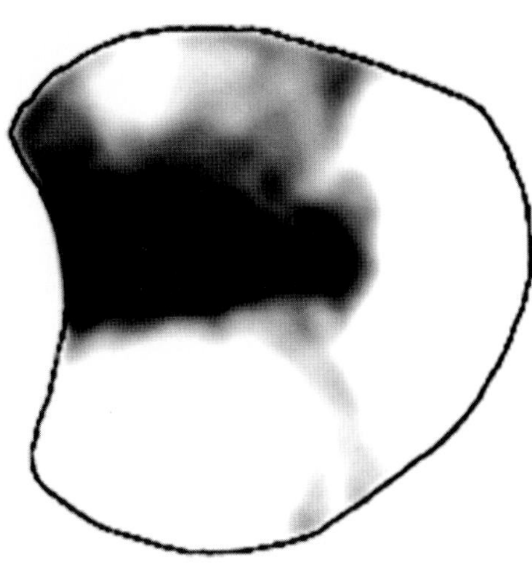

Figure 20–1: **A, Pilon fracture map. Primary fracture lines (blue) of 40 Orthopaedic Trauma Association (OTA) type 43C3 fractures, the most common and classic pilon variant. These primary fracture lines were mapped by the senior author from axial computed tomography (CT) cuts 3 mm above the plafond after an external fixator had been applied to the ankle. Appreciate the very consistent "Y" pattern creating three main articular fragments. B, Pilon comminution pattern. Zones of comminution were outlined from those same CT scan cuts detailed in panel A. The zones of impaction most commonly occur at the dome between the three main fracture fragments. Also, anterolateral comminution is commonly encountered with high-energy fractures. These are sites the surgeon typically must address with a bone void filler. Collectively, these two maps aid the surgeon in predicting necessary surgical tactics and approaches. (Presented at the OTA, 2004.)**

- The superficial peroneal nerve pierces the fascia of the lateral compartment approximately 12 cm proximal to the ankle joint en route to provide sensation to a majority of the dorsum of the foot.
- Sensation of the first dorsal web space is supplied by the deep peroneal nerve.
- The tendons of the distal anterior compartment from medial to lateral include the tibialis anterior, extensor hallucis longus, extensor digitorum longus, and peroneous tertius. Tendons of the anterior compartment are covered in paratenon, which should be preserved with surgical exposures to the distal tibial plafond.
- Anterolateral exposures for pilon fractures risk injury to the superficial peroneal nerve.
- The dorsalis pedis and deep peroneal nerve are at risk with an anterior exposure, and are found running together in the pericapsular fat between the tibialis anterior and extensor hallucis longus tendons.

Understanding the Injury

Context and Mechanism

- The tibial pilon fracture is a rare yet devastating injury. Despite the best treatment, patients sustaining high-energy pilon fractures generally do not return to their previous state of general health or function. After recovery from pilon fractures, many patients continue to have debilitating pain and ankle stiffness (Babis et al. 1997, Sands et al. 1998, Pollak et al. 2003).
- Fortunately, pilon fractures compose a minority of tibia or lower extremity fractures, occurring in approximately 7 and 1% of all cases, respectively.
- Pilon fractures can occur from both low- and high-energy mechanisms. Lower energy fractures typically occur due to rotational forces imparted to the distal tibia. High-energy fractures are generally associated with a component axial force that drives the talus into the tibial plafond, causing an "implosion" of the articular surface.
- In the most severe plafond fracture patterns, the articular segment is fractured into numerous pieces, with certain segments driven proximally into the metaphysis, creating marked joint incongruity and associated metaphyseal defects.
- An associated fibula fracture is often present in pilon fractures.
- The most common fracture pattern occurs with the ankle in dorsiflexion (i.e. the foot on the break pedal during a motor vehicle accident). When the ankle is dorsiflexed at the time of injury, pilon fracture patterns involve the anterior articular surface of the tibial plafond.
- Central articular (implosion) injury is the result of an axial load on the foot in neutral position.
- A severely traumatized soft tissue envelope accompanies the higher energy pilon fractures. Although many pilon fractures are open injuries, closed fractures have significant soft tissue compromise as well (Fig. 20–2).

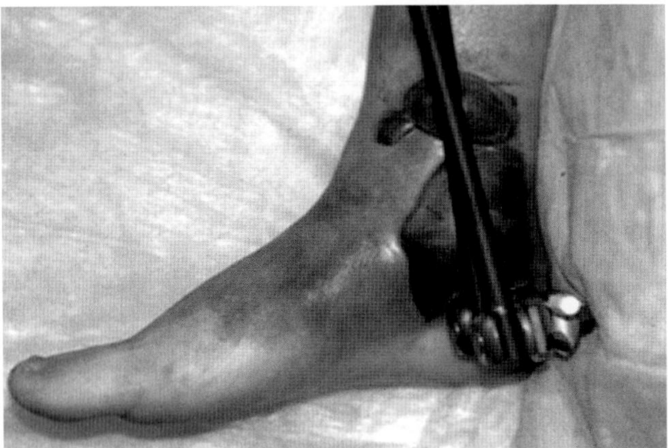

Figure 20–2: **Soft tissue injury associated with a 43C pilon fracture at 72 hours. On the evening of injury, the ankle was reported as "not swollen" and appropriate for a surgery. Skin incisions for fracture management are not advisable at this time due to wound healing and infection risk. Blood-filled blisters represent injury of dermoepidermal junction.**

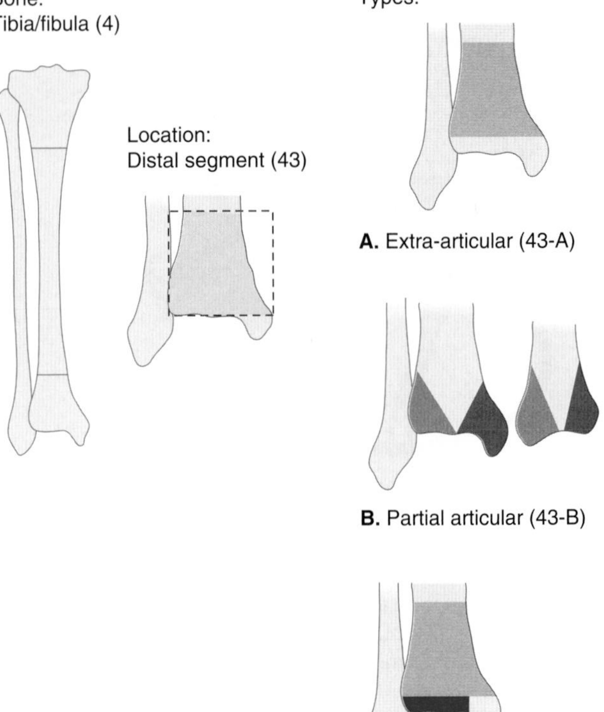

Figure 20–3: **Arbeitsgemeinschaft für Osteosynthesefragen/ Orthopaedic Trauma Association pilon fracture classification system.**

- Initial management of pilon fractures depends more on the soft tissue rather than the bony injury. Understanding the soft tissue injury accompanying pilon fractures is of utmost importance for providing optimal treatment while minimizing complications.

Classification

- Classification systems have been developed to stratify both severity of fracture pattern and soft tissue injury.
- Although the Arbeitsgemeinschaft für Osteosynthesefragen (AO)/Orthopaedic Trauma Association (OTA) classification system is the most widely accepted fracture classification system, the Ruedi-Allgöwer system is the classic fracture scheme often known and used for this injury throughout the world (Fig. 20–3).
- Ruedi-Allgöwer type 1 fractures are minimally displaced cleavage fractures, in contrast to type 2 injuries, which are displaced. Type 3 injuries portend the worst prognosis as a consequence of articular comminution and metaphyseal impaction.
- Moderate interobserver reliability makes the AO/OTA system reliable for classifying pilon fractures (Swiontkowski et al. 1997). The distal tibia is designated as #43 (4 = tibia, 3 = distal segment). The fractures are divided into types, and further into groups then subgroups.
- 43C patterns invariably represent high-energy injuries with a compromised soft tissue envelope. Irreversible damage to the articular cartilage, and at times the soft tissue anatomy, occurs at the time of injury.
- Soft tissue injury has been standardized using the method of Tscherne for closed fractures, and the Gustilo-Anderson classification for open injuries. The Tscherne scheme has four grades of increasing severity for soft tissue injury in closed fractures. Tscherne grades 0 and 1 have negligible soft tissue injury and superficial abrasions/contusion, respectively. Type 2 Tscherne injury describes advanced muscle contusion and deep, potentially contaminated abrasions. Pilon fractures with extensive crush, degloving, or vascular injury are considered type 3.
- The most widely accepted open fracture classification is credited to Gustilo and Anderson. Gustilo type 1 open fractures are generally clean with a less than 1 cm skin laceration. Type 2 open fractures have more extensive soft tissue injury with minimal to moderate crushing, typically with a laceration greater than 1 cm.
- Open pilon fracture with extensive soft tissue injury and a severe crush component are graded as type 3. Type 3A open fractures have adequate soft tissue coverage over the fracture. Type 3B are usually contaminated, with extensive periosteal stripping and bone exposure necessitating flap coverage. Open fractures with vascular injury requiring repair along with extensive soft tissue compromise are considered type 3C.

Evaluation

- In view of the fact that most pilon fractures usually occur as the result of violent trauma (i.e. motor vehicle accident), associated bodily injuries must be considered in the work-up of these patients.
- After more urgent injuries are stabilized, further work-up of the pilon fracture should be methodically performed.
- Examination should document the presence of both closed and open soft tissue injury, as well as location and extent of lacerations, abrasions, and contamination.
- A systemic motor and sensory examination is warranted in addition to documentation of distal pulses. Leg compartment syndrome should be diagnosed based on clinical examination, and confirmed if necessary with compartment pressures.
- Radiographs are critical for characterization of the bony injury and joint position, and must include an ankle anteroposterior, mortise, and lateral view. Traction views may be valuable for further characterization of the pilon fracture.
- Computed tomography (CT) examination is best delayed until restoration of length in shortened fractures, because ligamentotaxis helps to better approximate fragments closer to their native position, making interpretation easier.
- Initial splinting in the emergency room decreases further soft tissue trauma, and fracture dislocations should be reduced with adequate anesthesia to restore joint alignment.
- Open wounds are covered with moist gauze, and antibiotic and tetanus protocols are employed.

Historical Discussion

- Ruedi and Allgöwer revolutionized the management of pilon fractures after reporting their operative strategy in 1969.
- The series reported by Ruedi and Allgöwer described superior outcomes after formal open reduction and internal fixation (ORIF) in a majority of their patient population, with few major complications.
- The operative principles described by the AO group for operating pilon fractures serves as a working paradigm for ORIF of these injuries.
  - Length and rotation is restored by ORIF of the fibula.
  - Anatomical reconstruction of the articular surface of the tibial plafond is performed after the acute phase of the injury.
  - Metaphyseal bone defects are bone grafted to buttress the articular surface.
  - Buttressing of the tibial metaphysis is then required while connecting the articular block to the diaphysis.
- The results of the classic study from the Swiss AO group could not, however, be reproduced by all surgeons. Reports describing ORIF of tibial pilon fractures recognized a concerning complication rate with higher energy pilon fractures, including wound problems, deep infection, non-union, and malunion (McFerran et al. 1992, Teeny and Wiss 1993).
- Recognition of a different category of higher energy pilon injuries emerged, which was quite different than those treated by Ruedi and Allgöwer, who treated lower energy injuries primarily in healthy skiers—so called "boot top injuries."
- New research was undertaken to determine the best way to manage higher energy fractures of the tibial plafond, as traditional ORIF was fraught with devastating complications from open treatment of these injuries. External fixation alone became popular for managing complex pilon fractures associated with both closed and open compromised soft tissue envelopes.
- The rate of deep infection decreased with external fixation; however, at a great cost. The quality of reduction with external fixation alone was suboptimal, leading to poor outcomes secondary to joint arthrosis.
- Initial external fixator constructs spanned the ankle joint until fracture union, resulting in unacceptable ankle stiffness. Small wire epiphyseal-diaphyseal ring fixators were then employed to treat pilon fractures to allow for early ankle motion, in an effort to minimize long-term ankle stiffness. Limited ORIF to improve articular reductions without formal operative exposures was then employed to supplement external fixation strategies.
- Unsatisfied with the limitations of external fixation strategies, including compromised articular reduction, pin tract complications, and patient dissatisfaction, new strategies to allow for ORIF were investigated. Protocols developed to enhance soft tissue recovery prior to definitive operative fracture fixation, including greater waiting time for such recovery, became the mainstay.
- External fixation can be employed as a temporary treatment modality by regaining length, stability, and alignment of both the fracture and the surrounding tissue envelope. Tissue oxygen tension in the injury zone improves with increasing time, supporting the wisdom of greater waiting periods. Formal ORIF can be performed safely after soft tissue recovery, most often between 10 and 21 days after the initial pilon fracture.
- Staged ORIF is currently the "gold standard" practice for managing pilon fractures.

Management of Pilon Fractures

Non-operative Treatment

- Indications for closed reduction and cast treatment of pilon fractures are limited. Certain low-energy, non-displaced pilon fracture patterns may fare well with cast application as long as vigorous follow-up is scheduled to monitor for fracture displacement.

- No articular displacement should be accepted unless the patient is not an appropriate surgical candidate.
- Patients with medical infirmity precluding operative intervention may be candidates for conservative fracture management.
- Pilon fractures treated with a cast have led to poorer outcomes than those managed operatively.
- After closed reduction, maintaining lower limb alignment is very difficult in a cast, particularly due to a propensity for the fracture to fall into varus.
- The ability to impart a closed reduction relies on the principle of ligamentotaxis. Impacted joint segments, found in most plafond fractures, do not have capsular attachments and will not reduce with closed reduction techniques.
- Prolonged immobilization of the ankle joint after fracture can lead to "cast disease." Cast immobilization until fracture union promotes ankle stiffness, dystrophic changes, muscle atrophy, and disuse osteopenia. Cartilage nutrition is promoted by early ankle joint motion after articular injury, and arthrosis is hastened with cast treatment for pilon fractures.
- Furthermore, monitoring/managing the traumatized soft tissue envelope associated with high-energy pilon fractures cannot be efficiently performed if cast treatment is utilized.

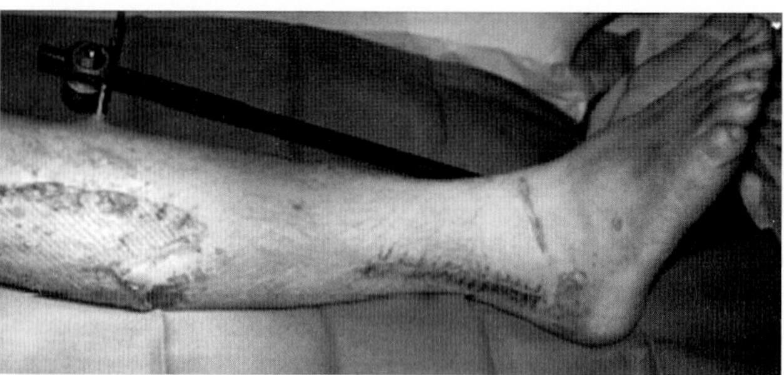

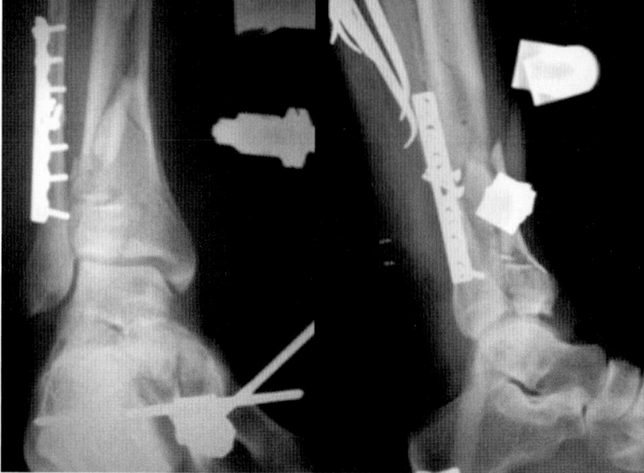

Figure 20–4: **Management of pilon fractures: Definitive fracture reconstruction of high-energy injuries is delayed until the soft tissue envelope has matured. Initial management goals consist of achieving length and skeletal alignment. A common strategy employed includes restoring the lateral column with open reduction and internal fixation of the fibula through a posterolateral approach. Medial stability can be achieved with a spanning medially based external fixator.**

External Fixation

Bridging External Fixation

- Definitive ORIF is not advisable through a compromised soft tissue envelope. An ankle-spanning external fixator can be used for both temporary as well as definitive management of distal intraarticular tibia fractures.
- Spanning external fixation as a temporary strategy can serve as so-called "traveling traction."
- The fixator can be applied so that the soft tissues and fracture fragments are held out to appropriate length, allowing for recovery of the traumatized tissue envelope.
- Many different frame configurations have been used to effect stability. A delta frame may be the most popular, and this configuration forms a triangle with a calcaneus transfixion pin attached medially and laterally to two pins placed in the tibia, proximal to the zone of injury.
- A medially based external fixator can also be used, typically employing half-pins placed in the tibia, talar neck, and calcaneus, in concert with anatomical restoration of the associated fibula fracture (Fig. 20–4).
- The bridging external fixator is best used in conjunction with a openly fixed and well-reduced ipsilateral fibula fracture, to aid in restoring length.
- External fixator application should be placed in such a way to allow for easy management of soft tissues, including access for flap procedures.
- Although fracture union can be achieved with external fixation, malunion rates are higher than with ORIF, as is dissatisfying and morbid articular incongruity.

External Fixation with Limited Internal Fixation

- The most important limitation of external fixation alone as definitive management for pilon fractures is incomplete articular reduction, which portends a worse clinical outcome.
- Limited open approaches to impart an improved reduction of the distal tibia joint surface can be used in conjunction with external fixation. The rationale of this approach is based on minimizing iatrogenic periarticular soft tissue injury.
- Strategic screws are used in an attempt to restore joint incongruity of the tibial plafond. In the absence of

comminution or displacement at the joint surface, lag screw techniques are utilized to impart compression and stability across joint fragments.

- External fixation decreases the incidence of wound dehiscence while imparting length, alignment, and rotation.
- But some degree of major and minor pin site problems and septic arthritis is inevitable with the use of external fixation.
- The incidence of malunion may be increased with external fixation, as stability is not as reliably imparted.
- Most concerning is the compromise of the articular reduction, in the name of "minimally invasive" or "biologic" surgery.
- Early joint motion, a basic goal of definitive internal fixation, is not possible with spanning frames with or without limited internal fixation.

Non-spanning External Fixation With or Without Limited Internal Fixation

- Joint immobilization has detrimental articular effects, at least in adults with intraarticular fractures. Non-bridging external fixators have been used for the management of high-energy pilon fractures to promote the possibility of early motion and weight bearing.
- Frame constructs consist of thin wire fixation into the epiphyseal or articular block, with attachment to the diaphyseal segment via rods that are connected to either thin wires (Ilizarov frame) or larger half-pins (hybrid designs) (Fig. 20–5).
- The distal fixation consists of tensioned wires connected to a ring.
- "Olive" wires can be placed strategically in the distal segment to assist in compression of articular fragments if open reduction is not performed. The olive part of the wire impinges against the cortex of an articular fragment, which is then pulled toward an adjacent joint segment, imparting an indirect reduction.
- If limited ORIF is used, direct articular reduction can be performed with screw fixation, and then a non-spanning external fixation can be placed to align the articular segment with the tibial shaft.
- Standard position of wires after limited open techniques consists of a posterolateral to anteromedial technique (transfibular) as well as a posteromedial to anterolateral placement.
- Encouraging clinical outcomes have been realized with non-spanning fixators by experienced surgeons using Ilizarov techniques.
- However, pin site problems, septic arthritis, patient dissatisfaction with external frames, sacrifices in articular reduction, and high-maintenance follow-up care are inherent challenges that complicate the care of these patients.

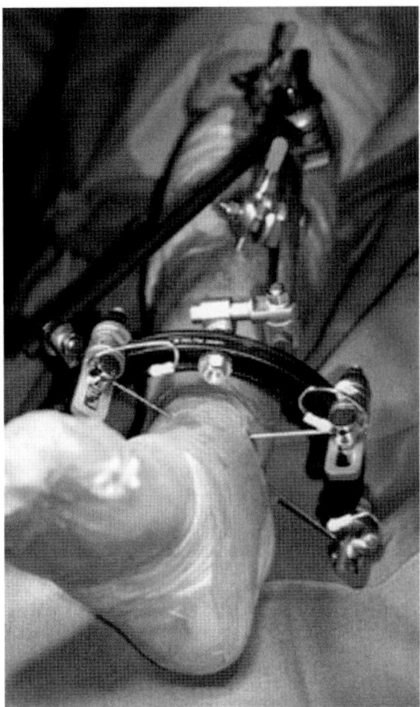

Figure 20–5: **Although not the authors' preferred treatment, a non-spanning external fixator is a definitive treatment method for pilon fractures. Typically, tensioned thin wires attached to a ring are placed in the articular segment. Proximal to the fracture, conventional Shantz pins can be placed in the tibial shaft. The fracture is then spanned with bars from the proximal Shantz pins to the distal ring. This is referred to as a hybrid design. As compared with open reduction and internal fixation, definitive treatment with external fixation is associated with suboptimal articular reduction and increased rates of metaphyseal-diaphyseal malunion. Also, pin tract infection is common. However, this technique is acceptable for Arbeitsgemeinschaft für Osteosynthesefragen/Orthopaedic Trauma Association type A (extraarticular) patterns. Also, external fixation is a good treatment consideration in severely compromised soft tissue envelopes that do not resolve within appropriate time periods to allow for open approaches.**

Staged Open Reduction and Internal Fixation

Principles

- Respect for the soft tissue envelope is paramount if considering ORIF. This includes conservative timing for definitive incisions, external fixation for the recovery phase from soft tissue trauma, carefully chosen incisions developing periosteocutaneous flaps, preservation of blood supply to major fracture fragments, gentle soft tissue handling during the case, and meticulous skin closure technique.
- Low-energy pilon fractures do occur and can be safely managed with traditional ORIF, but high-energy injuries require attention to the fracture itself as well as to the soft tissue anatomy.

- Numerous reports detail the serious complications encountered after untimely ORIF of high-energy tibial plafond fractures, including skin necrosis, wound dehiscence, deep infection, non-union, malunion, and amputation.
- During the period of temporary external fixation, the surgeon can get to know the patient and his or her injury.
- Understanding the patient's resources for assistance, job status and personality, recreational preferences and avocations, and comorbidities and bad habits can play a role in decision making.
- Staged reconstruction also allows the surgeon to develop a relationship with the patient, and begin the process of education of what is sure to be a difficult period for the patient.
- Education should cover everything from smoking cessation to injury perspective; it uses the patient's "negative circumstance" for an extraordinary opportunity, often beginning a process of healthy personal discipline—working on compliant preoperative care and postoperative rehabilitation.
- This period of time affords the surgeon the opportunity to study the injury pattern, obtaining appropriate studies and formulating a surgical tactic. An anteroposterior, mortise, and lateral ankle radiograph in a non-splinted ankle is obtained first in the emergency setting. It is optimal to wait on CT until after the first stage of surgery (ORIF of fibula and ankle external fixation).
- Early intraoperative consultation with a microvascular surgeon is particularly important in the management of open Gustilo type 3B pilon fractures (Fig. 20–6).
- On presentation of a pilon fracture, regaining length, stability, and alignment is necessary to give the tissue envelope time to recover from the initial traumatic event before definitive fracture fixation.
- In the presence of a fibula fracture, plating the fibula accurately first helps restore length, alignment, rotation, and stability to the lateral column. This sequence also allows for a more simplified external fixation scheme.
- Mature clinical judgment is required to determine when the definitive reconstruction should be performed. This stage is enhanced and expedited by strict limb elevation and mechanical pneumatic compression. Clinical signs of a maturing soft tissue envelope include return of the skin "wrinkle sign" and reepithelization of fracture blisters. Typically, this process of soft tissue recovery takes 2-3 weeks; however, it is not uncommon to wait 4-5 weeks for safe timing of definitive ORIF.

Technique: ORIF of Fibula

- ORIF of an ipsilateral fibula fracture and bridging external fixation are both performed as the initial management of high-energy pilon fractures.
- The external fixator should not be locked into position until the fibula is anatomically reduced, to avoid a fibular malreduction.

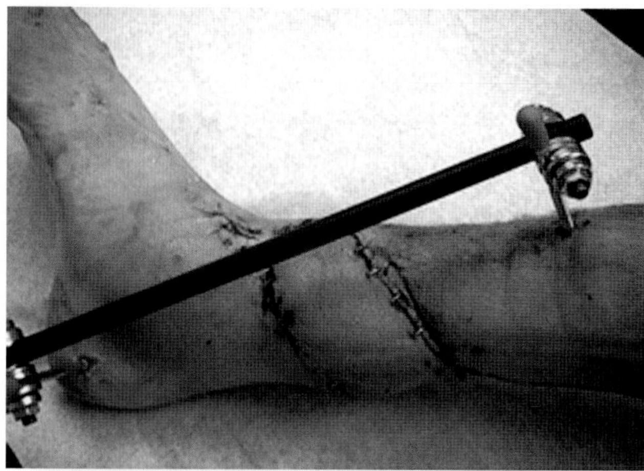

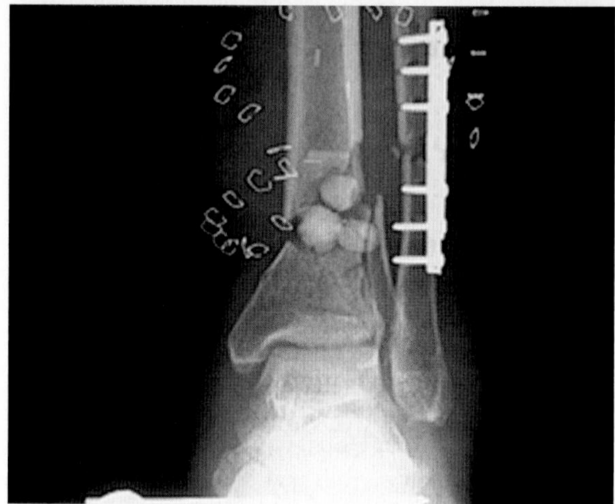

Figure 20–6: Open pilon fracture management consists of meticulous debridement, irrigation, and sometimes insertion of antibiotic beads. External fixator placement at the first debridement allows access for early flap coverage when necessary. Better outcomes and lower complication rates are associated with flap coverage within 72 hours. Use of a vacuum-assisted closure dressing technique is useful between presentation and flap coverage.

- Surgeons should study the radiographs to try to understand where it is that they will need to make an optimal incision based on the tibia fracture pattern.
- The incision for ORIF of the fibula fracture should be made posterolaterally, if possible, in order to maximize the eventual skin bridge after staged distal tibia reconstruction.
- It is a fallacy, however, that a 7-cm skin bridge is necessary between incisions. The healthy ankle tolerates parallel incisions very well.
- Occasionally, traumatic lacerations must be incorporated into the surgical approach to minimize insult to soft tissue flaps.
- For rotational injury patterns, the fibula fixation is typically achieved with a lag screw(s) and a neutralization plate. If the fibula is comminuted, a stiffer plate choice is

most appropriate for fixation, particularly if above the plafond (such as in Weber C fractures).

- If the fibula has significant comminution, stacked one-third tubular plates allow necessary plate malleability but adequate strength for these circumstances.
- Ensuring fibula length in the presence of comminution may require templating from the patient's contralateral ankle radiographs.
- There are times in the setting of osteoporosis, comorbid conditions such as severe diabetes, a patient with low activity demands, or high fibula fractures, when a fibular "nail" is the best option. A skinny rush rod or Steinman pin, placed through a small stab incision 1 cm below the lateral malleolus, in the midaxial line of the fibula, can be used in such circumstances.

Technique: ORIF of Tibia

- A comprehensive operative plan includes proper setup and positioning, choosing an operative exposure, planning a surgical tactic (order of steps), choosing hardware necessary to achieve rigid fixation, addressing the need for a bone void filler, and ensuring the availability of specialized equipment and personnel.
- Preoperative CT scanning assists the surgeon in defining the number and size of fracture fragments, orientation, and sites of articular impaction.
- A prepared surgeon operates efficiently, limiting both operative and tourniquet time.
- The most direct operative exposure reduces the need for excessive periosteal stripping, which would further denude the fracture segments of their critical blood supply.
- Only full-thickness flaps should be raised, and delicate soft tissue handling is performed.
- Self-retaining retractors should be used sparingly, if at all, for pilon fracture surgery.
- Although the classic operative exposure is an anteromedial approach, medial to the tibialis anterior tendon, current thinking is that the surgeon should be prepared for whatever interval gets the surgeon to the fracture plane with the least dissection.
- In the anterior approach, care must be exercised with the neurovascular bundle, which is hidden in the pericapsular fat between the tibialis anterior and extensor hallucis longus.
- The Böhler approach facilitates exposure of the anterolateral distal tibia with medial retraction of the extensor digitorum longus and peroneus tertius. When using the Böhler approach, the superficial peroneal nerve must be isolated and protected.
- Visualization of the tibial plafond articular surface is paramount for achieving an anatomical reduction. A "femoral" distractor, as well as a head light, should be a standard part of the pilon fracture surgeon's armamentarium to facilitate the view of the fractured joint surface (Fig. 20–7).
- The distractor can be strategically placed along the medial surface, perpendicular to the shaft of the tibia and parallel to the floor. Distractor pin placement includes a talar body pin placed one thumb's breadth distal to the medial malleolus, as well as a pin in the proximal medial tibial shaft.
- Fracture reduction should proceed in a stepwise manner, typically building from the posterior to anterior.

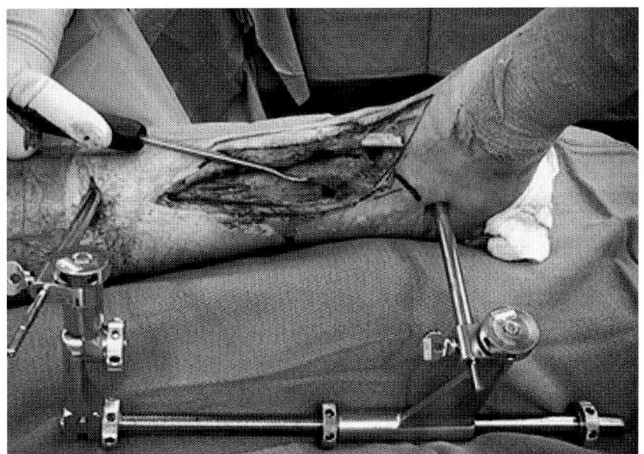

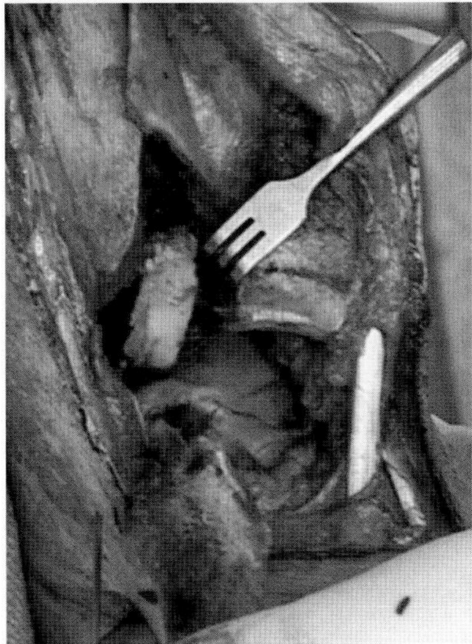

Figure 20–7: A femoral distractor is a useful tool during the definitive reconstruction of a pilon fracture. One proximal Shantz pin is placed in the medial tibia cephalad to the zone of injury, and a distal pin is typically placed in the talar body (one finger's breadth below the medial malleolus). Distraction allows for maintenance of longitudinal alignment while the articular surface is reconstructed. The distractor allows for superior joint visualization during plafond reduction. The talus serves as a perfect template for determining the position of comminuted articular segments. Also, the surgeon should use a head lamp to visualize the articular reduction, particularly in the context of the concave plafond.

The lateral fragments will typically be out to length due to their attachments to the fibula through the tibiofibular ligaments (assuming that the fibula length and rotation have been restored).

- Impacted articular fragments must be brought into their appropriate position, and some bone void filler should be packed behind the associated metaphyseal defect.
- Provisional K wires and bone reduction forceps should maintain the reduction before definitive fixation is placed.
- The articular reduction needs to be critically assessed with visual inspection in addition to intraoperative fluoroscopy. It is imperative to have a large fluoroscopy field of view, which allows for analysis of ankle alignment as well as articular reduction.
- The talar articular surface can be used as a template for judging the accuracy of the tibial plafond after the traction from the femoral distractor is let down.
- Strategic lag screws are placed to rigidly fix, and if appropriate to compress, the articular fragments.
- In many cases, the surgical tactic dictates that an anterolateral plate is applied, usually as a buttress for the often comminuted anterior surface. In other cases, a medial plate can bridge from the articular surface to the tibial shaft proximally.
- The plate can be slid under the soft tissues, with small stab incisions for proximal screw placement. This keeps the main incision and dissection limited to the articular surface.
- Low-profile implants are ideal for pilon fracture reconstruction, but the plate stem must be suitably sized for the typical metadiaphyseal extension (Fig. 20–8).
- The wound closure is of critical importance, and should be conducted after meticulous hemostasis, and over a deep suction drain to prevent excess skin tension.
- After capsular repair, the investing distal fascia and extensor retinaculum should be reapproximated to the best degree possible.
- Independent subcutaneous closure is avoided, and the skin is closed using a meticulous Allgöwer-Donati technique to maximize blood flow to the wound edges (Fig. 20–9).

Postoperative

- A splint is generally applied for 7-10 days to allow for sufficient wound healing prior to instituting a protocol of passive and active assisted range of motion exercise.
- Active range of motion exercise is encouraged after 6 weeks, during which time it is reasonable to consider partial weight bearing at 50 lbs and adding 10-15 lbs per week until the 3-month office visit.
- Generally, full weight bearing is encouraged at 3 months.
- A formal gait-training program is the best context in which to learn to wean crutches and transition to a cane.
- Pool therapy is a helpful adjunct for patients during the phase of increasing weight bearing.

Special Considerations in Open Fractures

- An open fracture is typically the result of high-energy trauma, implying significant bone and soft tissue injury.
- Prompt surgical debridement and irrigation is the mainstay of early operative management, with the chief goal of preventing septic complications.
- Bridging external fixation is appropriate management at the first debridement, to allow for soft tissue recovery and wound management.
- As an adjunct to surgical strategies, antibiotic and tetanus protocols should be administered in all open plafond fractures.
- Muscle flap coverage, when necessary, should be performed soon after the first debridement, and coordinated with the second look and debridement, ideally immediately after the definitive fixation.
- Although with modern surgical techniques, limb salvage is typically the best option for open pilon fractures, amputation should be considered in the mangled extremity, in non-ambulators, and in the multiply injured elderly patient with comorbidities.
- Elective bone grafting procedures to fill bone voids from open fracture management should be planned at 6-12 weeks.

Complications

Soft Tissue

Wound Problems and Infection

- Historically, an alarmingly high percentage of pilon fractures have developed wound complications, reported in the range of 12-40%. Wound complications after pilon fracture management often are a precursor to the development of deep infection.
- Partial and full-thickness skin necrosis, wound dehiscence, superficial infection, and deep infection are all reported complications of pilon fracture management.
- Application of the principles described above should help to decrease such problems to a manageable incidence somewhere below 5% in closed fractures. Early soft tissue coverage, ideally within 7 days, will minimize such complications in open injuries.

Arthrofibrosis

- Ankle function rarely returns to normal, even with superior operative strategies.
- Periarticular scar formation limits the final range of motion in high-energy pilon patterns.
- Temporary bridging external fixation, which immobilizes the ankle joint, may contribute to ankle arthrofibrosis.

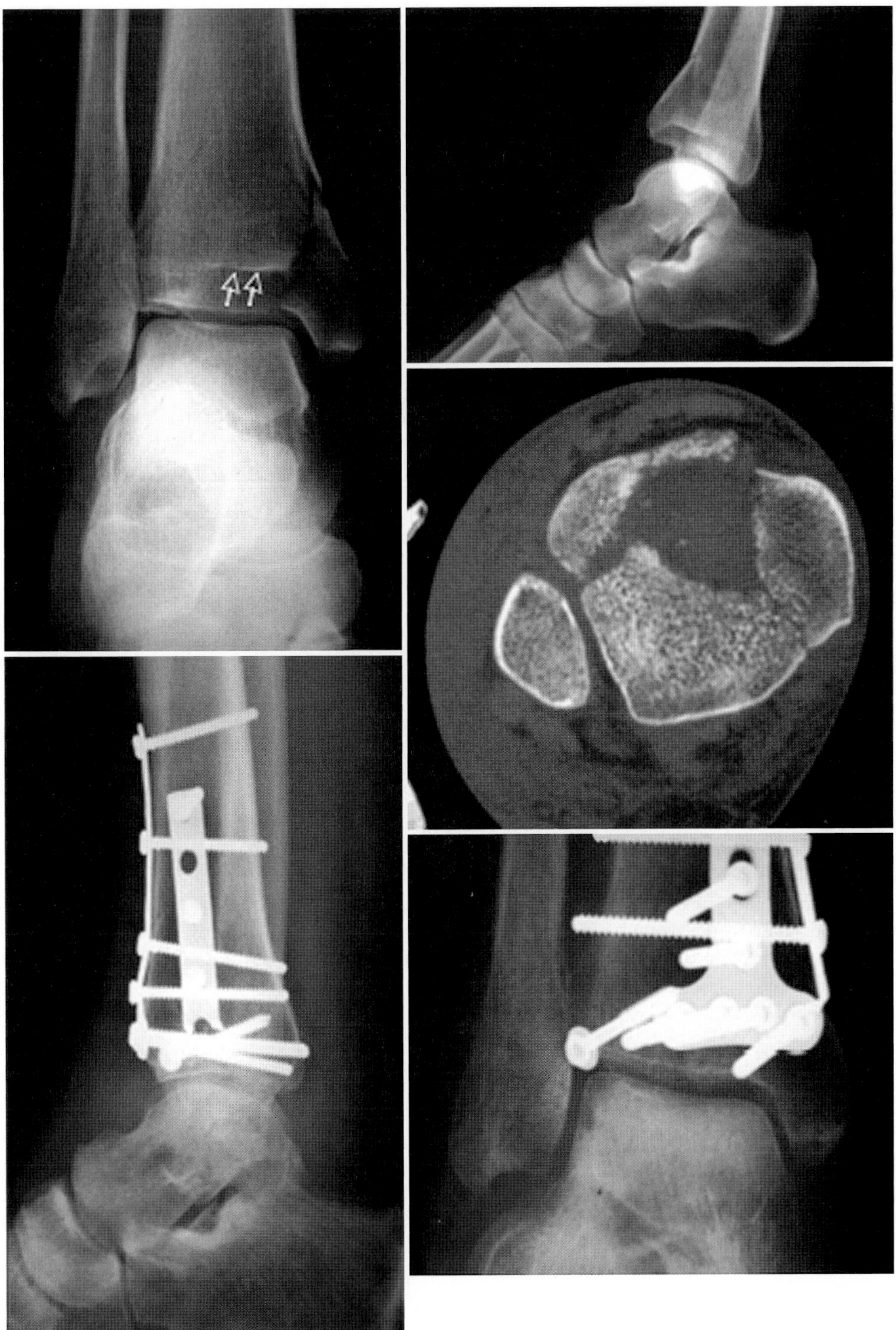

Figure 20–8: Definitive reconstruction of a 43B pilon fracture after a staged protocol. An anterior approach was utilized to anatomically reduce the anterior plafond impaction injury (arrows), as noted on plain radiography as well as with post-external fixation CT scan. In this fracture pattern, buttress plate fixation both anterior and medial is necessary, in addition to lag screw fixation of the joint surface. Bone void filler was used to fill the metaphyseal defect left after disimpaction of the articular segment.

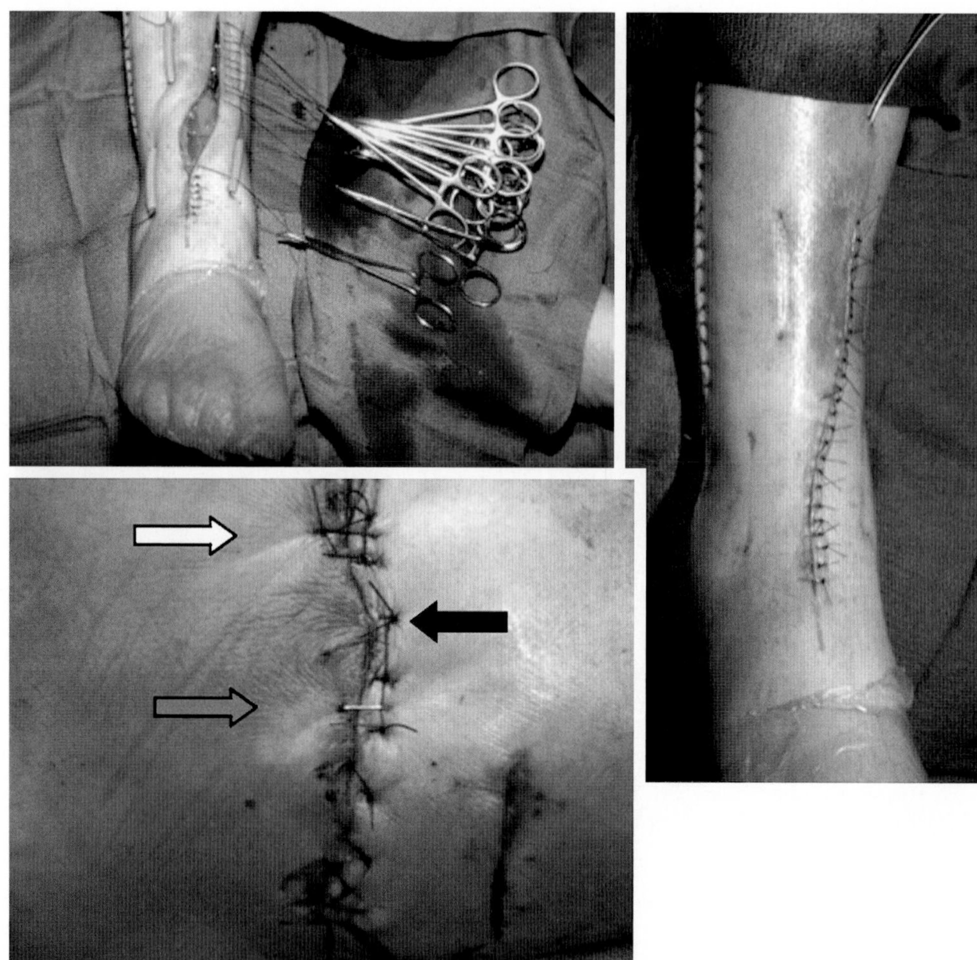

Figure 20–9: **Recommended closure technique for pilon fracture open reduction and internal fixation: The Allgöwer-Donati technique maximizes blood flow to the wound edges. Allgöwer-Donati technique (black arrow) compared with simple suturing (white) and skin stapling (grey). Note that with the other techniques, the skin edges are not perfectly opposed, and significant blanching of the skin is evident.**

- Early motion protocols after treatment with non-spanning external fixation or ORIF improves ankle range of motion at union. However, in the typical case with initial external fixation and then short-term postoperative splinting (after definitive ORIF), motion exercises do not begin until more than a month after injury.

Osseous

- Quality of articular reduction positively correlates with clinical outcome. Non-anatomical reductions with articular step-offs and gaps predispose the ankle joint to pain as well as early arthrosis.
- However, a perfect-looking joint on x-ray does not equate to a perfect or even good outcome, and an imperfect reduction does not always guarantee bad results.
- In cases of anatomical joint reductions after high-energy pilon fractures, degenerative joint disease may still occur. At the time of plafond fracture, an unpredictable percentage of the cartilaginous surface is irreversibly damaged. Impacted articular segments are often devascularized at the time of injury, occasionally resulting in osteonecrosis of the joint segment and cartilage loss.
- Injudicious periosteal or capsular stripping during ORIF can also devascularize segments of articular surface, leading to iatrogenic-induced focal osteonecrosis and resultant joint arthrosis.
- Particular emphasis should be given by the surgeon to preserve the blood supply to the major fragments, particularly the vulnerable anterolateral fragment and its soft tissue hinge that receives blood supply from the anterolateral sleeve of tissue corresponding with anterior syndesmotic attachments.
- This anterior fragment, often associated with the greatest degree of comminution, is vulnerable to avascular necrosis and thus susceptible to collapse with premature loading.
- First-line treatment for symptomatic ankle arthritis includes non-steroidal antiinflammatory medication.

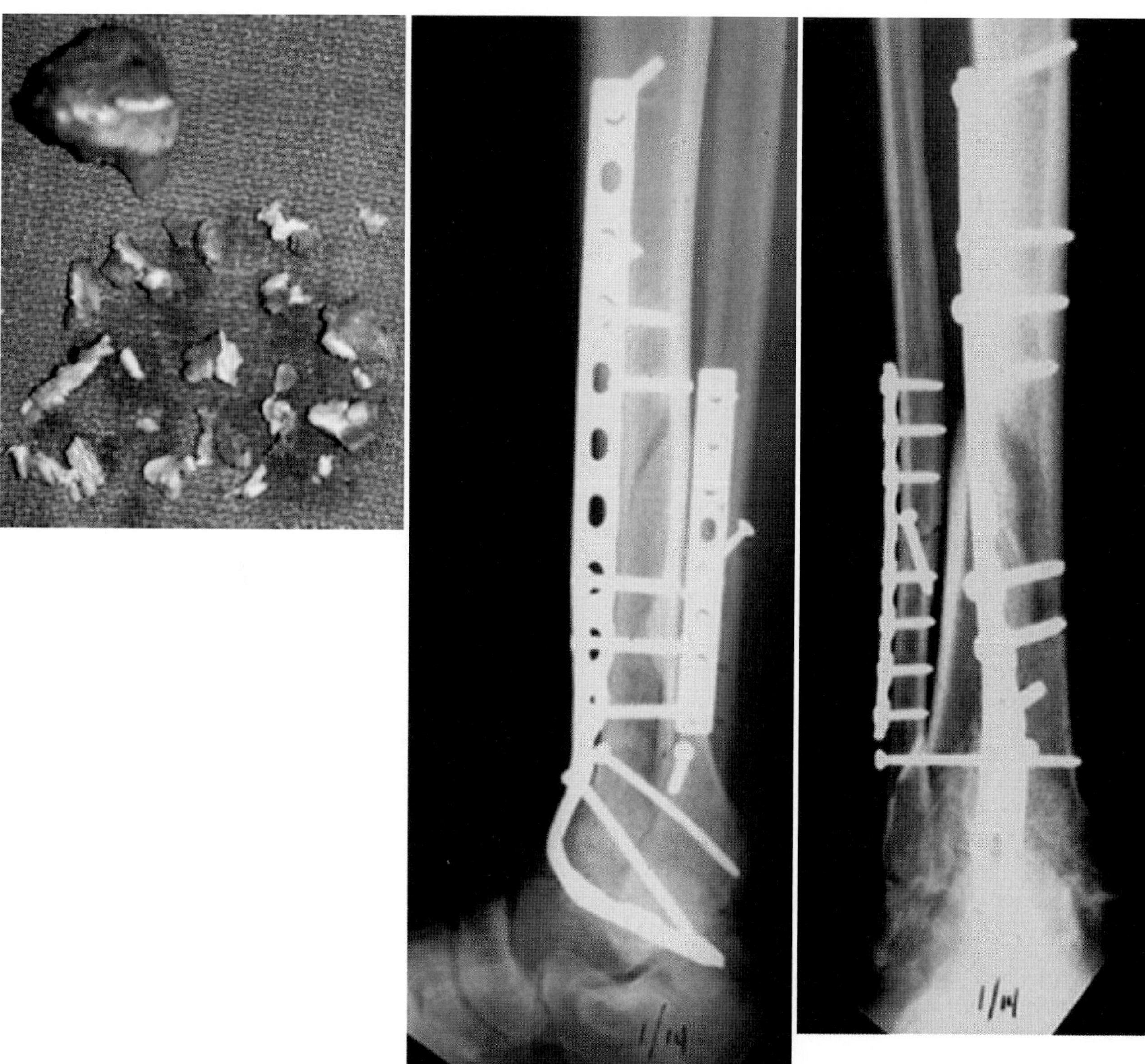

Figure 20–10: Ankle arthrodesis is both a primary as well as a later reconstruction option for pilon fractures. Extremely rare, consideration for primary fusion surgery should be contemplated when extensive comminution of the articular surface precludes stable reduction and anatomical restoration of the joint surface. However, more commonly arthrodesis is indicated for posttraumatic ankle degenerative joint disease. Fusion was chosen as a primary treatment option in this severely comminuted pilon fracture.

- An ankle orthosis, such as a double upright brace, functionally prevents ankle motion and may decrease arthritis symptoms.
- A cane used in the opposite hand decreases ankle joint reactive forces, which may decrease the symptoms of posttraumatic degenerative joint disease.
- Ankle fusion is the gold standard salvage procedure for the treatment of posttraumatic ankle arthrosis (Fig. 20–10). A properly performed ankle arthrodesis can restore the mechanical alignment of the hindfoot and achieve solid union across the tibiotalar interface.

References

Outcomes After Pilon Fracture

Babis GC, Vayanos ED, Papaioannou N et al. (1997) Results of surgical treatment of tibial plafond fractures. Clin Orthop 341: 99-105.

Retrospective study of 82 pilon fractures, of which 67 fractures were available for long-term follow-up (average 8 years). Fractures studied included Ruedi-Allgöwer types 1 (8), 2 (33), and 3 (26). Formal ORIF was performed in the majority of cases (50). The other 16 fractures were managed by limited ORIF (9) or external fixation (8). Clinical outcomes measured by the method of Burwell and Charnley were superior for the more simple fracture patterns (i.e. type 1 versus 3). Clinical results were correlated with the quality of reduction obtained at the index operation. Patients treated with traditional ORIF fared better than those treated with other techniques. Despite encouraging patient outcomes, serious complications were reported, including infection (11), skin necrosis (2), non-union (4), malunion (2), and deep vein thrombosis (1).

Pollak AN, McCarthy ML, Bess RS et al. (2003) Outcomes after treatment of high-energy tibial plafond fractures. J Bone Joint Surg Am 85A(10): 1893-1900.

Validated general health and functional outcome measurements were utilized to retrospectively determine the impact after treatment for a pilon fracture (2- to 5-year follow-up). Patients studied (n = 80) were treated with either ORIF or external fixation with or without limited ORIF. As reflected by the 36-Item Short-Form Health Survey, patients after pilon fracture have worse scores than the general population norms, especially for role disability due to physical health problems and physical function. Patients have difficulty returning to work after pilon fractures (43%). Patients reported persistent pain (33%), stiffness (35%), and swelling (29%). Patients also required orthotics (25%) and walking aids (13%). Superior results were obtained with patients treated with ORIF versus external fixation in terms of pain, range of motion, and ambulatory dysfunction ($P < 0.05$).

Sands A, Grujic L, Byck DC et al. (1998) Clinical and functional outcomes of internal fixation of displaced pilon fractures. Clin Orthop 347: 131-137.

Outcomes and complications following ORIF for 64 pilon fractures (50 closed, 14 open fractures) were retrospectively studied. Deep infection occurred in 5% of patients. Other complications included non-union (2%), delayed union (5%), malunion (6%), fixation failure (6%), and deep vein thrombosis (5%). Two patients required early salvage with ankle arthrodesis within 4 years of injury. 36-Item Short-Form Health Survey outcome scores were performed on 27 patients, revealing that patients after ORIF for plafond fractures fare worse than the general population as well as patients treated for tibial plateau fractures in terms of physical function.

Classification of Pilon Fractures

Swiontkowski MF, Sands AK, Agel J et al. (1997) Interobserver variation in the AO/OTA fracture classification system for pilon fractures: Is there a problem? J Orthop Trauma 11(7): 467-470.

Although many classification schemes have been used to describe pilon fracture patterns, the AO/OTA comprehensive system is currently the preferred method for both clinical and research purposes. The authors in this study determined that medical personnel with varied levels of expertise display a "moderate agreement" when asked to classify AO/OTA 43 injuries. For the 84 pilon fracture radiograph set, the raters agreed on fracture type, group, and subgroup 57%, 43%, and 41% of the time, respectively. The authors note that invariably, the inherent flaw in any classification system is "forcing a continuous variable [fracture], into a dichotomous variable [classification system]."

Work-up of Pilon Fractures

Tornetta P III, Gorup J. (1996) Axial computed tomography of pilon fractures. Clin Orthop 323: 273-276.

Twenty-two pilon fractures were studied prospectively to determine whether CT provided the surgeon with fracture pattern data that was not ascertained from plain radiography alone (anteroposterior, lateral, oblique, and traction anteroposterior). Compared with plain x-ray alone, CT scan predicted an increased number of fracture fragments, impaction, and increased comminution in 12, 6, and 11 patients, respectively. Precise location of the major fracture line with CT determined the most efficient operative approach (anteromedial versus anterolateral). Operative plan was influenced by CT scan in 64% of cases. Fracture pattern determination was enhanced with CT in 82% of pilon fractures studied. The operative experience in this series was more efficient in 77% of cases as a direct result of preoperative CT scan use.

Complications After Untimely ORIF of Pilon Fractures

McFerran MA, Smith SW, Boulas HJ et al. (1992) Complications encountered in the treatment of pilon fractures. J Orthop Trauma 6(2): 195-200.

Fifty-two pilon fractures were studied retrospectively to determine complication rates after surgical management. Fracture patterns defined by the Ruedi-Allgöwer classification included 27% type 1, 33% type 2, and 40% type 3 pilon fractures. Eleven fractures were open. Early ORIF was the index procedure in 88% of fractures. The overall complication rate was 40%, accounting for 77 additional procedures on 21 patients. Wound breakdown and/or deep infection occurred in 14 cases (27%). A majority of complications occurred within 3 weeks of the primary procedure.

Teeny SM, Wiss DA. (1993) Open reduction and internal fixation of tibial plafond fractures: Variables contributing to poor results and complications. Clin Orthop 292: 108-107.

A retrospective review. Sixty pilon fractures managed with ORIF were studied, highlighting the complications encountered in higher energy injuries. The fracture patterns included a majority of Ruedi-Allgöwer type 2 (27) and 3 (30) injuries, of which 12 were open fractures. Index surgery was performed at an average of 5.6 days for closed injuries. Quality of reduction correlated with clinical scores. However, despite an "anatomic reduction" in 22 fractures, good-excellent results were recorded in only 41% of these cases. Overall, 50% of patients had a major complication. However, in type 3 fractures a rate of 70% was reported, including wound problems and deep infection (37%), malunion (23%), and non-union (27%). Sixty percent of type 3 fractures required at least one reoperation, including a 26%

conversion rate to ankle arthrodesis over an average 2.5-year follow-up period.

Cast Treatment of Pilon Fractures

Bourne RB, Rorabeck CH, Macnab BA. (1983) Intra-articular fractures of the distal tibia: The pilon fracture. J Trauma 23(7): 591-596.

Retrospective review of 42 pilon fractures (11 type 1, 12 type 2, and 19 type 3) with an average follow-up of 53 months. Nine fractures were open injuries. ORIF was performed in 33 cases. Nine cases were managed with closed reduction and cast immobilization. Poor results (according to the Burwell and Charnley criteria) were reported for a majority of cases treated with plaster immobilization (7/9). ORIF predictably yielded good to fair results in fractures that were reduced anatomically. However, the ability to achieve an anatomical reduction in type 3 injuries was more difficult (2/19 cases), yielding only 44% good-fair results with these higher energy fractures. Furthermore, significant complications occurred in patients with type 3 injuries treated with ORIF, including infection, non-union, malalignment, and early ankle arthrosis. Seven pilon fractures (6/7 type 3) were salvaged with arthrodesis.

External Fixator Management of Pilon Fractures

Bone L, Stegemann P, McNamara K et al. (1993) External fixation of severely comminuted and open tibial pilon fractures. Clin Orthop 292: 101-107.

Twenty pilon fractures were treated with limited open osteosynthesis followed by application of a spanning external fixator as a neutralization device. All injuries were a result of high-energy mechanisms (Ruedi-Allgöwer type 3), with 12 open fractures. All fractures eventually healed, although three fractures required further intervention for a delayed or non-union. One malunion occurred. No wound problems or deep infections were reported. Pin tract problems occurred in two cases. Within the follow-up period (average 1.5 years), two patients underwent ankle arthrodesis for severe joint arthrosis, while an additional four patients had radiographic evidence of ankle arthritis.

McDonald MG, Burgess RC, Bolano LE et al. (1996) Ilizarov treatment of pilon fractures. Clin Orthop 325: 232-238.

Thirteen pilon fractures treated with the diaphyseal-epiphyseal Ilizarov external fixator were retrospectively studied at an average of 16-month follow-up. Fracture types included one type 1, eight type 2, and four type 3 fractures. The surgical strategy involved indirect joint reductions when possible (10). Complications included one non-union, one delayed union, one malunion, and nine superficial pin tract infections. One ankle fusion was required after initial Ilizarov frame management. No deep infections were reported.

Pugh KJ, Wolinsky PR, McAndrew MP et al. (1999) Tibial pilon fractures: A comparison of treatment methods. J Trauma 47(5): 937.

Two different methods of limited ORIF with external fixation including hybrid (n = 15) and spanning external fixation (n = 21) were compared with ORIF (n = 24) in this retrospective study of 60 pilon fractures. Sixty-eight percent of cases were AO/OTA 43C, with 26 open fractures. Major complications in the ORIF cohort included three deep infections resulting in two infected non-unions. Serious complications encountered in the external fixator group included three deep wound infections, one wound slough, three non-unions, and two ankles requiring fusion. However, the only statistically significant difference with regard to postoperative complications was an increased rate of malunion in the external fixator versus ORIF group (P = 0.03).

Tornetta P III, Weiner L, Bergman M et al. (1993) Pilon fractures: Treatment with combined internal and external fixation. J Orthop Trauma 7: 489-496.

A prospective study reported the outcomes of 26 patients treated with limited internal fixation and application of a hybrid non-spanning external fixator. Seventeen fractures were intraarticular, with 76% Ruedi-Allgöwer type 3 (13). Sixty-nine percent of fractures were associated with severe soft tissue injury (open fixation or Tscherne 2-3). Definitive surgical stabilization was delayed to allow for healing of the soft tissue envelope. At surgery, length was achieved with fibula plating or with an AO distractor. Non-displaced fractures were managed with percutaneous screws. Formal incisions were made over the primary fracture line to minimize iatrogenic soft tissue injury. The joint surface was reconstructed with screw fixation while the fixator served as a neutralization device. Eighty percent excellent/good results were reported overall, and 69% for type 3 fractures according to Tornetta's grading system. Only one deep infection in this series.

Watson JT, Moed BR, Berton R et al. (2000) Pilon fractures: Treatment protocol based on severity of soft tissue injury. Clin Orthop 375: 78-90.

One hundred seven pilon fractures were managed according to a prospective protocol based on grade of soft tissue compromise. Formal ORIF was the approach used for closed fractures Tscherne grades 0-1. Tscherne grades 2-3 and all open fractures were treated with a small wire ring fixator with or without limited ORIF. A majority (75% ORIF, 81% external fixation) had a good or excellent result according to the modified Mazur score considering all pilon fracture types (average 4.9-year follow-up). However, only 60% of AO/OTA type C fractures had favorable outcomes treated with either ORIF or external fixation. In the ORIF group, complications included non-union (11%), malunion (4%), symptomatic hardware (27%), and arthrosis requiring fusion (8%). Wound problems (14%) occurred in only 43C fractures after ORIF, resulting in two deep infections (5%). Pin tract problems occurred in all patients treated with external fixation, but no deep infections were reported. Non-union (3%), malunion (5%), and arthrosis requiring fusion (7%) were reported only in type C injuries managed with a fixator.

Two-stage Pilon Fracture Protocol

Anglen JO. (1999) Early outcome of hybrid external fixation for fracture of the distal tibia. J Orthop Trauma 13(2): 92-97.

A retrospective review was performed to determine the early results of patients treated by protocol with either staged ORIF (n = 19) or hybrid external fixation (n = 29) with or without limited ORIF. According to protocol, cases with severe soft tissue injury or "highly comminuted or longitudinally extensive fracture patterns" were managed with external fixation. Complications were more frequent in the external fixator group, including six non-unions, seven wire infections, three pin infections, three wound problems, one joint sepsis, one flexor tendon tethering, and one nerve injury. In the ORIF cohort, delaying surgery until soft tissue recovery resulted in 100% union rate, with only minor complications.

Helfet DL, Koval K, Pappas J et al. (1994) Intraarticular "pilon" fracture of the tibia. Clin Orthop 298: 221-228.

Thirty-four pilon fractures were reported, including 26 type 2 and 8 type 3 injuries managed with formal ORIF (28), external fixation (3), and limited internal and external fixation (3). Eighteen cases were open fractures, and eight were managed with muscle flap coverage. Fifteen fractures were initially managed with preliminary external fixation and fibula plating (11) before definitive management, which occurred at an average of 7.3 days (0-35 days) from injury presentation. Excellent-adequate clinical results were reported in 77% and 62% of type 2 and 3 fracture patterns, respectively. Complications included delayed union (1), malunion (4), and deep infection (2) and post-traumatic arthritis (3). One infection occurred in a patient treated with ORIF on the day of injury. The authors advocated delaying formal ORIF until the soft tissue envelope is optimized to accept surgical fixation.

Patterson MJ, Cole JD. (1999) Two-staged delayed open reduction and internal fixation of severe pilon fractures. J Orthop Trauma 13(2): 85-91.

Twenty-two consecutive AO/OTA 43C3 pilon fractures were managed with a staged protocol consisting of immediate fibula fixation (n = 20) and placement of an external fixator in an effort to restore length, alignment, and stability to the soft tissue and bony anatomy. ORIF was delayed until soft tissue recovery from the initial trauma (average 24 days). This operative strategy avoided wound problems and deep infection, which were frequent complications of premature ORIF reported in earlier literature. Clinical grades reported according to the criteria of Burwell and Charnley demonstrated good results in 77% of cases at an average of 22-month follow-up. Outcomes correlated with accuracy of reduction. In this series, complications included one non-union, one malunion, and two cases of early ankle arthrosis necessitating arthrodesis.

Sirkin M, Sanders R, DiPasquale T et al. (1999) A staged protocol for soft tissue management in the treatment of complex pilon injuries. J Orthop Trauma 13(2): S32-S38.

In an effort to minimize the soft tissue complications frequently reported after untimely ORIF of high-energy pilon fractures, the authors retrospectively studied the wound complications after a staged approach. Fifty-six fractures were initially managed with lateral column stabilization (in the presence of an associated fibula fracture) and a spanning external fixator, followed by delayed ORIF once the soft tissue envelope had matured. Forty-eight AO/OTA type C fractures (29 closed, 19 open) were available for a minimum of 1-year follow-up. In the closed fracture group, five cases of partial skin necrosis occurred, which resolved with local skin care and oral antibiotics. Only one case of deep infection was reported in the closed pilon fracture cohort. In the open fracture group, partial skin necrosis (10.5%) and deep infection (10.5%) were reported.

CHAPTER 21

Calcaneus Fractures

Rahul Banerjee* and Florian Nickisch§

*M.D., Clinical Instructor, Department of Orthopaedic Surgery, Texas Tech University Health Sciences Center, Interm Chief of Orthopaedic Trauma, William Beaumont Army Medical Center, El Paso, Texas, and Chief of Orthopaedics, 49th Medical Group, Holloman Air Force Base, New Mexico.

§M.D., OL Miller Foot and Ankle Institute at OrthoCarolina, Charlotte, NC

- Calcaneus fractures account for approximately 2% of all fractures. The calcaneus is the most frequently fractured tarsal bone, representing 60% of all tarsal fractures.
- A high-energy calcaneus fracture is often a life-altering event for the affected individual. The socioeconomic burden of calcaneus fractures is significant, as 90% of these fractures occur in working individuals of ages 20 to 40.

Historical Perspective

- Surgical treatment of the calcaneus was discouraged through most of the early twentieth century (Fig. 21–1). The treatment of acute fractures was all but abandoned, with a focus instead on late reconstruction of healed malunions. In 1916, Cotton and Henderson concluded that, "The man who breaks his heel bone is done." Similarly, in 1926 Conn wrote, "Calcaneus fractures are serious and disabling injuries in which the end results continue to be incredibly bad."
- Böhler advocated open reduction of calcaneus fractures as early as 1931. However, due to the limitations of poor diagnostic tools and the lack of appropriate implants to achieve stable fixation, the complication rate (i.e. wound problems, infection, and loss of reduction) was high.
- Throughout North America, primary triple or isolated subtalar arthrodesis was popularized during the 1930s and 1940s. The results of those treatments continued to be poor. In 1942, Bankart concluded that "the results of crush fractures of the os calcis are rotten." In 1958, Lindsey and Dewar studied the long-term outcome of calcaneus fractures and concluded that non-operative treatment provided the best outcome. Throughout the 1960s and 1970s, non-operative treatment continued to be the treatment of choice.
- Treatment options for calcaneus fractures remain controversial. However, advances in radiographic imaging, surgical technique, and a better understanding of the pathoanatomy of calcaneus fractures have led to improved results with surgical treatment of these challenging fractures over the past 20 years.

Mechanism of Injury

- Most intraarticular calcaneus fractures are the result of an **axial load** applied directly to the heel. High-energy intraarticular calcaneus fractures are usually the result of a fall from height or a motor vehicle accident. The actual fracture pattern is influenced by the position of the foot and the subtalar joint, the force of the impact, and the quality of the patient's bone.
- Extraarticular fractures are more frequently the result of a twisting or an avulsive force. Isolated fractures of the anterior process of the calcaneus may be the result of forced inversion of the plantar flexed foot, resulting in an avulsive force created by the insertion of the bifurcate ligament. Alternatively, forced dorsiflexion and eversion may compress the anterior process between the cuboid and the talus. Avulsion fractures of the tuberosity may be caused by a sudden forceful contraction of the

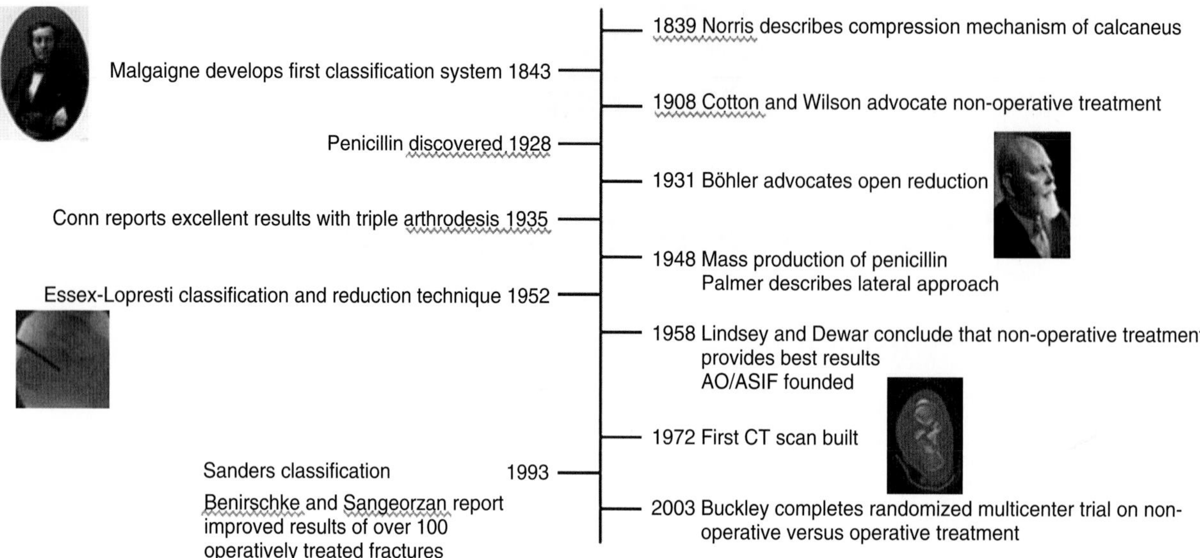

Figure 21–1: The history of calcaneus fractures demonstrates an oscillation between non-operative treatment and surgical intervention. Advances such as antibiotic therapy, the discovery of the computed tomography scan, and improved surgical techniques have led to improved outcomes for surgical treatment in the past two decades. AO, Arbeitsgemeinschaft für Osteosynthesefragen; ASIF, Association for the Study of Internal Fixation; CT, computed tomography.

gastrocnemius-soleus muscle complex, and may occur in patients with a previously tight heel cord (e.g. diabetics).

- In intraarticular fractures, the energy imparted to the calcaneus during axial loading results in two characteristic primary fracture lines (Fig. 21–2). The first fracture line usually starts at the crucial angle of Gissane (Fig. 21–3). The lateral process of the talus acts as a wedge, dividing the calcaneus into an anterior and a posterior half. The anteromedial fragment, also called the constant fragment, usually maintains its relationship with the talus, tethered by the strong interosseous and medial ligaments. The posterolateral fragment usually displaces laterally and into varus alignment. Secondary fracture lines travel in the sagittal plane along the length of the bone in an anterior and a posterior direction. These fracture lines can travel into the calcaneocuboid joint, split the anterior facet, or exit the body of the calcaneus medially or laterally.
- In higher energy fractures, additional secondary fracture lines develop, resulting in higher degrees of comminution.

Initial Evaluation and Management

- Initial evaluation of all patients with calcaneus fractures involves a thorough physical examination. The mechanism of injury (**axial loading**) often results in concomitant injuries to the lower extremities and the spine (Box 21–1). Therefore careful examination is warranted.
- Lumbar spine fractures may be associated with calcaneus fractures, especially when bilateral. Some would argue for routine lumbar spine radiographs in any patient with a calcaneus fracture from a fall.
- The injured foot is placed into a bulky dressing or a foam boot and is elevated. Often, even in cases of isolated calcaneus fractures, the patient may require admission for pain management.
- The neurovascular status of the fractured extremity should be carefully tested and documented. Numbness or a subjective decrease in sensation may be an early warning sign of impending compartment syndrome.
- Evaluation for **compartment syndrome** is essential on initial evaluation, and serial examination should follow. Compartment syndrome occurs in up to 10% of patients with displaced calcaneus fractures. Compartment syndrome may present as excruciating pain, an alteration in sensation, or pain with passive motion of the toes.
- Of course, many patients with calcaneus fractures will have pain with passive toe motion, because the origin of the flexor digitorum brevis is on the calcaneus. It is also common to see plantar nerve paresthesias with high-energy injuries, so the entire clinical picture must be taken into account when evaluating for compartment syndrome.
- Any patient with suspected compartment syndrome should undergo invasive measurement of the compartments of the foot (Fig. 21–4 and Box 21–2). Absolute compartment pressure > 30 mmHg or a 40 mmHg difference between the measured pressure and the patient's diastolic pressure is an indication for foot fasciotomies.

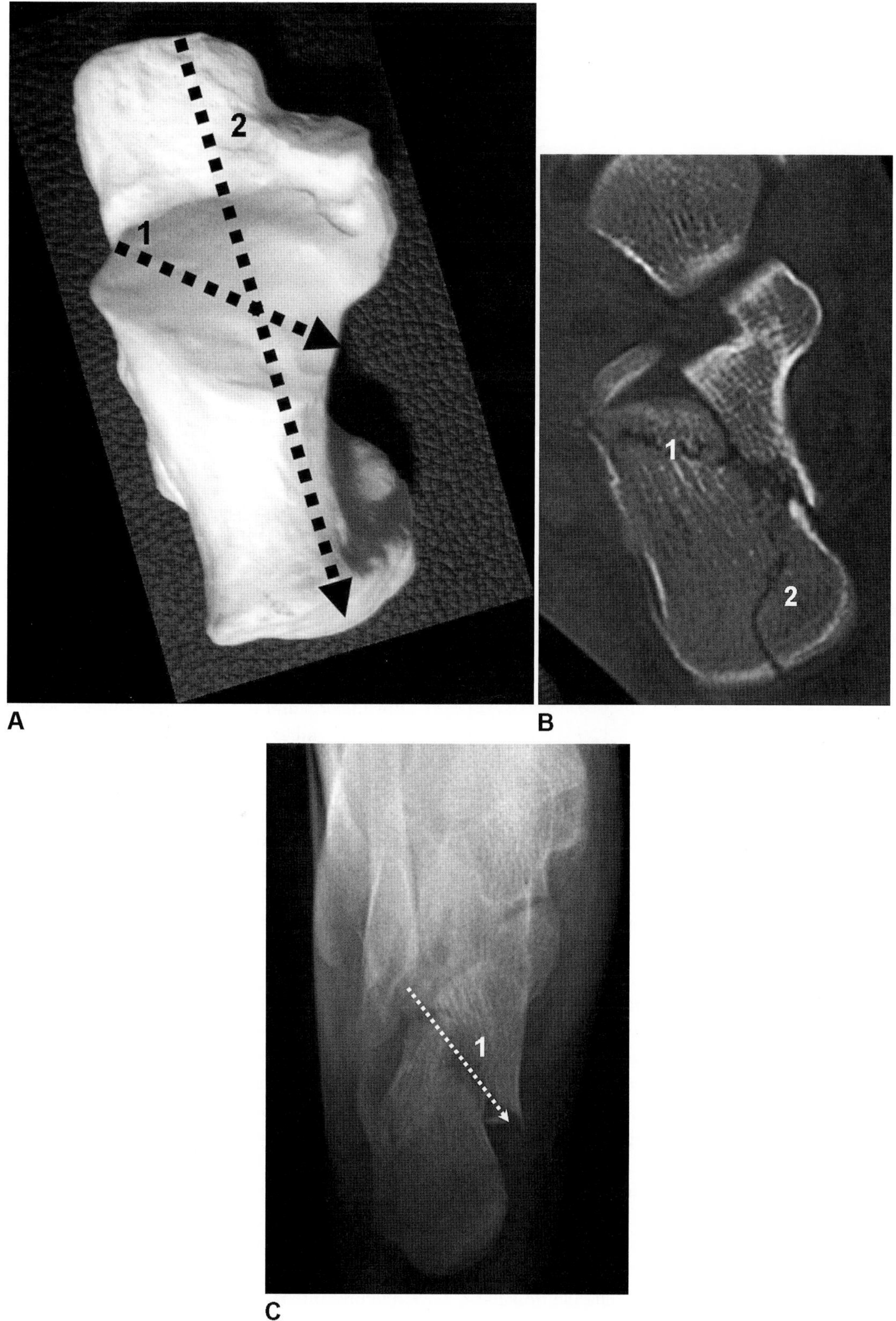

Figure 21–2: Examination of intraarticular calcaneus fractures demonstrates two characteristic fracture lines as described by Carr et al. These fracture lines are depicted in the diagram **A**, and seen on axial computed tomography scan **B**, and a Harris axial x-ray of the calcaneus **C**.

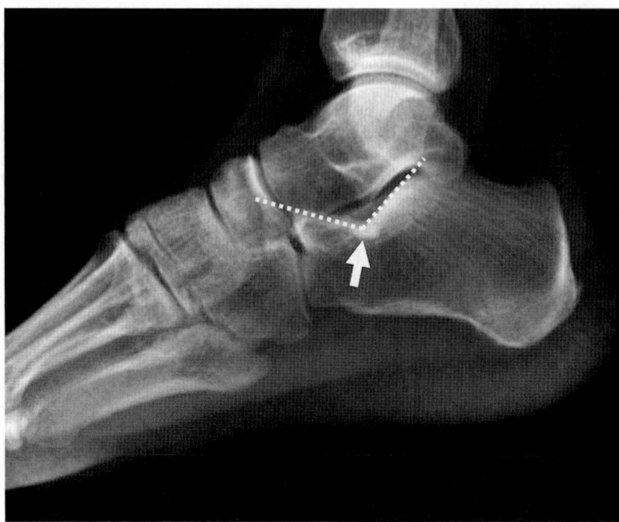

Figure 21–3: The primary fracture line usually begins at the crucial angle of Gissane (white arrow). The angle is subtended by a line drawn along the anterior process and the posterior facet (dotted line).

Box 21–1 Associated Skeletal Injuries

- Lumbar spine fracture
- Tibia fracture (pilon, plateau)
- Ankle fracture
- Additional foot fracture
- Acetabular fracture

- The energy imparted to the foot in calcaneus fractures is shared equally by the bone and soft tissues. Therefore evaluation and close monitoring of the soft tissues is important. Patients will often present with fracture blisters (Fig. 21–5), which result when there is cleavage at the dermal-epidermal junction. Blisters should be covered with sterile dressings and allowed to drain on their own. If the patient is to undergo surgical treatment, the operation is delayed until the blisters have reepithelialized and skin wrinkles are visible over the lateral aspect of the hindfoot. Sequential compression devices for the foot may be of some use in helping to control edema in the preoperative phase.
- An exception to delayed treatment is in cases where the soft tissue may be threatened by a displaced fracture (Fig. 21–6). Tuberosity avulsion fractures may result in pressure over the skin of the posterior heel. The surgeon should consider urgent reduction to prevent additional soft tissue injury, which may quickly lead to full-thickness skin necrosis.
- Severe injuries may result in open fractures (Fig. 21–7). Open calcaneus fractures are rare and account for less than 10% of all calcaneus fractures. The traumatic wound tends to be on the **medial** side, caused by the sharp spike of the medial wall created by the primary fracture line. The tuberosity is dislocated laterally.
- Open fractures should be treated with urgent debridement. The medial wound is debrided. Closed or minimally invasive techniques to realign the calcaneus can be performed at the time of debridement, but given the severe soft tissue injury, extensile approaches should be avoided until the soft tissues have recovered. Occasionally, higher energy injuries will result in fractures with open wounds laterally. Care must be taken in the debridement of these wounds, as the lateral exposure may be later utilized for stabilization of the fracture.
- Inspection and palpation of the **peroneal tendons** should also be performed on initial examination. Often, the initial examination is difficult due to swelling and patient discomfort. The examination is repeated under anesthesia. Dislocated tendons usually reduce to their anatomical location with adequate reduction of the fracture.

Radiographic Evaluation

- Initial radiographic examination of the injured foot should include a lateral of the foot and ankle, a mortise view of the ankle, and dorsoplantar and oblique x-rays of the foot. In addition, an axial (Harris) view is obtained. The Harris view is obtained with the foot in maximal dorsiflexion and the x-ray beam angled 45° cephalad. A lateral and axial view of the contralateral foot should be obtained for comparison (Fig. 21–8).
- All patients with calcaneus fractures should undergo axial computed tomography (CT) scan of the foot. Coronal images can be obtained by flexing up the knee and resting the foot plantigrade on the CT table. Alternately, coronal and sagittal reconstructions can be created with appropriate software (Fig. 21–9).

Classification

- Several systems have been developed for classification of calcaneus fractures. Calcaneus fractures can be divided into two broad categories: intraarticular and extraarticular. Thirty percent of calcaneus fractures are extraarticular. Anterior process fractures represent the majority of extra-articular injuries and account for 10–15% of all calcaneus fractures. They are more common in women. Intraarticular fractures comprise 70% of all calcaneus fractures.
- In 1952, Essex-Lopresti classified intraarticular calcaneus fractures into two broad types: tongue-type and joint depression (Fig. 21–10). Essex-Lopresti's classification was primarily descriptive but also helps to distinguish those fractures that could be approached through percutaneous techniques (Essex-Lopresti maneuver).
- In 1993, Sanders classified calcaneus fractures based on the number and location of articular (posterior facet)

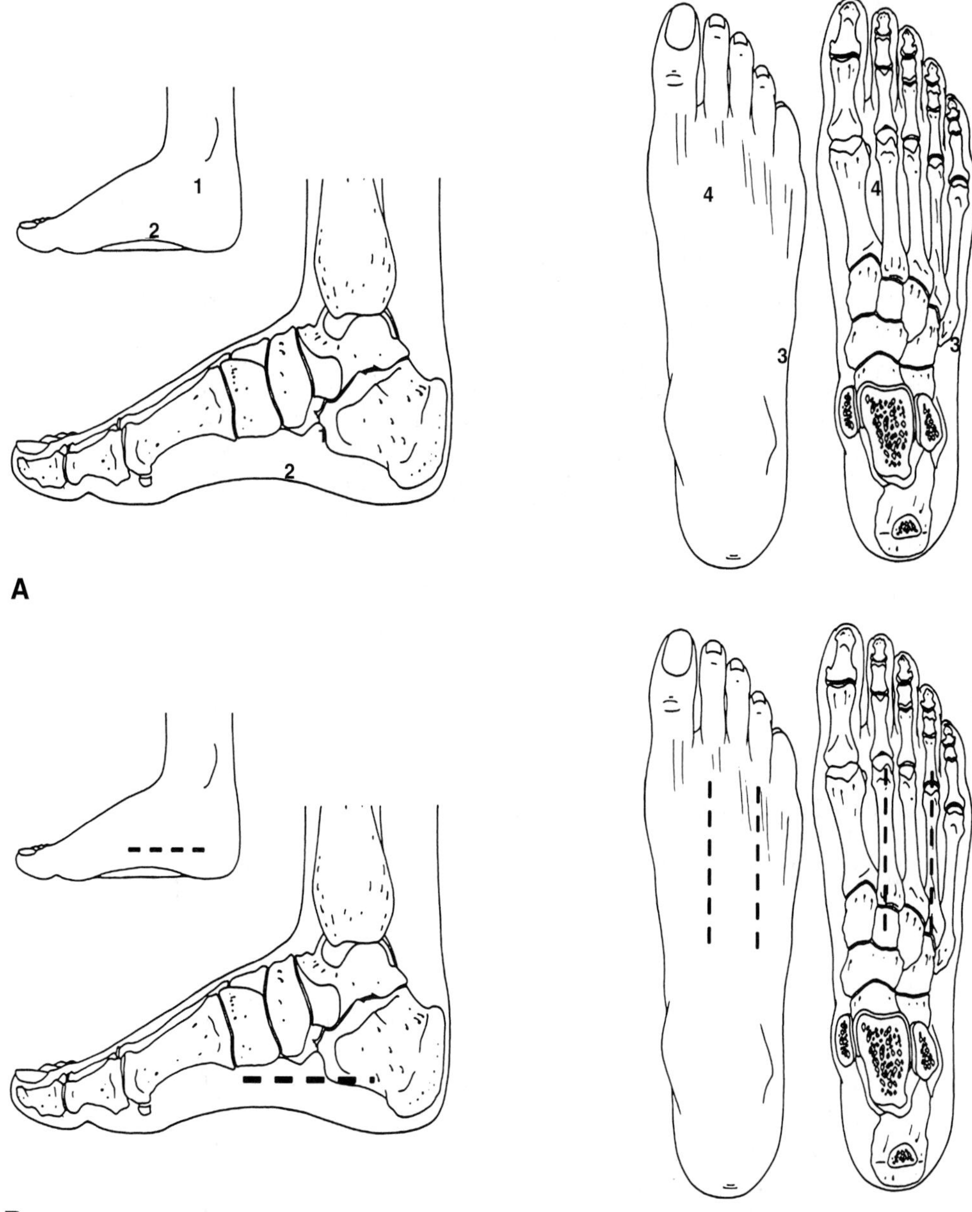

Figure 21–4: There are at least nine compartments in the foot. **A**, Compartment pressures are measured in four different locations in the foot. The needle of the pressure monitor is first inserted 4 cm inferior to the medial malleolus (1), which allows for measurement of the medial compartment in the hindfoot. The needle is then advanced through the medial intermuscular septum into the deep calcaneal compartment, and the pressure is measured. Next, the needle is inserted near the medial arch of the foot (2) in order to measure the superficial compartment. The needle is then inserted just inferior to the base of the fifth metatarsal (3) to measure the lateral compartment pressure. Finally, the needle is inserted in between the first and second metatarsals distally on the dorsum of the foot (4) in order to measure the interosseous compartment. The needle is then advanced deeper to measure the adductor compartment in the forefoot. Additional interosseous compartment measurements can be made by inserting the needle between the other metatarsals. **B**, If compartment releases are indicated, three incisions should be utilized. Two incisions are made over the dorsum of the foot, centered over second and fourth rays. The skin is divided, and the interosseous compartments are released on both sides of the metatarsal through each incision. An additional medial incision is also made. Through this medial incision, the fascia overlying the abductor hallucis muscle is released. The muscle is then retracted superiorly, and the dense fascia of the medial intermuscular septum is divided in order to release the deep calcaneal compartment. Care is taken in the release of this layer, as the lateral and medial plantar nerves lie just below the intermuscular septum. (From Cull P, ed. (1989) Sourcebook of Medical Illustration. Nashville: Parthenon Publishing Group.)

Box 21–2 Compartment Syndrome of the Foot

- Compartment syndrome of the foot should be suspected in all patients with calcaneus fractures.
- The most sensitive sign of compartment syndrome in the foot is severe pain with passive motion of the toes. An altered neurologic examination (diminished sensation) is also an early sign of compartment syndrome.
- The surgeon should not be deterred by the presence of pulses. If a compartment syndrome is suspected, compartment pressures of the foot should be measured using catheterization or a portable pressure monitor.
- Indications for fasciotomies are:
  - an absolute compartment pressure > 30 mmHg, or
  - a difference of less than 40 mmHg between the compartment pressure and the patient's diastolic blood pressure.

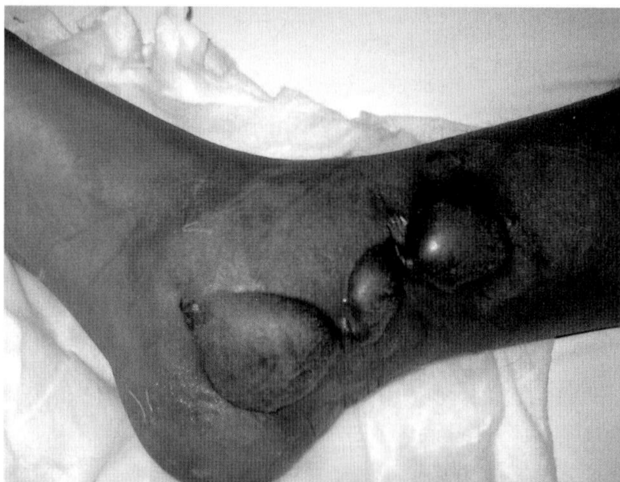

Figure 21–5: Fracture blisters around a calcaneus fracture following a motorcycle accident.

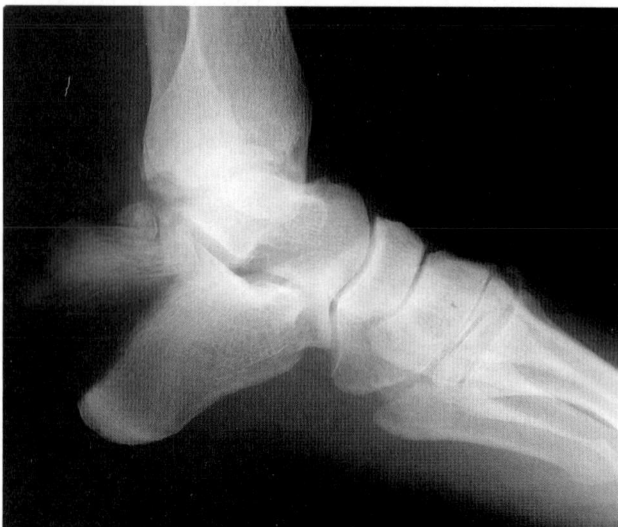

Figure 21–6: This patient suffered a displaced tuberosity fracture that was tenting the skin over the posterior heel. Urgent percutaneous reduction and fixation was performed to prevent skin necrosis.

fracture fragments (Fig. 21–11) as seen on CT scan. The Sanders classification is unique in that it is prognostic as well as descriptive. One of the limitations of the Sanders classification is that it is based purely on the posterior facet and does not address injuries to the remainder of the calcaneus.

- More recently, the Foot and Ankle Study Group of the Arbeitsgemeinschaft für Osteosynthesefragen (AO) has

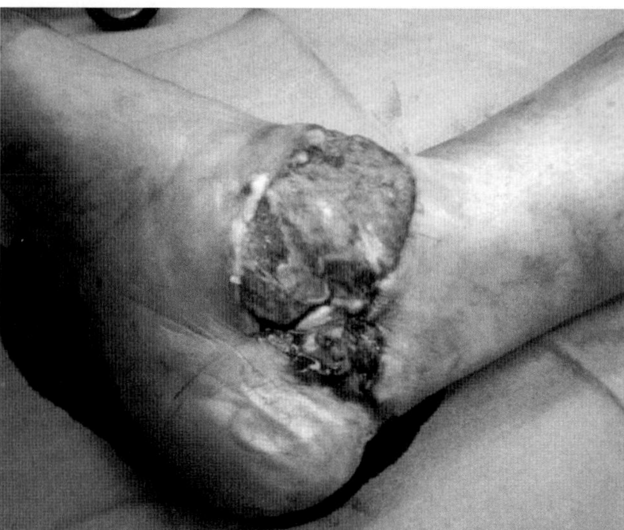

A

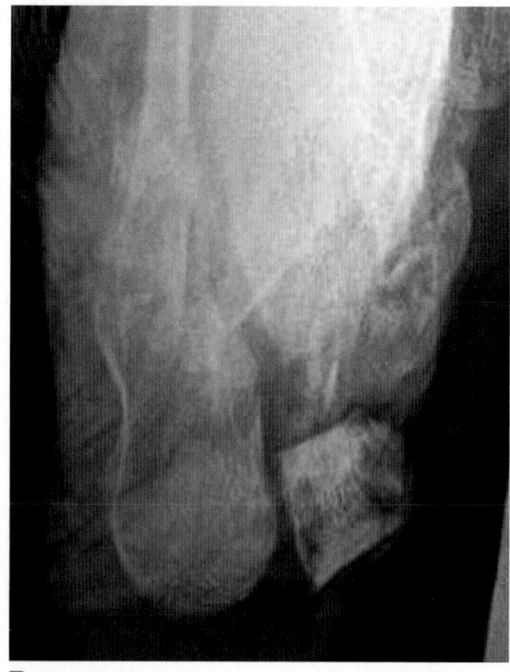

B

Figure 21–7: A 48-year-old woman sustained this open calcaneus fracture with an associated tibial pilon fracture in a motor vehicle accident. The photograph **A,** demonstrates the severe soft tissue injury. The axial **B** and lateral **C** x-rays demonstrate a fracture dislocation of the calcaneus. The patient underwent open reduction and internal fixation of the calcaneus through the open wound using K-wire fixation and with minimal additional soft tissue damage

Continued

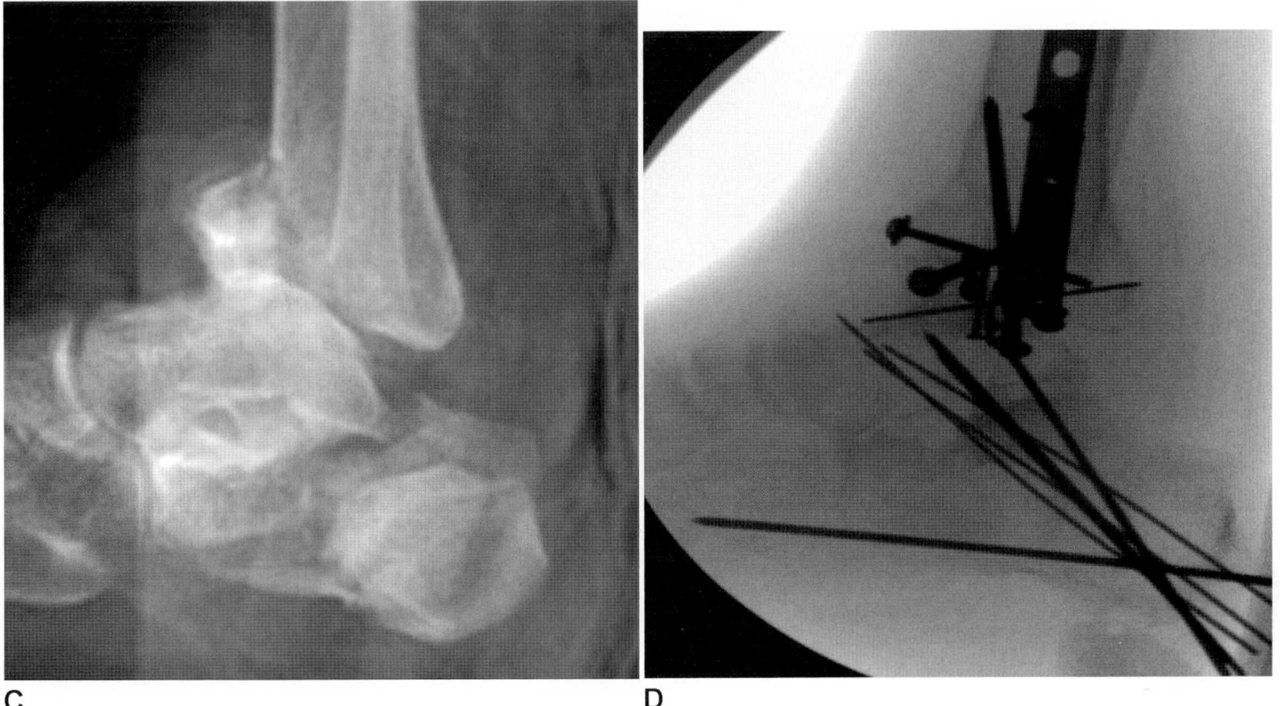

Figure 21–7: Cont'd (D). This case illustrates the importance of management of the injured soft tissues in open calcaneus fractures.

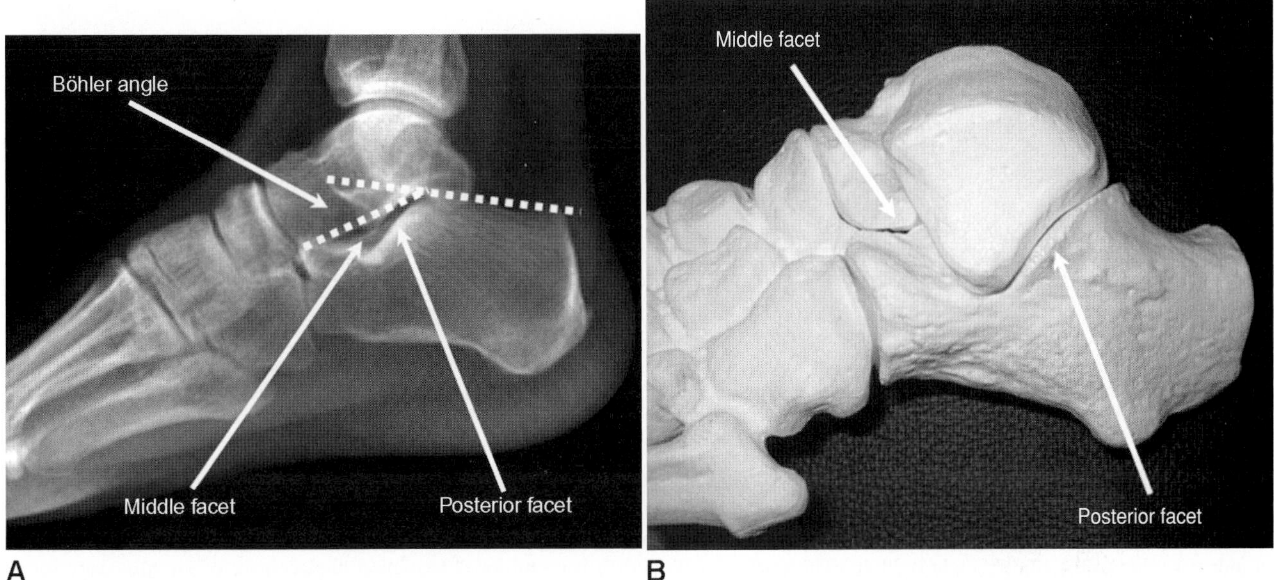

Figure 21–8: Normal (A and C) and pathologic (E and F) radiographic anatomy of the calcaneus. The lateral (A and E) and Harris axial (C and F) views of the calcaneus are useful in assessing the shape and alignment of the calcaneus.

Continued

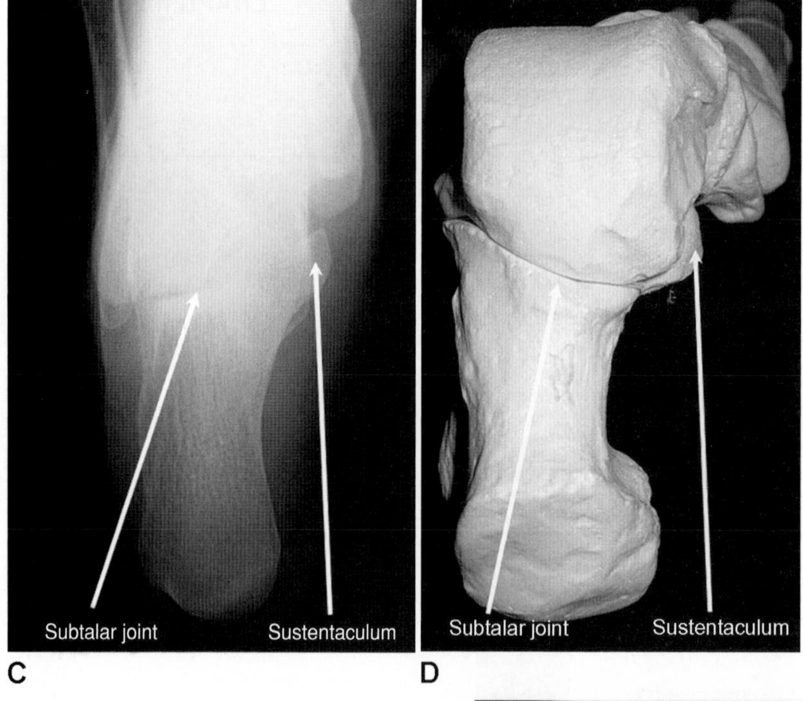

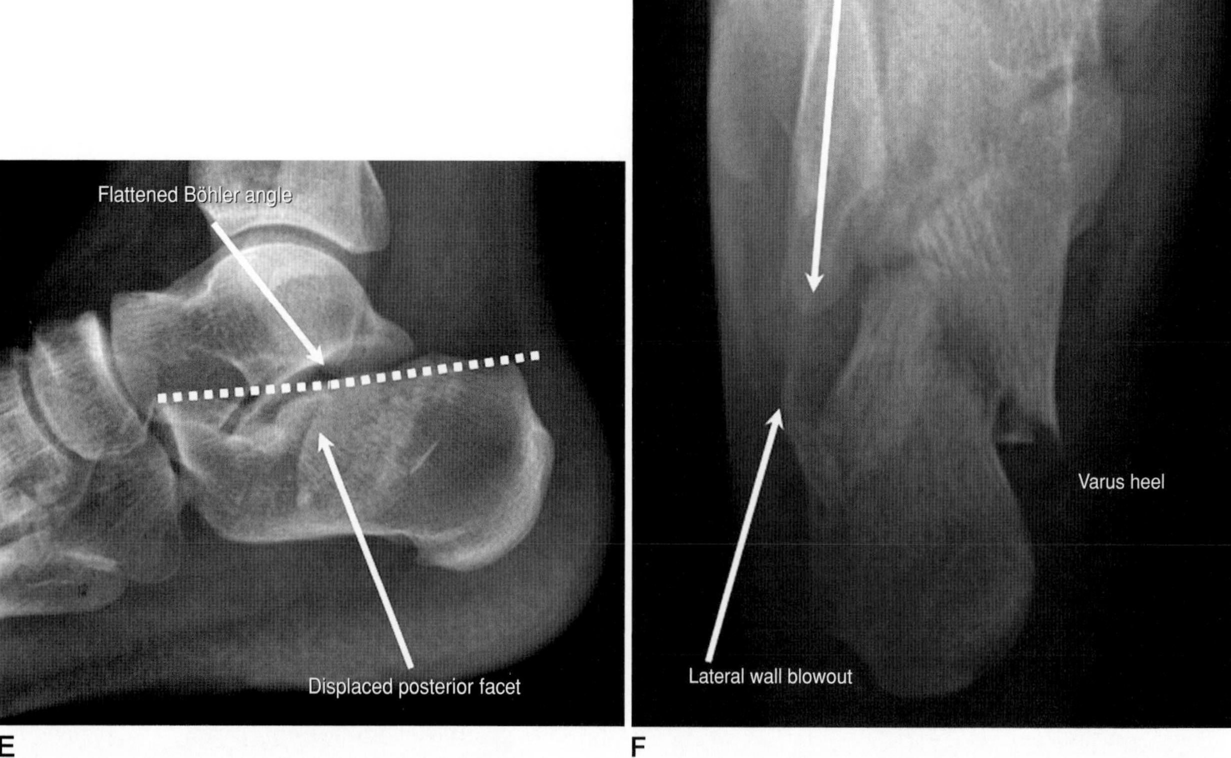

Figure 21–8: Cont'd The lateral view (A and E) allows for the assessment of the posterior and middle facet positions as well as an assessment of calcaneal height (Böhler angle). The Böhler angle is formed by drawing two lines. The first is drawn from the highest point on the anterior process to the highest point on the posterior facet. The second line is tangential to the superior edge of the tuberosity. The normal value of the Böhler angle is 20-40°. The axial view (C and F) is useful for determining displacement of the tuberosity, varus angulation, fibular abutment, and displacement of the lateral wall. A dorsoplantar view of the foot (not shown) assesses the calcaneocuboid joint for possible extension of the fracture.

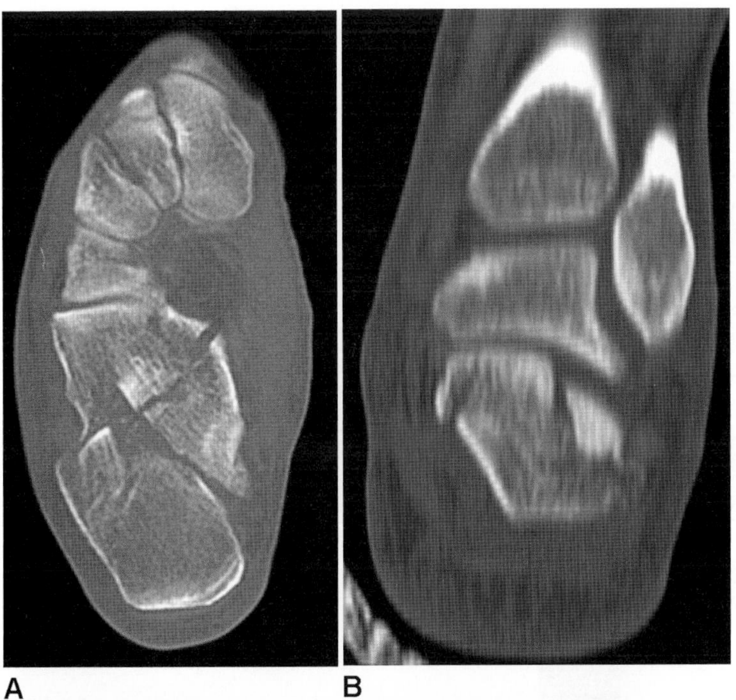

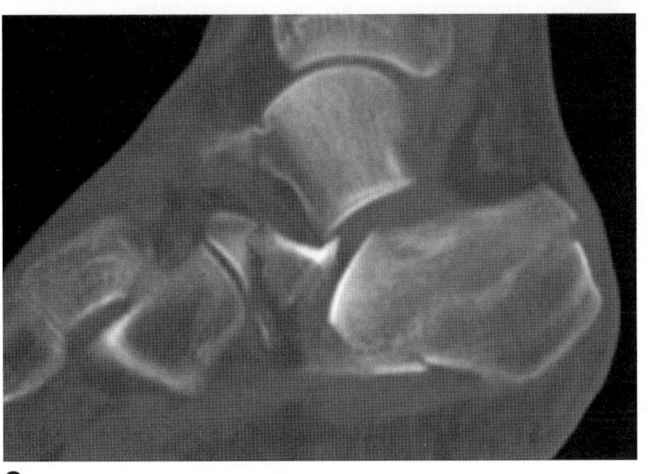

Figure 21–9: Computed tomography (CT) scan of the calcaneus is useful for preoperative planning. Axial CT scan **A**, is obtained in the transverse plane parallel to the sole of the foot. Coronal **B**, and sagittal **C**, reconstructions are also useful, but limited by the quality of the original axial images. Each image provides unique information relevant to the treatment of calcaneus fractures. The Axial CT scan provides information on the extent of lateral wall blowout, the calcaneocuboid joint, and the sustentaculum. The coronal CT scan allows for the assessment of heel width, subfibular impingement, and the extent of comminution and displacement of the subtalar joint, particularly the posterior facet. In addition, the location of the peroneal tendons can be verified in the soft tissue windows. The coronal CT scan is also the basis for the Sanders classification (see Fig. 21–11). The sagittal CT provides additional information about the anterior process and the subtalar joint, and is useful in distinguishing joint-depressed fractures from tongue-type fractures (see Fig. 21–10).

developed the Integral Classification of Injuries (ICI) to the bones, joints, and ligaments. This system provides a precise descriptive classification for injuries to the foot, including calcaneus fractures. In this fracture classification scheme, the foot is divided into three zones (hindfoot, midfoot, and forefoot), and a numeric system is used to describe the location of the fracture. 81.2 is the number used to designate the calcaneus. The fracture is then determined to be A (extraarticular), B (intraarticular), or C (fracture-dislocation). Additional subgroups are included for direction of dislocation, number of joints involved, and soft tissue injury. Although this system provides a comprehensive classification scheme, its reproducibility and usefulness remain to be seen.

Operative Versus Non-operative Treatment

- Definitive management of intraarticular calcaneus fractures consists of either operative or non-operative treatment. Several factors determine which method of treatment is used, including patient factors, type of fracture, and surgeon experience.
- A number of patient-related factors can affect the outcome of intraarticular calcaneus fractures, and therefore will impact the decision to pursue operative or non-operative treatment. Patients with drug and alcohol addiction, organic brain disease, or other forms of mental

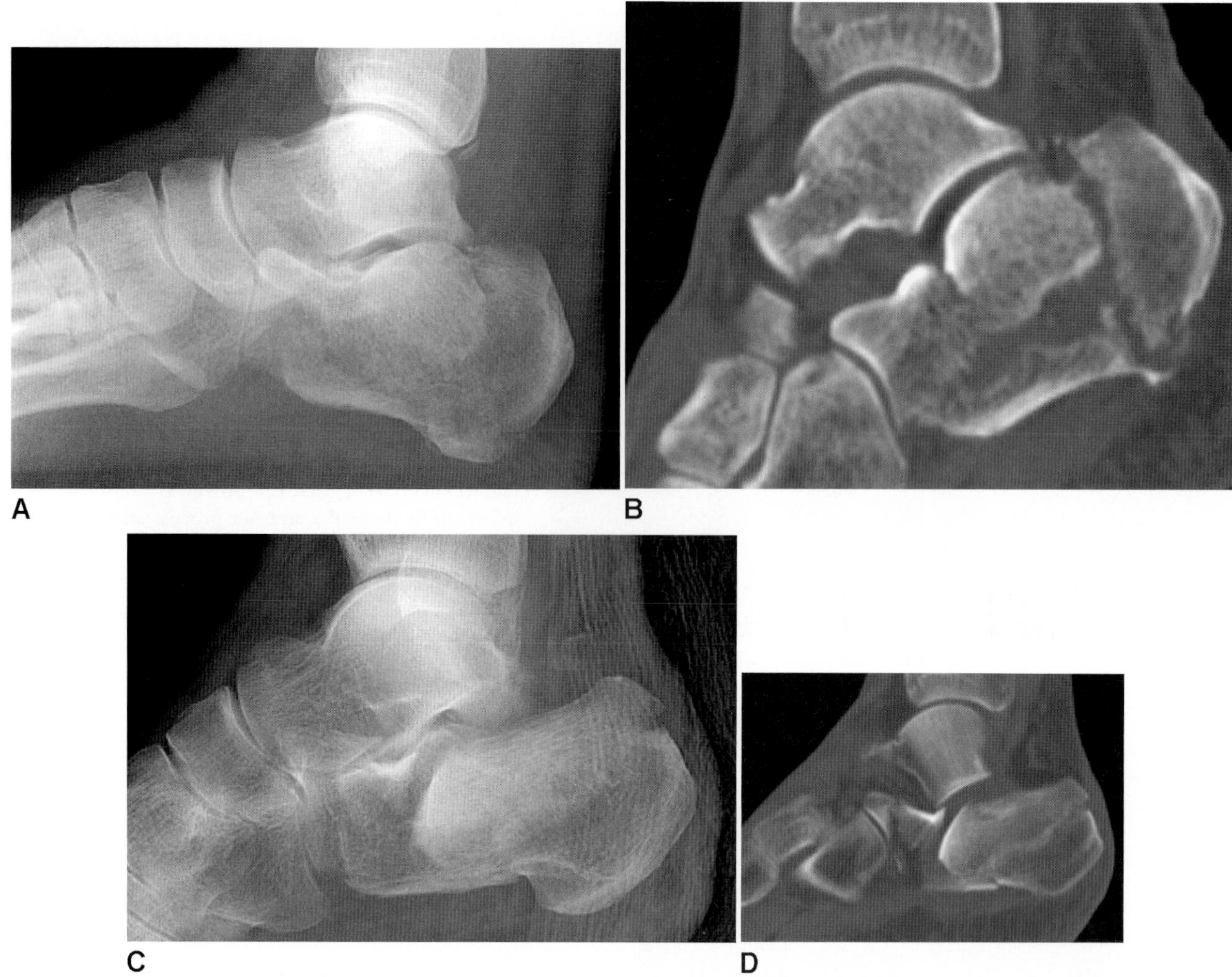

Figure 21–10: **In 1952, Essex-Lopresti described two distinct fracture patterns. In the tongue-type fracture A, and B, the tuberosity is continuous with the articular surface. In the joint depression fracture C, and D, the tuberosity fragment is separated from the articular fragment by an additional fracture line. Essex-Lopresti based his classification on plain radiographs. However, the classification is aided by sagittal computed tomography images. This classification system is useful in determining treatment but does not provide prognostic information.**

incapacitation, and who are unable to cooperate with the postoperative rehabilitation plan, are probably better treated non-operatively.

- Patient factors that may result in an inability to heal surgical wounds are also considered to be relative contraindications for operative treatment. Smoking or other regular nicotine use impairs wound healing. Patients with diabetes mellitus or peripheral vascular disease carry a higher risk of complications with surgery.
- The specific nature of the fracture also influences this decision. Minimally displaced fractures can be treated without surgery. There is some evidence that dramatically displaced fractures (particularly those with a negative Böhler angle) may have a poor outcome regardless of the treatment.
- Occasionally, the fracture type may supersede other factors in determining operative versus non-operative approach. For example, an Essex-Lopresti tongue-type fracture that can be reduced and stabilized through percutaneous methods may be treated operatively, with a low risk of complications, even in a smoker with diabetes mellitus.
- Finally, surgeon experience plays an important role in the operative treatment of calcaneus fractures. The learning curve for surgical repair of the calcaneus is well documented. Complications and poor results may occur more frequently if complex fractures are managed by inexperienced surgeons.
- In 2002, Buckley et al. reported the results of a prospective randomized study of operative versus non-

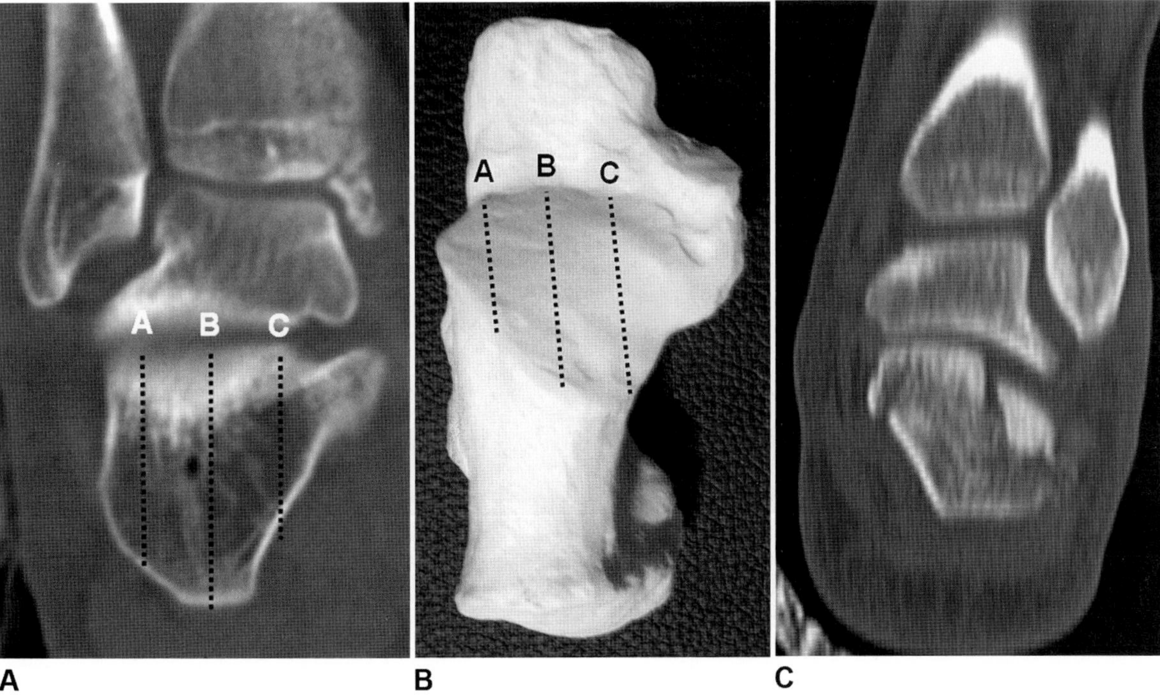

Figure 21–11: The Sanders classification is based on the fracture pattern through the posterior facet as seen on coronal computed tomography scan. Type 1 fractures are non-displaced. Type 2 fractures are two-part fractures of the posterior facet. Type 3 fractures are three-part fractures of the posterior facet. Type 4 fractures are highly comminuted, with four or more fragments to the posterior facet. Type 2 and type 3 fractures are further classified based on the location of the fracture lines (A–C), as seen above (left and center). Based on this classification system, the fracture on the right would be a Sanders type 3AC. The prognosis for calcaneus fractures worsens as the comminution of the posterior facet worsens.

operative treatment of calcaneus fractures (Box 21–3) at 2 years' follow-up. Three hundred and nine patients with 371 calcaneus fractures were randomized to receive a standardized operative or non-operative treatment conducted at four trauma centers. Based on 36-Item Short-Form Health Survey and visual analog scores, there was no difference in outcome based on treatment groups.

Box 21–3 Operative Versus Non-operative Treatment of Calcaneus Fractures[a]

Factors Associated With Improved Outcome in Operated Patients

- Female gender
- Non-workers' compensation status

Factors Associated With Improved Outcome in the Non-Workers' Compensation Group

- Younger age (age < 29)
- Low injury Böhler angle (0-14°)
- Light workload occupation
- Comminuted fracture
- Anatomical reduction (< 2-mm step-off)

[a] Buckley et al. (2002)

- However, when the treatment groups were stratified, operative treatment was shown to be superior in women and patients who were not on workers' compensation. Within the non-workers' compensation group, younger patients, patients with an injury Böhler angle of 0-14°, and patients with a lighter workload all had better results with operative treatment.
- This study is helpful in identifying patients who may have an improved outcome with operative treatment. However, the decision for operative or non-operative treatment must be made on an individual basis. Although Buckley contends that non-operative treatment may provide better outcomes at 2 years in certain cases, the surgeon should also consider the long-term effects of a malaligned calcaneus on the remainder of the joints in the foot and ankle. Later foot reconstruction is easier and safer with a well-aligned foot.

Treatment of Extraarticular Calcaneus Fractures

- Extraarticular calcaneus fractures are often missed on initial evaluation and often result in a painful foot and delayed diagnosis. The most common extraarticular

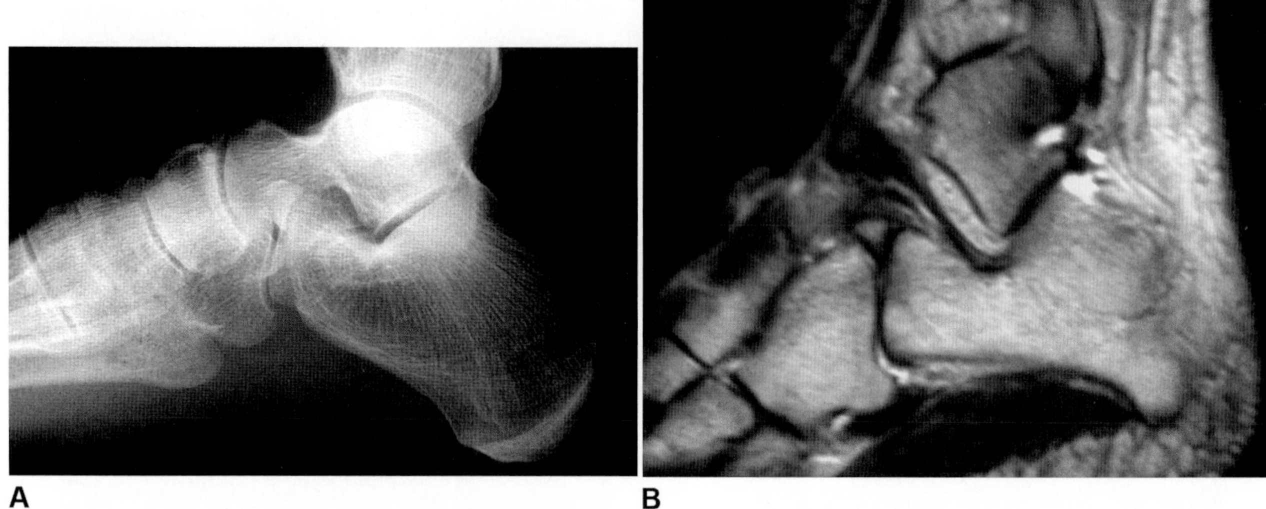

Figure 21–12: **Lateral x-ray and selected magnetic resonance imaging scan of a patient with an anterior process fracture of the calcaneus. The patient's fracture was not diagnosed at the time of injury, and he went on to develop a painful non-union of the fracture. He was treated with simple excision of the fragment.**

calcaneus fracture is the anterior process fracture (Fig. 21–12). Depending on the extent and symptoms of the fracture, treatment consists of non-operative treatment with functional rehabilitation, open reduction and internal fixation (ORIF), or excision of symptomatic fracture fragments.

- Extraarticular fractures of the calcaneal tuberosity often are minimally displaced, and can be treated non-operatively in the majority of cases. Displaced fractures, however, may threaten the thin posterior soft tissue envelope and lead to full-thickness necrosis. Fractures with soft tissue compromise must be reduced emergently to prevent potentially devastating wound complications and infection.

Treatment of Intraarticular Calcaneus Fractures

Non-operative Treatment

- Patients treated non-operatively are splinted in a neutral position. After initial discomfort improves and soft tissue swelling diminishes, patients are treated with early range of motion of the ankle, subtalar joint, and intrinsic muscles of the foot. Dorsiflexion splints are useful in preventing plantar flexion contracture. Weight bearing is delayed until radiographic fracture consolidation is evident, roughly 2 months.

Operative Treatment

- Operative treatment for intraarticular calcaneus fractures is divided into open and percutaneous techniques. Additional options include external fixation and primary subtalar arthrodesis.

Open Treatment

- Surgical approaches for open treatment include medial, lateral, or combined approaches.
- The medial approach allows for the direct visualization of the medial wall and direct reduction of the tuberosity fragment. This approach does not allow for direct visualization of the subtalar joint, and therefore reduction is performed indirectly using manipulation through the primary fracture line with the aid of fluoroscopy. Furthermore, this approach does not allow for decompression of the lateral wall.
- The major risk of the medial approach is damage to the neurovascular structures. The main nerve at risk from this approach is the medial calcaneal sensory branch, which is reported to be injured in up to 20% of cases. As the medial soft tissues are often severely compromised by the extreme shear forces produced by the fracture displacement, the risk of wound complications is high with this approach.
- The extensile lateral approach is the most commonly utilized approach for ORIF of the calcaneus. The approach utilizes a lateral flap based on the lateral calcaneal artery. An L-shaped incision (on the left foot, it is more like a "J" than an "L") is made over the lateral calcaneus, and a full-thickness flap containing the skin, peroneal tendons, sural nerve, and periosteum is elevated sharply off the lateral calcaneal wall. The lateral approach allows for direct visualization of the entire subtalar joint from the anterior process of the calcaneus to the tuberosity.
- The major risks for the extensile lateral approach are wound complications related to healing of the lateral

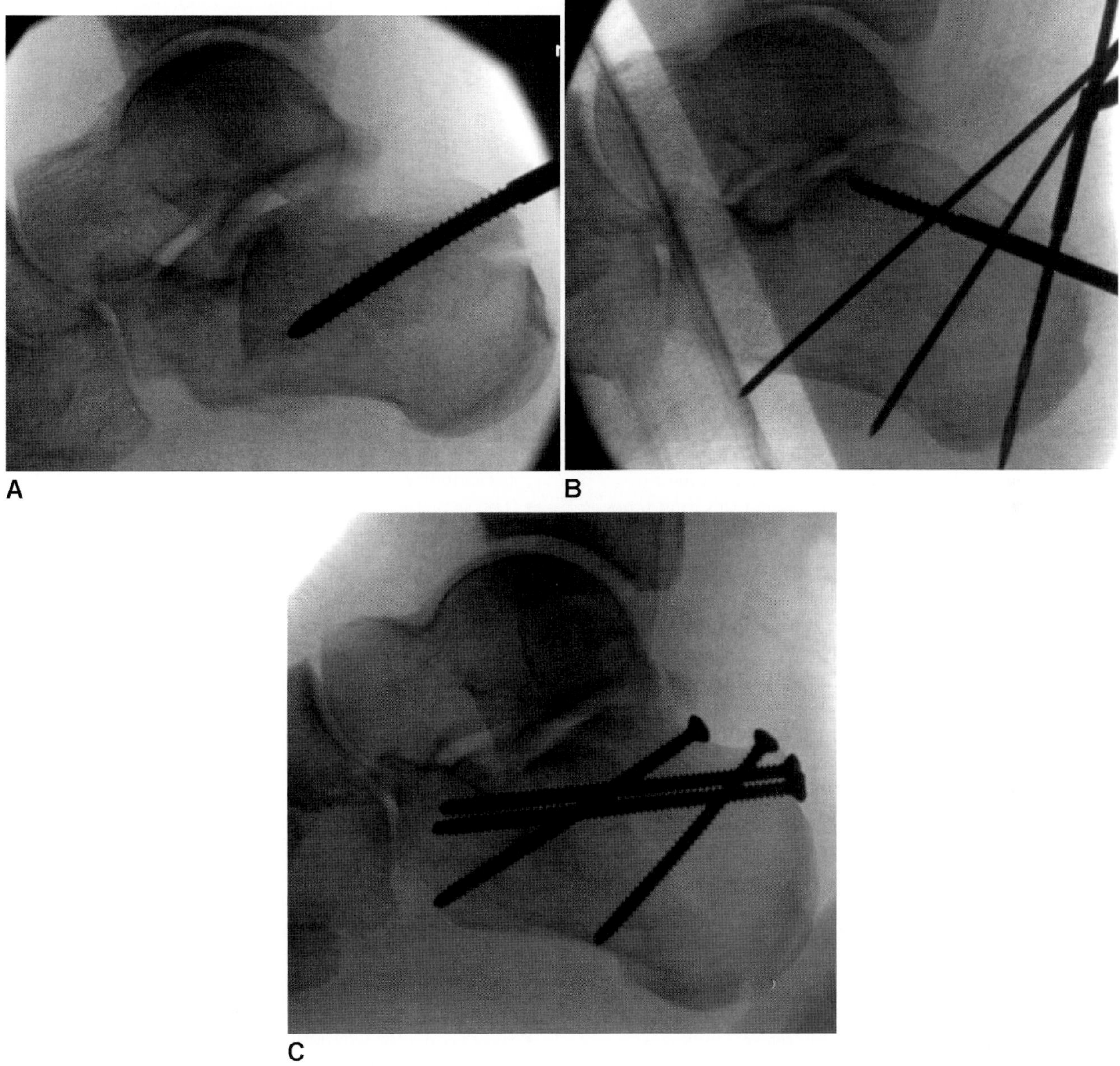

Figure 21–13: **The percutaneous reduction and fixation described by Essex-Lopresti is shown in these x-rays. A, Initially, a Steinmann pin is inserted into the tongue fragment. The fragment is then reduced using the Steinmann pin. B, Provisional K-wire fixation holds the fragment reduced. C, Definitive fixation is carried out with percutaneous screws.**

calcaneal flap. However, if performed carefully, the complication rate is low. Benirschke and Kramer reported a 1.8% infection rate in closed fractures, and a 7.7% infection rate in open fractures, in 379 cases with an extensile lateral approach.

- Combined medial and lateral approaches can be utilized to access both sides of the calcaneus. Although a combined approach allows for improved visualization, it also adds significant risk.
- The fragments are stabilized with strategically placed lag screws and bridging plates. Several different plates are available from different manufacturers, but the reduction is more important than the plate.
- Locking plates have recently been introduced, and may provide better fixation for the highly comminuted fracture. Locking plates are probably not necessary for most calcaneus injuries.
- The use of bone graft is controversial. Once reduction is achieved, there is consistently a void below the critical angle bone. Depression of the posterior facet crushes the loose cancellous bone normally found in this location at the time of injury. Cancellous autograft or allograft can be packed into the defect prior to plate application. In theory, the graft provides better support and makes a better construct, although no studies have shown an advantage to grafting.

- Recently, calcium phosphate cements have been developed to provide better buttressing than cancellous graft. Better constructs raise the possibility of earlier weight bearing. It is unclear whether the use of locked plates or calcium cements will allow earlier weight bearing.

Percutaneous Technique

- Minimally invasive or percutaneous techniques allow for an alternative approach to calcaneus fractures. These techniques are particularly useful in patients who have contraindications or significant risk factors that preclude open approaches. The technique (Fig. 21–13) was originally described by Essex-Lopresti, and is best indicated for fractures that fall into the tongue-type variety of Essex-Lopresti's classification scheme.
- Fractures treated by this method must be approached early (less than 2 weeks), as organized hematoma can interfere with fracture reduction beyond this time frame.
- The potential advantages of this technique include decreased wound complications, improved early postoperative motion, and decreased stiffness. Tornetta (1998) reported 87% good or excellent results utilizing this technique.
- Percutaneous reduction techniques usually do not achieve an anatomical reduction. But the decrease in wound complications and postoperative scarring may actually lead to better outcomes. Some skilled surgeons are using percutaneous techniques for some joint depression injuries. It is hoped that a comparative study will define the exact role of percutaneous surgery in the future.

External Fixation

- External fixation is rarely used to treat fractures of the calcaneus. However, external fixation may play a role, particularly in the definitive treatment of some open calcaneus fractures or in patients with a severely compromised soft tissue envelope. Two recent series (Ebraheim et al. 2000, Emara and Allam 2005) reported good results with external fixation, particularly in cases of soft tissue injury.
- A pin through the tuberosity holds the bone out to length. Other pins may be placed in the tibia and midfoot.
- When holding the reduction of an open calcaneus fracture temporarily while awaiting definitive surgery, a transfixion pin through the calcaneus should not be used, because the pin site will compromise definitive exposure. The displaced tuberosity should be maintained with axial K wires, with or without a bridging external fixator (tibia to midfoot—no pins in calcaneus).

Primary Arthrodesis

- In cases of severe comminution, the surgeon may consider primary subtalar arthrodesis for the treatment of calcaneus fractures. Although no randomized, controlled studies exist to date, subtalar fusion is a treatment option often proposed for patients with Sanders type 4 fractures. When performing subtalar fusion, the shape and alignment of the calcaneus must be restored prior to proceeding with fusion.
- One study suggested a faster return to work for comminuted fractures treated with early fusion.

Complications

- The historical aversion to operative treatment of the calcaneus was related to the severe complications that are often encountered with these complex fractures. Complications of calcaneus fracture treatment include compartment syndrome, nerve injury, wound-healing problems and infection, malunion, subtalar arthritis, and nerve injury.
- The sequelae of compartment syndrome (see Fig. 21–4) in the foot can be debilitating in patients with calcaneus fractures. Complications include clawing of the lesser toes, chronic pain, and atrophy.
- Nerve injury can occur during surgical approach or may be the result of the injury. The sural nerve is at risk for injury during the extensile lateral approach. Injury to this nerve may result in loss of sensation or the development of a painful neuroma near the proximal or distal end of the incision. In open fractures or high-energy calcaneus fracture-dislocations, the posterior tibial nerve may be at risk. The posterior tibial nerve may also become entrapped medially.
- Wound-healing problems and infection are the result of a multifactorial process including the subcutaneous nature of the calcaneus, the injury imparted to the soft tissues, and patient factors. Improper soft tissue handling and surgical technique can result in additional injury to the tissues at the time of surgery.
- Risk factors for wound healing include smoking, high body mass index, single-layered closure, peripheral vascular disease, diabetes mellitus, and open fractures. These patient factors have been shown to have an additive effect. With multiple risk factors, the rate of complications approaches 100%. Wound-healing problems tend to occur at the apex of the extensile lateral approach.
- Mild cellulitis can be treated with antibiotics. Wound drainage or severe cellulitis warrants a return to the operating room.
- Chronic osteomyelitis may require hardware removal, and soft tissue defects are best treated with a free flap.
- The rare case of unresolved osteomyelitis with soft tissue loss may be best treated by amputation.
- Malunion of the calcaneus may be the result of operative or non-operative treatment. The most common deformities are heel widening, varus of the hindfoot, and loss of heel height with subsequent

Achilles tendon contracture. Every effort should be made during surgery to restore the normal anatomy of the hindfoot to avoid these complications. Malunion resulting in a wide heel and subfibular impingement may also result in pain and irritation of the peroneal tendons and sural nerve.

- Subtalar arthritis may result despite anatomical reduction of the calcaneus. The development of posttraumatic arthritis is dependent on a number of factors, including initial injury and quality of reduction. Risk factors for subsequent subtalar fusion include a low Böhler angle (< 0°), comminution, workers' compensation status, and non-operative treatment.

Late Reconstruction

- Pain following a calcaneal fracture can arise from plantar fat pad atrophy, subtalar or calcaneocuboid arthritis, prominent hardware, or peroneal tendon problems. There also may be nerve damage from the original injury, or rarely sural neuromas from the surgical approach.
- If the previous treatment restored the overall shape and height of the calcaneus, posttraumatic arthritis can be treated with in situ arthrodesis.
- But if the calcaneus is shortened, subsequent surgery is more complex. Loss of calcaneal height will allow the talus to drop down and become less plantar flexed. It is very common to see anterior tibiotalar impingement from the loss of talar plantar flexion.
- In these cases of calcaneal malunion, reconstruction is performed with subtalar distraction arthrodesis. A structural block of bone is inserted into the posterior facet to "jack up" the talus and restore more normal anatomy. Because this increases the height of the heel acutely, it is common to see wound-healing problems following surgery.
- Even with successful subtalar fusion, varying degrees of discomfort and disability will remain. Calcaneus fractures often include injury to the plantar fat pad, the calcaneocuboid joint, and other surrounding soft tissues. Treating orthopaedists have been guilty of focusing too much attention on the posterior facet. Attention to all aspects of the injury, both osseous and soft tissue, will yield the best results.

References

Abidi NA, Dhawan S, Gruen GS et al. (1998) Wound-healing risk factors after open reduction and internal fixation of calcaneal fractures. Foot Ankle Int 19: 856-861.

Retrospective review of 64 calcaneus fractures treated with ORIF. Risk factors for wound complications included single-layered closure, high body mass index, extended time between injury and surgery, and smoking.

Aldridge JM, Easley M, Nunley JA. (2004) Open calcaneal fractures: Results of operative treatment. J Orthop Trauma 18: 7-11.

The authors report the results of 19 open calcaneus fractures. Two patients developed chronic osteomyelitis, and one required subsequent below-knee amputation. The overall complication rate was 11%. These results are better than those of previously reported series.

Barei DP, Bellabarba C, Sangeorzan BJ et al. (2002) Fractures of the calcaneus. Orthop Clin North Am 33: 263-285.

A good review of the modern controversies in treatment of calcaneus fractures.

Benirschke SK, Kramer PA. (2004) Wound healing complications in closed and open calcaneal fractures. J Orthop Trauma 18: 1-6.

Three hundred forty-one closed and 39 open calcaneus fractures were treated with ORIF utilizing an extensile lateral approach by Benirschke; 1.8% of closed and 7.7% of open fractures developed infections that required intervention beyond oral antibiotics. The paper demonstrates that the extensile lateral approach does not increase the risk of infection.

Böhler L. (1931) Diagnosis, pathology, and treatment of fractures of the os calcis. J Bone Joint Surg 13: 75-89.

An article of historical interest.

Buckley R, Tough S, McCormack R et al. (2002) Operative compared with nonoperative treatment of displaced intra-articular calcaneal fractures: A prospective, randomized, controlled multicenter trial. J Bone Joint Surg Am 84-A: 1733-1744.

This study is one of the few randomized prospective studies of a surgical technique. The authors identified subgroups of patients who benefited from surgery, although the entire population as a whole did not show clear benefits. Most of the surgeries were done by one surgeon, and critics have appropriately stated that the results of one surgeon should not be extrapolated to others. However, it remains to be proven whether other surgeons can show more dramatic results with surgery.

Carr JB. (2005) Surgical treatment of intra-articular calcaneal fractures: A review of small incision approaches. J Orthop Trauma 19: 109-117.

Carr provides a comprehensive review of small incision and percutaneous techniques of intraarticular calcaneus fractures. The paper reviews indications and provides technical tips for utilization of these techniques.

Csizy M, Buckley R, Tough S et al. (2003) Displaced intra-articular calcaneal fractures: Variables predicting late subtalar fusion. J Orthop Trauma 17: 106-112.

The authors report that the primary determinant of subsequent subtalar fusion was the amount of initial injury. Patients with low Böhler angles, those with Sanders type 4 fractures, workers' compensation patients, and patients treated non-operatively were more likely to require late subtalar fusion.

Emara KM, Allam MF. (2005) Management of calcaneal fracture using the Ilizarov technique. Clin Orthop Relat Res 439: 215-220.

The authors report the results of 12 patients with Sanders type 3 fractures who were treated with limited open reduction combined with Ilizarov technique. These patients were then compared with a control group treated with ORIF. Both groups had similar outcomes, but the control group had a higher rate of complications.

Essex-Lopresti P. (1952) The mechanism, reduction, technique, and results in fractures of the os calcis. Br J Surg 39: 395-419.

A classic article. A modern description of the percutaneous technique is found in the article by Tornetta.

Miric A, Patterson BM. (1998) Pathoanatomy of intra-articular fractures of the calcaneus. J Bone Joint Surg Am 80: 207-212.

The authors review 220 radiographs of intraarticular calcaneus fractures and characterize the pathoanatomy of the fracture lines. The review demonstrates a consistent anterolateral fracture fragment consistent with previous work by Böhler.

Sanders R, Fortin P, DiPasquale T et al. (1993) Operative treatment in 120 displaced intraarticular calcaneal fractures. Results using a prognostic computed tomography scan classification. Clin Orthop Relat Res 290: 87-95.

The authors describe a CT-based classification for intraarticular calcaneus fractures. The Sanders classification is descriptive and prognostic.

Tornetta P. (1998) The Essex-Lopresti reduction for calcaneal fractures revisited. J Orthop Trauma 12: 469-473.

Twenty-six patients with Essex-Lopresti tongue type (Sanders 2C) fractures were treated with percutaneous reduction and fixation as originally described by Essex-Lopresti. Twenty-three out of 26 achieved an acceptable reduction with closed methods. Three required open reduction. At 2.9 years' average follow-up, 87% of patients reported good or excellent results.

Zwipp H, Baumgart F, Cronier P et al. (2004) Integral Classification of Injuries (ICI) to the bones, joints, and ligaments—Application to injuries of the foot. Injury 35(suppl 2): SB3-SB9.

Report of the AO Foot and Ankle Group on the application of the ICI to injuries of the foot.

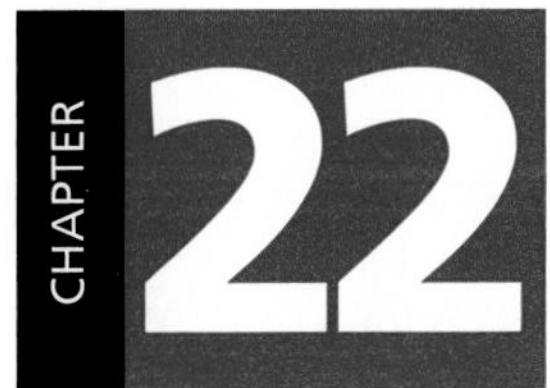

Talus Fractures

Michael P. Swords*, Jason Cochran§, and Jason Heisler†

*D.O., Assistant Clinical Professor, Michigan State University College of Osteopathic Medicine; Department of Orthopaedic Surgery, Sparrow Health System, Ingham Regional Medical Center, Lansing, MI; and Mid Michigan Orthopaedic Institute, East Lansing, MI
§D.O., Department of Orthopaedic Surgery, Michigan State University College of Osteopathic Medicine, Ingham Regional Medical Center, Lansing, MI
†D.O., Department of Orthopaedic Surgery, Michigan State University College of Osteopathic Medicine, Ingham Regional Medical Center, Lansing, MI

- The talus is the second most commonly fractured tarsal bone (after the calcaneus).
- Injuries are typically high energy, such as a fall from a height or a motor vehicle accident. As with any high-energy injury, initial evaluation consists of a thorough clinical examination with a search for other injuries.
- Because the talus is mostly articular, any significant fracture displacement requires a joint subluxation or dislocation. In other words, most displaced talar fractures are also dislocations.
- All dislocations should be reduced emergently to prevent further soft tissue injury. Prompt reduction also improves blood supply to the bone, possibly reducing the chance for avascular necrosis (AVN), as discussed more below.
- Radiographic examination consists of anteroposterior, lateral, and mortise images of the ankle, and anteroposterior, lateral, and oblique views of the foot. Canale views are beneficial and can increase the ability to visualize the talar neck.
- Computed tomography (CT) scanning of talus fractures is crucial; it aids in understanding the extent of injury as well as being critical for surgical planning. Imaging studies should be carefully reviewed for the presence of other fractures of the foot or ankle.

Skeletal Anatomy

- "Talus" comes from the word *talo*, Old French, meaning ankle, but the root of the word comes from *taxillus*, Latin, which means dice. The Romans used the heel bone of the horse to make dice. The Greeks used the second cervical vertebrae of sheep to make dice, and *astragalus* is vertebra in Greek.
- Two-thirds of the talus is covered by articular cartilage. There are no tendon or muscular attachments to the talus, but many muscles cross the talus. Because all these muscles insert distal to the talus, all muscles that act on the ankle joint also influence the subtalar and other hindfoot joints.
- It is a weight-bearing bone that transfers all the weight from the foot to the tibia and fibula. For descriptive purposes, it is divided into the body, neck, and head.

Body

- The body includes the talar dome and posterior facet, which make up the ankle and subtalar joints, respectively.
- The superior portion of the body is articular. It is shaped like a pulley in the coronal plane, with the trochlear portion lying offset more medially. In the axial plane, the superior surface is shaped like a keystone, with the anterior portion wider than the posterior.

- The lateral talus becomes somewhat triangular and articulates with the fibula. The perimeter of the lateral articular portion is called the lateral process. It serves for attachment of the lateral talocalcaneal ligament as well as the anterior and posterior talofibular ligaments. The undersurface of the lateral process makes up the lateral portion of the posterior facet of the subtalar joint, so that most lateral process fractures are intraarticular.
- The medial portion of the talus has a large articular surface for the medial malleolus. In the anterior non-articular area, there are vascular foramina. The posterior body serves as insertion for the deep deltoid ligament.
- The posterior process of the talus is made up of posteromedial and posterolateral tubercles, between which lies a groove for the flexor hallucis longus tendon.

Head

- The head primarily articulates with the navicular anteriorly.
- Inferiorly in the head are the anterior and middle subtalar facets. The subtalar facets on the calcaneus combine with the articular surface of the navicular to make the acetabulum pedis. These joint surfaces make a socket in which the talar head rotates (or, more accurately, the socket rotates around the talar head).
- There are attachments for the spring ligament, deltoid ligament, and sustentaculum tali.

Neck

- The neck lies between the body and head, and has multiple ligamentous attachments.
- It is oriented 15-20° medial to the talar body.
- The neck is the region most vulnerable to fracture.
- It lies directly over the sinus tarsi and tarsal canal.
- This region has numerous capsular attachments and vascular foramina.

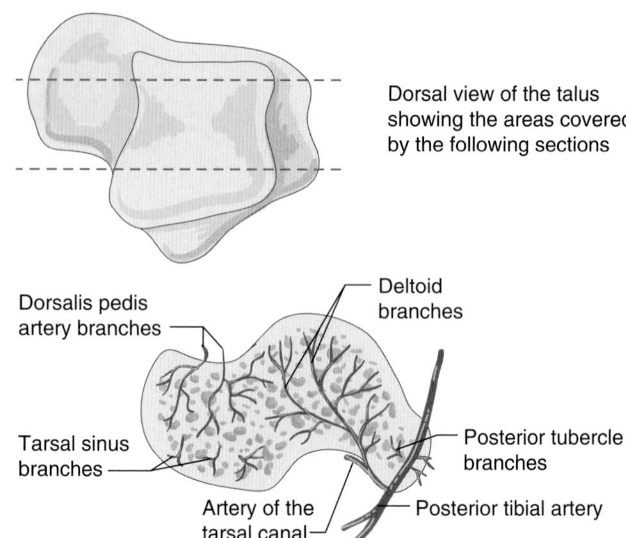

A. Blood supply to the medial one-third of the talus

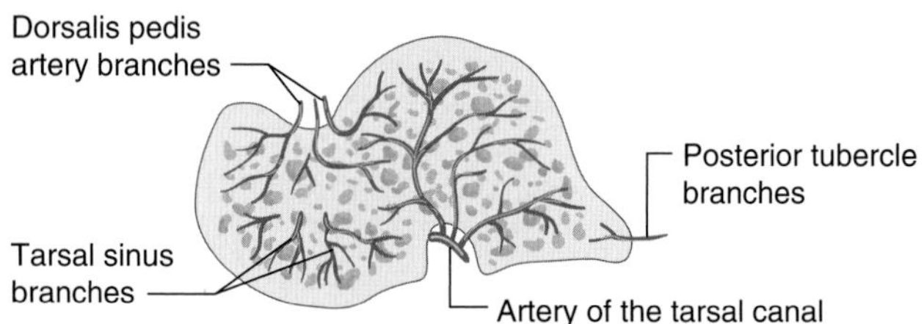

B. Blood supply to the middle one-third of the talus

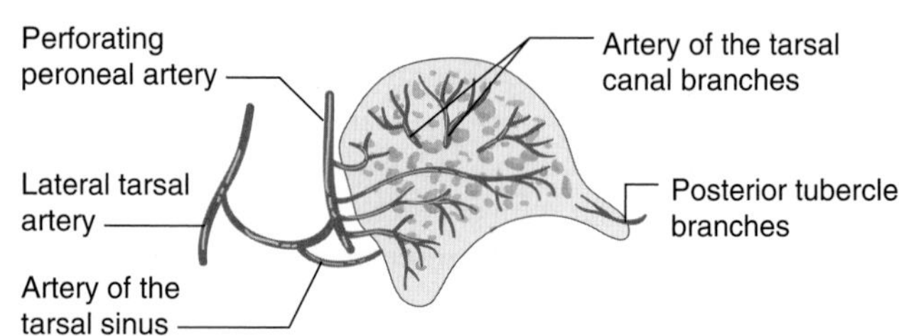

C. Blood supply to the lateral one-third of the talus

Figure 22–1: The blood supply to the talus. (From Mulfinger GL, Trueta J. (1970) The blood supply of the talus. J Bone Joint Surg Br 52: 160-167. Reproduced with permission and copyright of the British Editorial Society of Bone and Joint Surgery.)

Vascular Anatomy

- Historically, the vascular supply of the talus has been of special interest due to association of AVN with talus injuries.
- Because two-thirds of the talus is covered by articular cartilage and there are no muscular attachments, the blood supply is limited.
- There are contributions from the capsular and ligamentous attachments to the tibia, calcaneus, and navicular.

Extraosseous Arterial Supply

- Branches of the posterior tibial, dorsalis pedis, and peroneal arteries contribute to the talus; however, there are multiple variants on the branches (Fig. 22–1).
- There is a delicate network of anastomoses between the arteries, which envelops all the non-articular areas of the talus.
- The posterior tibial artery gives off the artery to the tarsal canal and a vascular plexus for the posterior process. The deltoid branch of the artery to the tarsal canal supplies the medial talar body.
- The dorsalis pedis leads to the anterior lateral malleolar artery and branches over the superior surface of the neck to supply the head. The anterior lateral malleolar artery anastomoses with the peroneal artery supply to form the artery of the tarsal sinus.
- The peroneal artery sends branches to the posterior process to anastomose with the posterior tibial vessels.

In addition, it contributes to the artery of the tarsal sinus via the perforating peroneal artery.

- The arteries of the tarsal canal and sinus anastomose, forming the artery of the tarsal sling. This supplies the inferior neck and lateral body.
- The arteries of the tarsal canal and sinus, along with the medial periosteal vessels, are the most essential supply to the talus.

Intraosseous Blood Supply

- The head receives its blood supply from the dorsalis pedis superiorly and artery of the tarsal sling inferiorly.
- The talar body gets it blood supply from five sources:
  - the anastomosis between the posterior tibial and peroneal branches at the posterior process
  - the superior surface of the talar neck
  - the inferior surface of the talar neck
  - the anterolateral surface of the talar body
  - the medial surface of the talar body (from the deltoid ligament).
- The artery of the tarsal canal supplies the lateral two-thirds of the talar body, while the deltoid branch supplies the medial third.
- There are also multiple intraosseous vascular anastomoses between the supplying arteries.

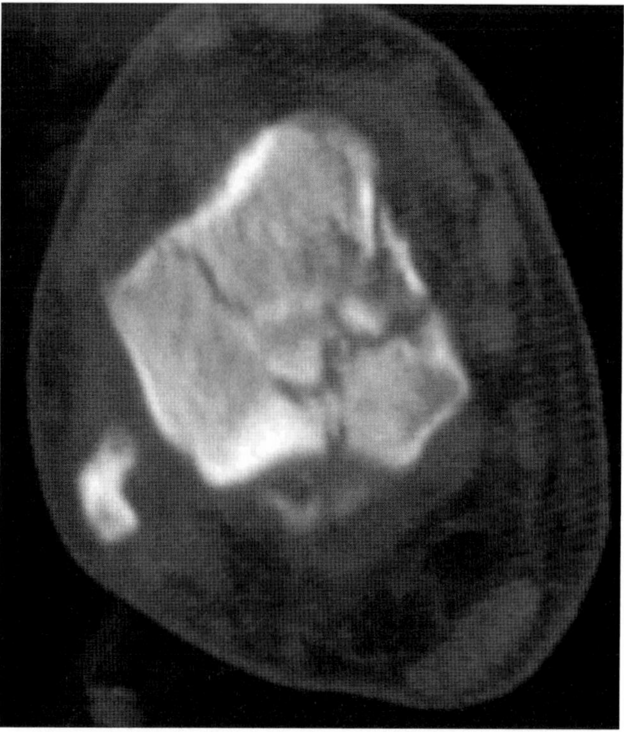

Figure 22–2: Computed tomography imaging demonstrates a comminuted injury to the talar dome sustained in a motor vehicle accident.

Talar Body Fractures

- Mechanism of injury is generally a fall from a height with axial loading or a motor vehicle accident. Associated injuries and fractures of other tarsal bones are common.
- Inokuchi et al. (1996) defined the difference between talar neck and body fractures based on the inferior articular surface of the talus. If the major fracture line exits at or posterior to the lateral process, it is considered a body fracture. Thus talar body fractures are intraarticular ankle and subtalar joint injuries. Fractures that exit anterior to the lateral process are neck fractures.
- Radiographs typically do not demonstrate the full extent of articular injury and comminution, therefore CT imaging is required (Fig. 22–2).
- Classification systems have been described by Sneppen, Boyd and Knight, and Fortin.
- Fortin (2001) divided talar body injuries into three major groups:
  - group 1 are proper or cleavage fractures (sagittal, horizontal, or coronal)
  - group 2 are talar process or tubercle fractures
  - group 3 are compression or impaction fractures.
- Treatment can be non-operative for non-displaced fractures, but more commonly open reduction and internal fixation (ORIF) is required.
- Closed reduction of all dislocations should be attempted after plain radiographs, usually before CT imaging.
- Emergent surgical treatment is necessary in all open injuries and in all dislocations that cannot be reduced, with irrigation and debridement of open wounds, and reduction of dislocations. Definitive reduction and fixation can wait.
- Delayed surgical treatment when the soft tissues recover is warranted in all other injuries.
- Fractures with more significant soft tissue injuries may require external fixation as a temporizing measure.
- For the definitive surgery, anatomical reduction with stable fixation is the goal. In the recent past, fixation with one or two large screws was favored, but with recognition that these fractures are often comminuted with small pieces, there has been a shift to fixation with small or mini fragment screws and sometimes plates. Bioabsorbable pins may also be useful occasionally (Figs 22–3 and 22–4).
- Multiple surgical exposures exist. Surgical approach is dictated by the area of injury.
- A medial approach through the interval between the tibialis anterior and the tibialis posterior is usually required. This approach can be extended proximally to incorporate a medial malleolar osteotomy for greater visualization of the medial talar dome (Fig. 22–5). The medial malleolus is predrilled for lag screws prior to the osteotomy, to ensure an anatomical repair of the malleolus.

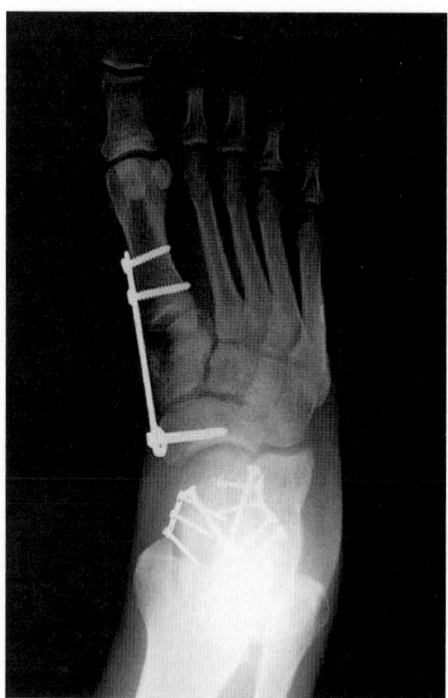

Figure 22–3: **In this case, the talus fracture was stabilized with medial and lateral mini fragment plates and screws. Note the medial midfoot injury stabilized with a bridge plate.**

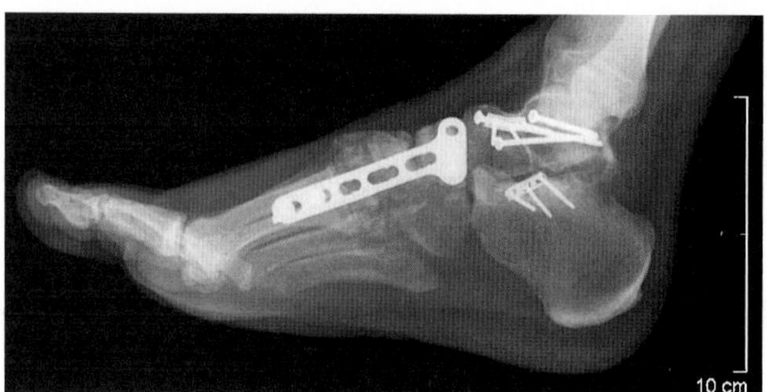

Figure 22–4: **Lateral view of the same patient as in Figure 22–3. The patient also sustained a crushing injury to his midfoot and a fracture of the sustentaculum tali.**

- The anterolateral approach is just lateral to the extensor digitorum longus and peroneus tertius tendons, and extends from anterior to the lateral malleolus toward the fourth toe. Care is taken to avoid injury to the superficial peroneal nerve, which is typically seen during the dissection. The extensor digitorum brevis may need to be elevated a bit to facilitate exposure.
- The fragments should be reduced perfectly to restore normal joint kinematics. Small non-viable cartilage debris may need to be resected.
- After provisional fixation with Kirschner wires, the reduction should be critically assessed. Once anatomical reduction is confirmed, final fixation is placed. It is occasionally necessary to countersink screw heads into the articular cartilage.

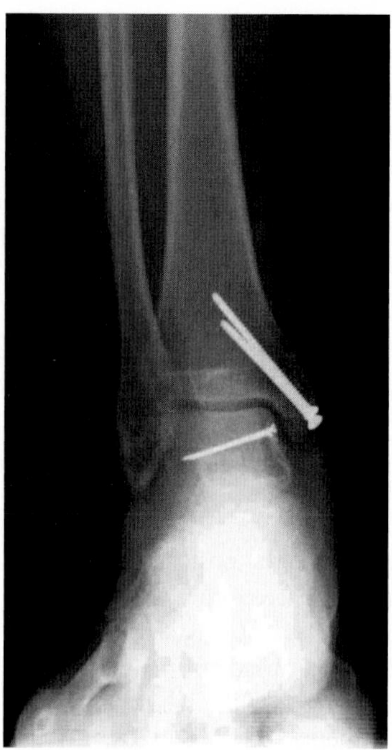

Figure 22–5: **A medial malleolus osteotomy was used to provide greater visibility and for placement of hardware in this sagittal split body fracture.**

- Definitive fracture fixation is achieved with screws and/or plates. Screws are typically inserted in lag fashion, but in areas of extensive comminution or bone loss, position screws should be used to prevent alteration of normal bony anatomy. Small plates may act as a washer for multiple lag screws, or may bridge comminution.
- Bone grafting is occasionally required to support articular segments that have been disimpacted.
- Postoperatively, the patient is splinted for 2 weeks, then a short leg non-weight-bearing cast is applied. A fracture boot is applied, and ankle and subtalar motion is initiated at 8 weeks. With stable fixation, it may be better to start motion at 2 or 3 weeks after surgery, using a brace and not a cast. All patients should remain non-weight bearing for 10–12 weeks.
- Outcomes are often dictated by the severity of the initial injury, joint reduction, and articular injury.
- Posttraumatic arthrosis, malunion, and AVN are more common in severe crush injuries, and are associated with the severity of the initial injury.
- In a prior study of talar body fractures, 21 patients with talar body fractures were reviewed. Eighteen of these fractures were treated with non-operative treatment, and three underwent ORIF. In this series, 60% of the patients had malunion of the fracture. The subtalar and ankle joints were found to have very high rates of posttraumatic arthritis. Ninety-five percent of patients had moderate to severe complaints (Sneppen et al. 1977).
- In a more recent series, Vallier et al. (2003) reviewed clinical, radiographic, and functional outcomes of

operative treatment of talar body fractures. Osteonecrosis was observed in 10 of 26 patients, 5 of which advanced to collapse and 5 showed signs of revascularization. Higher rates of osteonecrosis were observed in open fractures and those with associated talar neck fractures. Posttraumatic arthritis was reported in 65% of tibiotalar joints and 35% of subtalar joints. Mean Musculoskeletal Function Assessment (MFA) was 29.3 for isolated talar body fractures compared with a published reference value of 22.1 for hindfoot injury, indicating a worse functional outcome when compared with other hindfoot injuries. Twenty of 30 patients returned to prior level of employment. Eight patients did not return to work. Worse outcomes were found with fractures with open injuries and associated talar neck fractures.
- Lindvall et al. (2004) found no difference in union rate, AVN, posttraumatic arthritis, or American Orthopaedic Foot and Ankle Society (AOFAS) outcome score between fractures of the talar neck and body.

Posteromedial Talar Body Fractures

- Fractures of the posteromedial aspect of the talus represent a rare variant of talar body fractures. The radiographic findings are subtle and can be missed without thorough review of the radiographs (Fig. 22–6). In several case series, more than 50% were missed initially.
- Results of non-operative treatment for this injury are poor, with arthrodesis rates as high as 83%.
- Like all talar body fractures, they involve both the tibiotalar and the subtalar joints.
- CT evaluation greatly improves understanding of the extent of injury (Figs 22–7 and 22–8).
- Because of unacceptably high rates of posttraumatic arthritis with conservative treatment, displaced fractures should be treated with ORIF.
- The fracture cannot be adequately visualized with a medial malleolar osteotomy, as the majority of the injury is further posterior than can be visualized with this surgical approach.
- One option is to position the patient prone and approach the posteromedial aspect of the talus through the interval between the Achilles tendon and the flexor hallucis longus. Alternatively, they can be approached with the patient supine, through the interval between the posterior tibialis and flexor digitorum longus.
- Because of the limited area of extraarticular surface on the posterior talus, fixation is usually performed with minifragment plates or screws (Figs 22–9 and 22–10).
- A simple two-pin external fixator or a femoral distractor can aid in the ability to adequately visualize the tibiotalar and subtalar joint surfaces.
- Postoperative care consists of non-weight bearing for 12 weeks, with initiation of ankle and subtalar range of motion exercises at 6 weeks, or sooner with a reliable patient.

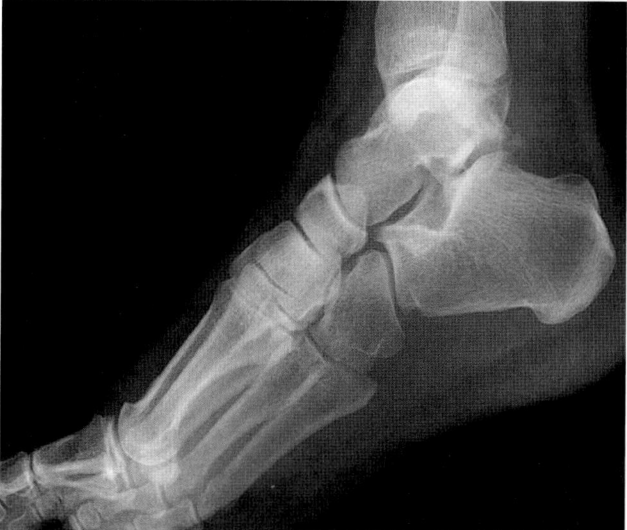

Figure 22–6: The radiographic appearance of a posteromedial talar body can be unimpressive, and is often incorrectly interpreted as an os trigonum.

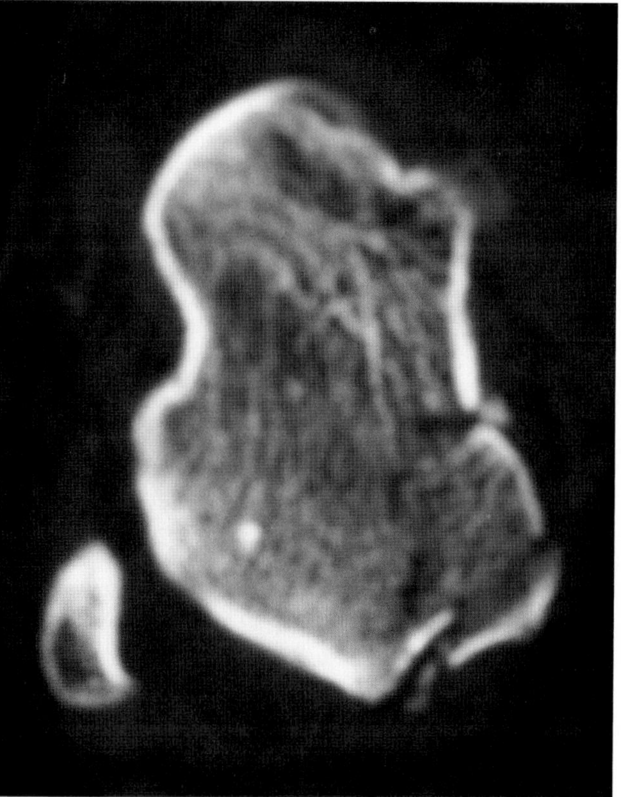

Figure 22–7: Axial computed tomography scan of the fracture in Figure 22–6, showing significant intraarticular involvement and displacement.

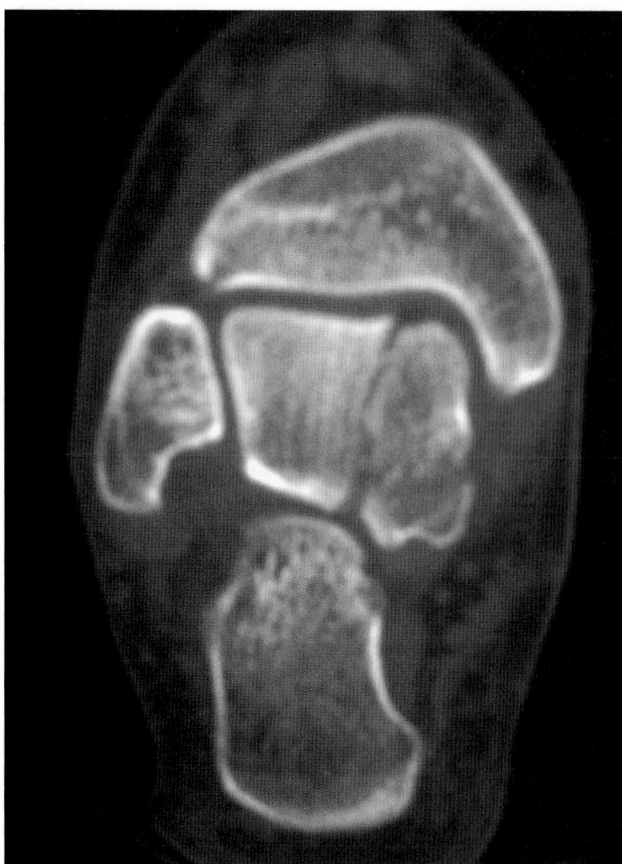

Figure 22–8: Coronal computed tomography scan of the posteromedial talar body fracture seen in Figure 22–5.

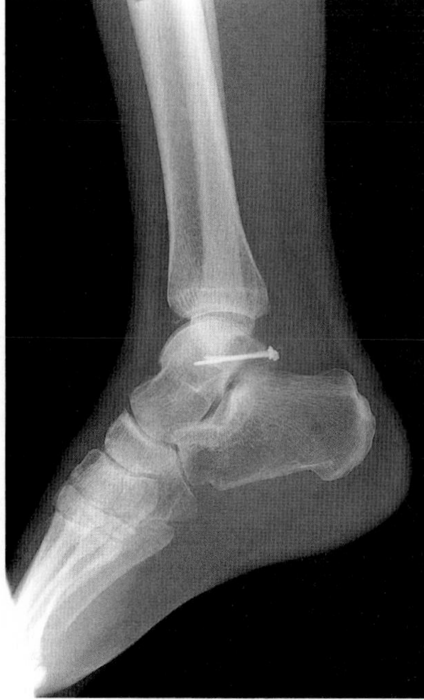

Figure 22–9: Fixation of a posteromedial talar body fracture using a posterior 2.0-mm plate and lag screws.

- Long-term results of this subset of body fracture are not currently known.

Talar Neck Fractures

- Fractures of the neck of the talus account for 50% of all talus fractures.
- While neck fractures are not intraarticular, they disrupt the normal relationships between the articular facets of the subtalar joint. The fracture line divides the posterior facet from the anterior and middle facets. For this reason, it is essentially an intraarticular injury, and anatomical reconstruction is critical. An in vitro study showed that displacement of the talar neck by 2 mm greatly increases contact pressures in the posterior facet (Sangeorzan et al. 1992).
- Injury begins with forced dorsiflexion, rupturing the posterior capsular ligaments of the subtalar joint, followed by impaction of the neck on the anterior distal tibial crest. As the forces progress, the posterior capsular structures and the deltoid tear and the talar body can dislocate posteriorly.
- Most talar neck fractures occur as a result of a motor vehicle accident or a fall. Historically, talar neck fractures were seen with early airplane crashes, thus the name "aviator's astragalus."
- Patients typically present with swelling and gross deformity. Skin and soft tissues should be carefully assessed, as major displacement can compromise tissue perfusion and lead to necrosis.
- All obvious dislocations should be reduced emergently (Fig. 22–11).
- Radiographic evaluation should include anteroposterior, lateral, and oblique images of the foot and three views of the ankle. Canale views can increase the ability to visualize the talar neck. CT evaluation is required in all talus fractures
- The most widely used classification is the Hawkins classification (Table 22–1). Higher rates of AVN are seen as the Hawkins group number increases, providing prognostic value. The original classification divided fractures into group 1, 2, or 3.
- In 1978, Canale and Kelly reported on their series of fractures, and referred to the Hawkins classification groups as types. A type 4 was also described. (The terms *group* and *type* have been confused in the literature from that time forward.)
- Group 1 fractures are non-displaced. These are uncommon injuries. If any displacement is present, even 1 mm, it is by definition a group 2 injury (Fig. 22–12).
- If, after CT review, the fracture is truly non-displaced and there is no fracture debris present in the subtalar joint, then the injury can be treated with a non-weight-bearing cast for 8 weeks. Fractures treated conservatively need to be monitored closely for any late displacement, which would require operative fixation.

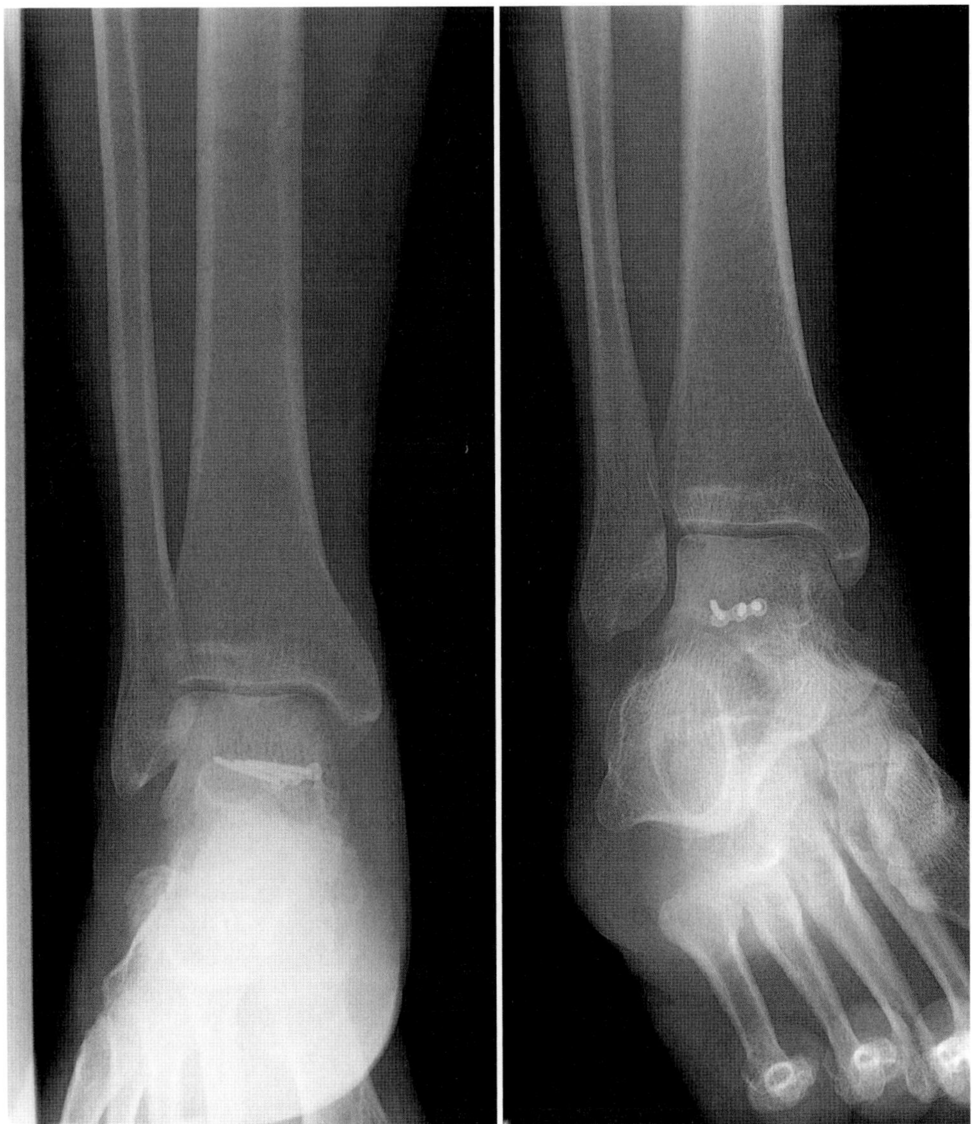

Figure 22–10: Mortise radiograph shows that reduction of articular surface is anatomical.

- Group 2 fractures of the talar neck demonstrate some subluxation or dislocation of the subtalar joint. The neck of the talus is typically malaligned in varus and has rotational deformity.
- Group 3 fractures have dislocation of the talar body at both the ankle and the subtalar joints. This usually required disruption of most or all soft tissue from the talar body. Closed reduction of the dislocation (to get the talar body back under the tibia) should be attempted. Failure with closed reduction requires emergent open reduction. It is helpful to use a distractor between the tibia and calcaneus to create room for the talar body. In many cases, the body dislocates posteromedially and can compress the neurovascular bundle. Associated medial malleolus fracture is not uncommon and can be used to facilitate reduction. The talar head is still well aligned with the navicular in group 3 fractures. This implies that some soft tissue remains attached to the talar neck, so that at least one fragment will have a viable blood supply.
- Group 4 fractures have all the characteristics of group 3 with dislocation of the talar head at the talonavicular joint. There may not be any soft tissue attachments left on any fragment of talus. The series reported by Canale and Kelly, who first reported this injury, found that only 3 of 71 fractures were group 4, and all had unsatisfactory results.
- Operative approach should be by two incisions in most fractures.
- A medial incision between the anterior tibialis and posterior tibialis tendons will provide exposure to the

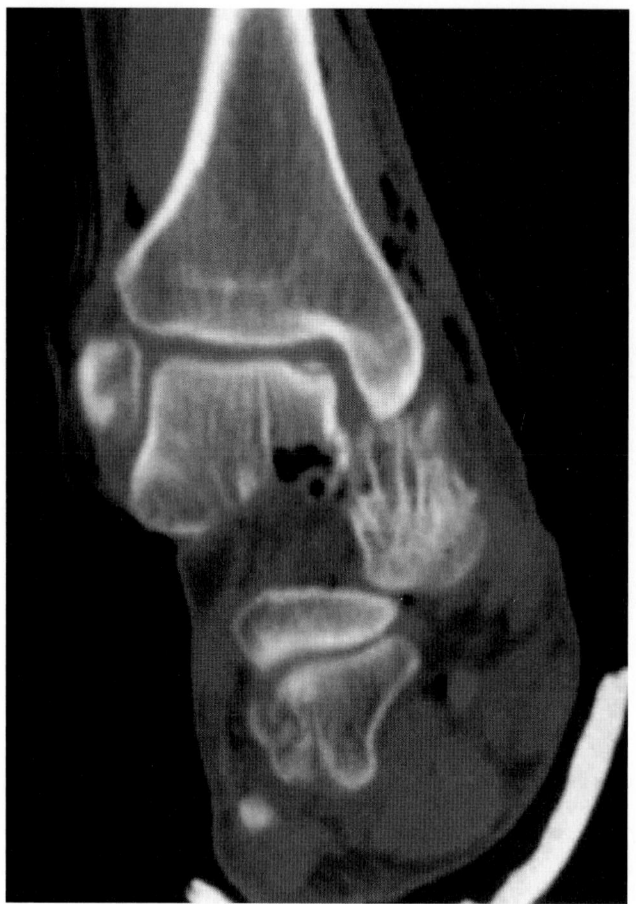

Figure 22–11: Coronal computed tomography imaging of an open talar neck fracture dislocation as a result of a motorcycle accident. Emergent reduction was performed, allowing reperfusion of the foot.

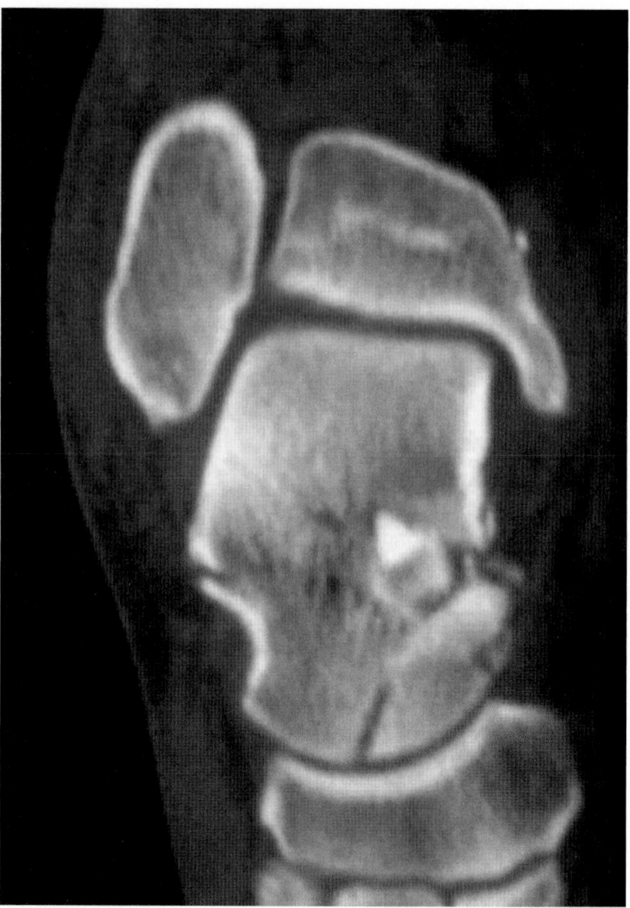

Figure 22–12: Computed tomography scan of another talar neck fracture demonstrating increased medial neck comminution, characteristic of neck fractures. The lateral cortex is quite dense and allows for accurate reconstruction of the neck.

Table 22–1: Hawkins Classification as Modified by Canale and Kelly

CLASSIFICATION	CHARACTERISTIC	RISK OF AVASCULAR NECROSIS (%)
1	Non-displaced	0
2	Displaced with subtalar subluxation	42
3	Displaced with subtalar and ankle subluxation	91
4[a]	Displaced type 3 with talonavicular subluxation	100

[a] Canale modification.
(From Hawkins LG. (1970) Fractures of the neck of the talus. J Bone Joint Surg Am 52: 991-1002.)

medial side of the neck. The incision can be carried proximally to incorporate a medial malleolar osteotomy. The lateral incision is from just anterior to the fibula, lateral to the peroneus tertius and common extensor tendons, and is directed toward the fourth toe. Care should be taken to prevent injury to the superficial peroneal nerve.

- Stripping of any remaining soft tissue should be avoided to preserve the remaining blood supply to the talus.
- Fractures are typically more comminuted medially, as the neck commonly displaces into varus. Comminution is evaluated through the medial incision.
- Length and alignment are assessed from the lateral incision, as typically there is less comminution laterally (see Fig. 22–12).
- Fixation can be inserted from distal to proximal. Screws can be countersunk into the head of the talus. For a simple neck fracture, two lag screws are adequate. With comminution, it may be better to not lag, but rather place position screws, to avoid shortening the length of the neck (Fig. 22–13).
- Alternatively, screws may be inserted from the posterior process back into the neck, but area for screw insertion is more limited. In an in vitro study, posterior to anterior screw placement had better mechanical strength when compared with standard anterior to posterior screws (Swanson et al. 1992).

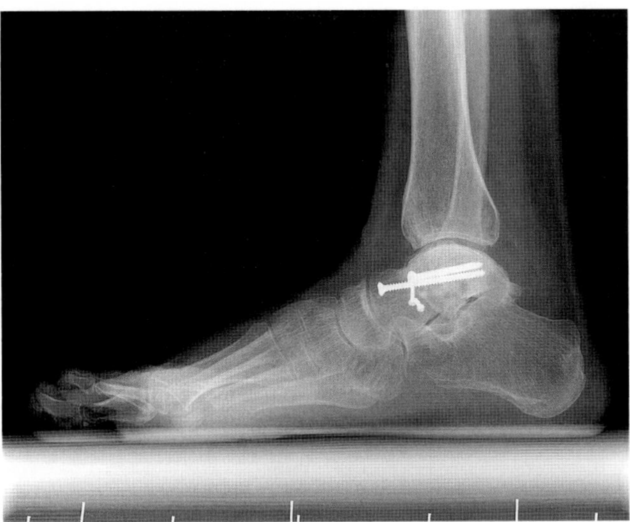

Figure 22–13: Anterior to posterior lag screws obtained stable fixation in this talar neck fracture. Two 2.0-mm lag screws secured an area of comminution in the talar head.

- Minifragment plating has also been used successfully in treating talar neck fractures, particularly in injuries with higher levels of comminution (Figs 22–14 and 22–15). As in body fractures, these plates may be used as washers for multiple lag screws, or may bridge fracture comminution.
- Postoperatively, the patient is placed in a splint for 2 weeks. Sutures are then removed and a cast is applied. At 6-8 weeks, motion of the tibial talar and subtalar joint is begun. With stable fixation, range of motion can begin at 2 weeks. Weight bearing is not allowed before the 12-week mark and is held until fracture union is present.

Outcomes of Talar Neck Fractures

- Traditionally, talar neck fractures have been associated with high complication rates (Box 22–1). There are many contributing factors, including the odd shape of the bony anatomy, relatively poor vascularity, high energy of the injury, comminution, and associated fractures and soft tissue injuries. Most surgeons rarely treat these injuries, so inexperience can also contribute to poor outcomes.
- Higher rates of osteonecrosis are seen with increasing displacement. Hawkins found no osteonecrosis in group

Box 22–1 Factors That Contribute to Poorer Outcomes of Talar Neck Fractures

- Talar neck comminution
- Open fractures
- Avascular necrosis with collapse
- Posttraumatic arthritis

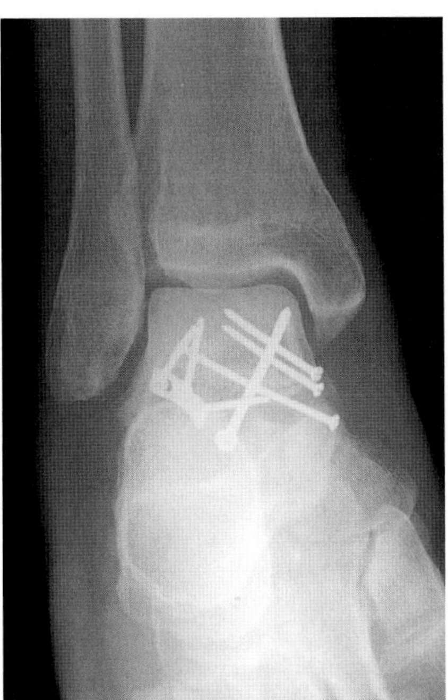

Figure 22–14: A lateral minifragment plate was placed as additional fixation in this more comminuted neck fracture.

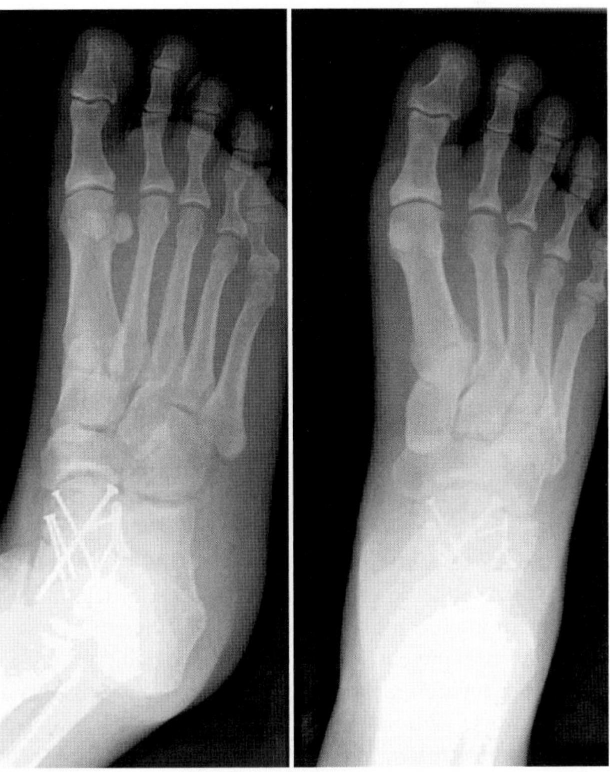

Figure 22–15: Anteroposterior and oblique films demonstrating fixation with a minifragment plate.

1 patients, but it was present in 42% of group 2 and 91% of group 3 patients.
- Historically, surgical delay was believed to lead to higher rates of osteonecrosis. However, recent literature has shown no difference in complication rates with delayed treatment (Lindvall et al. 2004, Vallier et al. 2004). The key is to reduce dislocations emergently, but wait until soft tissues are appropriate for definitive reduction.
- Vallier et al. (2004) published a retrospective study of 102 fractures in 100 patients. Each fracture was treated with ORIF. Functional outcomes were evaluated using the Foot Function Index (FFI) and the MFA. FFI scores were worst in this series for pain, disability, and activity when compared with values for the normal population. The mean MFA score was 24.6, which was worse than scores reported in uninjured patients (9.3) and in patients with other hindfoot injuries (22.1). For both outcome scores, fracture comminution was associated with a poorer result. No correlation was found with the age of the patient, Hawkins classification, or associated talar body fractures. Of the 45 patients who completed outcome questionnaires, 32 returned to work, 6 with job modifications.
- AVN is associated with open fractures and increased comminution.
- Posttraumatic arthritis is common after talar neck fractures. Vallier et al. (2004) reported evidence of arthritis in 54% of their patients. Lindvall et al. (2004) reported arthritic changes in the subtalar joint in 100% patients at final follow-up.

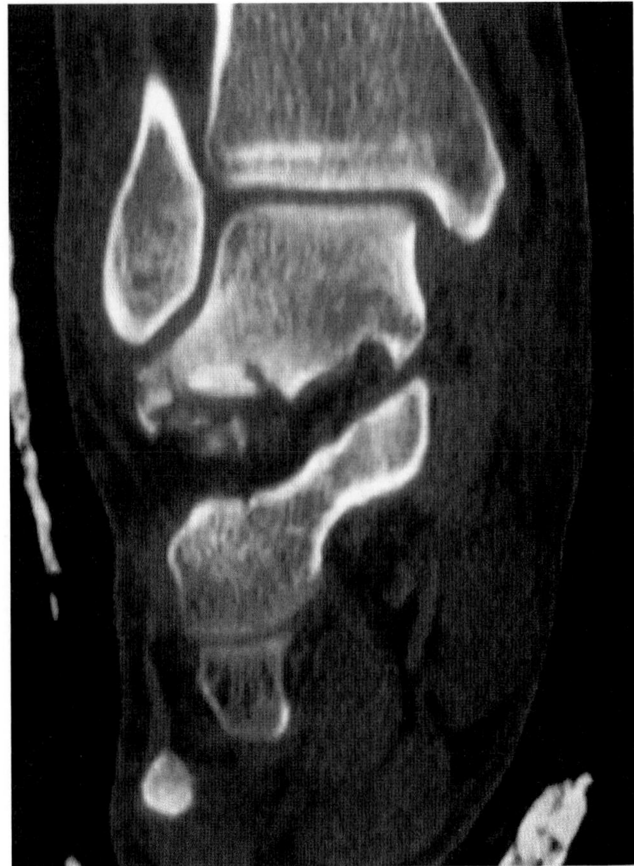

Figure 22–16: Computed tomography scan of a young female patient thrown from a horse, demonstrating a highly comminuted lateral process talus fracture.

Lateral Process Fracture

- Fracture of the lateral process occurs in less than 1% of all ankle injuries. Two common mechanisms of injury have been reported. The first is with acute dorsiflexion and inversion of the foot. The second, common in snowboarding injuries, is dorsiflexion and eversion.
- Because of similarity in mechanism of injury and location of pain, these fractures are often mistaken for ankle sprain injuries, and the diagnosis is missed approximately 30% of the time.
- High-energy mechanisms such as a fall from a height or a motor vehicle accident can also lead to this fracture pattern.
- On examination, the patient will have swelling and tenderness to palpation over the lateral side of the foot just distal to the tip of the fibula. The anterior talofibular ligament inserts on to the lateral process, therefore these patients may present with symptoms of instability.
- Late presentation often consists of lateral-sided ankle pain made worse with uneven walking surfaces and prolonged standing. Decreased subtalar range of motion can be seen clinically in fractures presenting late for treatment.
- Fractures often are not readily apparent on plain radiographs.
- In cases with a high index of suspicion for this injury and negative plain radiographs, a CT scan should also be obtained. All lateral process fractures should be evaluated by CT scan. This improves fracture understanding, evaluates for comminution, and can also identify any fracture debris in the subtalar joint (Fig. 22–16).
- Hawkins (1965) classified these injuries into three groups.
  - Type 1 is an extraarticular avulsion fracture.
  - Type 2 is a large fragment with a single fracture line that traverses both the superior (ankle) and inferior (subtalar) articular surfaces.
  - A type 3 fracture is comminuted and involves both articulations.

Treatment

- Acute fractures that are non-displaced or small in size can be treated in a short leg non-weight-bearing cast for 6 weeks.
- Displaced fractures, fractures of larger size, and fractures with debris present in the subtalar joint require operative treatment to restore congruity to the talofibular and subtalar articular surfaces.

- Subtalar joint debridement should be performed in all cases with intraarticular debris identified on CT scans (Fig. 22–17).
- Fixation can consist of either simple screw fixation or minifragment plating, depending on the fracture size and extent of comminution (Figs 22–18 and 22–19).
- It is imperative to restore congruity to the posterior subtalar facet. If the fracture is comminuted and not amenable to internal fixation, then the fragment should be excised to minimize the risk of subtalar arthrosis.
- Small fragments that present late can be treated by simple excision if symptomatic.
- Larger fragments should be treated by standard ORIF, as described above, after all fibrous and calcified material is removed from the fracture plane.
- Lateral process fractures identified and treated early have better results than those with delay in diagnosis.
- In a study of nine patients by Heckman and McLean (1985), three patients presented late and six presented acutely. Better outcomes were achieved with acute treatment versus late. All three patients who presented late had persistent symptoms after treatment. (Of course, any study evaluating late presentations may be biased toward worse outcomes, because those patients with missed injuries and no symptoms will never be detected.)

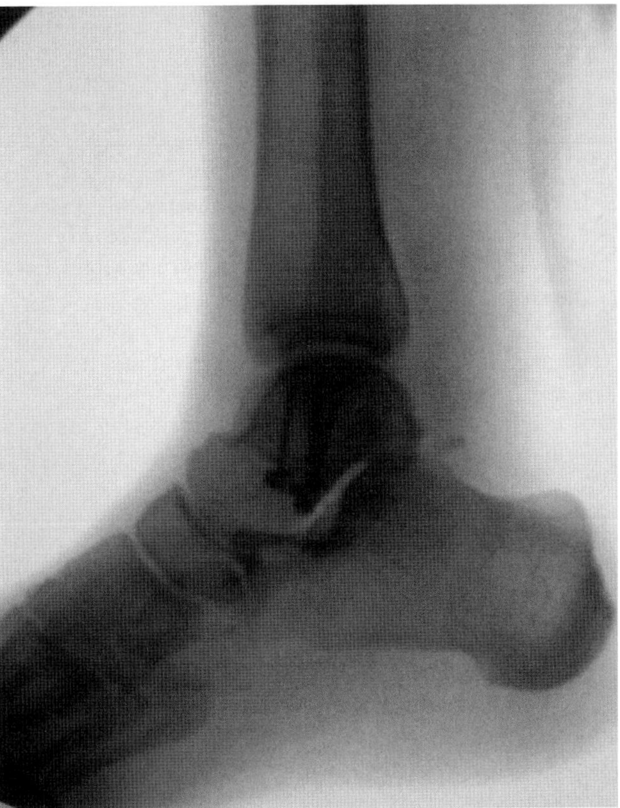

Figure 22–18: Lateral radiograph of a comminuted lateral process fracture treated by plate fixation.

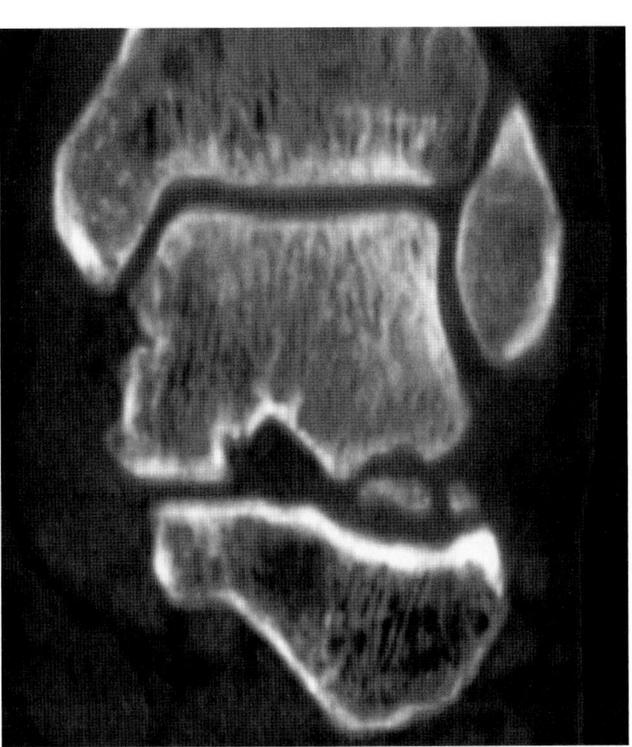

Figure 22–17: A lateral process fracture treated non-operatively in a 22-year-old man. Notice the large bone fragments, which have been free in the subtalar joint for greater than 1 year. The patient had complaints of pain and stiffness.

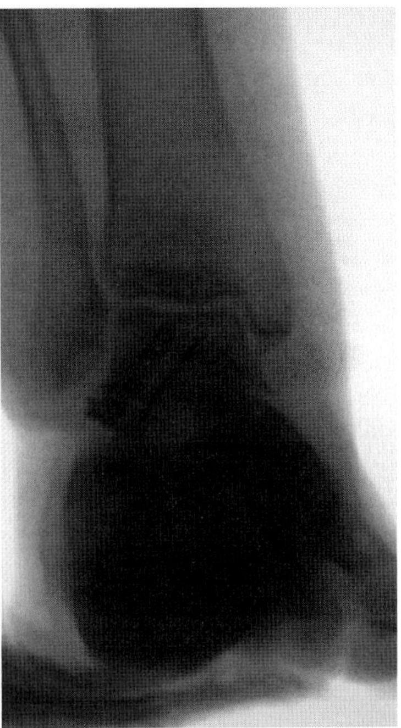

Figure 22–19: Mortise image of a comminuted lateral process fracture treated by minifragment plate fixation.

Avascular Necrosis

- AVN is a common complication of talus fractures. AVN is also reported as osteonecrosis or aseptic necrosis in the literature.
- Talar neck or body fractures, or dislocations without fracture, are all susceptible to developing AVN.
- AVN is directly related to the displacement at the time of injury and disruption of the tenuous vascular supply to the talar body.
- AVN is not always easy to recognize. Onset of AVN is generally within 8 weeks, but the diagnosis may be delayed until 12 weeks.
- Radiographs should be obtained 6-8 weeks after injury or surgery to assess for the presence or absence of a *Hawkins sign*.
- Hawkins sign is relative osteopenia of the subchondral portion of talar dome on the anteroposterior and mortise views, and can be used as a prognostic sign.
- A positive Hawkins sign is an indicator that the vascularity is retained (the body is developing disuse osteopenia) and development of AVN is unlikely.
- A negative Hawkins sign does not confirm that AVN will occur, but serial radiographic assessment should be performed.
- Magnetic resonance imaging can be of benefit in evaluating AVN; however, false negatives have been reported.
- Hawkins' classic paper reported risk of AVN by fracture type (Table 22–1).
- Increased initial fracture displacement, comminution, and open fractures are associated with higher AVN rates.
- AVN can lead to collapse of the talar dome, with painful ankle and subtalar arthritis. But there are multiple reports of patients with AVN who lack significant clinical symptoms. Currently, there is no way to predict if a patient with a negative Hawkins sign (early AVN) will go on to develop symptoms.
- The best prevention of AVN is prompt reduction of all dislocations, anatomical reduction and internal fixation, and avoiding unnecessary stripping of the talar neck.
- Historically, surgical delay was believed to lead to higher rates of osteonecrosis. However, recent literature has shown no difference in complication rates with delayed treatment.
- Both Hawkins and Canale found that even prolonged non-weight bearing does not prevent collapse. Additionally, it may take up to 36 months for revascularization to occur, and non-weight bearing for this duration is impractical.
- Vallier et al. (2004) found that 37% of their patients with AVN after a talar neck fracture demonstrated revascularization without limitations in weight bearing or bracing.
- Fracture healing should be assessed to determine weight bearing status. If union has been achieved, weight bearing should be advanced even if concern exists for AVN. Continued non-weight bearing is recommended if union has not been achieved.
- Core decompression and bone grafting have been performed for AVN of the talus, mainly in atraumatic AVN, and long-term results are not available. The results of these procedures in the traumatic population are largely unknown.
- AVN can occur without trauma, particularly in patients on steroids (or with other risk factors for AVN of the hip). Limited case series have shown some benefit to core decompression prior to collapse.
- Once the talar dome collapses, or for those with persistent pain after decompression, combined ankle and subtalar arthrodesis can be performed. Non-union rates are higher than normal because the talus is not viable. The non-viable talar body can be replaced with a tricortical iliac crest graft. Alternately, Blair fusion (fusion of the viable talar neck to the anterior tibia) or tibiocalcaneal fusion can be done. Both these result in shortening of the leg. For the rare active, young patient, transtibial amputation may be the most functional choice.

Non-union and Malunion

- Non-union is a rare complication of talus fractures. Reported rates vary from 0 to 12%. Non-union is more common in open fractures and fractures with extensive comminution. Traditional nonunion techniques are applicable, including bone graft, rigid fixation, and prolonged non-weight bearing.
- Malunion is probably more common than is reported. It is difficult to assess rotational and varus angulation on plain radiographs. Varus malunion is most common.
- Malalignment in the talar neck by as little as 2 mm alters joint contact characteristics in the subtalar joint (Sangeorzan et al. 1992).
- Varus malalignment can be corrected by osteotomy of the talar neck and bone grafting. This procedure is technically difficult.
- Arthrodesis is another salvage option, appropriate once posttraumatic arthritis develops. In cases with varus malunion, the medial column of the foot is shortened. At the time of arthrodesis, the medial column needs to be lengthened by bone grafting to obtain prior length, or the lateral column needs to be shortened. This can be done by removing a wedge out of the cuboid, or alternatively the anterior process of the calcaneus.
- The determination of which joints to fuse is made by assessing the status of the tibiotalar, subtalar, and talonavicular. Whenever possible, joints are left mobile.

- Dorsal malalignment can cause anterior impingement of the ankle.
- If identified early, impingement can be treated by removing the prominence off the talar neck with an osteotome to create more room for the anterior tibial plafond.
- Ankle arthroplasty is an option in patients who have tibiotalar arthritis from anterior impingement and concomitant subtalar arthritis. However, arthroplasty should probably not be performed in cases of unresolved AVN, because the necrotic talus will not grow into the pores of the implant.

Osteochondritis Dissecans

- Berndt and Harty in 1959 described a cadaver model for creating transchondral fractures of the talus. Although not all osteochondritis dissecans lesions are transchondral fractures, their results have been applied to all osteochondral lesions of the talus.
- Their paper described the transchondral fracture of the talus, including the mechanism and the location of injury and position of the foot at the time of injury. Lateral dome lesions are secondary to combined inversion and dorsiflexion forces impacting the anterolateral talar dome on to the tibial plafond. Medial dome lesions are secondary to a combined inversion, plantar flexion, and external rotation force impacting the posteromedial talar dome on to the tibial plafond.
- Osteochondritis dissecans of the talus is fairly common. The ankle is the most commonly injured joint of the body among athletes. There are approximately 23 000 ankle sprains per year that require medical attention, and perhaps 6.5% of ankle sprains result in osteochondritis dissecans lesions.
- It is likely that the etiology is not simple trauma in some cases, but may include ischemia and/or repetitive injury.
- Lateral lesions are more common than medial. Most or all lateral lesions are secondary to trauma. However, it should be noted that only 64% of medial lesions have an identifiable trauma.
- The characteristics of the lesions vary also. Lateral lesions are often shallow and wafer-shaped. These lesions rarely heal spontaneously and often need surgery. Medial lesions may have a familial history and are bilateral in 10-25%. They are often deep and cup-shaped, and frequently heal spontaneously with a low incidence of arthritis.
- Classification and treatment of osteochondritis dissecans is discussed further in Chapter 27.

References

Canale ST, Belding RH. (1980) Osteochondral lesions of the talus. J Bone Joint Surg Am 62: 97-102.

Canale ST, Kelly FB. (1978) Fractures of the neck of the talus. Long-term evaluation of 71 cases. J Bone Joint Surg Am 60: 143-156.
Describes group 4 talus neck fractures.

Chateau PB, Brokaw DS, Jelen BA et al. (2002) Plate fixation of talar neck fractures: Preliminary review of a new technique in twenty-three patients. J Orthop Trauma 16: 213-219.
Reports the technique of minifragment plate fixation for talar neck fractures and successful outcomes in 23 patients.

Fortin PT, Balaszy JE. (2001) Talus fractures: Evaluation and treatment. J Am Acad Orthop Surg 9(2): 114-127.
An excellent overview of talus fractures.

Giuffrida AY, Lin SS, Abidi N et al. (2003) Pseudo os trigonum sign: Missed posteromedial talar facet fracture. Foot Ankle Int 24: 642-649.
High rate of complications with missed posteromedial body fractures. Four of six fractures missed initially. Five of six required arthrodesis. Early recognition and treatment are key.

Hawkins LG. (1965) Fracture of the lateral process of the talus. J Bone Joint Surg Am 47: 1170-1175.
Classification system for lateral process fractures.

Hawkins LG. (1970) Fractures of the neck of the talus. J Bone Joint Surg Am 52: 991-1002.
Most widely used neck classification, and reports association with AVN.

Heckman JD, McLean MR. (1985) Fractures of the lateral process of the talus. Clin Orthop 199: 108-113.
Early treatment of lateral process fractures leads to better results than late treatment.

Inokuchi S, Ogawa K, Usami N. (1996) Classification of fractures of the talus: Clear differentiation between neck and body fractures. Foot Ankle Int 17: 748-750.
Reports using the inferior surface fracture line to differentiate between neck and body fractures.

Lindvall E, Haidukewych G, Dipasquale T et al. (2004) Open reduction and stable fixation of isolated, displaced talar neck and body fractures. J Bone Joint Surg Am 86: 2229-2234.
Posttraumatic arthritis seen in all fractures; osteonecrosis rates and AOFAS outcome score reported. Delay in surgical treatment did not affect outcome.

Mulfinger GL, Trueta J. (1970) The blood supply of the talus. J Bone Joint Surg Br 52: 160-167.
An overview of the blood supply, with great illustrations.

Sangeorzan BJ, Wagner UA, Harrington RM et al. (1992) Contact characteristics of the subtalar joint: The effect of talar neck misalignment. J Orthop Res 10: 544-551.
Changes in alignment as little as 2 mm alter the contact characteristics of the subtalar joint.

Sneppen O, Christensen SB, Krogsoe O et al. (1977) Fracture of the body of the talus. Acta Orthop Scand 48: 317-324.
A series of talar body fractures treated conservatively, leading to poor results.

Swanson TV, Bray TJ, Holmes GB Jr. (1992) Fractures of the talar neck: A mechanical study of fixation. J Bone Joint Surg Am 74(4): 544-551.

Posterior to anterior placed hardware is mechanically superior to anterior to posterior placement.

Vallier HA, Nork SE, Barei DP et al. (2004) Talar neck fractures: Results and outcomes. J Bone Joint Surg Am 86: 1616-1624.
An excellent paper looking at neck fractures. MFA outcome scores and factors leading to worse functional outcomes discussed. Fifty-four percent posttraumatic arthritis rate.

Vallier HA, Nork SE, Benirschke SK et al. (2003) Surgical treatment of talar body fractures. J Bone Joint Surg Am 85-A(9): 1716-1724.
Rates of posttraumatic arthritis, osteonecrosis, and open fractures are compared with functional outcomes. Worse outcomes in open fractures, with comminution, and with associated neck fractures.

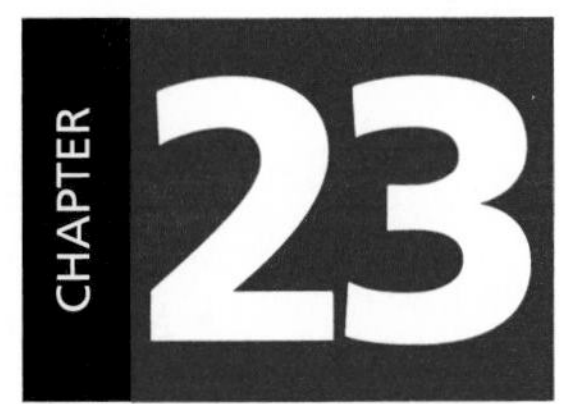

Navicular and Midfoot Injuries

Gregory J. Della Rocca* and Bruce J. Sangeorzan§

*M.D., Ph.D., Acting Instructor, Department of Orthopaedic Surgery, Harborview Medical Center, Seattle, WA
§M.D., Professor, Department of Orthopaedic Surgery, Harborview Medical Center, Seattle, WA

Anatomy and Function of the Midfoot

- The midfoot includes five tarsal bones: navicular, cuboid, and three cuneiforms (medial, first; middle, second; and lateral, third). It forms the transverse arch of the foot and part of the longitudinal arch.
- The navicular articulates in a mobile relationship with the talus proximally. The articulation distally is with three cuneiforms, where stability is more important than flexibility.
- The cuboid articulates in a mobile relationship with the anterior process of the calcaneus proximally. Articulation distally is with the fourth and fifth metatarsal bases and is also a mobile articulation.
- The cuneiforms articulate with navicular proximally, first through third metatarsal bases distally, and cuboid laterally (with lateral or third cuneiform). These articulations are rigid.
- The second metatarsal meets the middle cuneiform in a rigid joint, more proximal than the first and third joints, and is referred to as the "keystone" of the midfoot.
- The transverse tarsal, or Chopart, joint is formed by the talonavicular and calcaneocuboid joints. This complex is stiff with hindfoot varus, as in the toe-off phase of gait, and provides a rigid lever for ambulation. Hindfoot valgus "unlocks" the transverse tarsal joint.
- Mobility at the transverse tarsal joint is necessary for normal gait, and fusions are not well tolerated. Temporary spanning fixation of the talonavicular and calcaneocuboid joint in the setting of trauma will not be durable, and is often removed once healing of the traumatized foot has occurred.
- Fixation from fourth or fifth metatarsals into cuboid also restricts normal foot motion and is not well tolerated. Fixation across these joints is often removed once healing has occurred in the traumatized foot.
- The remaining midfoot joints (naviculocuneiform and medial three metatarsocuneiform) are relatively stable and non-mobile articulations and tolerate permanent fixation well.

Navicular Fractures

Introduction

- Navicular injuries include avulsion fractures of the tuberosity and fractures of the body, either extra- or intraarticular.
- Avulsion fractures may be present medially, dorsally, or plantarly. Medial avulsions may be caused by the posterior tibial tendon or the plantar calcaneonavicular (spring) ligament.
- Navicular body fractures are less common than avulsion fractures, but may be greater in severity. They can result from a direct mechanism ("crush") or an indirect mechanism (axial load through foot).

Evaluation

- History for an avulsion fracture typically involves a low-energy twisting injury, with pain at the medial midfoot and inability to bear weight afterward.
- Navicular body fractures may present with similar complaints, although a higher energy mechanism may result in a more diffuse midfoot injury in addition to the navicular fracture, and symptoms may correspond to the extent of the injury.
- Physical examination will reveal varying degrees of edema, ecchymosis, and tenderness over the proximal midfoot. Patients will often have significant pain with resisted adduction of the foot.
- Diffuse edema and ecchymosis about the foot do not negate the possibility of navicular injury; rather, they may be indicative of multiple midfoot injuries.
- Rule out compartment syndrome in any patient with significant foot swelling.
- Screening radiographs should include anteroposterior, oblique, and lateral foot radiographs. Navicular avulsion fractures will demonstrate a fleck of avulsed cortex, which is sometimes visualized on only one view (increasing the possibility of the injury being missed). This should be differentiated from an accessory navicular, which will be well corticated.
- Computed tomography (CT) scans can be obtained to further delineate anatomy and pick up subtle findings when plain films fail to show adequate detail.
- Classification of displaced navicular fractures:
  - type 1—transverse coronal plane fracture
  - type 2—sagittal plane fracture that often runs dorsolateral to plantarmedial, with the medial fragment often subluxed and the lateral fragment often comminuted
  - type 3—fractures with central or lateral comminution and associated with lateral displacement of the forefoot and/or occasionally disruption of the calcaneocuboid joint or fracture of the cuboid.

Treatment

- Dorsal avulsion fractures can usually be treated similar to an ankle sprain, with progressive weight bearing and functional rehabilitation.
- Non-displaced navicular body fractures are treated with limited weight bearing (usually non-weight bearing) and immobilization in a well-padded short leg splint or cast. Avulsion of the posterior tibial tendon, however, requires surgical correction.
- Type 1 displaced navicular body fractures can be reduced and fixed through a dorsomedial exposure and lag screw fixation from dorsal to plantar.
- Type 2 and 3 fractures require more extensive surgical intervention. The medial fragment, which is often subluxed, must be reduced. An aid to reduction is a medially placed minidistractor. This may also restore the alignment of the medial border of the foot in type 3 fractures.
- Medial to lateral lag screws may be used when there is no lateral fragment comminution. Screws may also maintain reduction by being placed across the naviculocuneiform joints or into the cuboid. Temporary Kirschner wire fixation from the navicular into the talar head may also prove helpful in difficult injuries.
- Temporary bridge plating across the medial midfoot can be used as an aid to maintaining reduction (Fig. 23–1).

Rehabilitation

- Postoperative well-padded short leg plaster splint immobilization, with a toe plate, is indicated for these injuries.
- Non-weight bearing is maintained for up to 12 weeks.
- Suture removal should occur at 2 weeks, followed by reapplication of a well-padded short leg splint or cast with a toe plate. For injuries with stable fixation, early range of motion exercises are begun, and the foot is splinted in a removable brace.
- Temporary Kirschner wires, as necessary, are removed at approximately 6 weeks.
- Removal of implants spanning multiple joints after severe injuries should not occur until healing is complete. Implants spanning naviculocuneiform joints need not be removed, but preservation of motion at the talonavicular joint is desirable.
- Navicular fracture outcomes are shown in Box 23–1.

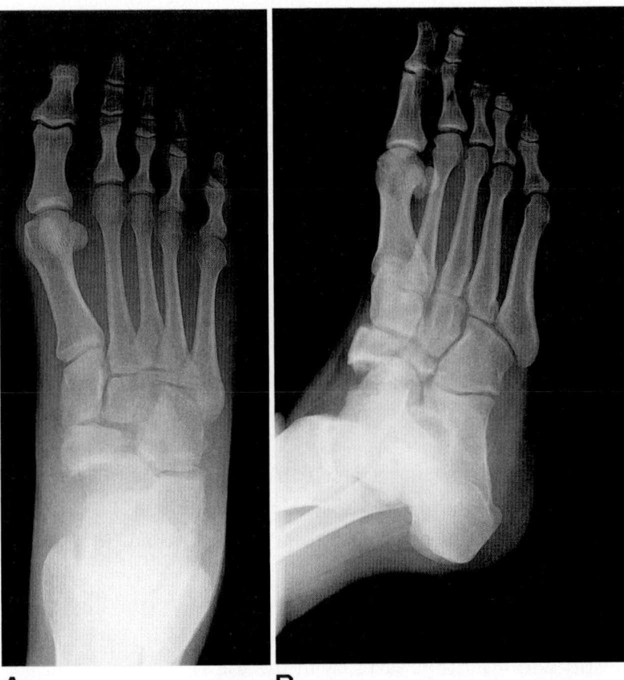

Figure 23–1: Navicular fracture. This patient sustained a type 3 navicular fracture in a motor vehicle crash. A-B, Anteroposterior and oblique injury radiographs.

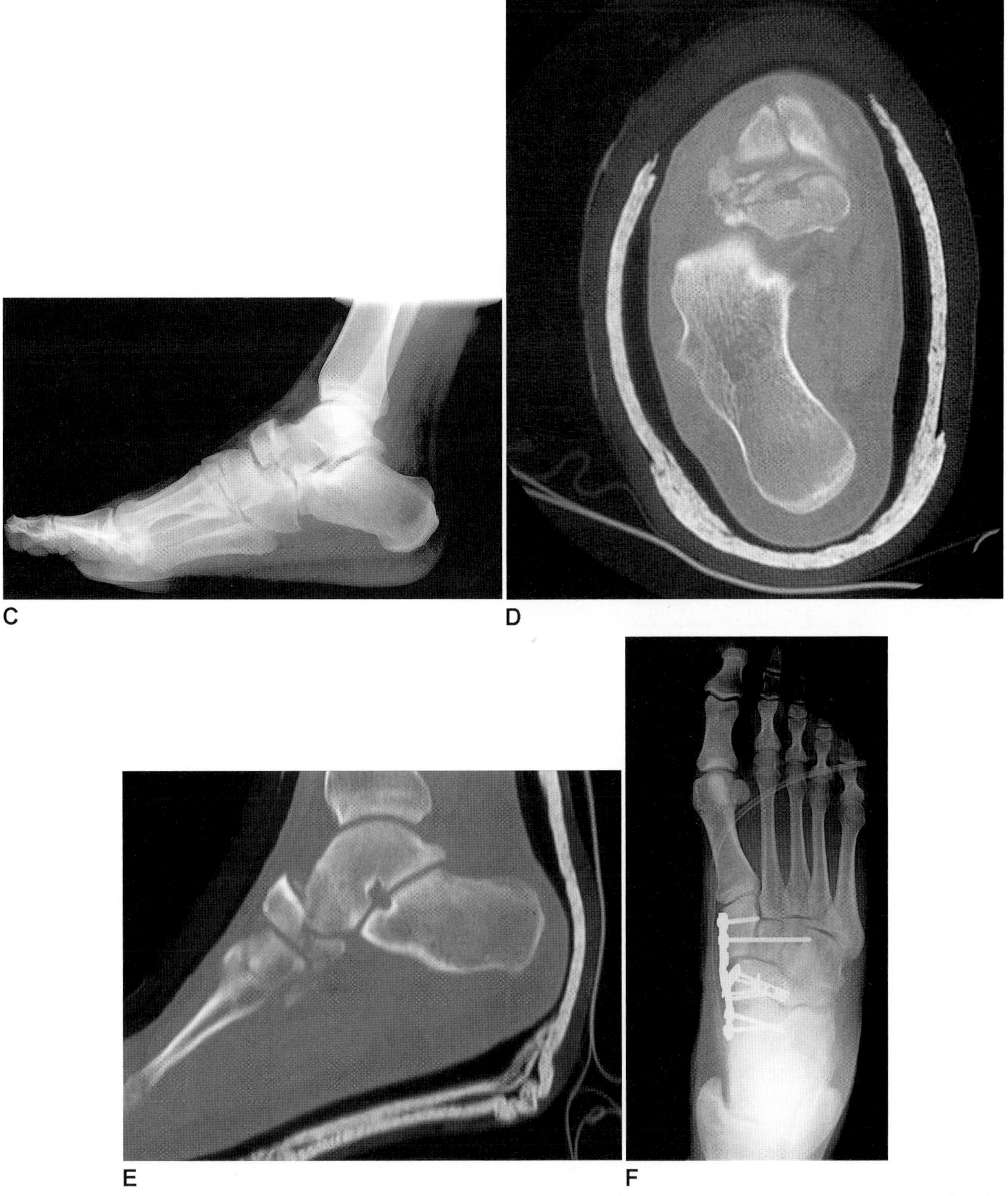

Figure 23–1: Cont'd C, Lateral injury radiograph. D and E, Coronal and sagittal computed tomography images, respectively, which demonstrate greater detail of the navicular fracture pattern. F, Anteroposterior and lateral postoperative radiographs demonstrating internal fixation of anatomically reconstructed navicular, with supporting bridge plate across medial column of forefoot. The bridge plate was removed approximately 3 months postoperatively.

Continued

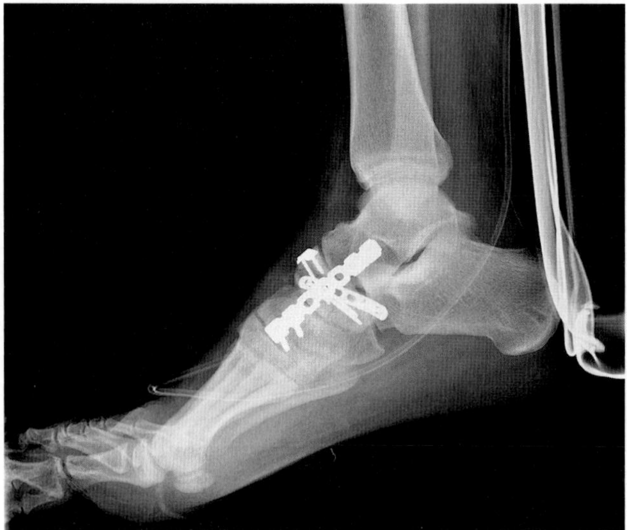

G

Figure 23–1: Cont'd G, Anteroposterior and lateral postoperative radiographs demonstrating internal fixation of anatomically reconstructed navicular, with supporting bridge plate across medial column of forefoot. The bridge plate was removed approximately 3 months postoperatively.

Box 23–1 Navicular Fracture Outcome

- Restoration of normal anatomical alignment leads to better outcomes in displaced fractures.
- Increasing comminution tends to result in more frequent poor outcomes.

Navicular Stress Fractures

Introduction

- Unusual injuries in the general population, but perhaps quite common in high-caliber athletes.
- Characteristic in athletes participating in sports that require cutting movements (basketball and soccer players) and explosive activity (sprinters and high jumpers). Not common in endurance-type of activity (distance runners and soldiers).
- Possible mechanism: Repetitive force during toe-off phase of gait that is channeled through the rigid lever of the second metatarsal-middle (second) cuneiform to the central navicular may cause fracture.
- Other risk factors may include a long second metatarsal or a short first metatarsal.

Evaluation

- History often includes an insidious onset of midfoot pain. The pain will characteristically be exacerbated by explosive athletic activity and relieved by rest.
- Physical examination findings will not often include edema or ecchymosis. Tenderness is often localized to the lateral aspect of the navicular. Maintaining a single-limb stance can often be quite difficult.
- Radiographic evaluation should include standard anteroposterior, oblique, and lateral foot plain radiographs. The fracture line is often invisible, however, on these films. Other conditions should be ruled out.
  - Callus is not always apparent.
- Radionuclide bone scanning can be diagnostic, especially in the absence of plain film findings. Marked uptake will be noted in the navicular alone.
- CT or magnetic resonance imaging (MRI) scan will often confirm a diagnosis of stress fracture. Fracture lines may be incomplete or non-displaced, making initial plain radiographs somewhat unreliable.

Treatment

- The mainstay of treatment for navicular stress fractures is rest. Weight bearing is protected for 6 weeks. Cast, splint, or walker boot immobilization is utilized as desired.
- Failed conservative treatment indicates operative intervention. A dorsal approach is often used. Sclerotic fracture margins are debrided. Autogenous iliac crest bone graft is then placed into the fracture gap, and the navicular is secured with interfragmentary screws.

Rehabilitation

- Postoperative regimen may include immobilization at the surgeon's discretion. Early range of motion exercises are often allowed for the ankle and hindfoot.
- Suture removal occurs at 2 weeks.
- Weight bearing is restricted for 4-6 weeks, and athletic activities for 3 months.

Cuboid Fractures

Introduction

- Often termed *nutcracker* fractures, these are uncommon injuries.
- The nutcracker injury results from violent abduction of forefoot on hindfoot, compressing lateral aspect of cuboid between the anterior process of the calcaneus and the bases of the fourth and fifth metatarsals.
- Fracture can occur with direct trauma (e.g. crush injury to midfoot).
- Distraction forces on the medial aspect of the foot may result in associated tear of the posterior tibial tendon or avulsion fracture of the medial tubercle of the navicular (insertion of posterior tibial tendon).

Evaluation

- History may reveal a foot injury with substantial force having been applied to the foot (e.g. motor vehicle crash, fall from a substantial height, crushing injury). Patients may complain of lateral foot pain and inability to bear weight.
- Examination often reveals substantial lateral foot edema, ecchymosis, and tenderness. Deformity in this location

may be a consequence of frank cuboid dislocation (rare) or of a complete transverse midfoot disruption (e.g. Lisfranc injury).

- Medial foot edema can occur, especially with associated navicular or posterior tibial tendon or Lisfranc injury.
- Any patient with significant foot edema or deformity should be carefully evaluated, especially if a decreased level of consciousness impedes history taking and physical examination.
- Remember to assess ipsilateral ankle for associated injury.
- Compartment syndrome should be ruled out.
- Radiographic evaluation should include anteroposterior, lateral, and oblique views. A 30° medial oblique view will allow for full visualization of the cuboid without overlapping structures. CT scanning may be helpful in comminuted fractures or in the absence of adequate plain radiographs.

Treatment (Fig. 23–2)

- Non-displaced isolated cuboid fractures are treated with well-padded short leg splinting or casting and protected weight bearing.
- Cuboid dislocations should be reduced and splinted. Open reduction through a lateral or dorsolateral incision is usually necessary. Instability after reduction may be treated with Kirschner wires from the base of the fifth metatarsal, spanning the cuboid, and terminating in the anterior process of the calcaneus.
- Displaced fractures (including comminuted crush injuries resulting in lateral column shortening) are treated with open reduction and internal fixation (ORIF). Failure to treat these fractures appropriately can lead to persistent deformity and pain.
- Exposure of the fracture is accomplished through a lateral longitudinal incision in the interval between extensor digitorum brevis and peroneal tendons.
- Articular reduction is accomplished first, and provisionally stabilized with Kirschner wires.
- A laminar spreader then may be used to correct lateral column length, if necessary. Alternatively, a lateral small joint distractor, with half-pins placed in the fifth metatarsal diaphysis and the anterior process or tuberosity of the calcaneus, can assist in reestablishing lateral column length.
- If distraction is necessary, then the resulting defect should be filled with tricortical autogenous iliac crest bone graft or other structural graft as necessary. Structural graft can be held with Kirschner wires, cortical screws, and/or a lateral buttress plate.
- A plate spanning the calcaneocuboid joint and/or the fifth tarsometatarsal joint may be considered if no purchase can be gained in the cuboid itself.

Rehabilitation

- Initially, the operative foot is immobilized in a well-padded short leg plaster splint. Sutures are removed after

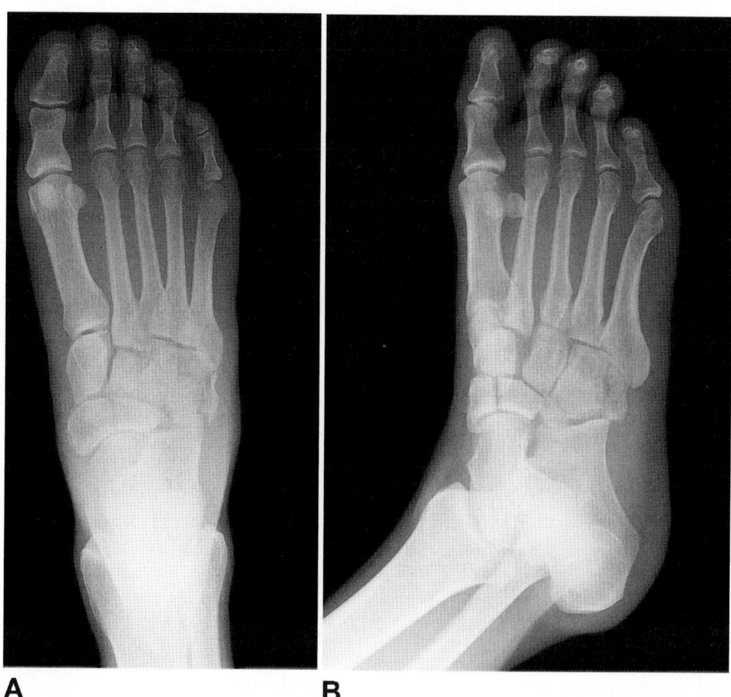

Figure 23–2: Navicular and cuboid fractures with middle (second) cuneiform dislocation. This patient sustained these injuries in a motor vehicle crash. **A-B**, Anteroposterior and oblique injury radiographs.

Continued

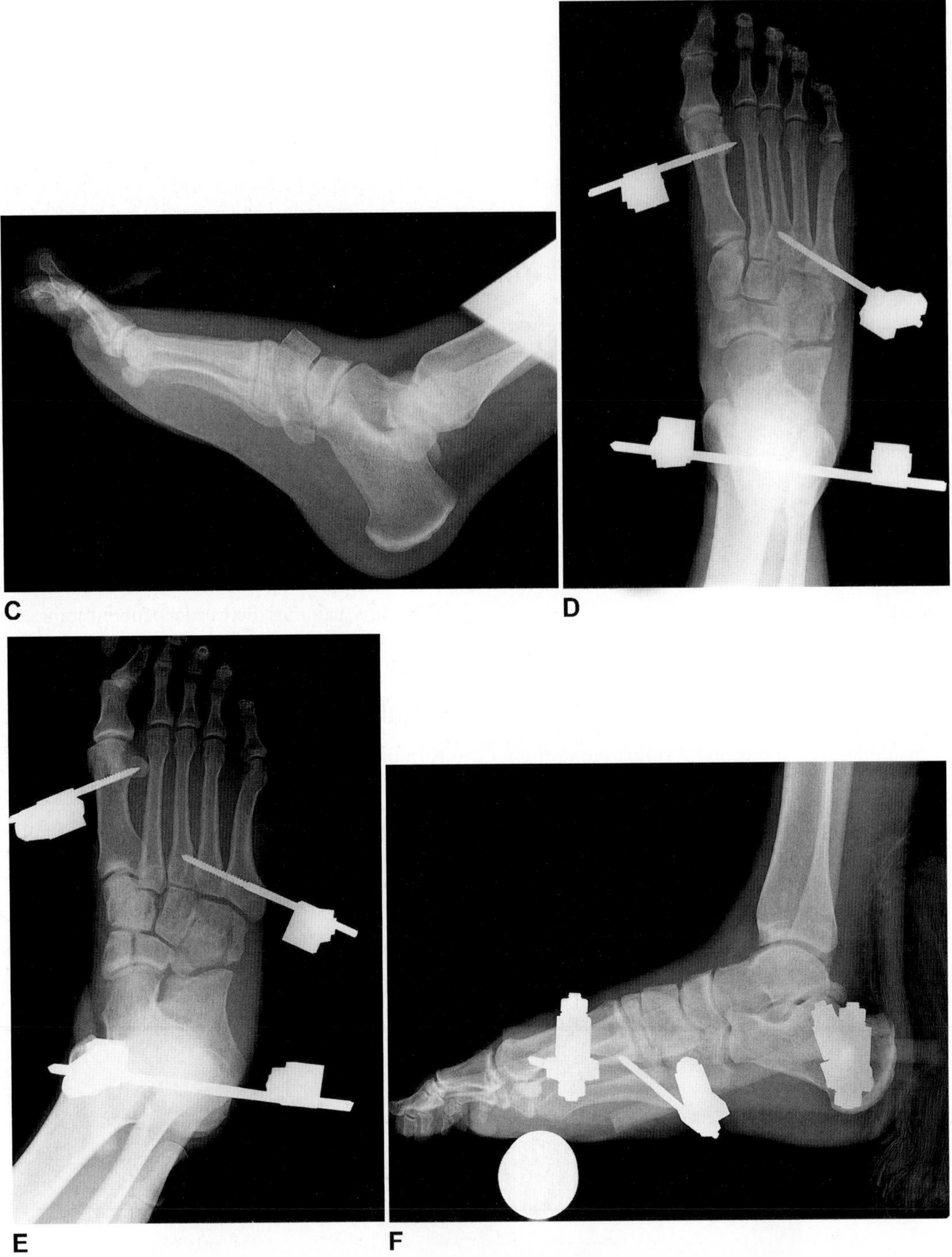

Figure 23–2: Cont'd C, Lateral injury radiograph. D-F, Definitive open reduction and internal fixation (ORIF) of this patient's injuries could not be accomplished acutely due to profuse edema. Closed reduction of middle (second) cuneiform dislocation and of foot alignment was accomplished, and held utilizing a through and through calcaneal tuberosity pin, attached via carbon fiber rods to a distal first metatarsal pin medially and a proximal fourth and fifth metatarsal pin laterally.

2 weeks, and further immobilization with splinting or casting is continued for a total of 6-8 weeks.

- Weight bearing is protected for a minimum of 6 weeks.
- At the 6- to 8-week mark, the patient may be placed into a walker boot, and range of motion exercises are initiated for the ankle and subtalar joints. Weight bearing is progressed as the clinical situation allows. Any Kirschner wires present can be withdrawn in the clinic at the 6-week mark.
- Implant removal can be accomplished due to irritation of skin or underlying structures, or to restore calcaneocuboid and/or fifth tarsometatarsal joint motion

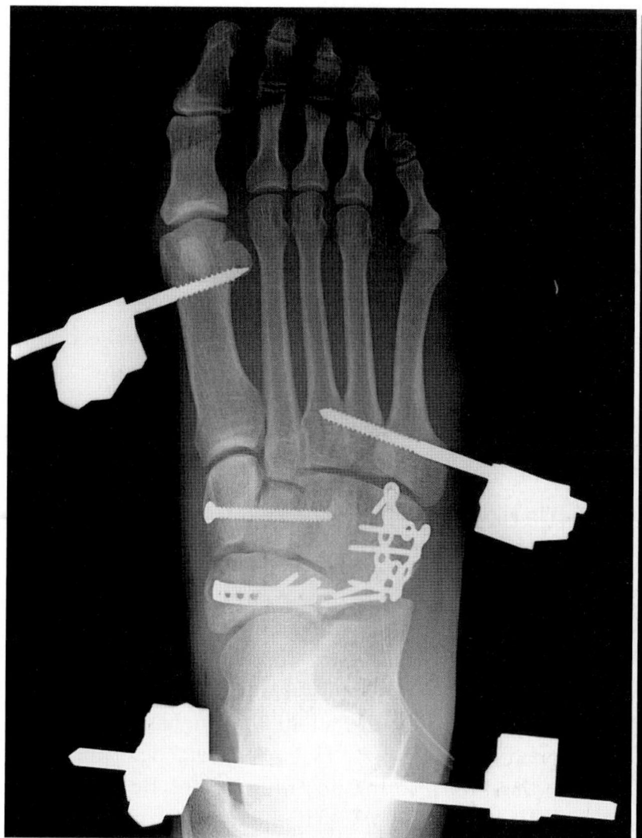

G

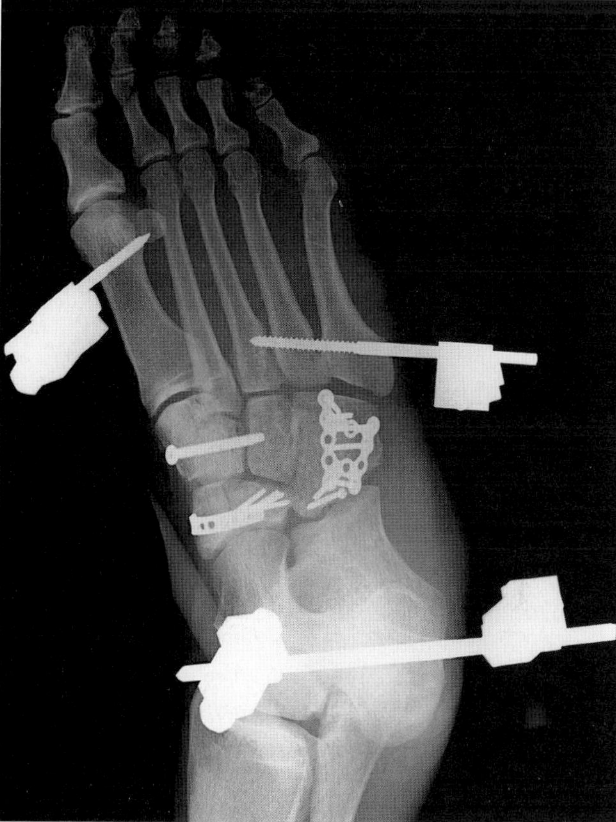

H

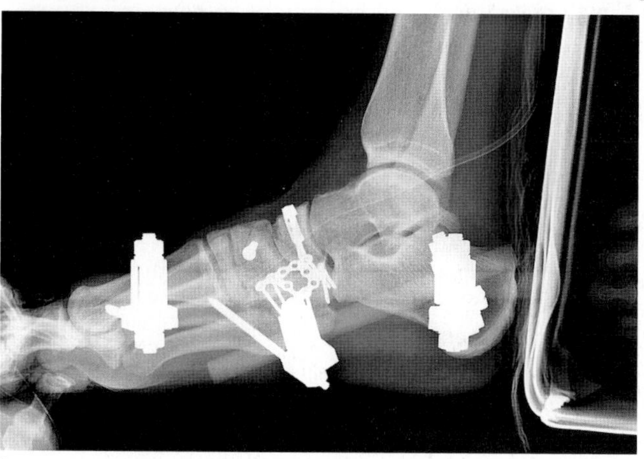

I

Figure 23–2: Cont'd **G-I**, Definitive ORIF was accomplished after foot edema was controlled. A single intercuneiform screw holds the middle (second) cuneiform reduced. Plate fixation is noted on the navicular and cuboid, maintaining anatomical reduction. The medial and lateral external fixator was left in place for 6 weeks to supplement fixation support.

(in the case of bridging plates), once healing of the fracture is accomplished.

Cuneiform Fractures

Introduction

- Isolated fractures are rare.
- Often occur in conjunction with other midfoot injuries (e.g. Lisfranc injuries, cuboid fractures, navicular fractures).
- Most commonly involve the medial (first) cuneiform.
- Injuries may occur via a direct mechanism (direct blow) or an indirect mechanism (violent forefoot abduction or adduction).

Evaluation

- Patients may complain of generalized midfoot pain or may isolate their area of maximal pain to the medial midfoot. They will often be unable to bear weight on the injured foot.
- Physical examination may reveal signs of typical midfoot injury: edema, ecchymosis, and tenderness. Skin examination

is necessary to rule out impending compromise by bony deformity, which is more likely in the setting of multiple bony or ligamentous injuries (such as a Lisfranc injury).
- Be suspicious of compartment syndrome with severe swelling and high-energy mechanisms.

Treatment

- Non-displaced cuneiform fractures, especially without associated midfoot injuries, may be treated conservatively with a well-padded short leg splint. Protected weight bearing is maintained acutely.
- Displaced cuneiform fractures require ORIF. Interfragmentary compression, if possible, may be employed for non-comminuted fractures.
- Incision is often centered dorsally over the interspace between first and second metatarsal bases and the medial (first) and middle (second) cuneiforms.
- Comminuted fractures may be stabilized to adjacent, uninjured cuneiforms with intercuneiform screw fixation.
- Associated midfoot injuries, such as Lisfranc injuries, should also be treated accordingly.
- Temporary bridge plating, from the base of the first metatarsal to the navicular or talus, may be employed for severely comminuted medial cuneiform fractures in order to maintain medial column length.

Rehabilitation

- Initial postoperative care should entail immobilization in a well-padded short leg plaster splint with a toe plate and non-weight bearing on the operative foot.
- Suture removal should occur at about 2 weeks.
- Support is maintained after 6 weeks in a removable walker boot. The boot may be removed for range of motion exercises for the hindfoot and ankle.
- Weight bearing is progressed as clinically indicated, beginning 6-12 weeks after surgery, in the walker boot. Extensive midfoot reconstructions will often require longer periods of protected weight bearing, approximating 12 weeks.

Lisfranc Injuries

Introduction

- Injury to the tarsometatarsal joint includes a wide spectrum of soft tissue and bony injuries.
- The injury may be purely ligamentous or purely fracture, or a combination of both (fracture-dislocations). Purely ligamentous Lisfranc injuries may lack radiographic abnormality, but they may also be characterized by fleck of bone apparent near base of second metatarsal, representing avulsion of the Lisfranc ligament, which normally courses from medial cuneiform to base of second metatarsal.
- Mechanism determines spectrum of injury: Lower energy, indirect (axial load on plantar flexed foot) or direct (athletic) mechanisms can cause ligamentous injury, while higher energy mechanisms (motor vehicle crashes) more often result in fractures or fracture-dislocations.
- Purely ligamentous injury may often be missed or diagnosis delayed due to lack of radiographic abnormality.
- Injury may involve entire forefoot dislocating laterally ("homolateral" type) on the midfoot, or may involve dissociation of metatarsals from one another ("dissociative" type). Common dissociative injury pattern includes a reduced (but injured) first tarsometatarsal joint with lateral dislocation of second to fifth tarsometatarsal joints.
- Lack of adequate treatment of these injuries can result in loss of stability of both transverse and longitudinal arches, leading to deformity, pain, and arthrosis.

Evaluation

- History: mechanism important, complaints of pain over midfoot.
- Examination: areas of ecchymosis (check plantar foot), midfoot tenderness. Global midfoot tenderness may indicate more severe injury than lateral tenderness alone. Skin evaluation for lacerations, fracture blisters, and impending compromise by gross skeletal deformity are important for prioritization of treatment. Be suspicious of compartment syndrome with high-energy mechanism, even in the setting of open fracture.
- Compartment syndrome may occur when dislocation leads to disruption of the deep perforating branch of the dorsalis pedis artery.
- Radiographic evaluation: weight bearing anteroposterior, lateral, and 30° oblique views. Comparison views with uninjured contralateral foot may be helpful in subtle injuries.
- Radiographic clues of purely ligamentous injury:
  - loss of alignment of medial border of middle (second) cuneiform and medial border of base of second metatarsal
  - widening between bases of first and second metatarsals and/or between base of second metatarsal and medial (first) cuneiform
  - flattening of longitudinal arch (on lateral view).
- Fractures of multiple metatarsal bases, medial cuneiform, and/or cuboid should alert examiner to the possibility of complete tarsometatarsal joint disruption (analogous to transradial, transscaphoid, and/or transcapitate perilunate wrist injury).
- Stress radiographs, perhaps under anesthesia, should be utilized when index of suspicion is high and diagnosis is not apparent on normal screening radiographs. Stress view obtained with an anteroposterior view while abduction force is applied to the forefoot against a stabilized hindfoot and midfoot.
- Positive stress radiograph may show disruption of line that intersects medial borders of navicular, medial (first)

cuneiform, and base of first metatarsal. Intercuneiform instability may also be detected.

- Routine use of CT and MRI for further evaluation of these injuries is controversial and may not add to evaluation.

Treatment

- Weight bearing and abduction stress radiographs, under anesthesia if necessary, should be considered in all cases of suspicious midfoot injuries and prior to electing non-operative therapy of these severe foot injuries. The role of non-surgical therapy for injuries apparent on stress radiographs is unknown at this time. Definitive surgical therapy should be delayed until swelling allows (often 1-2 weeks).
- Frank deformities should be urgently reduced to prevent skin compromise. Often, closed manipulative reduction can be employed under sedation in the emergency department. Postreduction non-stress radiographs are appropriate. A well-padded short leg plaster splint with toe plate is appropriate immobilization. Use "RICE" (rest, ice, compression, elevation) to assist with edema control.
- Surgical therapy usually requires two incisions over dorsum of foot: the first in the interval between metatarsals 1 and 2, and the second in the interval between metatarsals 3 and 4.
- Order of reduction: medial to lateral. Reduce first metatarsal to medial cuneiform in both transverse and sagittal planes. Treat intercuneiform instability next to provide a good "mortise" for reduction of the second metatarsal base. Debride soft tissues (scar, ligament remnants, bony debris) as necessary to allow for anatomical second metatarsal base reduction.
- Provisional fixation is provided with strategically placed Kirschner wires, such that they do not obstruct screw placement. Neutralization (not lag) screw fixation of the first and second tarsometatarsal joints is appropriate at this juncture, along with a single intercuneiform screw if necessary for stabilization of intercuneiform stability (Fig. 23–3).
- Treatment of the third tarsometatarsal joint is next performed, with Kirschner wires for provisional fixation, and stabilization with a neutralization screw.
- Comminuted metatarsal base fractures can be bridged with one-third or one-quarter tubular plates across the tarsometatarsal articulation, as necessary, to achieve stability (Fig. 23–4).
- Some researchers are investigating whether dorsal plating has mechanical and biologic advantages over transarticular screws.
- One recent study found improved early outcomes with formal metatarsocmeiform fusion, rather than simple

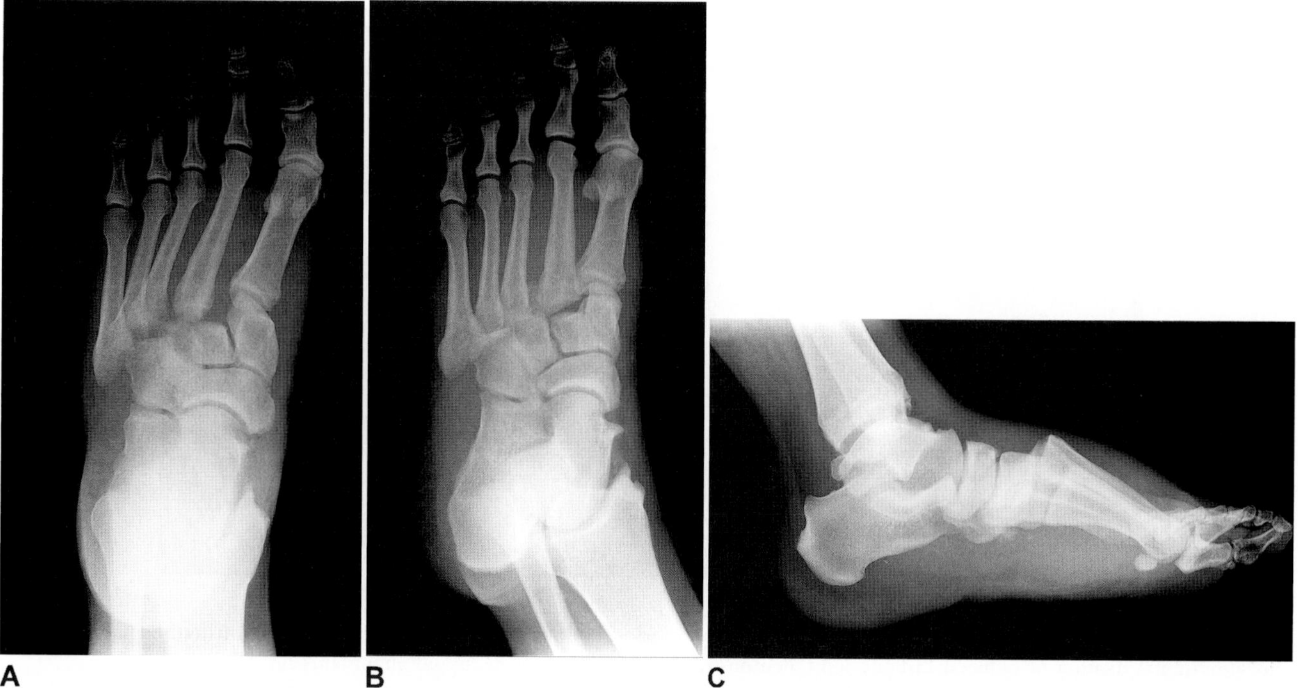

Figure 23–3: Ligamentous Lisfranc injury. This patient sustained this injury in a motorcycle crash. A-C, Anteroposterior, oblique, and lateral injury radiographs. Note wide disruption of first to second metatarsal interspace without disruption of medial alignment of first metatarsal with medial (first) cuneiform (A), disruption of medial alignment of third metatarsal with lateral (third) cuneiform and of fourth metatarsal with cuboid (B), and significant dorsal dislocation of lesser metatarsal bases relative to cuneiforms (C).

Continued

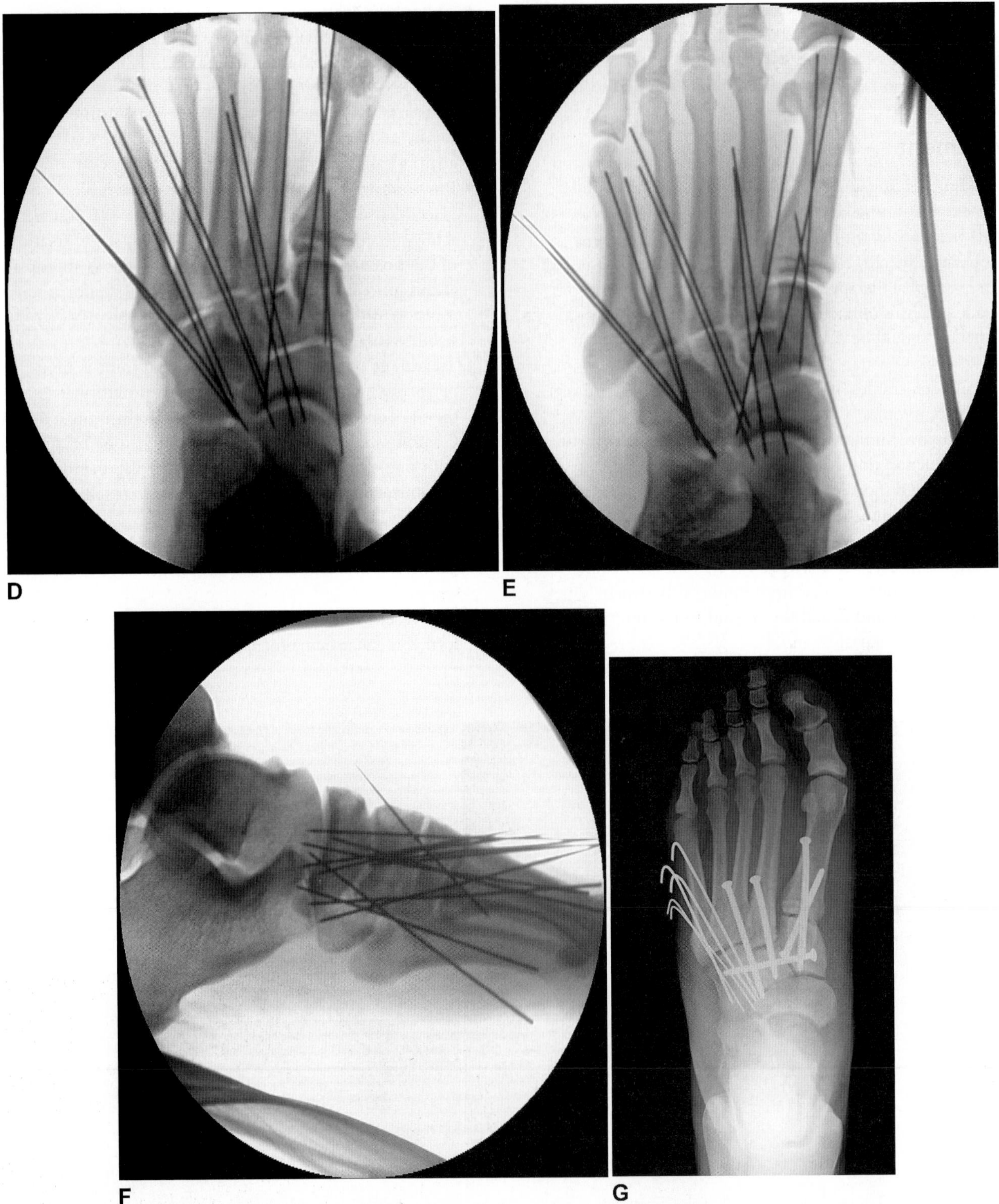

Figure 23–3: Cont'd **D-F,** Intraoperative fluoroscopic anteroposterior, oblique, and lateral radiographs demonstrating Kirschner wire provisional fixation of reduced Lisfranc joint, demonstrating restoration of disrupted alignments noted in panels A-C. **G,** Postoperative anteroposterior radiograph demonstrating definitive screw fixation constructs across first, second, and third tarsometatarsal joints, and Kirschner wire fixation across fourth and fifth tarsometatarsal joints. In most cases, one K wire across each of the fourth and fifth tarsometatarsal joints is sufficient. Also note medial to lateral intercuneiform screw, maintaining reduction of disruption between first and second ray. Kirschner wires were removed in the outpatient clinic at 6 weeks.

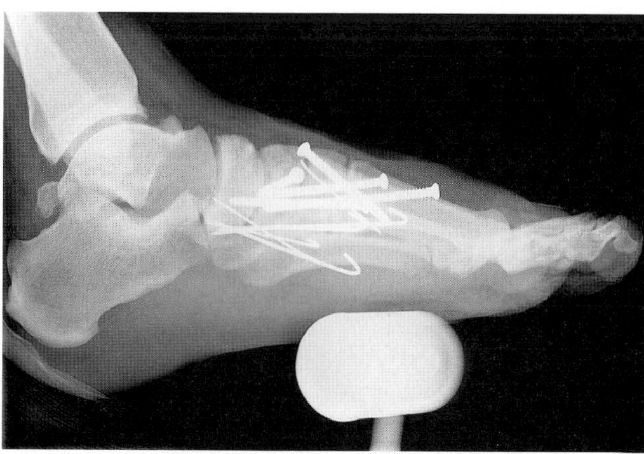

Figure 23–3: Cont'd **H,** Postoperative lateral radiograph demonstrating definitive screw fixation constructs across first, second, and third tarsometatarsal joints, and Kirschner wire fixation across fourth and fifth tarsometatarsal joints. In most cases, one K wire across each of the fourth and fifth tarsometatarsal joints is sufficient. Also note medial to lateral intercuneiform screw, maintaining reduction of disruption between first and second ray. Kirschner wires were removed in the outpatient clinic at 6 weeks.

reduction and fixation, of purely ligamenous Lisfranc injuries.

- As the fourth and fifth metatarsals are mobile on their proximal articulations, definitive fixation as necessary requires temporary (4-6 weeks) fixation with 0.062 Kirschner wires inserted percutaneously (after reduction under direct visualization through lateral incision and under fluoroscopic guidance) and left out of skin for removal in clinic.
- If early ORIF requires delay due to profuse foot edema, and deformity places skin at risk, emergent closed reduction is required. Failure to maintain this reduction with splinting may require spanning external fixation of the midfoot via medial and lateral frames.
- Complex midfoot injuries with combinations of fractures and dislocations may be treated definitively with a combination of internal fixation and spanning external fixation constructs.
- Well-padded short leg plaster splint with toe plate, with the ankle in neutral position, is an appropriate postoperative dressing.

Rehabilitation

- Rigid splinting/casting is utilized, with ankle in plantigrade position, for 6 weeks.
- Suture removal at 2 weeks, Kirschner wire removal (when placed) at 6 weeks.
- Patient is transitioned to a removable walker boot at 6-week time point, and is allowed to come out of boot for ankle and subtalar joint motion with physical therapy.
- Patient is maintained non-weight bearing on operative foot for 3 months, after which partial progressive weight bearing is initiated.
- Screw removal is indicated only for cutaneous irritation (from screw heads) or in setting of infection. There is no

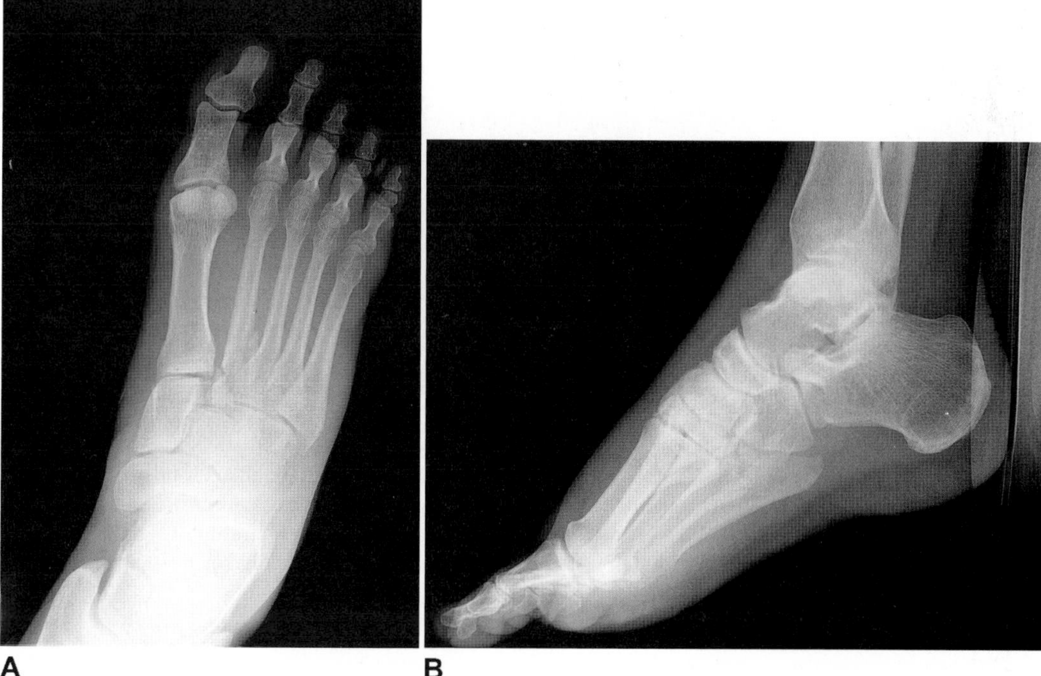

Figure 23–4: Bony Lisfranc injury. This injury was sustained in a motor vehicle crash. **A** and **B,** Relatively innocuous-appearing bony Lisfranc injury on anteroposterior and lateral plain injury radiographs.

Continued

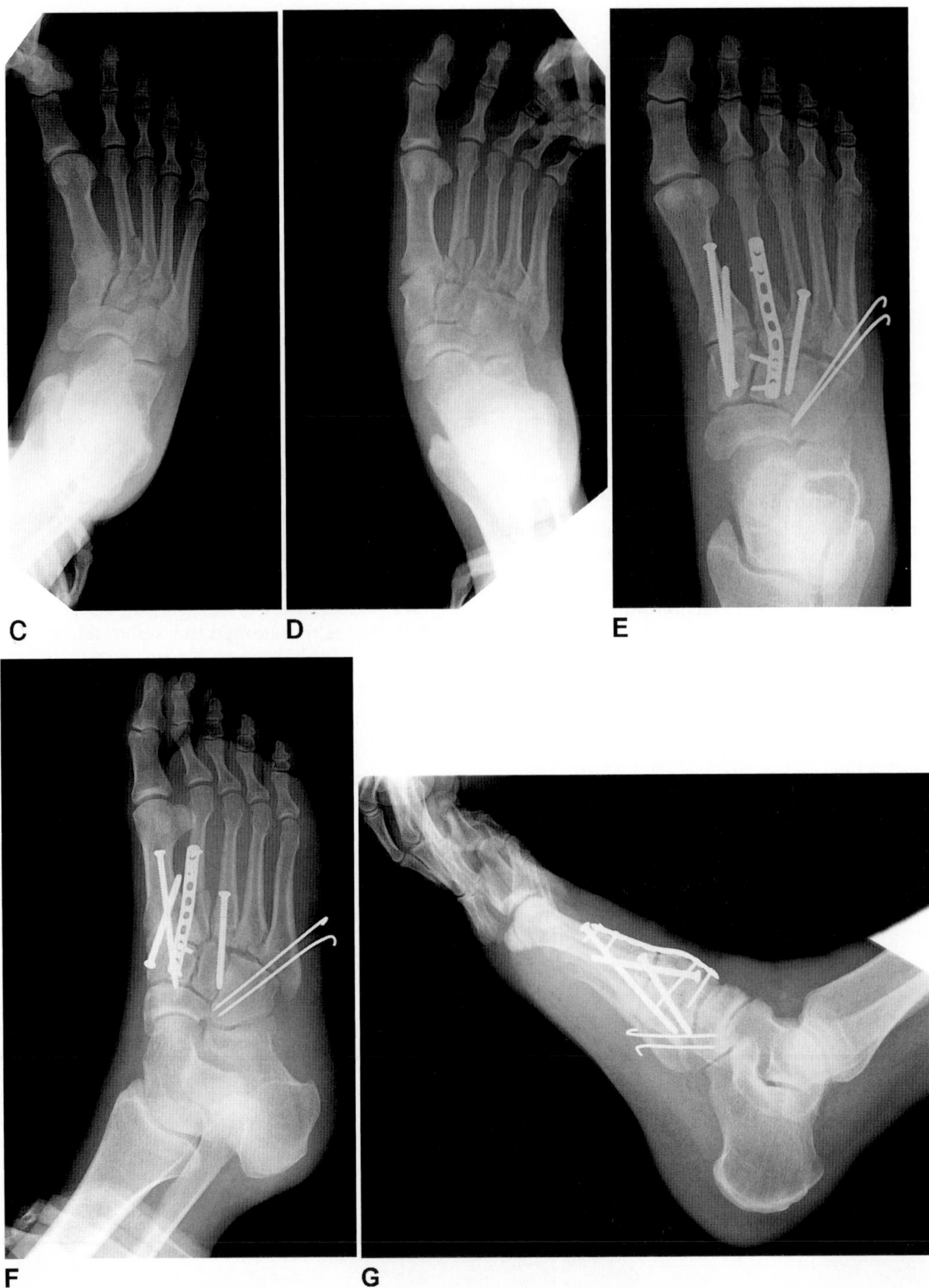

Figure 23–4: Cont'd **C** and **D**, Stress radiographs obtained with patient under general anaesthetic. Note disruption of first to second interspace. Also, note widening of medial aspect of first tarsometatarsal joint on lateral stress in panel D. **E–G**, Anteroposterior, oblique, and lateral postoperative radiographs demonstrating definitive fixation constructs after anatomical reduction of the midfoot. A bridge plate was utilized across the second metatarsal base fracture due to extensive comminution; this plate was not removed after healing. Kirschner wires were removed in the outpatient clinic at 6 weeks.

evidence that screw removal improves long-term outcome. If screw removal is required, a 9- to 12-month interval between fixation and removal is advocated to ensure adequate healing and prevent late collapse of longitudinal and transverse arches.

- Recent data in high-performance athletes has shown that early (3 month) screw removal can lead to recurrent midfoot subluxation.
- Final outcome correlates with reduction. In other words, poor alignment leads to poorer outcome.

References

Arntz CT, Veith RG, Hansen ST. (1988) Fractures and fracture-dislocations of the tarsometatarsal joint. J Bone Joint Surg Am 70: 173-181.

Consecutive series of 41 tarsometatarsal joint injuries treated with ORIF. Anatomical reduction achieved in 30 patients, of whom 28 had good or excellent outcomes. Six patients had fair or poor outcomes, of which five had open injuries. Posttraumatic arthrosis was associated with lack of an anatomical reduction and/or severe articular surface injury.

Coss HS, Manos RE, Buoncristiani A et al. (1998) Abduction stress and AP weightbearing radiography of purely ligamentous injury in the tarsometatarsal joint. Foot Ankle Int 19: 537-541.

Twenty patients without foot injuries underwent abduction stress and standing anteroposterior radiographs as control subjects. Nine feet from cadavers had Lisfranc and dorsal tarsometatarsal ligaments sectioned in a varying sequential manner, and the same radiographs were utilized. All cadaveric feet had disruption of the medial column line on radiographic evaluation after sectioning of both Lisfranc and dorsal tarsometatarsal ligaments. This study supports the use of stress views for identification of subtle, purely ligamentous Lisfranc injuries.

Kuo RS, Tejwani NC, DiGiovanni CW et al. (2000) Outcome after open reduction and internal fixation of Lisfranc joint injuries. J Bone Joint Surg Am 82: 1609-1618.

Average 52-month follow-up of 48 cases treated with ORIF. Twelve patients had posttraumatic arthrosis at follow-up, and six of these required arthrodesis. Anatomical reduction at index procedure correlated with best outcomes.

Myerson M, Fisher RT, Burgess AB et al. (1988) Fracture-dislocations of the tarsometatarsal joints: End results correlated with pathology and treatment. Foot Ankle Int 8: 225-242.

Fifty-two patients with 55 Lisfranc injuries evaluated at an average of 4.2 years. Twenty-seven feet had good to excellent results, and 28 feet had fair to poor results. Quality of reduction was the major determinant of unacceptable results. Recommendations are made for ORIF if displacement is greater than 2 mm or if talometatarsal angle is greater than 15°.

Sangeorzan BJ, Benirschke SK, Mosca V et al. (1989) Displaced intra-articular fractures of the tarsal navicular. J Bone Joint Surg Am 71: 1504-1510.

Series of 21 patients with navicular fractures evaluated at an average of 44 months. A classification scheme for navicular fractures is proposed. Satisfactory reduction is achieved less often with increasing grade of fracture. Fourteen patients had a good outcome. Quality of outcome correlates with fracture type and with accuracy of operative reduction.

Sangeorzan BJ, Swiontkowski MF. (1990) Displaced fractures of the cuboid. J Bone Joint Surg Br 72: 376-378.

Four cases of displaced cuboid fractures treated with ORIF are presented, with outcomes better than those reported for conservative management or for management with late midtarsal fusion.

Torg JS, Pavlov H, Cooley LH et al. (1982) Stress fractures of the tarsal navicular. J Bone Joint Surg Am 64: 700-712.

Nineteen patients with 21 navicular stress fractures were analyzed. They occur most commonly in young male athletes. Routine radiographs often fail to show the fracture, or the fracture is not recognized if shown. Radionuclide bone scintigraphy was required to locate 14 of the fractures, and 17 required tomography for diagnosis or to follow healing. The fracture is characteristically sagittal in orientation and located within the central one-third of the navicular. When treated with non-weight-bearing casting, healing occurred without complication.

Turchin DC, Schemitsch EH, McKee MD et al. (1999) Do foot injuries significantly affect the functional outcome of multiply injured patients? J Orthop Trauma 13: 1-4.

Twenty-eight polytraumatized patients with foot injuries were randomly matched to 28 polytraumatized patients without foot injuries. Three validated outcome measurement tools were utilized. Outcomes were significantly worse in patients with foot injuries, as assessed by all three outcome measurement tools. The authors recommend paying close attention to these foot injuries in this population of patients, and suggest that aggressive management may play a role in improving their outcome.

Weber M, Locher S. (2002) Reconstruction of the cuboid in compression fractures: Short to midterm results in 12 patients. Foot Ankle Int 23: 1008-1013.

Twelve patients with cuboid fractures treated with ORIF are evaluated at 1-4 years. Distracting external fixation was utilized to restore lateral column length. Good results were achieved with regard to lateral column length, articular congruity, and functional outcome. Residual symptoms appeared to correlate with associated midfoot injuries. Aggressive treatment of these fractures with ORIF with or without bone grafting is recommended to maximize odds of good outcomes.

CHAPTER 24

Metatarsal and Phalangeal Fractures

Niket Shrivastava[*] and Justin Greisberg[§]

[*]M.D., Department of Orthopaedic Surgery, Columbia University College of Physicians and Surgeons, New York, NY
[§]M.D., Assistant Professor of Orthopaedic Surgery, Columbia University College of Physicians and Surgeons, New York, NY

Introduction

General

- Toe and metatarsal fractures are the most common fractures of the foot.
- Toe fractures have an incidence of 140 per 100 000 per year.
- The majority are low-energy injuries suitable for closed treatment. The intact soft tissues splint the fracture.
- High-energy injuries, even when closed, have extensive soft tissue disruption and may require operative treatment.
- The fifth metatarsal is the most frequently fractured metatarsal (23%).
- The metatarsals are affected by stress fractures more commonly than all other sites in the body.
- Lawn mower injuries are common, with an incidence of between 50 000 to 160 000 each year, leading to significant morbidity and, rarely, even death.

Forefoot Structure

- The metatarsals are the major weight-bearing structure of the forefoot.
- The first metatarsal head and its two associated sesamoids bear approximately one-third of the body weight, while the remainder is distributed among the lesser four metatarsals, with the second and third frequently bearing more than the fourth and fifth.
- The metatarsal bases are rigidly stabilized to the cuneiforms and cuboid in the midfoot.
- The metatarsals are interconnected distally by stout transverse intermetatarsal ligaments between adjacent metatarsal necks that limit motion in the sagittal plane.
- A low-energy metatarsal shaft fracture does not disrupt these proximal or distal stabilizers, so the metatarsal head remains in the appropriate location for weight bearing.
- A higher energy injury, with disruption of the stabilizing soft tissue proximally or distally, will elevate or depress the metatarsal head. This may lead to metatarsalgia and painful plantar keratosis. Fractures of the metatarsals may thus disrupt the normal distribution of weight in the forefoot, resulting in metatarsalgia and intractable plantar keratoses.
- The second, third, and fourth metatarsals in particular have an abundant soft tissue envelope consisting of interosseous muscles and ligaments that helps to limit displacement of shaft fractures in those bones.
- The first metatarsal is intimately associated with the sesamoids, which are held fixed in relation to the lesser metatarsals by attachments to the intermetatarsal ligaments and the two heads of the adductor hallucis. Displacement of the first metatarsal head in any direction can alter the balance of the entire forefoot.
- The tibialis anterior works to elevate the first metatarsal, while the peroneus longus plantar flexes. Either of these muscles may act to deform a first metatarsal fracture.

- The flexor digitorum longus, flexor hallucis longus, and intrinsic muscles place plantar flexion stress on the metatarsal heads in distal fractures and can cause plantar flexion deformities.
- The fifth metatarsal, like the first, has less soft tissue coverage than the middle metatarsals and has extrinsic muscle attachments, the peroneus brevis and tertius, which attach at its base. It also has a strong attachment to the lateral band of the plantar fascia. It is the most mobile of the metatarsals.

Evaluation

- Patients with metatarsal fractures present with pain on ambulation or difficulty with weight bearing on the affected foot, swelling, deformity, and ecchymosis.
- Dorsal swelling is typical, because the plantar skin allows little swelling due to the thick fibrous septa within the skin pad.
- Each metatarsal and toe should be carefully and sequentially evaluated. Palpation of each digit and each metatarsal shaft usually will elicit point tenderness at the fracture site.
- Subungual hematoma is a hallmark of distal phalangeal fractures and may be associated with open fractures of the distal phalanx.

Imaging

- Radiographs should include anteroposterior, lateral, and oblique views of the foot.
- Metatarsal head alignment can be evaluated further with anteroposterior and lateral weight-bearing views of the whole foot and a tangential view of the metatarsal heads. Unfortunately, these views are difficult to obtain in a patient with a new injury.
- Stress fractures frequently do not appear initially on plain x-ray. Follow-up films 3-4 weeks later will usually demonstrate a resorption gap that confirms the diagnosis.
- Magnetic resonance imaging (MRI) can identify a stress fracture immediately but is not often needed, because the diagnosis can be made clinically.
- Bone scans also will detect a stress fracture after a few days of symptoms.

Metatarsal Fractures

Mechanism

- Metatarsal fractures result from a wide variety of mechanisms, and may range from an isolated single bone fracture to multiple fractures with severe soft tissue compromise.
- Direct trauma with a heavy falling object is common in industrial workers.
- Many low-energy injuries arise from indirect trauma, a twisting force with a fixed forefoot.
- Fractures of the fifth metatarsal base result from avulsion by the lateral band of the plantar aponeurosis.
- Stress fractures occur as a result of repetitive force on the metatarsals, and occur frequently in athletes, soldiers, and dancers.

Classification

- Metatarsal fractures can be classified according to the location, and thus include head, neck, shaft, and base fractures.
- It is useful to classify first and fifth metatarsal fractures separately from the rest, because the treatment options differ widely for these types.
- Second, third, and fourth metatarsal fractures can be grouped together, as the treatment options are similar.
- Proximal fifth metatarsal fractures can be categorized by zone (Table 24–1).
- Metatarsal base fractures can occur in isolation. However, it is important to recognize that many, perhaps all, such fractures represent an injury to the midfoot.
- An isolated, non-displaced metatarsal base fracture may be stable, but if any uncertainty exists, then further evaluation of the midfoot with stress x-rays is necessary.

First Metatarsal Fractures

- Non-displaced or minimally displaced fractures of the first metatarsal shaft or neck are generally stable and can be treated non-operatively.
- Non-operative options range from a short leg cast with progressive weight bearing over 4-6 weeks, to a CAM Walker boot, to a wooden rocker shoe for very stable fractures.
- Displacement, shortening, or angulation of the first metatarsal in any plane anywhere along the bone can significantly alter the weight-bearing distribution of the foot, and is therefore an indication for operative management.
- It is important to restore the length and the alignment of the bone anatomically in both the sagittal and transverse planes, in order to maintain normal weight bearing through the first ray.

Table 24–1: Fractures of the Fifth Metatarsal Classified by Zone

ZONE	LOCATION	DESCRIPTION
1	Fifth metatarsal tuberosity (most proximal)	Tuberosity avulsion fracture
2	Proximal metaphyseal-diaphyseal junction	"Jones" fracture (can be acute or chronic)
3	Diaphysis	Classic "dancer's fracture" of the shaft

- For shaft fractures, the types of fixation are limited due to the thin layer of soft tissue surrounding the bone, necessitating the use of a low-profile device. There is more room for plates on the plantar-medial side of the bone (Fig. 24–1).
- 3.5-, 2.7-, or 2.4-mm implants can be used. Long oblique fractures may be well treated with multiple lag screws, but most displaced shaft fractures will require a plate.
- Common approaches include a longitudinal approach between the first and second metatarsals, and the medial

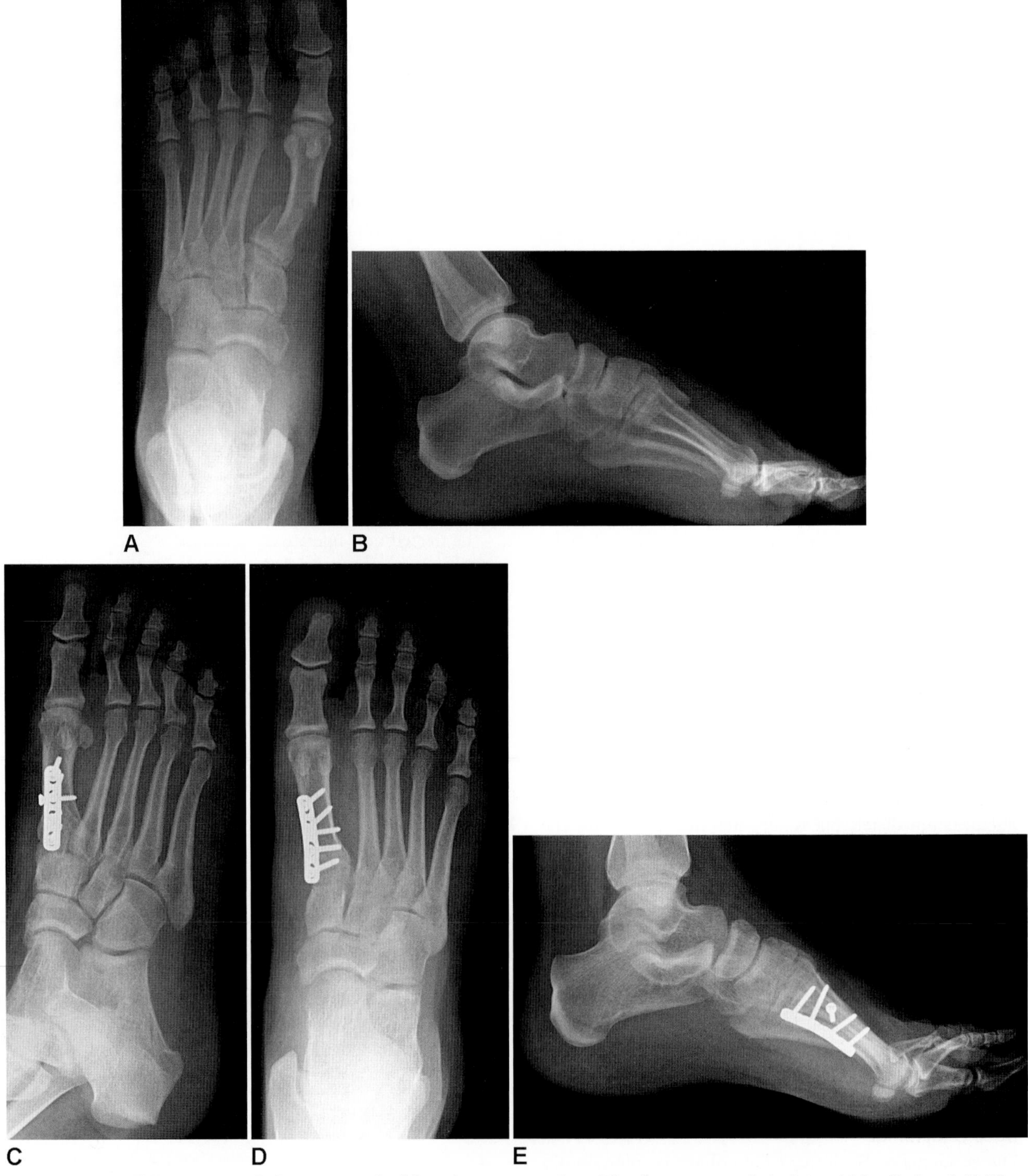

Figure 24–1: **A,** This young man's foot was crushed by a large garage door. The first metatarsal shaft is widely displaced. **B,** There is not much vertical displacement of the metatarsal head, suggesting that some of the soft tissue connections were intact between the first and second metatarsal heads. **C** and **D,** Open reduction was performed through a medial incision, with a lag screw and neutralization plate. **E,** After 6 weeks' non-weight bearing, he went on to a full recovery.

approach. The superficial peroneal nerve, deep peroneal nerve, and dorsalis pedis artery are at risk with the former approach, while the terminal branches of the saphenous vein and nerve are at risk with the latter.

- Comminuted base fractures may occasionally require bridging across the first tarsometatarsal joint to maintain proper alignment. Occasionally, fusion of the first tarsometatarsal joint may be necessary. So long as the fusion is performed with anatomical alignment of the metatarsal, no long-term consequences should be expected.

Second, Third, and Fourth Metatarsal Fractures

- Most low-energy fractures of the middle metatarsals are minimally displaced due to the soft tissue restraints previously described.
- Three to four millimeters of displacement in the sagittal plane (elevation or depression of the metatarsal head) can significantly affect the distribution of weight in the forefoot. This results in transfer of load to adjacent metatarsals (if the affected metatarsal is elevated), or overload of the fractured metatarsal (if it is plantar flexed).
- Similarly, shortening of a metatarsal can lead to adjacent metatarsal overload (transfer lesions or intractable plantar keratoses).
- Deformity in the transverse plane (medial or lateral angulation) does not have a large impact on weight-bearing distribution, and thus a higher degree of deformity, up to 4 mm of displacement and 10° of angulation, can be accepted in this plane.
- Non-operative treatment can be considered for shaft fractures with less than 2 mm of shortening, elevation, or depression of the metatarsal head in the sagittal plane.
- Such fractures in the lesser rays can be treated with cast immobilization, a wooden sole shoe, or a Cam Walker with progressive weight bearing over 4-6 weeks. The vast majority of low-energy fractures can be treated this way, with quite good results.
- Fractures that result in elevation or depression of the metatarsal head and alteration of the weight-bearing distribution should be treated surgically to maintain an anatomical reduction.
- Displaced shaft fractures can be treated with closed reduction and percutaneous pinning. The pins enter from the metatarsal head. However, the pins force the metatarsophalangeal (MTP) joints to remain extended while they are in place. This can result in extension contractures at the MTP joints, with claw toe deformity.
- To avoid clawing, the surgeon can place the pins more medially or laterally in the metatarsal head. This is technically more difficult. The pins could enter through the toe, and pass across the MTP joint and then across the fracture. This is also difficult.
- Shaft fractures can be treated with open reduction and internal fixation using mini implants (2.7, 2.4, or 2.0 mm).
- The rare displaced metatarsal head fracture should probably be treated with open reduction and internal fixation.

Multiple Metatarsal Fractures

- It is possible to fracture multiple metatarsals. In some cases, the proximal and distal soft tissues will remain intact, so metatarsal head alignment will not be affected. These injuries can be treated closed (Fig. 24–2).
- However, some injuries with multiple shaft fractures may represent a variant of a midfoot (Lisfranc) injury. In all cases of metatarsal fracture, especially when there are multiple fractures, midfoot stability should be assessed carefully.

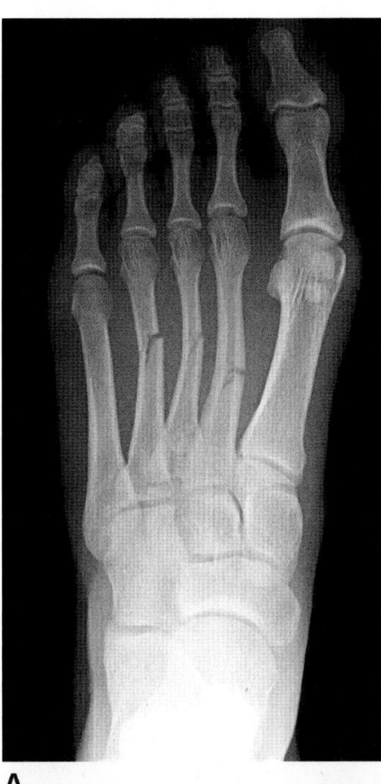

A

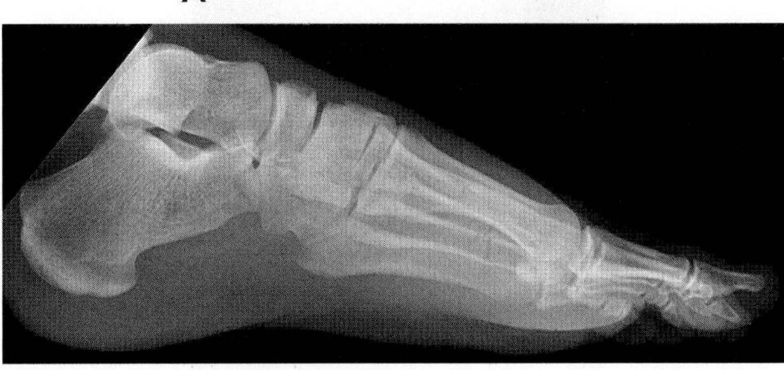

B

Figure 24–2: **A,** This young man twisted his foot while playing basketball. The fractures of the middle metatarsal shafts represent a variant of a midfoot injury, but the fractures are non-displaced and the midfoot is stable. **B,** The lateral view confirms good foot alignment. He went on to heal the injury well, with no restrictions.

Fifth Metatarsal Fractures

- There are four major types of fractures of the fifth metatarsal: tuberosity avulsion fractures, acute metadiaphyseal fractures, metadiaphyseal stress fractures, and acute diaphyseal fractures. Table 24–1 groups the fractures by geographic zone. Note that zone 2, the proximal metaphysis, includes both acute and chronic injuries (Table 24–1). Approximately 90% of fractures in this bone are tuberosity avulsion fractures (Fig. 24–3).
- Although it was once believed that the avulsion was due to the pull of the peroneus brevis during foot inversion, more recent studies implicate the lateral band of the plantar fascia.

Tuberosity Avulsion Fracture

- Almost all tuberosity avulsions can be treated non-operatively with a walking cast, boot, or hard-soled shoe, and weight bearing as tolerated. The majority will heal within 8 weeks, but symptoms may persist for several months. Radiographic non-union is not uncommon, but painful non-union is rare.
- The rare painful non-union can be treated with excision of the fragment and peroneus brevis repair, or bone grafting and intramedullary screw fixation for larger fragments.

"Jones" Fractures

- Jones fractures occur at the metaphyseal-diaphyseal junction, an area of poor vascularity and therefore reduced healing potential. A Jones fracture can be distinguished from tuberosity avulsions by its point of exit medially, which is in the intermetatarsal region just beyond the metatarsocuboid joint.
- Fractures in the Jones region can be acute injuries or chronic ones. The literature on these injuries is confusing, mostly because authors have pooled acute and chronic injuries together.
- Acute proximal metaphyseal fractures have no prodromal pain, and a clean appearance on x-ray.
- These acute fractures can be treated with limited (or non-) weight bearing in a cast or brace for 6-8 weeks. Most will heal uneventfully, although symptoms may last for months (Fig. 24–4).
- Some surgeons advocate immediate surgery (percutaneous screw fixation) for these acute fractures in high-level athletes to quicken return to sport. The precise role for surgery for these injuries is not clear.
- The chronic metadiaphyseal fracture is very different. The patient may present with the same history as for acute fracture: new pain in the foot after an injury. In some cases, there will be a history of mild aches or even previous fracture in this region.
- X-rays will show sclerosis at the fracture site, suggesting some chronicity to the injury (Fig. 24–5).

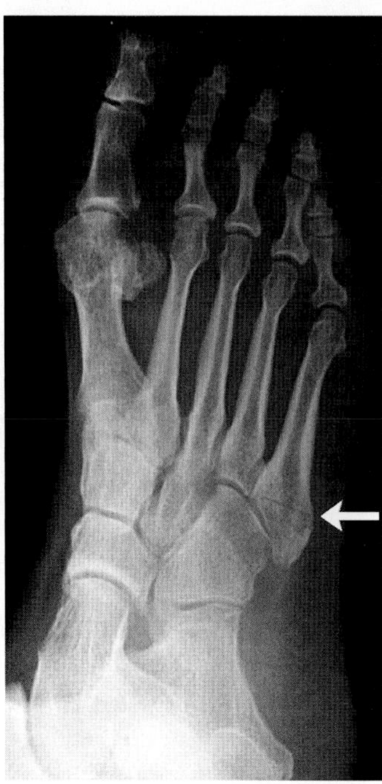

Figure 24–3: **Fifth metatarsal tuberosity fractures typically exit close to or in the metatarsocuboid joint. They usually are mildly displaced and heal well regardless of treatment.**

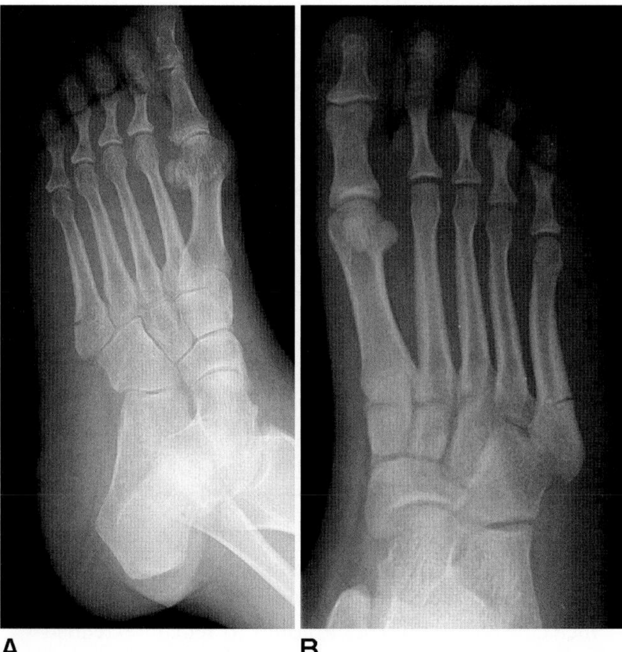

Figure 24–4: **A, This older woman had acute onset of pain in the lateral foot after a twisting injury. X-ray shows an acute fracture of the base of the fifth metatarsal. Many of these patients can be treated without surgery. B, The acute fracture must be distinguished from the patient with chronic pain and chronic radiographic changes. This patient presented with indolent pain and an x-ray showing cortical sclerosis. Early surgery may be more appropriate for this patient.**

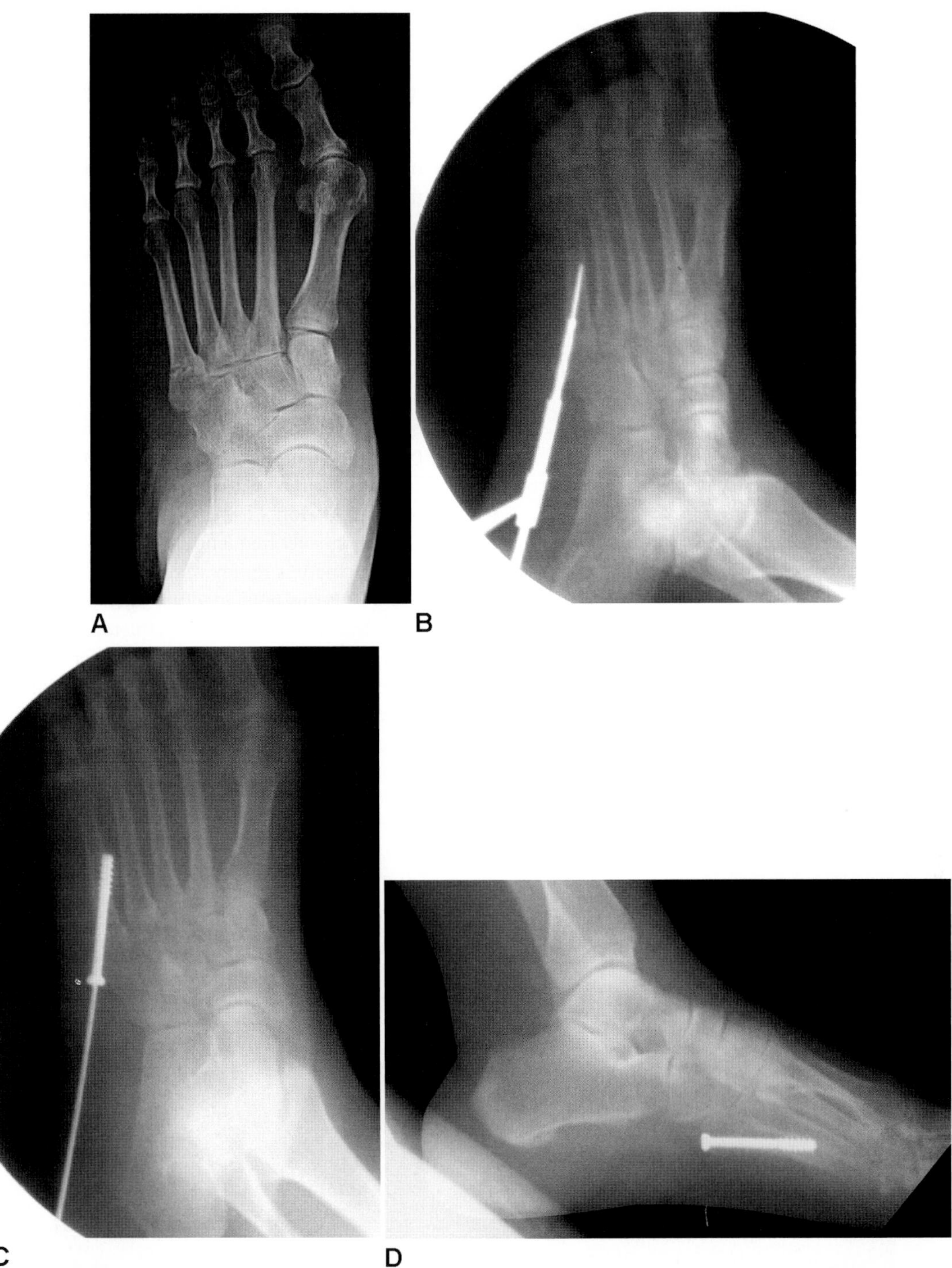

Figure 24–5: **A,** This woman presented with months of pain in the lateral foot. Her foot was straight and well balanced. The x ray reveals a chronic fracture of the proximal fifth metatarsal shaft, with sclerosis. **B,** During surgery, the non-union is "reamed" with a drill over a guide wire. **C,** A cannulated screw is passed across the fracture. Although most surgeons aim for an intramedullary screw, better distal purchase may be obtained in the medial cortex. Because of the small intramedullary canal, the screw violated the cortex of the shaft, but this presents no problem. **D,** On the lateral view, the screw is well placed.

- These chronic fractures can be expected to not heal quickly and to recur. Although a prolonged course of non-weight bearing with a cast can be attempted, most surgeons advocate operative treatment.
- The fracture is drilled to "ream" the canal and stimulate healing. A screw is then placed from the tuberosity across the fracture into the shaft.
- Some surgeons add bone graft as well.
- In cases of chronic injury, alignment of the foot must be assessed. Patients with a varus hindfoot will overload the fifth ray, leading to stress injury (Fig. 24–6). This can also be seen after varus tibial malunion. If the deformity causing fifth metatarsal overload is not corrected, the fracture may recur.

"Dancer's" Fractures

- Fractures of the fifth metatarsal shaft have been referred to as dancer's fractures.
- The treatment of shaft fractures in the fifth metatarsal differs slightly from that of the medial four metatarsals because of the increased mobility of this bone. Thus a larger degree of displacement and angulation of shaft fractures can be accepted.
- Often, these fractures appear to have significant displacement, especially on the oblique view (Fig. 24–7).
- Fortunately, most heal quite well. Patients can be treated non-operatively with a walking cast or boot.
- Surgery is indicated for the rare, highly displaced injuries.

Fifth Metatarsal Stress Fractures

- Fifth metatarsal stress fractures occur at the metadiaphyseal junction. Unlike acute Jones fractures, there will be a history of activity-related pain for weeks, months, or even years.
- Radiographs show sclerosis, medullary canal narrowing, or periosteal reaction at the fracture site at time of first presentation (suggesting longstanding bone injury).
- They are most frequently seen in young athletes who have a sudden increase in demand on the foot, or who have mild genu varum or heel varus deformities that overload the fifth metatarsal.
- Non-operative treatment with a short leg walking cast can take from 6 to 20 weeks and requires a long period of rehabilitation. However, refracture and non-union occur relatively frequently with non-operative treatment when activity is resumed.
- Most surgeons now advocate operative management for these fractures, especially in athletes, because of a lower refracture rate and a much quicker return to activity.
- Operative treatment consists of intramedullary screw fixation. The drilling for screw insertion is thought to increase healing potential, just as with reaming for intramedullary nailing in the tibia.

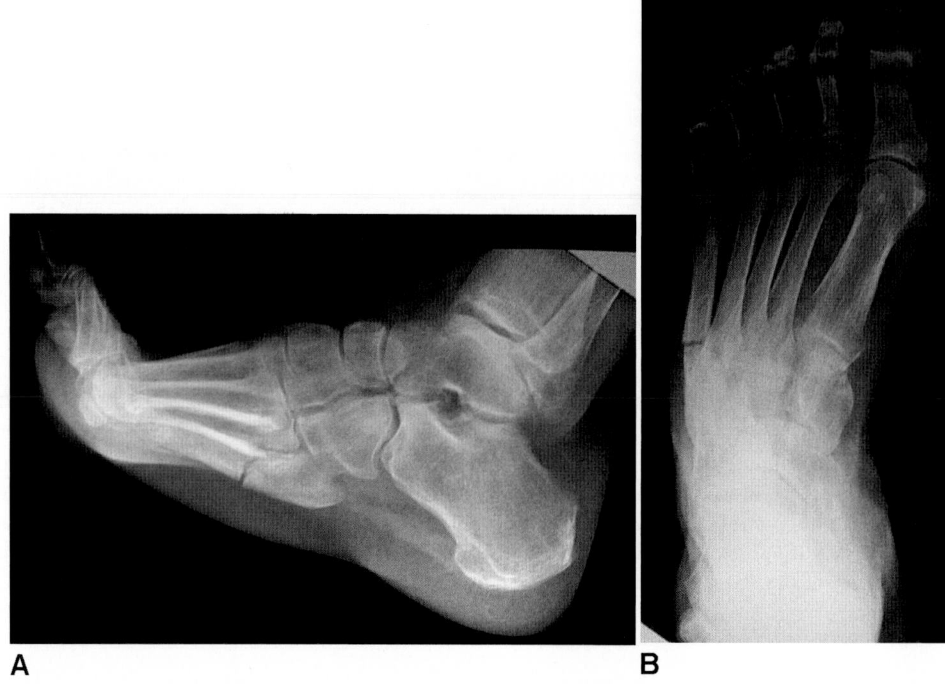

Figure 24–6: **A, Watch for the "Jones" fracture in the varus foot. This patient had a cavovarus foot deformity secondary to a stroke. Chronic lateral foot overload resulted in a fifth metatarsal fracture and subsequent non-union. B, The fracture appears incompletely healed after 6 months of symptoms. He underwent surgery, including intramedullary screw placement and hindfoot osteotomy with muscle transfers, to balance the deformity.**

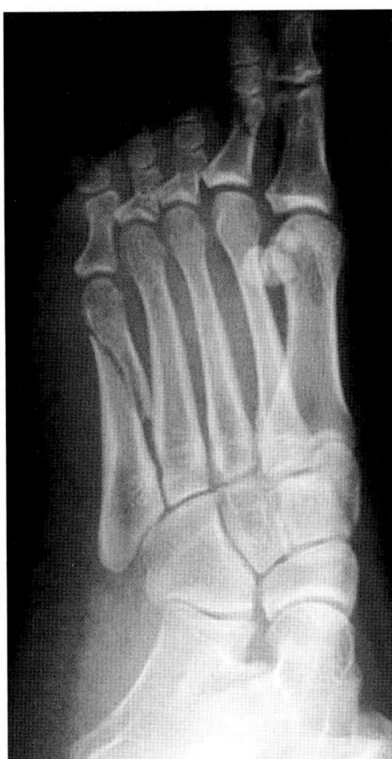

Figure 24–7: A spiral fracture of the fifth metatarsal shaft can follow a twisting injury, and is sometimes referred to as a "dancer's fracture."

- Some surgeons also advocate bone grafting of the dorsomedial surface of the fracture site.

Other Metatarsal Stress Fractures

- Stress fractures of the medial four metatarsals occur frequently. They are commonly referred to as "march fractures" because of their occurrence in new military recruits going for long marches.
- Treatment of these fractures is usually non-operative and focuses on unloading the affected metatarsal with altered shoe wear, orthotics, or a short leg cast for complete fractures (Fig. 24–8).
- It is important to look for underlying causes for the stress injury. Often, none will be found.
- As mentioned above, stress injuries can result from imbalance in the foot (osseous alignment). Metabolic causes are also common, such as in the amenorrheic female athlete (Table 24–2).

Phalangeal Fractures

First Proximal Phalanx Fracture

- Because of the role of the first toe in normal gait, deformity in the first toe may be less well tolerated than in the other digits.
- The flexor hallucis brevis muscles can act to plantar flex a proximal phalanx fracture. This will lead to a painful prominence on the bottom of the toe, a painful plantar keratosis.

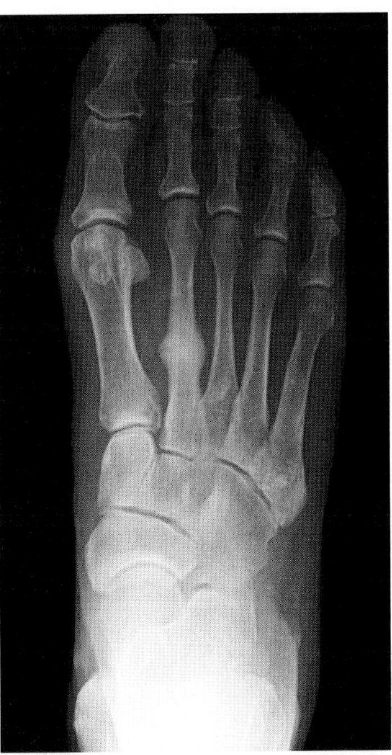

Figure 24–8: This young woman presented with forefoot pain and swelling without trauma. X-rays 6 weeks after the pain began reveal a stress fracture of the second metatarsal.

Table 24–2: Common Etiologies of Metatarsal Stress Fractures

CAUSE	EXAMPLES
Mechanical	First metatarsal instability Sudden increase in activity Shoe problems Malunion of another metatarsal Overall foot balance (cavus foot)
Metabolic	Osteoporosis Amenorrhea

- Non-displaced or minimally displaced fractures can be treated with buddy taping and a hard-soled shoe, and weight bearing as tolerated.
- Displaced fractures should be treated with closed or open reduction and fixation with crossed K wires, lag screws, or even plating with miniimplants.
- Displaced fractures of the MTP joint should be treated with reduction and stabilization. Such fractures often are quite comminuted, and anatomical reduction may be difficult.
- If the MTP joint is functioning normally, then the interphalangeal joint is less important. Posttraumatic arthritis of the interphalangeal joint can be easily treated with fusion, if it develops (Fig. 24–9).

Lesser Phalangeal Fractures

- Diaphyseal fractures in the middle and proximal phalanges are common, and usually are closed and occur

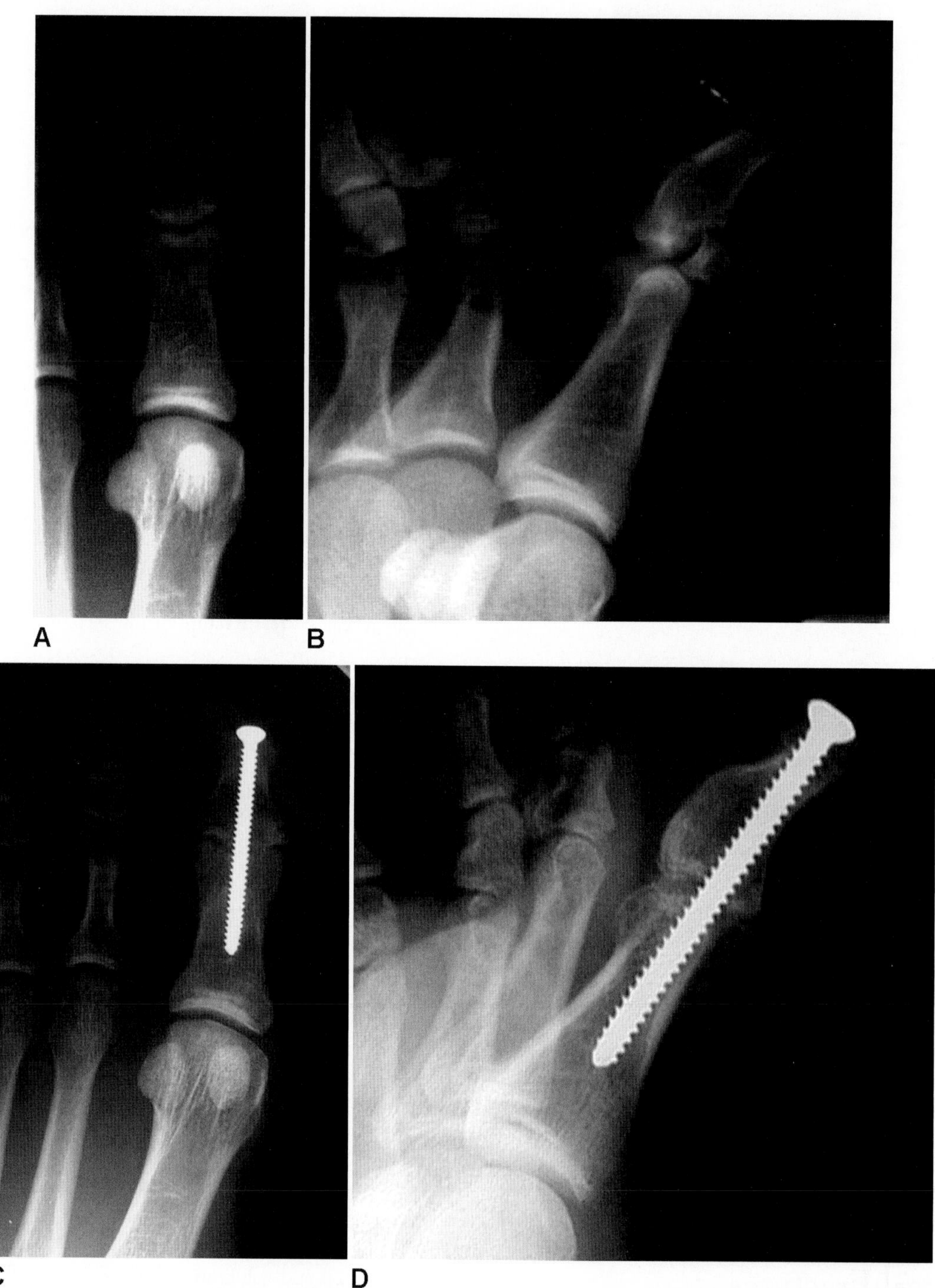

Figure 24–9: **A,** This young man sustained a trauma to his first toe 6 months ago. The anteroposterior view reveals good alignment, but **B,** the lateral view, reveals a displaced intraarticular fracture of interphalangeal joint. He was bothered by pain at the interphalangeal joint, and stiffness was noted on examination. **C,** Fusion of the interphalangeal joint led to a good functional result. **D,** The screw head was only slightly prominent at the tip of the toe.

as a result of kicking an object such as a leg of a table or chair while barefoot, a so-called "night walker" fracture.
- The vast majority of these fractures can be treated non-surgically with buddy taping, and weight bearing as tolerated.
- The fifth proximal phalanx is often fractured as a result of an abduction injury.
- For these fifth toe injuries, it is important to correct the lateral angulation with a closed reduction. Persistent angulation will be a problem when the patient goes back into shoes.
- Rarely, closed or open reduction with K-wire fixation is needed for severely displaced fractures.
- Although rare, toes that heal with excessive angulation or abundant callus can irritate adjacent toes (interdigital corn). This rare complication can usually be treated with exostectomy.

Distal Phalanx Fractures and Nail Bed Injury

- Injuries to the distal phalanx typically occur when an object is dropped directly on the digit, and are extremely common.
- The majority of distal phalanx fractures can be treated non-operatively with buddy taping and a hard-soled or wide toe box shoe until pain and tenderness subside.
- Distal phalanx fractures, however, are frequently accompanied by nail bed injuries due to the proximity of the skin and periosteum at the nail root.
- Nail bed lacerations and bleeding from the eponychium should lead to suspicion of an open fracture, which must be treated according to the principles of open fracture management to prevent infection.
- Nail bed injuries can occur without a fracture.
- Subungual hematoma, if painful and tender, can be treated with drainage through a hole bored in the nail plate with a small burr, heated paper clip, or electrocautery device.
- Nail bed lacerations should be carefully cleaned, debrided, and repaired using an absorbable suture material such as 5-0 or 6-0 catgut.

Open Fractures and Lawn Mower Injuries

Open Fractures

- Open fractures of the metatarsals and phalanges are not uncommon, because of the thin soft tissue envelope on the dorsum of the foot and the proximity of the distal phalanx to the skin at the root of the nail.
- As with any open fracture, they should be treated with antibiotic prophylaxis, debridement of non-viable or foreign material, and irrigation. Consideration should be given to osseous stabilization with wires to protect the soft tissues from further injury.

Lawn Mower Injuries

- Lawn mower injuries typically occur as a result of mowers that have tipped over, and frequently damage both the toe and the metatarsal regions of the forefoot.
- Children riding on the lap of an adult on a riding mower are another source of injury.
- Predisposing factors include a lack of shoe wear, insufficient soles, and use of a riding mower on a wet, sloped surface.
- Between 50 000 and 160 000 injuries occur each year. Significant morbidity occurs, with eventual amputation frequently becoming necessary. The injuries have extensive soft tissue destruction, severe contamination, and degloving of bone and soft tissue. By the Gustilo grading system, these are typically grade 3 injuries. Tetanus prophylaxis and appropriate antibiotics must be administered (first-generation cephalosporin plus aminoglycoside).
- The foot should be wrapped with a sterile dressing and splinted with abundant soft padding and/or plaster. Radiographs in the emergency department are appropriate, but further care should probably be given in the operating room.
- In the operating room, aggressive debridement of foreign material and non-viable tissue is performed, followed by copious irrigation.
- Skeletal stabilization can be achieved with wires, external fixators, or bridging plates (if soft tissue allows).
- Fasciotomies should be performed for those at risk for compartment syndrome.
- The wounds should be left open but protected from desiccation, and a return trip to the operating room for further wound care planned in 48-72 h.
- Flap coverage or skin grafting for soft tissue defects is required in approximately 50% of patients.
- Segmental bone loss can be splinted out to length with a bridging plate or wires, with structural bone grafting done later, once soft tissues are covered and healed.

References

Dameron TB. (1975) Fracture and anatomic variations of the proximal portion of the fifth metatarsal. J Bone Joint Surg Am 57(6):788-792.

A series of patients with fifth metatarsal fractures. The proximal tuberosity injuries uniformly fared well, while the Jones region posed many problems. The same author presented a modern opinion on these injuries in a similar publication in 1995.

DiGiovanni CW, Benirschke SK, Hansen ST. (2003) Foot Injuries: Skeletal Trauma, Basic Science, Management, and Reconstruction, vol. 2. Philadelphia: Saunders. pp. 2375-2492.

A comprehensive overview of injuries to the foot.

Konkel KF, Menger AC, Retzlaff SA. (2005) Nonoperative treatment of fifth metatarsal fractures in an orthopaedic suburban multispecialty practice. Foot Ankle Int 26(9): 704-707.

This series of 65 patients found uniformly good results with non-operative treatment of tuberosity, acute metaphyseal, and diaphyseal fractures. Healing time was long, though.

Rammelt S, Heineck J, Zwipp H. (2004) Metatarsal fractures. Injury 35(suppl 2): SB77-SB86.

An up-to-date review of the treatment of metatarsal fractures.

Theodorou DJ, Theodorou SJ, Kakitsubata Y et al. (2003) Fractures of proximal portion of fifth metatarsal bone: Anatomic and imaging evidence of a pathogenesis of avulsion of the plantar aponeurosis and the short peroneal muscle tendon. Radiology 226: 857-865.

This MRI-based study suggests that both the lateral band of the plantar fascia and the peroneus brevis may contribute to tuberosity fractures.

Vollman D, Khosla K, Shields BJ et al. (2005) Lawn mower-related injuries to children. J Trauma 59(3): 724-728.

The authors report their findings in a series of 85 children injured by lawn mowers.

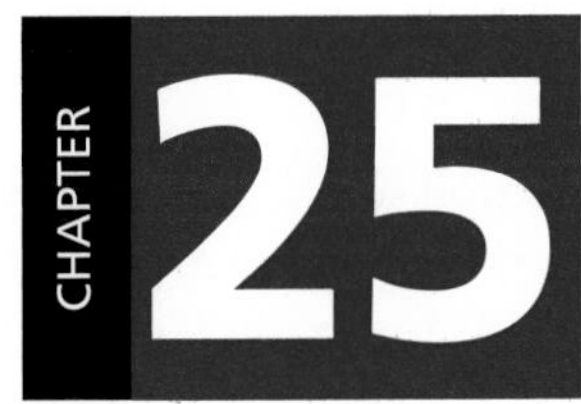

Tumors of the Foot and Ankle

Phillip R. Langer[*] and Richard M. Terek[§]

[*]M.D., M.S., Department of Orthopedic Surgery, Brown Medical School/Rhode Island Hospital, Providence, RI
[§]M.D., F.A.C.S., Associate Professor, Department of Orthopedic Surgery, Brown University, Providence, RI

- Foot and ankle tumors are rare entities but must be kept in the differential diagnosis of musculoskeletal complaints.
- Meticulous work-up of all lesions and/or suspicious masses must be undertaken.
- The overwhelming majority of bone and soft tissue tumors in the foot and ankle are benign, but occasionally a primary sarcoma will be present.
- It is imperative that all caregivers be knowledgeable of the common foot and ankle neoplasms—both bone and soft tissue in nature—such that accurate diagnoses, proper treatment, and patient education regarding expected prognosis can occur.
- This chapter will outline the common bone and soft tissue tumors of the foot and ankle, their classic characteristics, and their typical presentation, as well as current management protocols.

Clinical Evaluation

- Initial patient assessment must always begin with a thorough history and physical examination.
- A careful clinical evaluation is necessary to avoid delays in diagnosis and treatment, which are often detrimental to patient outcome and/or survival.
- Retrospective analysis of missed or improperly diagnosed malignant lesions often uncovers significant clues in both the clinical history and physical examination.
- Specific to the evaluation of musculoskeletal tumors, key data include pain during rest or at night, increasing pain, pain refractory to pharmacologic modalities, progressive neurologic deficit, alteration or increase in size of the mass, overlying swelling and/or erythema, loss of function, constitutional symptoms, history of prior malignancy or systemic disease, antecedent trauma, family history, and social history (i.e. tobacco use).
- A complete physical examination must be undertaken, with special attention paid to nodules, adenopathy, masses, skin changes, and local tenderness.
- In older patients, metastatic disease is more common than primary bone sarcomas, although metastases distal to the knee are rare. Potential primary lesions such as breast, lung, thyroid, renal, and prostate cancer should direct the examiner to systematically examine each of these organs.
- Although most malignant musculoskeletal tumors metastasize to the lung, some soft tissue sarcomas go to the draining lymph nodes. Consequently, a careful physical examination of both regional and systemic lymph nodes is required.
- Despite the importance of a thorough history and physical examination, there are some patients who present with an asymptomatic soft tissue mass that is a sarcoma, and conversely, the majority of patients with pain will have alternative diagnoses.
- Malignant neoplasms of the soft tissues are approximately 3-4 times more common than malignant tumors of the bone, but both are rare, with soft tissue sarcoma comprising less than 2% of all malignancies.

- Laboratory studies generally are not helpful in the work-up of soft tissue masses or bone tumors, with a few exceptions.
  - Complete blood count with differential, C-reactive protein, and erythrocyte sedimentation rate can help if infection is a possibility. However, these can be normal in the face of infection, and erythrocyte sedimentation rate can be elevated in tumors.
  - Serum calcium can be elevated in widespread metastatic disease and primary hyperparathyroidism. The characteristic brown tumor of hyperparathyroidism is often radiographically and histologically difficult to differentiate from a giant cell tumor of bone.
  - Any bone-forming process, including fracture healing and osteosarcoma, will elevate alkaline phosphatase.
  - Serum protein immunoelectrophoresis may be positive in patients with myeloma, but a primary presentation in the foot would be extremely uncommon.
- Imaging should begin with orthogonal radiographic views of the area of concern.
- Most bone tumors can be diagnosed with a conventional radiograph. Magnetic resonance imaging (MRI)/computed tomography (CT) can be used to determine complete anatomical extent and/or additional clues.
- Enneking et al. (1980) outlined four basic questions that should be asked when evaluating bone lesions on plain radiographs.
  - Where is the lesion?
  - What is the lesion doing to the bone?
  - What is the bone doing to the lesion?
  - Is there any characteristic within the lesion to suggest a specific diagnosis?
  - Specific to Enneking's second question, Lodwick (1966) found that radiographic patterns of bone destruction offer insight into the rate of growth. Geographic patterns imply a slow growth rate, and moth-eaten patterns indicate intermediate rates of growth, whereas permeative patterns point to rapid growth rates. More rapid growth implies infection or malignancy.
- Bone scan is sometimes helpful to identify a stress fracture, infection, reflex sympathetic dystrophy (complex regional pain syndrome), or difficult to find tumors such as osteoid osteoma. Bone scan is not useful for the evaluation of soft tissue masses.
- MRI is the most useful study for the evaluation of soft tissue masses.
- CT scanning can be useful to confirm the nidus of an osteoid osteoma identified with bone scanning, and for the evaluation of some fractures and dislocations of the hindfoot. It is less specific but can be used in patients for whom MRI is contraindicated.

Biopsy and Surgical Excision

- Before biopsy, local imaging should be completed.
- If a diagnosis cannot be made with imaging studies, then a biopsy should be performed.
- Biopsies can be performed via needle or open approach.
- Ideally, the surgeon and pathologist should work in concert.
- If an open biopsy is performed, which may be preferable in the foot so as not to contaminate normal structures, a frozen section analysis should be performed to ensure that diagnostic tissue has been obtained.
- For bone tumors with a soft tissue mass, the soft tissue component is usually diagnostic.
- Additional principles for performing a biopsy are as follow.
  - Use longitudinal as opposed to transverse incisions.
  - Maintain meticulous hemostasis with use of a drain brought out in line with the wound if necessary.
  - Submit all biopsy samples for bacteriologic analysis should frozen section fail to reveal a neoplasm.
  - Avoid neurovascular planes.
  - Keep soft tissue dissection and development of tissue planes at a minimum.
  - Use the smallest biopsy incision that will allow adequate tissue sampling and that can be incorporated into the definitive resection.
  - Do not use Esmarch to exsanguinate if a tourniquet is used.
  - Do not biopsy Codman's triangle (new subperiosteal bone that forms when a lesion such as a tumor lifts the periosteum away from the bone).
  - Close wound in layers.
  - Use the most direct approach to the lesion, through—not between—compartments/muscle.

Staging

- The most frequently employed staging system for musculoskeletal tumors was described by Enneking and is currently used for bone tumors.
- Table 25–1 shows the staging system of the Musculoskeletal Tumor Society (Enneking system).
- Although most bone sarcomas metastasize to the lungs, 5-10% do not. Therefore both a chest CT and a total body bone scan are used for systemic staging. The role of positron emission tomography scanning is yet to be determined.

Table 25–1: Staging System of the Musculoskeletal Tumor Society (Enneking System)

STAGE	EQUIVALENT	DEFINITION
1A	G1T1M0	Low grade, intracompartmental, no metastases
1B	G1T2M0	Low grade, extracompartmental, no metastases
2A	G2T1M0	High grade, intracompartmental, no metastases
2B	G2T2M0	High grade, extracompartmental, no metastases
3	G1/2T1M1	Any grade, intra/extracompartmental, metastases

- The American Joint Commission on Cancer system is used for soft tissue sarcoma, and incorporates the three most important prognostic factors, which are:
  - Grade
  - Size (> 5 cm = worse prognosis)
  - Relationship of tumor to the fascia (lesions deep to the fascia = worse prognosis).
  - Of the three, the tumor grade is most important.
- In soft tissue sarcomas, greater than 95% of metastases occur in the lungs. Consequently, a chest CT is obtained to stage the tumor. Bone scan is usually not necessary.
- The 5-year survival rate of high-grade soft tissue sarcoma is 50%; of all stages combined, it is 70%.
- The types of surgical margins and their associated local recurrence rates are as follow.
  - Intralesional: Dissection plane directly through the tumor; recurrence rate is 100% for sarcoma.
  - Marginal: Dissection plane through the reactive zone of the tumor; recurrence rate is 25-50% for sarcoma.
  - Wide: Dissection through a cuff of normal tissue; recurrence rate is 25%, but < 10% if radiation therapy is used for soft tissue sarcoma or chemotherapy for bone sarcomas.
  - Radical: Entire compartment containing the tumor is resected; recurrence rate near 0%.
- In practice, intralesional surgery is used for benign bone tumors, marginal surgery is used for benign bone and soft tissue tumors, wide margins are used for bone and soft tissue sarcomas, and radical surgery is of historical interest, except in the foot, since below knee amputation is frequently performed for sarcoma.
- Rougraff et al. (1993) presented a prospective study of diagnostic strategy in locating a primary tumor in a patient presenting with a skeletal metastasis. The following diagnostic yields were obtained.
  - History and physical: 8%.
  - Laboratory work (excluding multiple myeloma): 0%.
  - Chest x-ray: 43%.
  - CT scan abdomen/pelvis: 13%.
  - Biopsy of bone metastases: 8% diagnostic, 35% diagnostic or confirmatory.
- The basic work-up of an adult patient with possible metastatic disease is a bone scan; CT scans of the chest, abdomen, and pelvis; and a biopsy of the most accessible lesion. Lesions in the foot are unlikely to be metastatic, but if so, are usually lung or renal carcinoma.

Bone Lesions: Benign

Synovial Chondromatosis

- Synovial chondromatosis is a benign condition that involves the synovial lining of joints, bursae, or tendon sheaths.
- It is characterized by the development of multiple osteochondral loose bodies.
- It typically affects joints.
- It is a monoarticular condition. When it arises in the soft tissues from tendon sheaths, it is called soft tissue chondroma.
- In order of decreasing frequency, it is typically found in the knee, elbow, shoulder, and hip, yet may present in the foot and/or ankle.
- Case reports of primary synovial chondromatosis of the ankle have also been reported, and some have presented as tarsal tunnel syndrome.
- The offending entity is the synovium, which may appear hyperemic, thickened, and with fronds.
- Cartilaginous bodies are initially enveloped and then break free to form loose bodies. They are small grey-white shiny polyploid bodies.
- Immunohistologic studies show that these cartilaginous loose bodies are the result of metaplasia of the synovium.
- These loose bodies may go on to ossify. This has been described by Milgram (1977) to occur in three stages.
  - First, the synovium undergoes metaplasia. This is an active process of intrasynovial proliferation of cartilage nests. At this time, cartilage nodules are formed that remain attached to the synovium.
  - In the second stage, the nodules become detached and are present as loose bodies.
  - In the third phase, the synovium has burnt itself out. There is no longer evidence of metaplasia, but there are still loose bodies present. These may have become ossified by this time.
- The etiology of synovial chondromatosis is not known. Some suspect that it is due to synovial irritation. This may be from trauma or possibly from infection, but this is unclear. No organism has ever been cultured. No significant correlation has been made with trauma.
- Symptoms include swelling, pain, locking, stiffness, limited joint motion, crepitus, or giving way.
- Complaints are often tied to a traumatic event, but this may be coincidental.
- On physical examination, an effusion may be present. There may be tenderness of the joint or pain on range of motion. The range of motion may be limited. A palpable tender mass may be present.
- Evidence on imaging studies depends on the stage of disease.
- Until the loose bodies are ossified or calcified, they may be radiographically invisible (Fig. 25–1).
- Although the metaplastic changes of the synovium are reported to be self-limited, damage to the joint from multiple loose bodies may lead to early degenerative arthritis.
- The histologic appearance of this process shows well-defined cartilage nests embedded in a layer of synovium. There may be significant pleomorphism and/or evidence of advancing stages with maturation of the cartilage; mineralization and ossification are radiographic findings characteristic of maturation. Mitotic figures are not a prominent feature of the proliferating chondrocytes. There may, however, be some plump hyperchromatic nuclei.

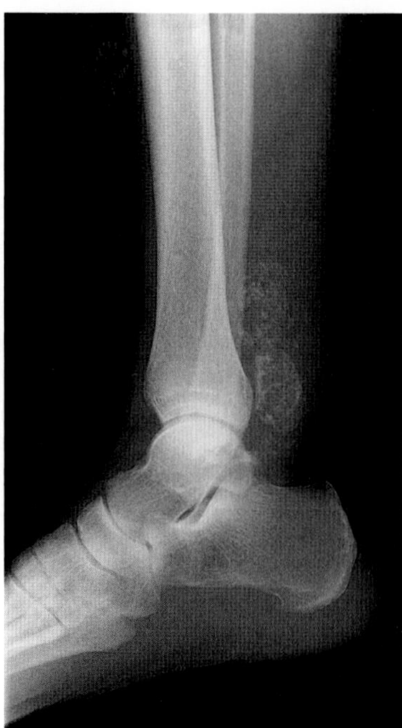

Figure 25–1: Synovial chondromatosis. Lateral ankle x-ray.

- Treatment includes arthroscopic or open debridement of loose bodies.
- Controversy exists as to whether a synovectomy should be performed. A retrospective study of 13 patients with synovial chondromatosis of the knee has lent argument in favor of a thorough synovectomy. Of the five patients who had removal of loose bodies alone, three had recurrence of loose body formation. None of the eight treated with initial removal of loose bodies and a thorough synovectomy had recurrence.
- Synovial chondromatosis is reported to be a benign, self-limiting disease process. Chondrosarcoma of synovium has been described. There is controversy as to whether malignant degeneration takes place leading to a secondary malignant process. There have been at least 19 well-documented cases of such a secondary malignant process. Unfortunately, there are no clear-cut radiologic studies that can differentiate the entities. Histologically, the malignant tumor can be differentiated by its loss of a solid matrix, a so-called "runny" matrix; hypercellularity, with crowding and spindling of the nucleus; and necrosis or local invasion. Metastasis is the hallmark of malignancy, and pulmonary spread was present in 7 of the 19 cases.

Giant Cell Tumor

- Giant cell tumor of the foot is rare.
- It is a benign yet locally aggressive tumor that typically occurs in the second and third decades of life, with a slight female predilection.
- It is usually a metaphyseal-epiphyseal, juxtaarticular lesion found most commonly about the knee (50%), shoulder, and distal radius, although it has been reported in virtually all the foot bones.
- It originates in the metaphysis and extends into the epiphysis following physeal closure.
- Radiographic analysis reveals a lytic, eccentric, expansile appearance. It typically thins out the cortex, has no internal matrix, and may have a sclerotic rim centrally (Fig. 25–2).

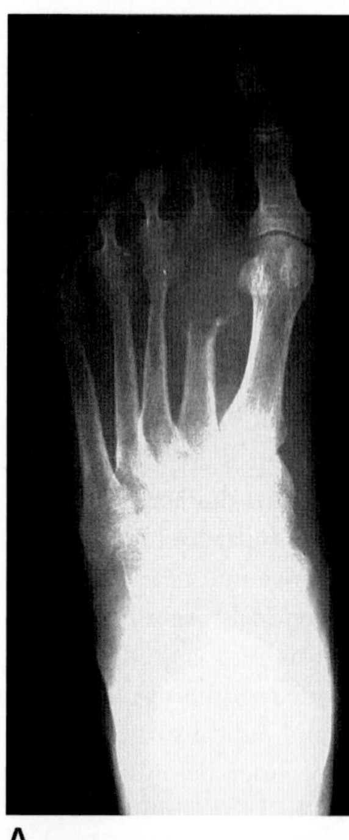

A

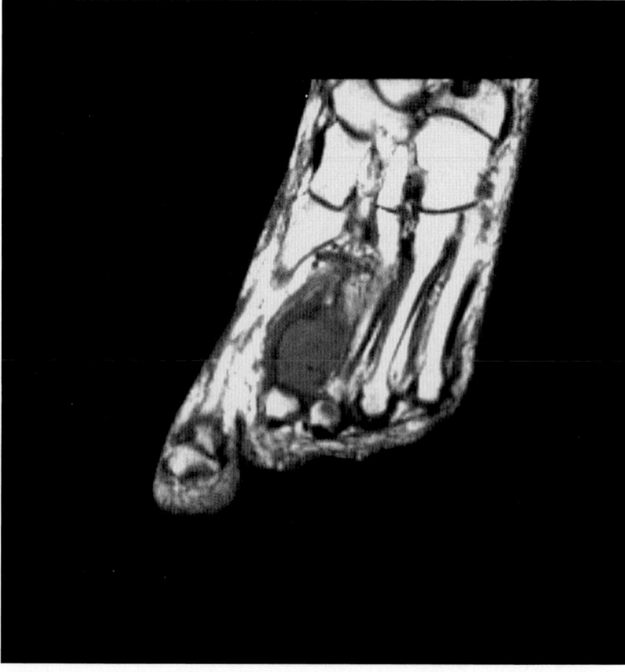

B

Figure 25–2: Giant cell tumor. A, Anteroposterior foot x-ray. B, Magnetic resonance imaging scan of foot.

- Less than 2% metastasize to the lungs. Biscaglia et al. (2000), in a retrospective review of 21 giant cell tumors of the foot, found no pulmonary metastases. These tumors were noted to be more aggressive than those of long bones.
- Treatment typically involves biopsy to confirm the diagnosis; intralesional curettage and mechanical burring; treatment with adjuvants such as phenol, cryosurgery, or hydrogen peroxide; and packing the resultant defect with bone graft or bone cement.
- When a metatarsal is involved, resection may be more expeditious than reconstruction, depending on degree of destruction and which metatarsal is involved.

Aneurysmal Bone Cyst

- Solitary, expansile osteolytic lesion with a thin wall, containing blood-filled cystic cavities.
- Occurs in patients aged 10-30 years; peak incidence is age 16.
  - About 75% are less than 20.
- Female:male ≈ 1.3-2:1.
- Develops in metaphyseal region of long bones, pelvis, vertebral posterior elements—in decreasing order of frequency:
  - lower leg (24%)
  - upper extremity (21%)
  - spine (16%)
  - femur (13%)
  - pelvis and sacrum (12%)
  - short tubular bones (10%)
  - clavicle and ribs (5%)
  - skull and mandible (4%)
  - foot (3%).
- Etiology is unknown; possibly traumatic (acute fractures? increased venous pressure) or secondary to preexisting bone tumors.
  - Approximately 30% are secondary to preexisting bone tumors, such as chondroblastoma, chondromyxoid fibroma, osteoblastoma, giant cell tumor, or fibrous dysplasia. Less frequently, it results from malignant lesions such as osteosarcoma, chondrosarcoma, and hemangioendothelioma.
- They present with acute, rapidly increasing pain, swelling, and/or decreased motion.
- Radiographs often have a "blown out" appearance with thin septations (Fig. 25–3A,B).
- CT characteristically demonstrates multiple fluid-fluid levels within cystic spaces.
- MRI classically reveals multiple fluid-fluid levels (Fig. 25–3C).
  - ABC appears on both T_1 and T_2 MRI, with a low-signal rim encircling the cystic lesion. A careful search for radiologic signs of the precursor lesion, if any, is recommended.
- Gross examination: Soft, fibrous walls separate blood-filled spaces.
- Histology reveals cystic spaces filled with blood. Typically, the fibrous septa have immature woven bone trabeculae

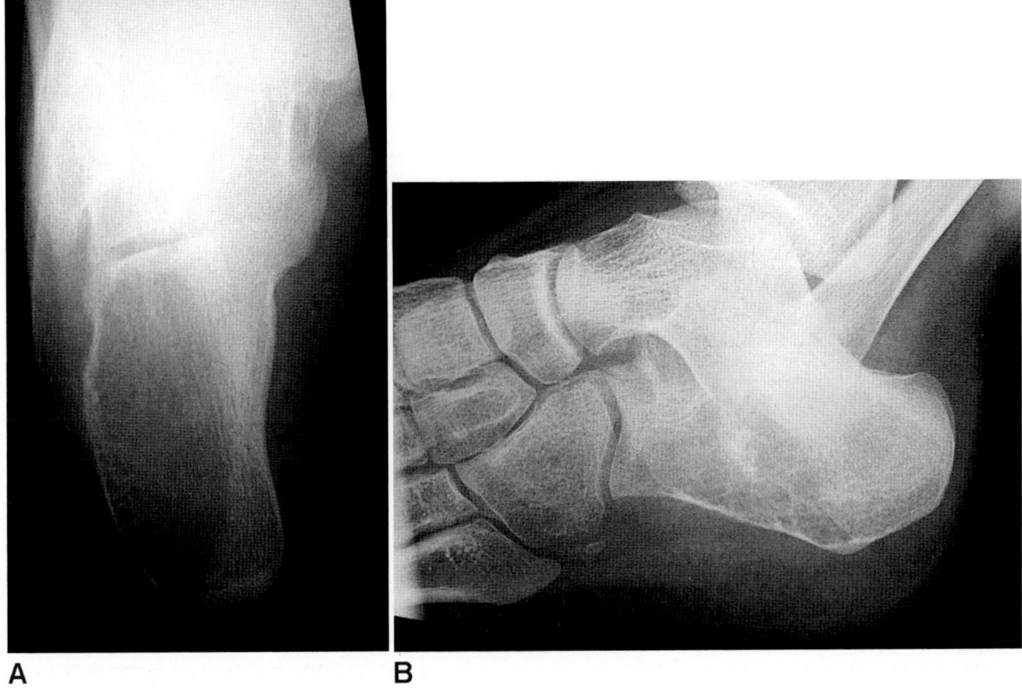

Figure 25–3: Aneurysmal bone cyst. **A**, Harris view. **B**, Lateral hindfoot x-ray.

Continued

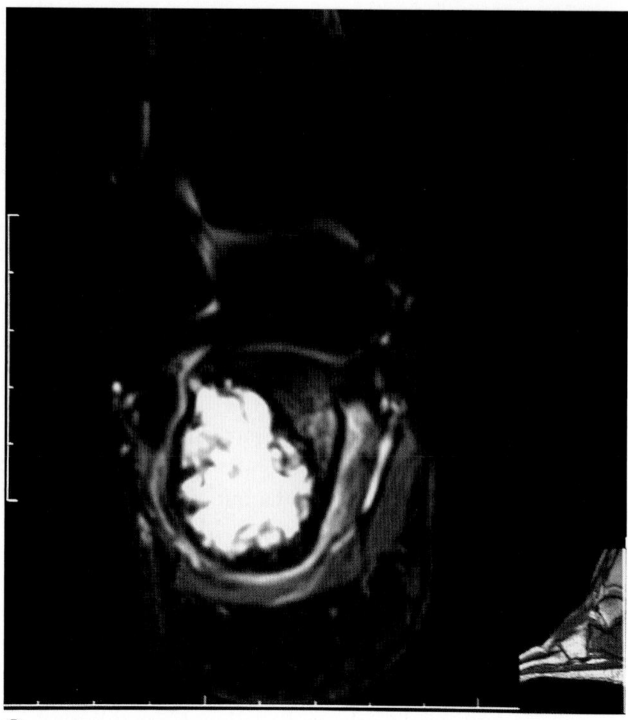

C

Figure 25–3: Cont'd **C, Magnetic resonance imaging scan.**

as well as macrophages filled with hemosiderin, fibroblasts, capillaries, and giant cells.

- ABC are active lesions that destroy bone, and therefore are almost always treated. Treatment consists of curettage and bone graft or rarely resection.
  - Local recurrence with curettage and bone grafting can be as high as 25% (Gibbs et al. 1999).
  - If a recurrence is detected, a thorough examination of the original radiographs and pathology specimens should be performed to ensure that the primary lesion, if any, is discovered, because this may alter the treatment plan. One unfortunate scenario is to biopsy an ABC, which then recurs and presumably evolves into a telangiectatic osteosarcoma. Once the precise diagnosis is known, local recurrences may be retreated by appropriate methods.
  - Occasionally, wide resection and limb-sparing reconstructions may be necessary to prevent progressively destructive recurrence. Other strategies include embolization and steroid injection.

Unicameral Bone Cyst (UBC or Simple Bone cyst)

- A benign radiolucent cavity found within a bone that is filled with straw-colored fluid.
- It is unifocal and affects patients who are skeletally immature, most frequently in children aged 5-15 years, with an average age of approximately 9 years.
  - The rarity of the lesion in adults supports a hypothesis of spontaneous resolution.
  - They enlarge during skeletal growth and become inactive, or latent, after skeletal maturity.
- Male:female ratio is 2:1.
- Predilection for the metaphysis of long bones.
- Most common location is the proximal humerus.
  - Proximal humerus (50%) and proximal femur (40%) account for 90% of UBCs.
  - Less common locations include the pelvis, talus, and calcaneus.
- Historically, location played a prognostic role. If the cyst is:
  - immediately adjacent to the physis, it is active
  - distant from the physis, it is latent.
  - Recurrence is high for active cysts (50%) and low for latent cysts (10%).
- Etiology is unknown.
  - Possible theories involve a growth defect or disturbance at the epiphyseal plate.
- Radiographs typically reveal a central lytic metaphyseal lesion with a sclerotic in and little to no bone expansion.
  - The "fallen fragment sign" is usually pathognomonic (Struhl et al. 1989).
- MRI/CT is not routine but may be helpful if the UBC is not typical in its appearance.
- Most UBCs are asymptomatic and incidentally discovered.
- Lesions usually remain asymptomatic unless complicated by fracture.
- If a UBC is thinning the bone, there may be pain with weight-bearing activities. If there is a pathologic fracture through the cyst, the affected extremity may have pain, swelling, and deformity.
- In contrast to ABCs, UBCs are sometimes not treated, such as in the absence of symptoms or mechanical compromise of the involved bone (i.e. extensive cortical thinning).
- Treatment should be considered for lesions that have resulted in fracture or marked weakening of bone. Spontaneous healing of a UBC may occur following fracture. Such healing occurs in only a minority of cases. Growth disturbance secondary to a UBC also is a concern.
- Calcaneal cysts reaching a critical size, defined as 100% in cross-sectional area in the coronal plane and at least 30% in the sagittal plane, are at risk for becoming symptomatic and at risk for fracture (Pogoda et al. 2004).
- A lesion with precarious cortical thinning (with or without pain) may demand surgical intervention. CT is used to assess cortical thinning.
  - Factors such as age and stress secondary to a weight-bearing location may strongly influence surgical decisions.
  - Goal of treatment is prevention of a pathologic fracture.

- Treatment options include open bone grafting, aspiration followed by injection of methylprednisone, demineralized bone matrix, autologous bone marrow, calcium phosphate bone cement or calcium sulfate pellets, or placement of a percutaneous cannulated screw.
  - Specific to the lesions of the calcaneus, curettage and bone graft has been found to be superior to steroid injection (Glaser et al. 1999).

Intraosseous Lipoma

- Intraosseous lipomas are rare tumors.
- Often confused with other benign tumors, such as ABC and UBC and/or bone infarction.
- Mean age is third to fourth decade.
- Most frequently occur in the lower limb; calcaneus is the most common site.
- Imaging (x-ray, CT, MRI) shows mineralization/calcification, fat necrosis, and cyst formation.
  - Blends in with normal marrow fat on MRI, which helps to distinguish them from ABC and UBC.
- May be subdivided into three groups depending on the degree of involution:
  - solid tumors of viable lipocytes
  - transitional cases with partial fat necrosis and focal calcification but also regions of viable lipocytes
  - late cases in which the fat cells have died, with variable degree of cyst formation, calcification, and reactive new bone formation of a characteristic morphology.
- Involution is spontaneous, therefore surgical management is often not necessary.
- An asymptomatic intraosseous lipoma without impending pathologic fracture can be treated conservatively.
- The adequate treatment of a symptomatic intraosseous lipoma is curettage and bone grafting. Phenolization showed no added benefit.

Enchondroma

- Enchondroma is a benign cartilaginous tumor of bone that is present in patients of all ages.
- The majority are asymptomatic unless associated with a pathologic fracture.
- Characteristically, they are found in the intramedullary canal of the central metaphysis.
- Enchondromas result from failure of normal endochondral ossification below the physis—representing a dysplasia of the aspect of the physis.
- Common sites of involvement include the small tubular bones of hands or feet (40-65%), and the metaphysis of the proximal and distal femur, as well as the proximal humerus. With respect to the feet, it most frequently involves the diaphysis of the proximal phalanx, followed by the middle phalanx and the metatarsals; it commonly spares the distal phalanx.
- The physical examination is unremarkable unless a pathologic fracture exists.
- Histologically, it is composed of hyaline cartilage.
- Radiographs reveal "speckled" or "popcorn" calcifications in this central radiolucent lesion, with well-defined margins, endosteal erosion, and no aggressive features (Fig. 25–4).
- The risk of transformation is low: < 2% of asymptomatic solitary enchondromas transform to chondrosarcoma.
- In contrast, enchondromatosis—i.e. Ollier disease—has a 10-30% risk of malignant transformation. Patients with Ollier disease often have problems with growth and angular deformity of the extremities.
- Multiple enchondromas plus soft tissue hemangiomas, known as Maffucci disease, are associated with an increased risk of astrocytoma and gastrointestinal cancer, as well as a higher risk of malignant transformation to chondrosarcoma than in Ollier disease.
- It is often difficult to distinguish an enchondroma from a low-grade chondrosarcoma. Differentiation requires the correlation of x-rays and clinical findings.
- Degeneration to chondrosarcoma is more common in the pelvis and proximal extremities.
- Treatment options are as follow.
  - Asymptomatic solitary enchondromas may be followed non-operatively with serial radiographs.
  - If an enchondroma becomes symptomatic or begins to enlarge, it may require biopsy to rule out malignancy; curettage and bone grafting is usually adequate for borderline lesions.

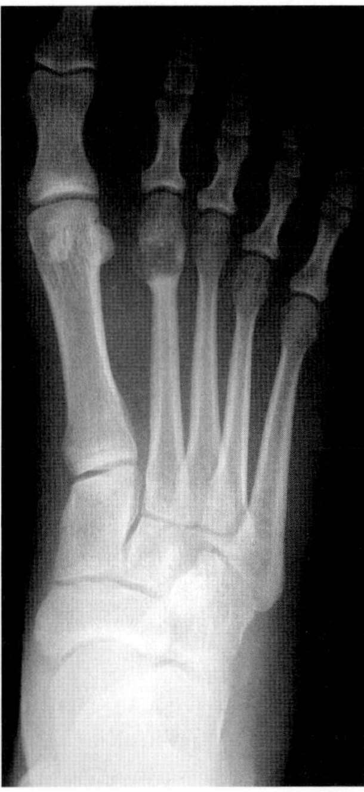

Figure 25–4: **Enchondroma. Anteroposterior foot.**

- Pathologic fractures are commonly allowed to heal with closed treatment, followed by curettage and bone grafting to prevent refracture.
- Recently, there have been reports that have found that the Ilizarov technique is successful in treating patients with Ollier disease despite some complications and the difficulty in using the technique. Jesus-Garcia et al. (2001) recently presented the results of treatment of 10 patients with Ollier disease using the Ilizarov technique. The Ilizarov device was used to treat leg length discrepancy and angular deformity, and to enhance the conversion of chondroma cartilage into normal mature bone, with no curettage and bone grafting. The mean duration of treatment was 9.4 months. This technique was found to be highly efficient in treating the disease, for it led to conversion of the abnormal cartilage into histologically mature bone in all patients. Complications included decreased knee mobility, which required prolonged use of the device.

Osteochondroma

- Osteochondroma is the most common benign bone tumor.
- It is a developmental dysplasia of peripheral growth plate, which forms a cartilage-capped projection of bone found near the metaphysis of long bones, pointing away from the joint.
- Characteristically, it grows via endochondral ossification of the proliferating cartilage cells.
- It often presents as a firm, non-tender, immobile mass arising near the end of a long bone.
- It frequently occurs in the distal tibia and metatarsals, as well as about the knee, proximal femur, and proximal humerus.
- Specific to the foot and ankle, they may cause angular deformities and/or limit the range of motion of the ankle via syndesmotic impingement.
- On radiographic analysis, it classically is continuous with the medullary canal of the underlying metaphyseal bone, growing away from the epiphysis.
- A cartilaginous cap of 2-2.5 cm or greater and growth after skeletal maturation may indicate malignant transformation.
- They may be solitary or multiple, as seen in hereditary multiple exostoses (HMEs), an autosomal dominant condition associated with mutations in EXT1 and/or EXT2 genes.
- Malignant degeneration is the most significant of potential complications. Less than 1% of solitary osteochondromas undergo malignant transformation to a low-grade, secondary chondrosarcoma. In patients with HME, the incidence is higher. The older literature suggests rates as high as 2-11%, but current studies indicate a rate of 2.8% (Wicklund et al. 1995).
- Management is as follows: Non-operative treatment if asymptomatic, versus marginal excision of the exostosis, cartilaginous cap, and overlying perichondrium if the lesion is symptomatic. If the osteochondroma continues to grow after skeletal maturity, chondrosarcoma must be ruled out with an MRI to measure the thickness of the cartilage cap and to look for an associated soft tissue mass. If chondrosarcoma is suspected, biopsy and resection will be necessary.
- In a recent study, ankle deformity, pain, and early arthritis were noted in approximately one-third of individuals with HME, most of whom had abnormal tibiotalar tilt. Early treatment of this deformity may prevent or decrease the incidence of late deterioration of ankle function (Noonan et al. 2002).
- Shawen et al. (2000) recently presented a case report in which symptomatic ankle valgus deformity secondary to HME was corrected with the Ilizarov technique. Two salient features of this case report were the age of the patient at presentation, and the success of the procedure. The authors learned that symptomatic valgus deformities of the ankle secondary to HME are normally corrected during adolescence, prior to physeal closure. Reducing the ankle mortise by distally displacing the fibula and correcting rotational and angular ankle deformities with Ilizarov external fixation improved their patient's ankle function and relieved his pain.

Subungual Exostosis

- Subungual exostosis radiographically resembles an osteochondroma.
- It typically develops on the distal phalanx, most commonly on the medial aspect of the great toe in young children.
- In contrast to osteochondroma, it is often associated with a history of trauma.
- Surgical excision is indicated if elevation of the nail leads to deformity and/or pain. The nail bed can usually be preserved, with amputation reserved for selected cases, such as recurrence (Landon et al. 1979).

Osteoid Osteoma

- Osteoid osteomas represent 11% of all benign bone tumors.
- It is a benign vascular osseous tumor, which occurs primarily in adolescents. Age range is 5-30 years old; classically, it is found in the second decade of life.
- The typical presentation is dull pain, often with increased severity at night, classically relieved by prostaglandin E_2 inhibitors such as aspirin or non-steroidal antiinflammatory drugs (NSAIDs).
- Alcohol may precipitate an acute painful crisis via vasodilatation.
- Most commonly, it is found in the proximal femur (femoral neck = 30% incidence). Other locations include the distal femur, distal humerus, phalanges of the hand, tibial shift, posterior spine (often causing painful

scoliosis), and the talus, navicular, and/or calcaneus of the foot.

- The pathognomonic radiographic finding is a nidus typically measuring < 1.5 cm in diameter. The nidus is best localized with CT scans with cuts set to 1-2 mm (Fig. 25–5).
- No cases of malignant transformation have been reported.
- Because they spontaneously resolve with time, treatment options include medical management with NSAIDs, en bloc excision or curettage, or percutaneous radiofrequency coagulation under CT guidance. The last option has become increasingly preferable, because it has resulted in near immediate pain relief and is the least invasive. Rosenthal et al. (1988) found that the success rate is comparable with that of the standard open technique (90%).

Osteoblastoma

- Osteoblastoma is a benign osseous tumor typically occurring in the second and third decade.
- Clinically, it presents as a dull, deep pain; however, unlike osteoid osteoma, it is not nocturnal, does not improve with NSAIDs, and is progressive in nature.
- The size of the nidus is > 1.5 cm (versus osteoid osteoma, which is < 1.5 cm).
- The foot, typically the talar neck, is the third most common location after the posterior spine and long bones. Other sites of involvement include the metatarsals, proximal humerus, and hip.
- There is a 7% incidence of pathologic fractures; most commonly in the forefoot. Secondary aneurysmal changes have been reported in 10% of cases.
- An associated soft tissue mass may be seen in about 25% of patients.
- Treatment typically involves excision and curettage; if it is aggressive in nature, wide excision is favored.
- Recurrence rate following curettage and bone graft is 10-20%.
- Recurrence should raise the suspicion of conversion to an aggressive or malignant osteoblastoma.

Chondroblastoma

- Chondroblastoma is considered a benign, aggressive tumor typically occurring in the second decade.
- Radiographically, it is a lytic lesion.
- In up to 50% of cases, cystic changes occur, which unlike a simple bone cyst, always efface the subchondral bone.
- It is commonly found in the epiphysis about the knee (50%), proximal humerus, triradiate cartilage of the pelvis, and/or the apophysis of long bones.
- In the foot and ankle, the talus and calcaneus are the most frequent locations.
- Histologically, it has "chicken wire calcification" and stains with S-100 antibody.
- It is associated with mutations in chromosomes 5 and 8.
- About 2% metastasize to the lungs.
- Treatment is curettage and bone graft.

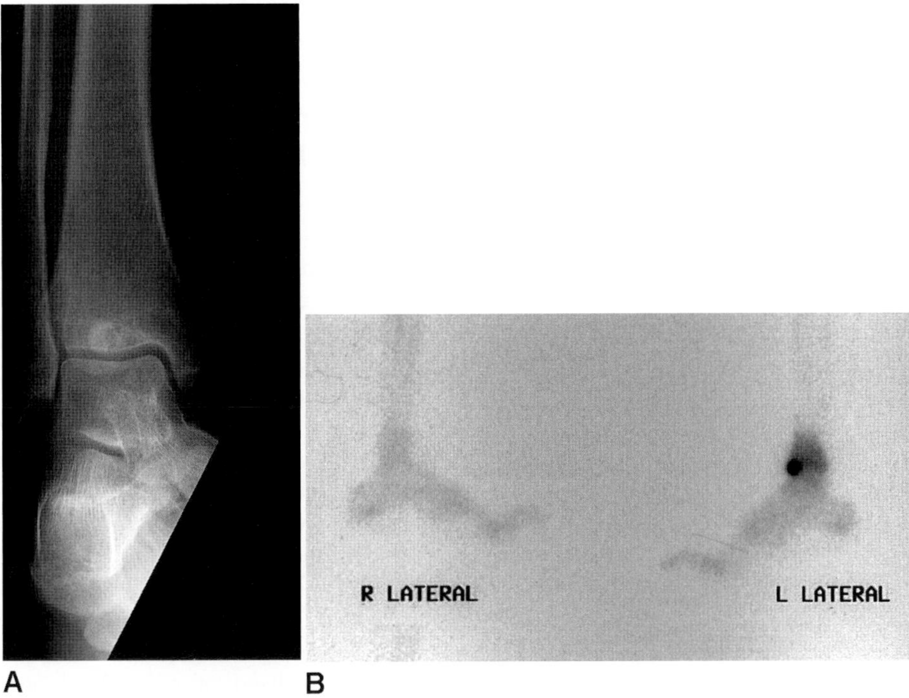

Figure 25–5: Osteoid osteoma. **A**, Anteroposterior ankle x-ray. **B**, Bone scan, ankle.

Giant Cell Reparative Granuloma

- Giant cell reparative granuloma is an uncommon benign reactive intraosseous lesion.
- The peripheral giant cell granuloma has an unknown etiology, with some dispute as to whether this lesion represents a reactive or a neoplastic process. Most favor the former etiology.
- It is solitary and osteolytic in nature. Expansion into surrounding soft tissues is rare.
- It is commonly found in the skull, jaw, hand, foot, and facial bones.
- Radiographically, the appearance is variable and appears aggressive, mimicking malignancy.
- Differential diagnosis includes ABC, giant cell tumor, or brown tumor of hyperparathyroidism.
- Histology shows fibrous stroma with spindle-shaped fibroblasts, multinucleated giant cells, inflammatory mononuclear cells, with areas of hemorrhage.
- Treatment is curettage and bone grafting.
- Recurrence is rare.

Bone Lesions: Malignant

Acral Metastases

- The incidence of skeletal metastasis to primary bone tumor is ≈ 25:1.
- Frequently, the metastatic bone lesion is found before the primary tumor (22% in some studies), and consequently it is occasionally mistaken for a primary bone lesion.
- From autopsy bone sampling, the overall incidence of skeletal metastasis from carcinoma has been rated as high as 70%.
- In general, bones distal to the knee and elbow are very exceptional sites for metastases.
- The majority of acral metastases (those distal to the knee or elbow) are from lung and renal carcinoma. Lung is more common than renal.
- The median survival time of patients with lung cancer metastasic to bone is 4 months, the shortest of all primary malignancies associated with bone metastasis.
- Many of the metastatic bone lesions are multiple, compared with primary bone tumors, which tend to be single lesions.
- Treatment should always involve consultation with an oncologist.
- Radiation can be used for palliative pain relief.
- Surgical treatment may require partial or complete amputation.

Osteosarcoma

- Osteosarcoma is the second most common primary bone malignancy after myeloma.
- Seventy-five percent occur in patients 10-25 years old.
- It is associated with mutations of the p53 and retinoblastoma tumor suppressor genes.
- This neoplasm typically has mixed lytic-blastic bone-forming lesions, with periosteal reaction and frequently a soft tissue mass characteristic of this tumor.
- It is usually a metaphyseal tumor. In the foot and ankle, it is commonly found in the distal tibia, with reports of lesions in the metatarsals and tarsals.
- In a retrospective review of 52 patients with osteosarcoma of the foot by Choong et al. (1999), the most common site was the calcaneus.
- Prior to current treatment regimens, long-term survival was 20%.
- With present treatment protocols, the mainstay being neoadjuvant chemotherapy and surgical resection, long-term survival is 60-70%.
- Specific to the foot and ankle, wide surgical resection in the face of close proximity of neurovascular structures can be difficult. Small tumors may be possible to resect with preservation of the foot. Larger tumors may require below-knee amputation.

Chondrosarcoma

- Chondrosarcoma is a malignant cartilage tumor typically found in patients 40-70 years old.
- In the foot and ankle, this tumor is most often a malignant transformation in patients with Ollier disease or multiple hereditary exostoses.
- Treatment involves wide excision, as radiotherapy and chemotherapy are ineffective.
- In a study by Fiorenza et al. (2002), survival following resection was 70% at 10 years and 63% at 15 years; survival was adversely affected by extracompartmental spread, development of local recurrence, and high histologic grade. Risk factors for local recurrence were inadequate surgical margins and tumor size > 10 cm.

Ewing Sarcoma and Peripheral Primitive Neuroectodermal Tumors

- Ewing sarcoma is a rare, malignant neoplasm in the small blue round cell family of tumors that is most common in children and adolescents.
- The peak incidence is between ages 10 and 20.
- While any bone of the axial or appendicular skeleton can be affected, it has rarely been reported in the bones of hands and feet.
- The characteristic radiologic findings include an "onion skin" and/or moth-eaten appearance of the lesion (Fig. 25–6A,B).
- Ewing sarcoma may occur entirely in soft tissue.
- The differential diagnosis includes round cell osteosarcoma, osteomyelitis, eosinophilic granuloma, extranodal lymphoma, and metastatic neuroblastoma.
- Histologically, it consists of sheets of round blue cells separated by bands of stroma. Metastases are common to lungs and other bones.

- Historically, treatment has consisted of chemotherapy and radiation therapy.
- Surgery is preferred to radiation therapy for resectable lesions. Radiotherapy is primarily used for unresectable lesions and cases with positive margins.
- Leeson and Smith (1989) reported a series of five consecutive cases of Ewing sarcoma of the forefoot treated with below-knee amputation for local tumor control. Four of five patients also had chemotherapy. The authors recommend below-knee amputation for Ewing sarcoma of the foot. Case reports exist for resection of small foot tumors with reconstruction. Figure 25–6C shows an ankle arthrodesis with an allograft/vascularized composite after resection of a distal tibia Ewing sarcoma reconstruction.
- Treatment consists of surgery and chemotherapy.
- Survival is highly dependent on the initial presentation of the disease. About 80% of patients present with localized disease, whereas 20% present with metastatic disease, most often to the lungs, bone, and bone marrow.
- The overall survival rate in patients with Ewing sarcoma is 60%; however, for patients with localized disease, it approaches 70%. If metastatic, the long-term survival rate is less than 25%.

Soft Tissue Lesions: Overview

- Soft tissue masses are common in the foot, and the vast majority are benign.
- A small number of these will be sarcomas.
- Kirby et al. (1989) retrospectively examined the cases of 83 patients who had a soft tissue tumor or tumor-like lesion in the foot or ankle to determine the relative frequency of the lesions and which factors, if any, could be used to identify them preoperatively. Seventy-two (87%) of the lesions were benign, with ganglion cysts and plantar fibromatoses being the most common, and 11 (13%) were malignant tumors, 5 (45%) of which were synovial sarcomas. For eight patients (12%), radiographs were helpful in identifying the nature of the lesion. The gender of the patient, a traumatic history, the duration of the symptoms, the size of the lesion, and the presence of pain or of neurologic symptoms were not useful in discriminating a benign lesion from a malignant tumor.
- It is important to have a diagnosis before embarking on treatment of a soft tissue mass.
- The diagnosis of a ganglion can be made by a simple aspiration.
- Lipomas, plantar fibromas, hemangiomas, and pigmented villonodular synovitis (PVNS) can usually be presumptively diagnosed with MRI (Table 25–2).
- Small masses (1-2 cm) can be primarily excised, but larger masses should be biopsied prior to removal, because there is a significant chance that a heterogeneous mass on MRI, which is large and deep, may be a sarcoma.

Soft Tissue Lesions: Benign

Pigmented Villonodular Synovitis/Giant Cell Tumor of Tendon Sheath

- PVNS is a proliferative disease of the synovium, which has a tendency to bleed and cause hemarthrosis and eventually destruction of a joint.

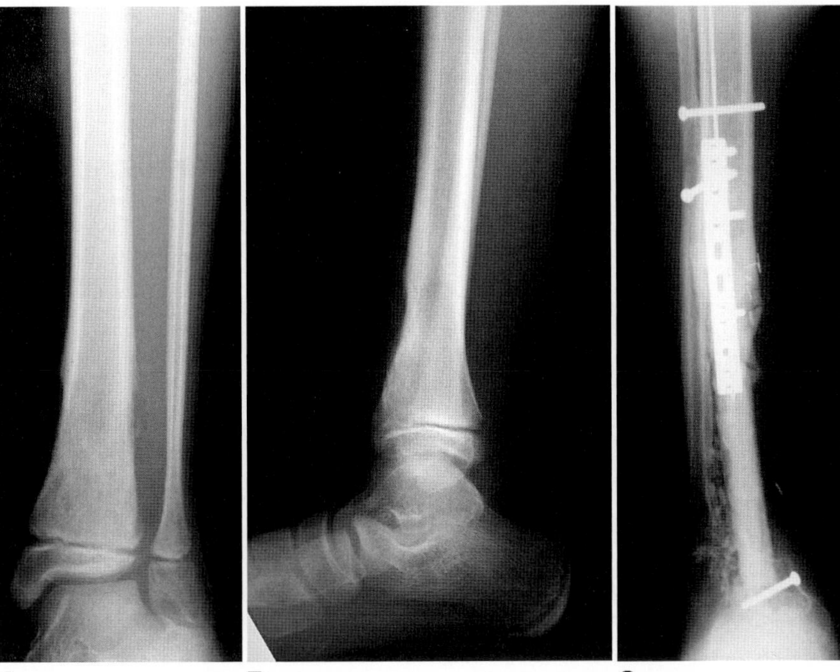

Figure 25–6: Ewing sarcoma. **A,** Anteroposterior distal tibia x-ray. **B,** Lateral distal tibia x-ray. **C,** Post reconstruction.

Table 25–2: Magnetic Resonance Imaging Characteristics of Benign Soft Tissue Lesions

MAGNETIC RESONANCE IMAGING	T_1	T_2	HOMOGENEOUS HETERO-OR	OTHER
Ganglion	Low	Bright	Homogeneous	Rim-enhanced gadolinium
Lipoma	Bright	Low	Homogeneous	Fat suppression
Hemangioma	Mixed	Mixed	Heterogeneous	Serpiginous tubular structures
Pigmented villonodular synovitis	Intermediate-dark	Intermediate-dark	–	–

- It is most common in the third through fifth decades of life, but has also occurred in the ankle in children under the age of 10.
- It is most common in the knee, with most series reporting < 5% occurrence in the foot and ankle.
- It may be localized (nodular) or diffuse, and can occur either extraarticularly or intraarticularly.
- It is one cause of periarticular bone erosions.
- Symptoms include swelling and stiffness, arthralgia, and a "popping" feeling with movement. The symptoms usually start slowly and may come and go over time.
- PVNS should be considered in patients with persistent ankle pain and swelling, particularly if bone erosions are visible on plain radiographs.
- The etiology is unclear, although a substantial proportion have chromosomal abnormalities.
- On gross examination, it may be nodular or globular, yellow-tan, with villous growths associated with synovial membranes. Microscopic findings include hemosiderin deposits, foamy histiocytes, giant cells, and large synovial cells.
- MRI is useful in delineating the extent of PVNS, as indicated by medium- to low-signal intensity lesions, often eroding bone and involving synovium of either joints or tendon sheaths (Fig. 25–7).
- Treatment generally consists of local resection.
- Recurrence is common and may be treated with radiation.

Hemangioma

- Hemangiomas are the most frequently seen tumors of childhood, and account for 7% of all benign tumors.
- Solitary capillary hemangiomas are the most common type.
  - Typically, they present as elevated, red-purple cutaneous lesions, most commonly on the head and neck.
- Cavernous hemangiomas are larger and less common.
  - The enlarged vascular spaces of this cavernous lesion give it the characteristic "cluster of purple grapes" appearance.
  - They can lie deep within the musculature of extremities, or even within the synovium of joints.
- Hemangioma of the tendon sheath is also rarely reported. Urguden et al. (2000) reported a case of a cavernous hemangioma in a 22-year-old man, which presented as peroneal tenosynovitis. Treatment consisted of complete excision.
- Case reports of intraosseous hemangiomas have been described in the foot and ankle. Sheth et al. (1994) reported an intraosseous hemangioma of the talus, which simulated an osteoid osteoma on the anteroposterior x-ray.
- Treatment of symptomatic lesions includes compressive stockings, embolization or sclerosis (which is usually performed by interventional radiologists), or excision.

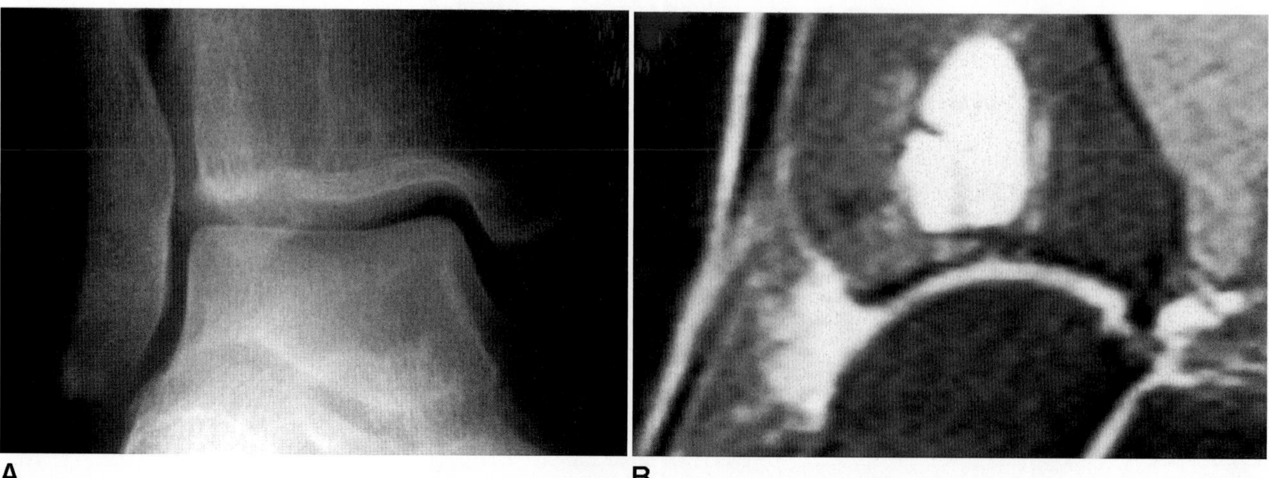

Figure 25–7: Pigmented villonodular synovitis. A, Anteroposterior ankle x-ray. B, Magnetic resonance imaging scan of ankle, sagittal view.

If the hemangioma cannot be completely resected, recurrence is likely. Debulking is unpredictable for pain relief, and therefore excision should be used selectively.

Ganglion

- Ganglions are mucinous-filled cysts found adjacent to a joint capsule or tendon sheath.
- Eleven percent are found in the foot and ankle.
- They are the most common lesions in the foot, and often arise from the tarsal joints.
- Ganglions should be aspirated to confirm the diagnosis. If the typical gelatinous fluid cannot be aspirated, MRI, biopsy, or excision should be performed to rule out other soft tissue tumors.
- Management typically begins with non-operative management—often employing aspiration and injection of corticosteroids. Those cysts that are refractory to non-operative modalities are excised.
- Rozbruch et al. (1998) reported, in a series of 40 patients treated with surgical excision, an 86% satisfaction rate and a 10% recurrence rate.

Lipoma

- Lipoma is the most common benign soft tissue tumor in adults.
- It is composed of lobules of mature fat.
- It usually presents superficial to the fascia; however, in the foot and ankle it is typically deep to the fascia.
- Case reports include occurrence on the plantar aspect of the toe.
- Treatment of symptomatic and/or enlarging lesions refractory to non-operative management is marginal excision. Recurrence is rare.

Fibromatosis

- Fibromatosis is a locally aggressive idiopathic proliferative fasciitis of the plantar aponeurosis that is often (50%) bilateral.
- The responsible cell is myofibroblast.
- It typically occurs in the second to fourth decades of life.
- Twenty percent of patients with Dupuytren contracture have plantar fibromatosis.
- If associated with Dupuytren contractures in the hand and/or Peyronie disease, it is referred to as Lederhosen syndrome, and presents as discrete plantar nodules often seen in non-weight-bearing areas (especially medial plantar).
- Radiographs typically reveal a non-specific soft tissue mass, and calcification is common only in juvenile aponeurotic fibroma.
- Imaging (ultrasound, CT, and MRI) demonstrates lesion extent. Involvement of adjacent structures is common, reflecting the infiltrative growth pattern often seen in these lesions.
- MRI scans may show characteristic features of prominent low to intermediate signal intensity and bands of low signal intensity representing highly collagenized tissue. However, fibromatoses with less collagen and more cellularity may have non-specific high signal intensity on T_2-weighted images.
- Non-operative management, consisting of NSAIDs and accommodating orthotics, is the first line of treatment.
- If surgery is elected, excision must include the entire slip of plantar fascia. Because of the aggressive nature of these fibromatoses, partial or subtotal fasciectomy results in recurrence rates nearing 60%.
- Some literature supports the judicious use of postoperative radiotherapy to decrease recurrence rates.

Nerve Sheath and Peripheral Nerve Tumors

- *Schwannoma*, *neurilemmoma*, or *neurinoma* is a benign nerve sheath tumor located within the epineurium, typically of spinal roots and superficial nerves on the flexor surfaces of extremities.
  - It commonly affects patients between the ages of 20 and 60 years.
  - Men and women are equally affected.
  - Eighty percent are solitary; multiple lesions have been reported and are associated with neurofibromatosis.
  - Clinical presentation typically involves a painful mass without neurologic impairment; supportive physical examination findings include a positive Tinel sign.
  - The schwannoma can usually be excised with preservation of nerve fascicles, unlike neurofibromas, which are more infiltrative.
- *Neurofibromas* are benign peripheral nerve tumors; 90% are solitary.
  - Multiple lesions, called neurofibromatosis, consist of two types: Neurofibromatosis type 1 (von Recklinghausen disease) involves peripheral nerves; type 2 neurofibromatosis involves acoustic nerves.
  - There is a 10% incidence of development of a malignant peripheral nerve sheath tumor in neurofibromatosis type 1. Fifty percent of neurofibrosarcomas are the result of malignant transformation.
  - Individuals afflicted with neurofibromatosis have 4 times the risk of developing malignant tumors versus the general population.
  - Treatment can be resection if the neurofibroma is sufficiently symptomatic and the functional loss will be minimal, understanding the risk of a painful neuroma; because of the intimate association with nerve fascicles, permanent injury to the nerve is likely.

Soft Tissue Lesions: Malignant

- Soft tissue sarcomas are neoplasms arising from mesenchymal tissues.
- The most common histopathologies for extremity soft tissue sarcoma are malignant fibrous histiocytoma and

liposarcoma. However, in the foot a disproportionate number are synovial sarcoma.
- From a practical point of view, the histopathology has minimal impact on treatment.
- All sarcomas are resected with a wide margin, and deep high-grade tumors are treated with radiation therapy, which decreases the local recurrence rate.
- Treatment of foot sarcomas is complicated by relative paucity of expendable soft tissues and the need for durable skin able to withstand weight bearing. These limitations may necessitate a more frequent use of amputation than is used for soft tissue sarcoma arising more proximally in the extremity, although free tissue transfer has been successfully used on the weight-bearing surface of the foot after sarcoma resection.
- Chemotherapy is considered for those with high-risk tumors (large, deep, high grade) and those with metastatic disease.

Synovial Sarcoma

- Synovial sarcoma is the most common malignant soft tissue mass in the foot and ankle.
- It most often occurs in adolescents and young adults, and presents as a slowly enlarging, painless mass. The goal is to diagnose a soft tissue while it is resectable. Figure 25–8 shows a large synovial sarcoma that required an amputation.
- It histologically resembles synovial tissue; it is usually found along fascial planes and in periarticular structures and, rarely, in joints; and it may involve the sheaths and bursae of the tendons.
- It is associated with gene translocation (X:18).
- Lymph node metastases are more common than for other sarcomas.
- On radiographic evaluation, it is typically a soft tissue density.
- Discrete intrinsic calcifications can be seen (30% incidence), often best on CT. This is not pathognomonic; the differential diagnosis includes chondroma and hemangioma.
- Histologic analysis reveals two forms: biphasic (epithelioid) and monophasic (spindle cell type) (Fig. 25-8C).
- The biphasic form is composed of both epithelial cell and spindle cell components, whereas the monophasic form is almost always the spindle cell type.
- The predominant spindle cell component (monophasic synovioma) contains cords of spindle cells, which may resemble *fibrosarcoma*.
- All synovial sarcoma are considered high grade, although prognostic variables that have been identified include nuclear atypia and the specific breakpoint of the translocation.
- Synovial sarcoma of the foot and ankle frequently is misdiagnosed, which leads to delays in treatment.

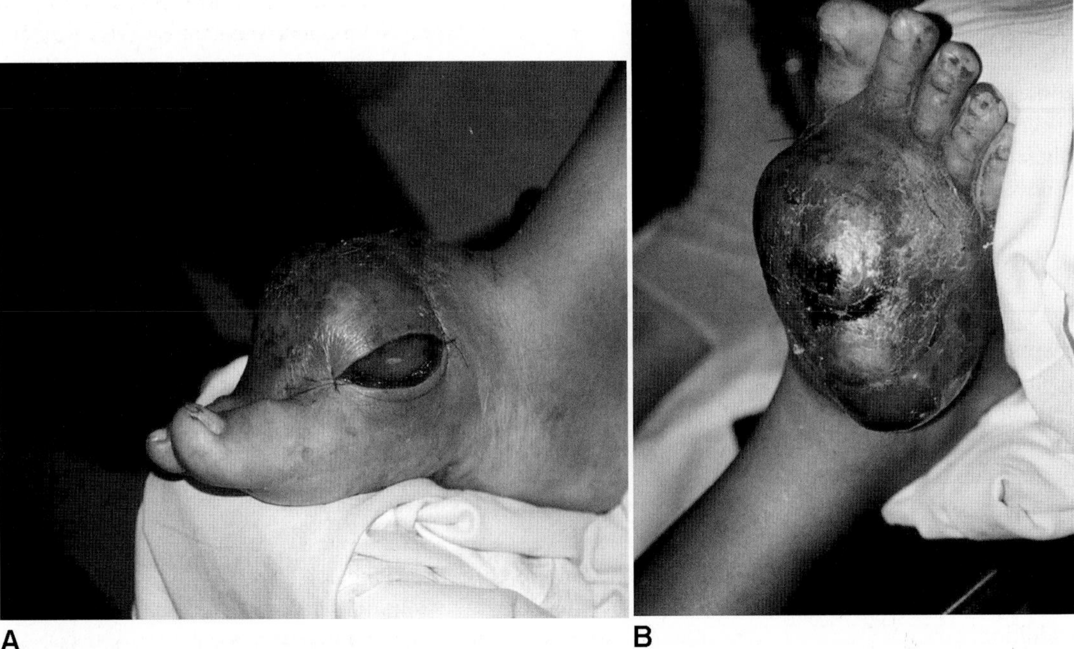

Figure 25–8: Synovial sarcoma. **A**, Foot, gross photo of extreme presentation. **B**, Foot.

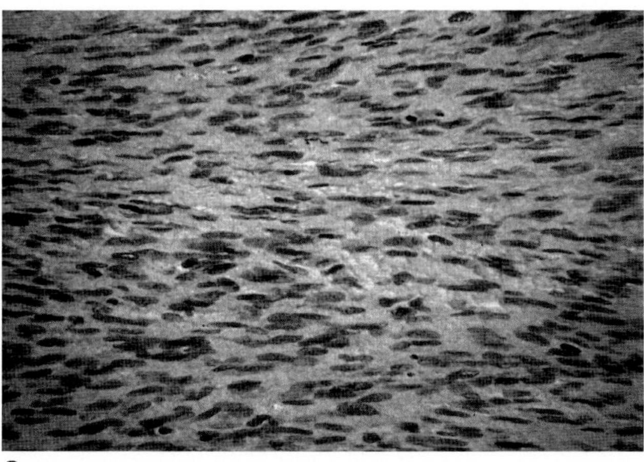

C

Figure 25–8: Cont'd **C, Histology, monophasic.**

- Treatment consists of wide resection and usually radiation therapy. Chemotherapy is considered for large, deep, high-grade tumors and for those with metastatic disease.
- Fifty percent metastasize to the lungs; 30% spread to regional lymph nodes. The 5-year survival rate ranges from 25 to 55%.
- Scully et al. (1999) reviewed the clinical records of 14 patients with synovial sarcoma of the foot and ankle. Of the 14 patients, 12 underwent an attempted curative surgical procedure. Ten patients had partial foot amputations or below-knee amputations, whereas two had an attempted limb salvage by wide resection. Of the 14 patients, 1 experienced regionally recurrent disease and 8 had pulmonary metastasis develop. All patients who developed metastases died of their disease. Tumor size was not observed to be a prognostic variable. Patients with a prolonged duration of symptoms before diagnosis had a better outcome, presumably because these tumors biologically were less aggressive. The authors concluded that wide resection could be considered in a select group of patients.

Clear Cell Sarcoma (Malignant Melanoma of Soft Parts)

- Clear cell sarcoma of tendons and aponeuroses is a slow and progressive tumor with poor prognosis, commonly found in young adults.
- It is commonly located in the extremities, specifically about the knee, feet, and ankle.
- Fifty percent occur in the foot, frequently the deep compartments.
- Tumor cells contain melanin, which is demonstrated by S-100 protein, HMB45, and microphthalmia transcription factor. In addition, Leu7, NSE, vimentin, and keratin are also found (Langezaal et al. 2001).
- The presence of melanin is responsible for slighty higher signal on T-1 images.
- Clear cell sarcoma and conventional malignant melanoma may demonstrate significant morphologic overlap at the light microscopic and ultrastructural level.
- Consequently, the clinically relevant distinction between primary clear cell sarcoma and metastatic melanoma in the absence of a known primary cutaneous, mucosal, or ocular tumor may occasionally cause diagnostic problems.
- A balanced translocation, t(12;22)(q13;q13), has been identified in a high percentage (50-75%) of clear cell sarcomas, and is presumed to be tumor-specific. It results in fusion of the EWS (Ewing sarcoma) gene and ATF-1.
- Large size of the tumor and presence of necrosis is indicative of poor prognosis.
- Metastasis occurs in more than 50% of cases. Common sites include bone, lymph node, and lungs.
- Treatment consists of wide local resection and radiotherapy.
- Local recurrence is common.

Melanoma

- Melanoma is the most common primary malignant tumor of the foot, occurring most frequently on the plantar skin.
- The skin and nails of the foot should be examined as part of the physical examination of the foot, with particular attention to the plantar skin.
- All pigmented lesions should be noted, and atypical lesions should be biopsied or referred to a dermatologist or general surgical oncologist.
- There are two types of melanoma:
  - superficial spreading—most common in caucasians
  - acral lentiginous—most common in Asian, Latin, and African ethnic groups.
- Malignant melanoma may begin as a benign lesion, the dysplastic nevus. Tumor thickness is the most important prognostic factor.
- Treatment involves excision, with a 3-cm margin, and radiation therapy for those with lymph node metastases.
- The overall 5-year survival rate is 80%; specific to the foot and ankle, it is 63% (subungual is 16-60%).
- Figure 25–9 shows a fungating subungual melanoma of the fourth toe.

Kaposi Sarcoma

- Kaposi sarcoma is present in 15% of HIV-positive homosexual men and can be found on the plantar surface of the foot in some (Montes et al. 1994).
- Treatment involves chemotherapy and radiation, with an 88% response rate.

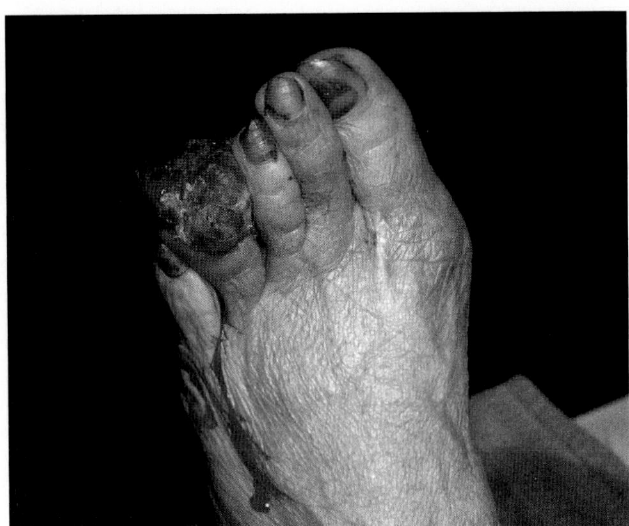

Figure 25–9: Melanoma, foot.

References

Biscaglia R, Bacchini P, Bertoni F. (2000) Giant cell tumor of the bones of the hand and foot. Cancer 88(9): 2022-2032.

Analysis of data gathered on giant cell tumors of the hands and feet over a 50-year time period at the Rizzoli Orthopedic Institute.

Campbell RS, Grainger AJ, Mangham DC et al. (2003) Intraosseous lipoma: Report of 35 new cases and a review of the literature. Skeletal Radiol 32(4): 209-222.

Metaanalysis of 145 cases of intraosseous lipoma—the common features of this fatty tumor were identified. The mean age was 43 years. Gender distribution was equal. The most frequent location was the lower limb (71%)—the calcaneus was the most common (32%). In the calcaneus, the lesions were centrally located and more often calcified with marginal sclerosis, fat necrosis, and cyst formation than those located in long bones. Lipomas located in long bones were typically eccentric.

Casadei R, Ruggieri P, Moscato M et al. (1996) Aneurysmal bone cyst and giant cell tumor of the foot. Foot Ankle Int 17(8): 487-495.

Retrospective review of 257 cases of benign bone tumors treated—authors offer a comparison of ABC versus giant cell tumor. The identifying characteristics of ABC are average age of patients (15 years); a rare propensity to small tarsal bones (6%); and sharp, trabeculated margins on x-ray, leading to cortical expansion. On the contrary, giant cell tumor was defined by an average patient age of 27 years; a higher localization to small tarsal bones (19%); and an eccentric, round, aggressive lytic appearance with ill-defined edges, leading to erosion and cortical penetration on x-ray. Septation was seen in both tumors.

Choong PF, Qureshi AA, Sim FH et al. (1999) Osteosarcoma of the foot: A review of 52 patients at the Mayo Clinic. Acta Orthop Scand 70(4): 361-364.

Review of 52 cases of osteosarcoma of the foot seen and treated at the Mayo Clinic.

D'Angelo G, Petas N, Donzelli O. (1996) Lengthening of the lower limbs in Ollier's disease: problems related to surgery. Chir Organi Mov 81(3): 279-285.

Comparison of Wagner's technique and the Ilizarov method in lengthening of the lower limbs in Ollier disease.

de Bree E, Zoetmulder FA, Keus RB et al. (2004) Incidence and treatment of recurrent plantar fibromatosis by surgery and postoperative radiotherapy. Am J Surg 187(1): 33-38.

After collecting data from nine patients (11 feet), the role of postoperative radiotherapy in prevention of recurrence was analyzed. Plantar fasciectomy was associated with the lowest recurrence rate. Adjuvant radiotherapy decreased the recurrence rate; however, it was associated with significantly impaired functional outcome in three cases.

Donley BG, Philbin T, Rosenberg GA et al. (2000) Percutaneous CT guided resection of osteoid osteoma of the tibial plafond. Foot Ankle Int 21(7): 596-598.

Case report of a juxtaarticular osteoid osteoma of the tibial plafond treated with CT-guided resection.

Enneking WF, Spanier SS, Goodman MA. (1980) A system for the surgical staging of musculoskeletal sarcoma. Clin Orthop 153: 106-120.

Classic article. Enneking details a surgical staging system for musculoskeletal sarcomas stratifying bone and soft tissue lesions of any histiogenesis by the grade of biologic aggressiveness, by the anatomical setting, and by the presence of metastasis.

Fiorenza F, Abudu A, Grimer RJ et al. (2002) Risk factors for survival and local control in chondrosarcoma on bone. J Bone Joint Surg Br 84(1): 93-99.

Report of 153 patients with non-metastatic chondrosarcoma of bone performed at a minimum follow-up of 5 years to determine the risk factors for survival and local tumor control.

Gibbs CP Jr., Hefele MC, Peabody TD et al. (1999) Aneurysmal bone cyst of the extremities. Factors related to local recurrence after curettage with a high-speed burr. J Bone Joint Surg Am 81(12): 1671-1678.

Retrospective study of 40 patients treated by the same surgeon for an ABC between January 1, 1976, and December 31, 1993, performed to identify the rate of local recurrence and the prognostic factors related to local recurrence after use of contemporary methods of curettage with a high-speed burr. There were four recurrences—recurrence was statistically related to young age and open growth plates, and may be less likely following wide excision than following intralesional treatment by curettage.

Glaser DL, Dormans JP, Stanton RP et al. (1999) Surgical management of calcaneal unicameral bone cysts. Clin Orthop Relat Res 360: 231-237.

This is one of the largest series of UBCs located in the calcaneus. It compares the efficacy of methylprednisolone acetate injection treatment with curettage and bone grafting in the treatment of 11 patients with 12 UBCs of the calcaneus. At a mean follow-up of 28 months, there were no recurrences of the cyst in the nine patients who underwent bone grafting, and persistence of the cyst in the two patients who underwent injection therapy. The results markedly demonstrate that curettage and bone grafting is a better option than aspiration and steroid injection in treating cysts in this location.

Holm CL. (1976) A case of primary diffuse synovial chondromatosis of the ankle with long-term follow-up. J Bone Joint Surg Am 58(6): 878-880.

Case report of primary diffuse synovial chondromatosis of the ankle, with long-term follow-up.

Jaffe HL. (1943) Hereditary multiple exostosis. Arch Pathol 36: 335-357.

Classic article outlining the features of HME.

Jesus-Garcia R et al. (2001) Use of the Ilizarov external fixator in the treatment of patients with Ollier's disease. Clin Orthop Relat Res 382: 82-86.

The results of a mean duration of 9.4 months of treatment of 10 patients with Ollier disease using the Ilizarov technique are detailed.

Kirby EJ, Shereff MJ, Lewis MM et al. (1989) Soft-tissue tumors and tumor-like lesions of the foot. An analysis of eighty-three cases. J Bone Joint Surg Am 71(4): 621-626.

A retrospective analysis of 83 cases of soft tissue tumor or tumor-like lesions in the foot or ankle. The relative frequency of the lesions and possible preoperative identifying factors are determined.

Landon GC, Johnson KA, Dahlin DC. (1979) Subungual exostoses. J Bone Joint Surg Am 61(2): 256-259.

Review of 44 patients with subungual exostoses seen at the Mayo Clinic from 1910 through 1975.

Langezaal SM, Graadt van Roggen JF, Cleton-Jansen AM et al. (2001) Malignant melanoma is genetically distinct from clear cell sarcoma of tendons and aponeurosis (malignant melanoma of soft parts). Br J Cancer 84(4): 535-538.

Detailed discussion outlining the distinctions between malignant melanoma and clear cell sarcoma of tendons and aponeurosis.

Leeson MC, Smith MJ. (1989) Ewing's sarcoma of the foot. Foot Ankle 10(3): 147-151.

Discussion of five consecutive cases of Ewing sarcoma of the forefoot treated with below-knee amputation.

Letts M, Davidson D, Nizalik E. (1998) Subungual exostosis: Diagnosis and treatment in children. J Trauma 44(2): 346-349.

Retrospective review of 21 children treated for subungual exostosis at the Children's Hospital of Eastern Ontario from 1975 to 1995.

Lodwick GS. (1966) Solitary malignant tumors of bone: The application of predictor variables and diagnosis. Semin Roentgenol 1: 293.

Mankin HJ, Mankin CJ, Simon MA et al. (1996) The hazards of the biopsy; revisited: Members of the MTS. J Bone Joint Surg Am 78(5): 656-663.

Multicenter study revisiting the 1982 and 1992 data compilations—found that errors, complications, and changes in the course and outcome were 2-12 times greater when the biopsy was done in a referring institution instead of in a treatment center.

Milgram JW. (1977) Synovial osteochondromatosis. J Bone Joint Surg 59-A: 792-801.

Clinical and pathologic study of 30 cases of synovial osteochondromatosis; details the observed temporal sequence of pathology characterized by three recognizable phases.

Montes C, Luepschen OM et al. (1994) Kaposi's sarcoma of the foot in the HIV patient. J Foot Ankle Surg 33(4): 341-345.

Discussion of etiology, classifications, histopathology, evaluation, and treatment of an AIDS-related Kaposi sarcoma.

Noonan KJ, Feinberg JR, Levenda A et al. (2002) Natural history of multiple hereditary osteochondromatosis of the lower extremity and ankle. J Pediatr Orthop 22: 120-124.

Thirty-eight subjects with an average age of 42 years completed a detailed subjective questionnaire and underwent clinical and radiographic evaluation of their ankles to evaluate the natural history of the ankle joint in patients with multiple hereditary osteochondromatosis.

O'Keefe RJ, O'Donnel RJ, Temple HT et al. (1995) Giant cell tumor of bone in the foot and ankle. Foot Ankle Int 16(10): 617-623.

Case report of 12 giant cell tumors arising in the foot and ankle followed for more than 2 years.

Papagelopoulos PJ, Mayrogenis AF, Badekas A et al. (2003) Foot malignancies: A multidisciplinary approach. Foot Ankle Clin 8(4): 751-763.

Excellent review of the multidisciplinary approach to treating malignancies specific to the foot and ankle.

Pisters PW, Pollock RE. (1999) Staging and prognostic factors in soft tissue sarcoma. Semin Radiat Oncol 9(4): 307-314.

Outline of the current American Joint Committee on Cancer staging system for soft tissue sarcoma, and summary of the available data on traditional clinicopathologic and molecular prognostic factors.

Pogoda P, Priemel M, Linhart W et al. (2004) Clinical relevance of calcaneal bone cysts: A study of 50 cysts in 47 patients. Clin Orthop Relat Res 424: 202-210.

Defines the risk factors of pathologic fracture resulting from UBC located in the calcaneus. Those cysts that reached a critical size, defined as 100% intracalcaneal cross-section in the coronary plane and at least 30% in the sagittal plane, were found to be at risk for becoming symptomatic and subsequent fracture.

Ramseier LE, Jacob HA, Exner GU. (2004) Foot function after ray resection for malignant tumors of the phalanges and metatarsals. Foot Ankle Int 25(2): 53-58.

Review of four patients with malignant tumors of the proximal toe phalanx treated with ray resection and reconstruction by free microvascular fibula transfer, intermetatarsal bony fusion, or soft tissue stabilization. Follow-up between 21 months and 8 years.

Ratner V, Dorfman HD. (1990) Giant-cell reparative granuloma of the hand and foot bones. Clin Orthop Relat Res 260: 251-258.

An excellent descriptive analysis of giant cell reparative granulomas of the hands and feet.

Rosenthal DI, Hornicek FJ, Wolfe MW et al. (1988) Percutaneous radiofrequency coagulation of osteoid osteoma compared with operative treatment. J Bone Joint Surg 80-A(6): 815–821.

Comparison of percutaneous radiofrequency coagulation of osteoid osteoma with operative management. A consecutive series of 87 patients treated operatively was compared with 38 patients treated with percutaneous ablation with radiofrequency.

Rougraff BT, Kneisl JS, Simon MA et al. (1993) Skeletal metastases of unknown origin: A prospective study of diagnostic strategy. J Bone Joint Surg Am 75(9): 1276-1281.
A prospective study of diagnostic strategy in 40 consecutively seen patients who had skeletal metastases of unknown origin, which was extremely successful for the identification of the site of an occult malignant tumor before biopsy in patients.

Rozbruch SR, Chang V, Bohne WH et al. (1998) Ganglion cysts of the lower extremity: An analysis of 54 cases and review of the literature. Orthopedics 21(2): 141-148.
A review of 54 consecutive patients with lower extremity ganglion cysts treated from 1981 to 1993 with surgical excision and postoperative histologic analysis.

Sammarco GJ, Mangone PG. (2000) Classification and treatment of plantar fibromatosis. Foot Ankle Int 21: 563-569.
A retrospective study of 18 patients (23 feet) with plantar fibromatosis treated with surgical excision between 1991 and 1998.

Saxena A, Perez H. (2004) Pigmented villonodular synovitis about the ankle: A review of the literature and presentation in 10 athletic patients. Foot Ankle Int 25(11): 819-826.
Review of 10 patients over a 10-year period, who were identified as having PVNS of the ankle. Authors concluded that PVNS should be considered in athletically active patients with persistent lateral ankle pain and swelling, particularly if bone erosions are visible on plain radiographs.

Scully SP, Temple HT, Harrelson JM. (1999) Synovial sarcoma of the foot and ankle. Clin Orthop Relat Res 364: 220-226.
Review of the clinical records of 14 patients with synovial sarcoma of the foot and ankle revealed that it is frequently misdiagnosed, leading to delays in treatment.

Shawen SB et al. (2000) Correction of ankle valgus deformity secondary to multiple hereditary osteochondral exostoses with Ilizarov. Foot Ankle Int 21: 1019-1022.
Case report of correction of ankle valgus deformity secondary to multiple hereditary osteochondral exostoses with an Ilizarov fixator.

Sheth D, Marcove RC, Healey J et al. (1994) Intraosseous hemangioma of the talus: A case report. Foot Ankle Int 15(1): 41-43.
Case report of an intraosseous hemangioma of the talus that initially simulated an osteoid osteoma.

Solomon L. (1963) Hereditary multiple exostoses. J Bone Joint Surg 45B: 292-304.
Classic article outlining the features of HME.

Spear MA, Jennings LC, Mankin HJ et al. (1998) Individualizing management of aggressive fibromatoses. Int J Radiat Oncol Biol Phys 40(3): 637-645.
One hundred seven fibromatoses presenting between 1971 and 1992 were analyzed to examine prognostic indicators in aggressive fibromatoses that may be used to optimize case-specific management strategy.

Struhl S, Edelson C, Pritzker H et al. (1989) Solitary (unicameral) bone cyst. The fallen fragment sign revisited. Skeletal Radiol 18(4): 261-265.
Reynolds is credited with describing the fallen fragment sign in 1969. Typically, the sign is identified when the patient with a UBC presents with a pathologic fracture. The interior of the bone cyst may have complete or nearly complete thin bony septations within the cyst. At the time of pathologic fracture, a portion of one of these bony segments actually may break free and float to the bottom of the cyst. This is possible because the UBC is fluid-filled and is not a solid tumor. Some authors have altered the original description of this sign and referred to it as the "fallen leaf sign," as they choose to imagine the broken fragment of bone gently wafting down from the top of the cyst to the bottom of the cyst as if it were a leaf slowly falling to earth from a tree. The fallen fragment sign is found in approximately 20% of patients who present with a pathologic fracture secondary to UBC.

Urguden M, Ozdemir H, Duygulu E et al. (2000) Cavernous hemangioma behaving like peroneal tenosynovitis. Foot Ankle Int 21(10): 856-859.
Case report of a cavernous hemangioma of the tendon sheath that presented as peroneal tenosynovitis.

Wicklund CL, Pauli RM, Johnston D et al. (1995) Natural history study of hereditary multiple exostoses. Am J Med Genet 55(1): 43-46.
Delineates the natural history of HMEs carried out through retrospective review of 43 affected probands and 137 of their affected relatives.

CHAPTER 26

Amputations

Mathieu Assal* **and Eric Gordon§**

*M.D., Médecin Adjoint du Chef de Service, Service de Chirurgie Orthopédique et Traumatologie de l'Appareil Moteur, University Hospital of Geneva, Switzerland
§M.D., Department of Orthopaedic Surgery, New York Orthopaedic Hospital, Columbia-Presbyterian Medical Center, New York, NY

General

- Amputation and disarticulation should be viewed as reconstructive procedures and not a failure of treatment. In this manner, one realizes that it is the initial step in getting patients back to their previous functional status.
- Indications for amputation include ischemia, trauma, infection, tumor, and painful dysfunction of the foot and ankle not amenable to further conservative management.
- The goal is to create a modified locomotor end organ that provides a comfortable interface with a prosthesis and offers the most efficient energy-conserving gait as possible. Preoperative planning and surgical expertise directly correlate with patient outcome, and therefore there is no excuse for a poorly fashioned stump.
- A team effort, with a team composed of different medical specialists, is the best way to ensure a good result and restore patients to their optimal level of function.
- It is important to be aware of the psychosocial recovery of the patient with an amputation (Fitzpatrick 1999).
- In 1996 in the USA, amputees numbered approximately 1.2 million or about 1 in 200 (Fig. 26–1).

Indications

Peripheral Vascular Disease

- PVD is the most common reason for amputation and affects mainly the geriatric patient and those with diabetes mellitus.
- Up to 20% of patients with diabetes mellitus will suffer from PVD, and at some stage will develop foot ulcers leading to lower extremity amputation.
- Diabetics have the added problem of peripheral neuropathy, where loss of protective pain sensation will further compromise the likelihood of healing their ulcers.
- Prior to considering amputation, vascular studies are mandatory in order to determine:
  - the possibility of revascularization by an experienced vascular surgeon, and
  - the level of amputation.
- If the limb can be revascularized by means of vascular surgery or angioplasty, it is best to wait several days to assess the benefit of the procedure before determining the level of amputation, provided that there is no threat of infection (wet gangrene).
- Twenty-five percent of patients with diabetes who undergo amputation will require an amputation on the contralateral limb within the following 3 years.
- Because of the complexity of the numerous morbidities in this fragile group of patients, management is best with a team approach with a team composed of primary care physician, internist, surgeon, physiatrist, physical therapist, prosthetist, and social worker. In addition, the input of an infectious diseases specialist may be required.
- PVD accounts for 90% of amputations, with 97% of dysvascular amputations performed on the lower limb.
- African American males are at greatest risk for dysvascular amputation. African Americans are 2-4 times more likely

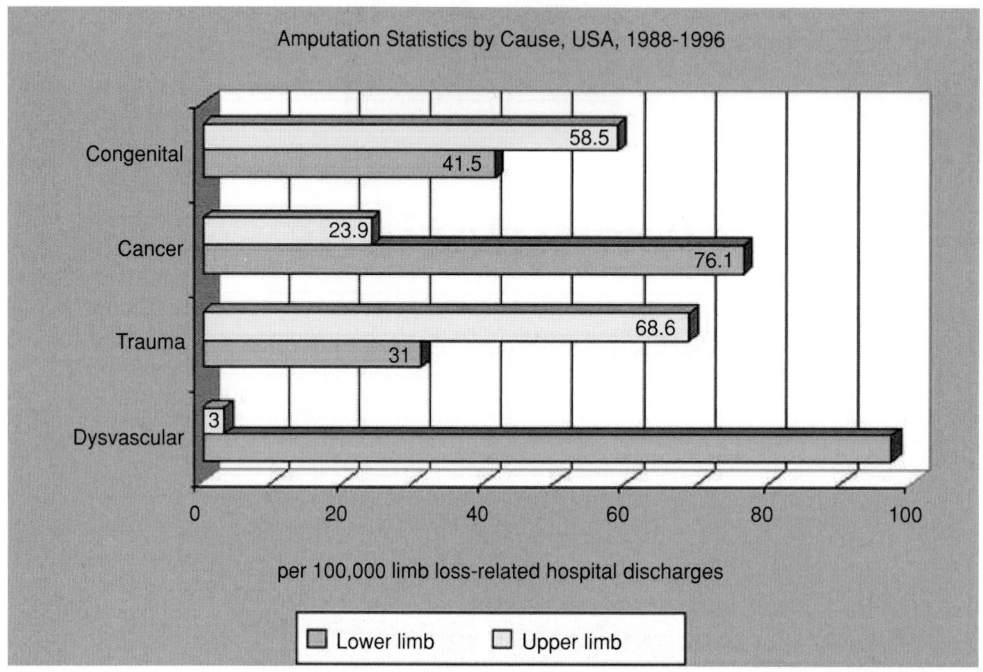

Figure 26–1: US amputation statistics by cause. (From Adams PF et al. (1999) Current estimates from the National Health Interview Survey, 1996. Vital Health Stat 10: 200.)

to lose a limb than white persons of similar age and gender (Dillingham et al. 2002).

- In amputees with PVD, the 5-year survival rate is between 70 and 90%, with heart disease as the leading cause of death (51%).
- Approximately 50% of dysvascular amputees are diabetic.

Trauma

- Several well-established scoring systems (Table 26–1) have been developed to help in arriving at a decision to perform an immediate amputation following lower extremity trauma.
- A commonly used scoring system is the Mangled Extremity Severity Score (MESS), which consists of four categories: skeletal/soft tissue injury, limb ischemia, shock, and age (Table 26–2). A lower number of points indicates a less severe injury, and a total score of 7 or below is almost always compatible with limb salvage (Helfet et al. 1990, Johansen et al. 1990).

Table 26–1: Scoring Systems for Severely Injured Limbs

REFERENCE	NAME OF SCORE	ACRONYM
Gregory et al. (1985)	Mangled Severity Extremity Index	MESI
Howe et al. (1987)	Predictive Salvage Index	PSI
Helfet et al. (1990)	Mangled Extremity Severity Score	MESS
Russell et al. (1991)	Limb Salvage Index	LSI
McNamara et al. (1994)	Nerve, Ischemia, Soft tissue, Skeletal, Shock, Age Index	NISSSA

Table 26–2: Mangled Extremity Severity Score Variables[a]

VARIABLE GROUP	DESCRIPTION	POINT(S)
Skeletal/soft tissue injury	Low energy (stab, simple fracture)	1
	Medium energy (open fracture, multiple fractures)	2
	High energy (high-velocity gunshot, crush)	3
	Very high energy (above + gross contamination)	4
Limb ischemia	Pulse ↓ or absent, perfusion normal	1[b]
	Pulseless, paresthesias, ↓ capillary refill	2[b]
	Cool, paralyzed, insensate	3[b]
Shock	Systolic blood pressure always > 90 mmHg	0
	Transient hypotension	1
	Persistent hypotension	2
Age	< 30 years	0
	30-50 years	1
	> 50 years	2

[a]A score of 7 or less is nearly always compatible with limb salvage.
[b]Score doubled for ischemia > 6 h.

- It is felt by some that soft tissue injury severity has the greatest impact on decision making regarding limb salvage versus amputation (MacKenzie et al. 2002).
- However, there are problems with all scoring systems. They frequently are difficult to apply and may not accurately predict outcome (Bosse et al. 2001).

- In cases of severe limb damage, primary amputation at first surgery may be best for the patient's physical and psychologic well-being.
- In other cases, it may be better to plan an initial attempt at limb salvage and observe. If it is thought that amputation is inevitable, it should be performed as a delayed primary amputation within the first 10-14 days after injury.
- But prolonged attempts at limb salvage lead to severe psychologic and economic burdens on the patient and the family.
- Almost 70% of trauma-related amputations are upper limb amputation.
- The most common causes of lower extremity trauma requiring amputation are lawn mower injuries and motorcycle accidents.
- Traumatic amputees have a better prognosis than dysvascular amputees.

Malignancies

- The most common malignant tumor found in the region of the foot and ankle is synovial sarcoma. While metastases to the feet are uncommon, any cancer can metastasize to bone, and any bone can be involved.
- The most common primary tumors that metastasize to the feet are carcinoma of the lung, adenocarcinoma of the colon, genitourinary carcinoma, melanoma, and other undifferentiated tumors.
- The development of limb salvage procedures for malignant tumors of the extremities, combined with chemotherapy, has reduced the incidence of amputation for primary malignancies of the lower extremity.

Infection

- Life-threatening infection of the lower extremity requires an open amputation. The stump can be closed only when it is certain that the infectious process is under control.
- In some circumstances, patients will require repeated debridement and lavage in the operating room until the stump is clear of infection and necrotic tissue.
- Chronic osteomyelitis is not an absolute indication for amputation, and can be managed with good preoperative planning and selective surgery including fistulectomy, sequestrectomy, and similar less invasive procedures. Plastic surgery is often required for coverage of soft tissue defects.
- The ultimate function of the salvaged limb should justify the physical and psychologic costs of the treatment.
- Recurrent infection points to the possibility of PVD, which prevents adequate perfusion of the infected area, leading to decreased efficacy of antibiotic therapy.
- Recurrent infection is most often seen in patients with diminished peripheral protective sensation combined with bony deformities leading to abnormal pressure points and recurrent ulcers.
- Charcot neuroarthropathy involving the foot and ankle is a major cause of recurrent infection.

Dysfunctional Limb

- Painful dysfunction of the limb following several attempts at reconstruction may result with severe foot and ankle disorders or trauma.
- In some cases, consultation with a pain management specialist and a psychiatrist is helpful.
- With the correct indication and a well-healed stump and a properly fitted prosthesis, most patients with painful dysfunction of the limb will benefit from amputation and regain excellent function, with significant pain relief.
- The most common level of amputation for a dysfunctional foot and ankle is a long transtibial amputation, provided that the soft tissues forming the stump are healthy.
- A well-functioning transtibial amputation in a healthy young person will lead to better function than a multiply fused foot and ankle (such as a pantalar fusion).

Level of Amputation

- Determining the appropriate level of amputation or disarticulation is the most important, and yet probably the most difficult, part in the treatment of a patient who has no hope for limb preservation.
- If the indication for amputation is a malignant tumor, a life-threatening infection, or an irreparably damaged body part, then the level of amputation must be done proximal to the lesion, in healthy tissues.
- If amputation is performed for PVD, a thorough evaluation of arterial blood flow is essential. Forefoot and toe blood pressure obtained using Doppler devices are of limited value in determining foot amputation levels in vascular patients, because artificially high values may be obtained from heavily calcified, hence incompressible, vessels.
- Transcutaneous oxygen measurements (tcPO_2) can assist in evaluating tissue oxygenation peripherally to the dorsal distal metatarsal level. Values > 30-40 mmHg indicate that wound healing is likely. A value < 20 mmHg indicates that wound healing is unlikely to occur at that level (Pecoraro et al. 1991).
- Hyperbaric oxygen chamber therapy with the patient breathing 100% oxygen at 2.5 atm may help wound healing for those patients who are able to increase their tcPO_2 to 40 mmHg under the administration of 100% normal baric oxygen via a snugly fitting mask for 20 min (Brakora and Sheffield 1995).
- The presence of palpable pulses does not guarantee healing of the stump, because the patient may have heavily calcified arteries or poor peripheral blood distribution due to microangiopathy.

- The presence of hair on the leg or the dorsum of the foot is a positive sign for adequate skin perfusion and secondary wound healing.
- The presence of a thermal gradient from proximal to distal, as well as skin trophic changes, is a clinical sign of poor vascular supply to the soft tissue envelope, which may predispose to failure of wound healing.
- Lack of protective sensation by itself should not be a factor in considering a more proximal amputation level.
- There is a 2.5 times higher complication rate of infection and reamputation in patients who continue to smoke after amputation (Lind et al. 1991).
- Perfusion should be optimized by avoidance of vasoconstrictors such as nicotine and caffeine. Platelet function and fibrinogen levels require approximately 1 week of smoking cessation to return to normal levels.
- Serum albumin level below 3.0 g/dL, total lymphocyte count < 1500/mm^3, and poor glucose control in patients with diabetes (Hb A1-C > 7%) significantly decrease wound-healing potential.
- Partial foot amputation is associated with major advantages over higher amputation levels, including preservation of weight bearing, improved proprioceptive function, and decreased disruption of body image. In addition, it requires only shoe modifications or a limited prosthesis (Table 26–3).
- A determined effort should be made to save maximum length to enhance function. At the same time, the likelihood of healing should be sufficiently high to avoid the need for a second surgery consisting of reamputation secondary to a non-healing stump.
- In cases of peripheral ischemia secondary to frostbite, vasoconstrictor administration for hypotension, and cryoglobulinemia, it is essential to allow time for completion of tissue demarcation and to keep the necrotic areas dry. In many cases, maximum tissue preservation can be achieved by allowing autoamputation of the necrotic portions. No urgent surgery should be done until the necrotic tissues are well demarcated and the ischemic wounds are dry.
- A contracted knee despite intensive physical therapy is an indication for a knee disarticulation instead of a transtibial amputation, because the prosthesis can only partially compensate for the lack of extension of the knee, thus making ambulation challenging.
- A non-ambulatory patient requires a level of amputation that will ensure the best chance of healing whenever a lower level might be questionable.
- Split skin grafts should be avoided, especially on surfaces that experience significant shear forces, such as at the end of the stump, where they may ulcerate.
- Patients with significant gangrenous changes of the heel pad should have a transtibial amputation.

Physiology of Amputation: Energy Expenditure

- The metabolic demands of walking are increased by the following factors:
  - decreasing residual limb length
  - increasing number of amputated joints
  - increasing number of amputated limbs
  - dysvascular amputation.
- The rates of metabolic energy expenditure ($\dot{V}O_2$, ml/kg per min) at various amputation levels were compared with those of non-amputees, demonstrating the increased metabolic costs shown in Table 26–4.

Table 26–3: Effect of Different Amputation Levels

LEVEL OF AMPUTATION	BODY IMAGE DISRUPTION	LEG LENGTH PRESERVATION	PRESERVATION OF END WEIGHT BEARING	PROPRIOCEPTIVE FUNCTION	ABILITY TO WALK WITHOUT A PROSTHESIS	LIMITED PROSTHESIS[a]	FULL PROSTHESIS	WALKING PACE ADAPTATION
Transmetatarsal	±	Y	Y	Y	Y	Y	N	Y
Lisfranc-Chopart	±	Y	Y	Y	Y	Y/N	Y/N	Y
Ankle (Syme)	+	N	Y	N	Y	N	Y	Y
Transtibial	+	N	N	N	N	N	Y	Y
Knee disarticulation	++	N	Y	N	N	N	Y	N
Transfemoral	+++	N	N	N	N	N	Y	N

[a]For example, a shoe filler.

Table 26–4: Increased Metabolic Costs at Various Amputation Levels

AMPUTATION LEVEL	INCREASE IN METABOLIC COST (%)
Syme	15
Traumatic transtibial	25
Traumatic transfemoral	68
Vascular transtibial	40
Vascular transfemoral	100

Surgical Technique (Box 26–1)

- A well-planned amputation or disarticulation conserves all tissue possible according to the diagnosis and good function.
- The skin is the most important tissue for the healing of the amputation wound. It therefore must be handled very carefully with the use of skin hooks.
- The transected muscles should provide an adequate soft tissue mantle for the residual extremity. The soft tissue envelope must be mobile, because it will absorb the normal and indirect shear forces during prosthetic usage.
- Myodesis consists of suturing the transected muscle to the bone through drill holes (Fig. 26–2).
- Myoplasty refers to the suturing of the cut ends of the antagonistic muscle groups and their fascias together (Fig. 26–3).
- Bony prominences, such as sharp edges and corners, must be removed and the cut surfaces properly contoured to prevent damage to the soft tissue envelope.
- All transected nerves develop a neuroma, which is painless in the vast majority of patients.
- Neuromas within the weight-bearing area can become painful. Therefore each nerve must be dissected free and sharply transected at a level well above the level of amputation.
- Arteries and veins must be dissected free and doubly ligated before transection. They must be independently ligated in order to prevent the development of an aneurysm or arterial venous fistula.

Box 26–1 Take Home Messages for Surgical Approach to Amputation

- Team assessment
- Atraumatic soft tissue handling
- Adequate skin flaps
- Myodesis or myoplasty whenever possible
- Nerve transection sharp, and at level well above amputation
- Artery and vein dissected free and double ligated
- Closure without tension
- No "dog ear" resection
- Accept delayed primary closure if there is tension

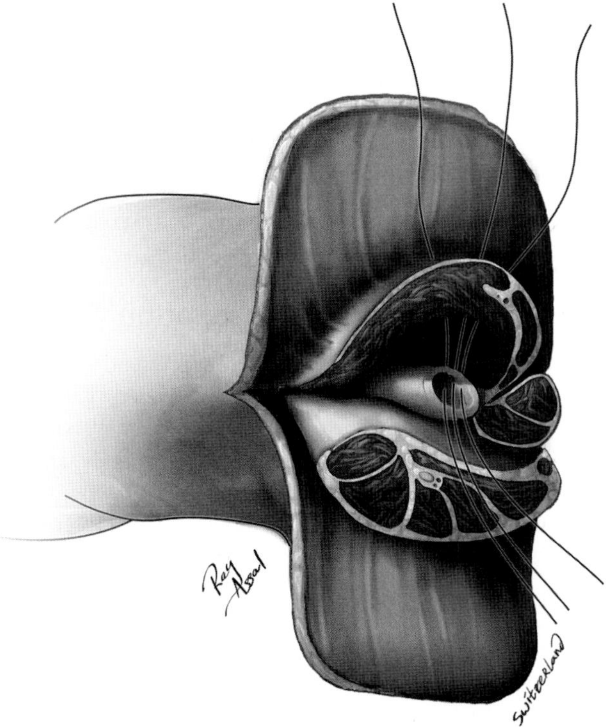

Figure 26–2: Myodesis consists of suturing the transected muscle to the bone through drill holes.

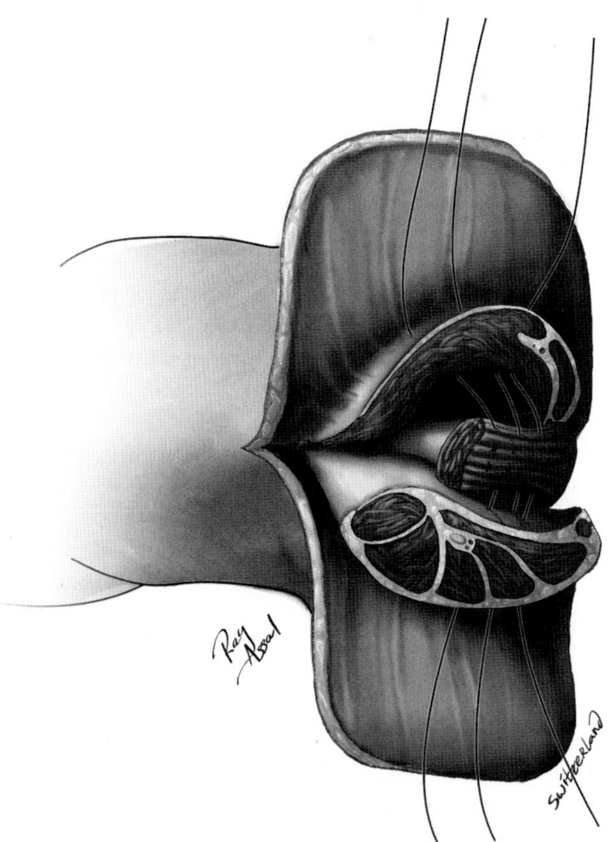

Figure 26–3: The cut ends of antagonistic muscle groups and their fascias are sewn together for myoplasty.

- Split thickness graft may be used occasionally, but only over soft tissues and not placed over bone or thick scars.
- Skin grafts are more successful in children than in adults.
- During wound closure, the flaps are trimmed to fit without tension.

Specific Levels of Amputation and Disarticulation

Toe Amputation or Disarticulation

- Before considering toe amputation, it is essential that the midfoot is sufficiently vascularized to allow for healing of the surgical wound. The tcPO_2, measured at the level of the midfoot, should never be less than 20 mmHg, and ideally greater than 30 mmHg.
- If more than one toe requires amputation in a vascular patient, one should consider performing a transmetatarsal amputation.
- Whenever possible, it is advisable to save the proximal phalanx of the first ray. This helps with balance, putting on a shoe, and results in a better gait than after disarticulation at the metatarsophalangeal joint, with its accompanying loss of the sesamoids and the flexor hallucis complex.
- Equivalent length dorsal and plantar full-thickness fish mouth-type skin flaps should be created, thus favoring the tougher plantar skin for the end of the stump (Fig. 26–4).
- Extensor and flexor tendons should be transected and allowed to retract.
- "Dog ears" should not be resected, as they will retract and assume a smooth contour.

Ray Resection of the Foot

- The most common indication for medial ray amputation is septic arthritis and osteomyelitis secondary to a penetrating ulcer under the first metatarsal head. First ray amputation should be as limited as possible for effective orthotic restoration of the medial arch.
- In first metatarsophalangeal joint septic arthritis with a viable great toe, the joint alone can be removed through a medial longitudinal incision.
- The cut first metatarsal should be beveled on its plantar and medial aspects to avoid a high-pressure area and permit appropriate fitting of shoes.
- Provided that there is good vascularity on the dorsum of the foot, single-ray amputations are feasible. Resection may be carried out through the proximal metaphysis, where the involved ray intersects with the adjacent metatarsals.
- The fifth metatarsal should be transected obliquely.
- It is not recommended to resect two or more central rays.
- If the length of the first metatarsal is too short due to excessive resection, a planovalgus position of the foot may occur secondary to loss of medial column support.

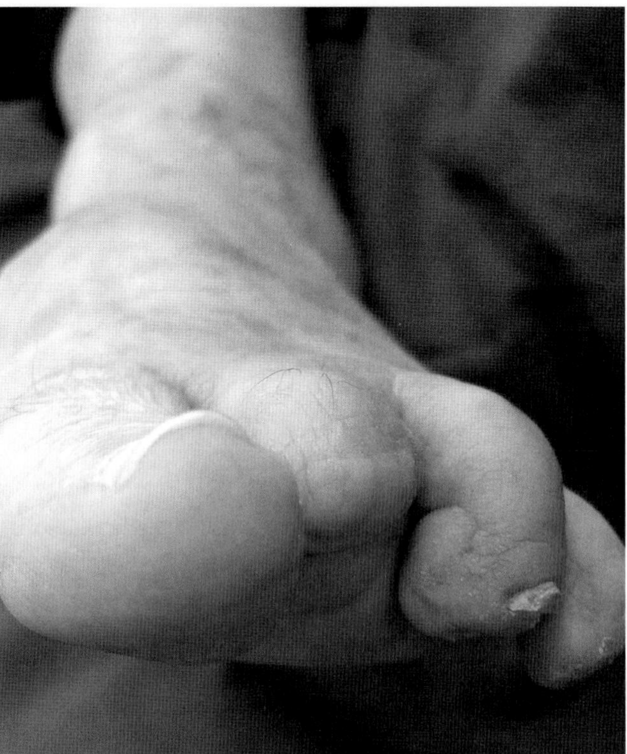

Figure 26–4: Equivalent length dorsal and plantar full-thickness fish mouth-type skin flaps should be created, thus favoring the tougher plantar skin for the end of the stump.

- Both strength and gait can be seriously impaired because of a too short first ray amputation.

Transmetatarsal Amputation

- Transmetatarsal amputation should be considered:
  - when most or all of the first metatarsal must be removed,
  - if two or more medial rays must be amputated, or
  - if more than one central ray must be amputated.
- It is the most proximal amputation where patients are able to walk with an almost physiological gait, because all the tendons that attach to the midfoot base of the metatarsals are left intact.
- Achilles tendon lengthening or gastrocnemius recession is recommended in order to further decrease distal plantar pressures.
- The longer the length of the shaft of the metatarsal, the better the function.
- Distal coverage of the metatarsal shafts with a durable plantar flap is of utmost importance (Fig. 26–5).
- To achieve maximum length, the transverse plantar incision is made at the base of the toes. The dorsal incision is made 3-5 mm distal to the metatarsal cuts.
- The metatarsal cuts must be performed in an elliptic manner (Fig. 26–6), starting with the first metatarsal and

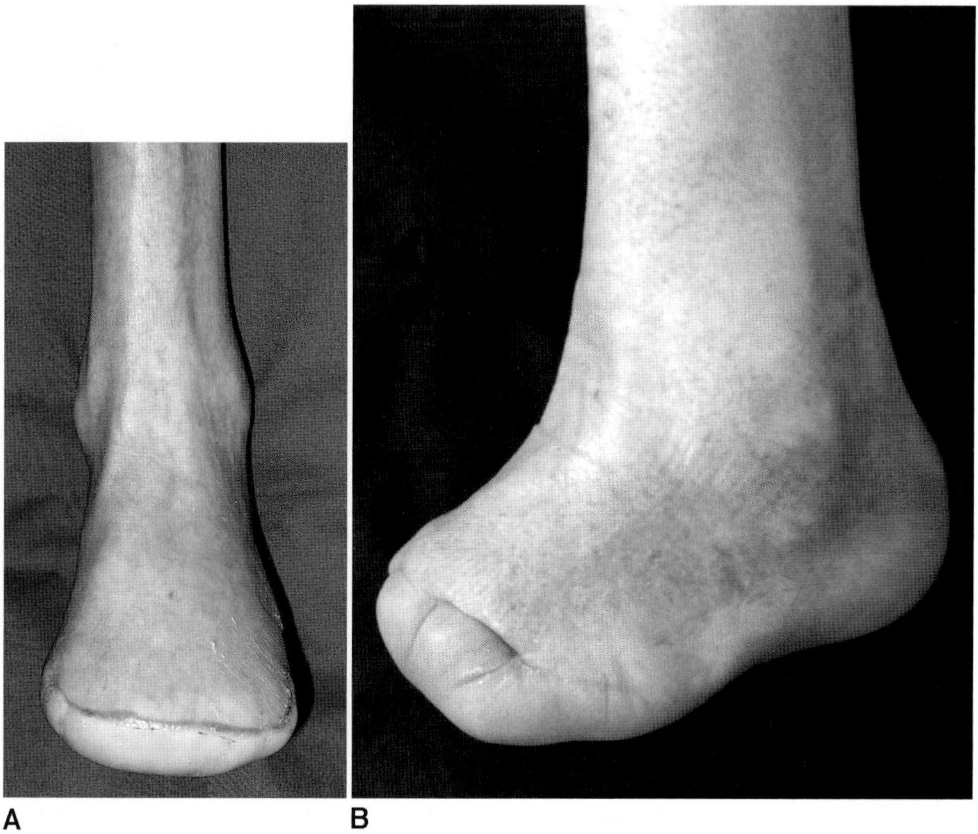

Figure 26–5: Transmetatarsal amputation. Distal coverage of the metatarsal shafts with a durable plantar flap is of utmost importance.

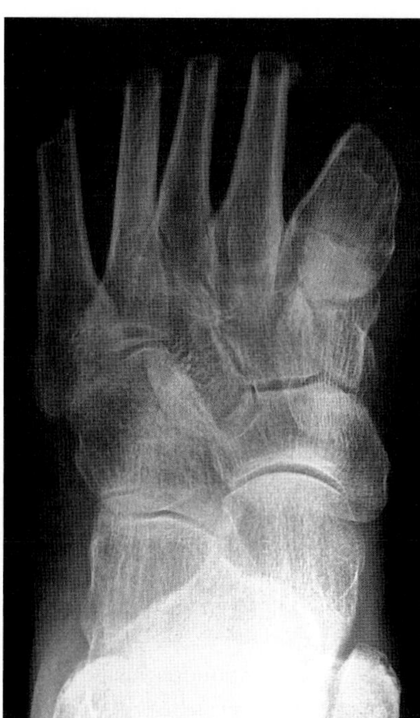

Figure 26–6: Transmetatarsal amputation. The metatarsal cuts must be performed in an elliptic manner, starting with the first metatarsal. Metatarsal length depends on the status of the plantar flap. Ideally, metatarsal length should be as long as possible to give the longest lever arm.

removing as little bone as possible. The lesser metatarsals should be cut roughly perpendicular to the shaft axis.

- Metatarsal shafts should be beveled on the plantar surface to decrease distal plantar pressures.
- Postoperative care should include a well-padded cast with the foot plantigrade or slightly dorsiflexed to prevent equinus, with regular cast changes until the wound is well healed.
- Change cast to shoe with filler and stiff rocker sole at about 6 weeks, when the wound is healed.

Metatarsal Disarticulation (Lisfranc)

- The indications for amputation at the level of the Lisfranc joint are limited, with trauma and selected cases of foot tumors as the main indications.
- The foot becomes unbalanced because of the loss of forefoot lever and the massive triceps surae overpowering the relatively weaker dorsiflexors, thus leading to an equinus contracture.
- Transfer of the distal insertion of the peroneus longus and the tibialis anterior to the medial cuneiform, and leaving a portion of the base of the fifth metatarsal to preserve the insertion of the peroneus brevis tendon, will improve residual foot balance.
- Preservation of the base of the second metatarsal helps maintain the proximal transverse arch.

- Percutaneous Achilles tendon lengthening is recommended to weaken the triceps surae relative to the ankle dorsiflexors.
- Compared with a long transmetatarsal amputation, the Lisfranc disarticulation results in a major loss of forefoot length, which correlates with impaired barefoot walking.
- Postoperative care should include a well-padded cast with the foot plantigrade or slightly dorsiflexed to prevent equinus, with regular cast changes until the wound is well healed.
- Change cast to shoe with filler and stiff rocker sole at 6 weeks.

Midtarsal Disarticulation (Chopart)

- The disarticulation is performed through the talonavicular and calcaneocuboid joints.
- Even more so than with the Lisfranc disarticulation, the stump has a tendency to develop an equinus posture over time because of severe muscle imbalance between dorsiflexor and plantar flexor muscles, leading to pain and/or ulceration.
- The tibialis anterior and long extensor tendons must be inserted into or around the talar neck in order to balance the foot in the sagittal plane. An Achilles tendon lengthening or even complete tenotomy is needed to prevent equinus.
- The main advantage over a more proximal amputation level is that it allows end bearing and does not sacrifice leg length. In addition, in some cases it requires only a filler in a regular shoe. In the more active patient, however, a formal prosthesis is required because the shoe is unstable.
- Postoperative care should include a well-padded cast in neutral to slight dorsiflexion.
- At 6 weeks, change to a close-fitting rigid ankle prosthesis/orthosis plus shoe with rigid rocker sole.

Syme Ankle Disarticulation

- Originally described in 1843 by James Syme, it provides an end-bearing stump that allows ambulation without prosthesis over short distances (Fig. 26–7).
- The heel pad is preserved. Therefore this level of amputation requires an adequate functioning posterior tibialis artery, the main source of flow to the heel pad.
- The limb will be approximately 4-6 cm shorter than the opposite leg.
- Contraindications include infection or severe traumatic damage to the heel pad, inadequate blood flow to the heel pad, uncompensated congestive heart failure with pedal and heel edema, psychosis, and patient non-compliance.
- In the presence of severe foot trauma or infection, a two-stage amputation is recommended. The wound is initially left open, and the viability of the heel flap is established prior to the definitive wound closure.

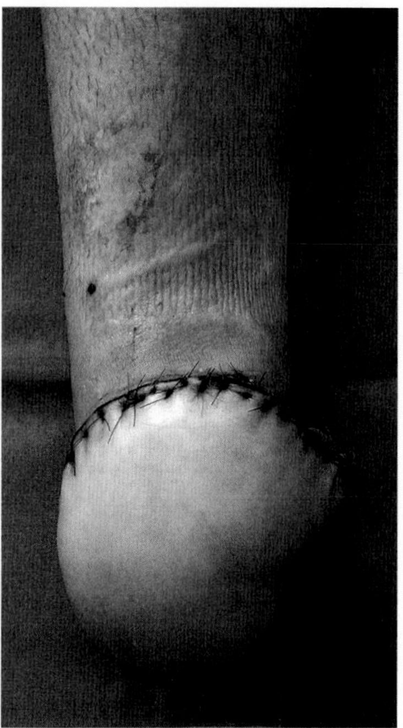

Figure 26–7: **The Syme ankle disarticulation (7 days postoperative) provides an end-bearing stump that allows ambulation without a prosthesis over short distances.**

- It is an excellent amputation for children, because it preserves the physes at the distal end of the tibia and fibula.
- Surgery must be done with great care so as to preserve the posterior tibial neurovascular bundle, and as well the integrity of the fat-filled fibrous chambers of the heel pad, which provide shock absorption on heel strike.
- Bruising of the posterior tibial vessels may lead to thrombosis and loss of the heel pad. Iatrogenic disruption of the integrity of the heel pad during dissection of the plantar aspect of the calcaneus will lead to heel pad atrophy and a dysfunctional weight-bearing stump over time.
- Before closure, the interior of the heel pad must be carefully palpated for flakes of residual cortical bone left from the calcaneus dissection. They must be meticulously removed to avoid painful bony growth.
- At closure, the heel pad flap must be perfectly centered under the leg and accurately secured to the anterior tibial cortex by suturing the plantar fascia through drill holes.
- This level of disarticulation is more energy-efficient than a transtibial level. The presence of an insensate heel is not a contraindication to a Syme ankle disarticulation.
- The medial and lateral redundant tissue always present at closure (dog ears) must never be trimmed, as it provides vascularity to the distal part of the flap.
- Patients will need a below-knee prosthesis. This can be a molded plastic socket with a removable medial window through which the stump is inserted, or a similar type of prosthesis, to which a foot unit is attached.

- Removal of the calcaneus from the heel pad creates a large empty space, and a drain should be inserted to prevent the formation of a large hematoma. It is removed 2 days postoperatively.
- Postoperative care should include a carefully molded cast placing the heel pad in a slightly forward and centered position. Weekly cast changes are performed until the wound is well healed at approximately 4-5 weeks. A temporary prosthesis is then fitted with a walking heel cast changed every 2 weeks (or whenever loose). Final prosthetic application is performed once the limb volume has stabilized.

Transtibial Amputation

- As compared with more distal levels of amputation, end weight bearing is no longer possible, and walking will not be feasible without a prosthesis.
- In comparison with a higher level of amputation, such as a knee disarticulation or transfemoral amputation, the knee joint is preserved. This greatly facilitates ambulation, balance, and walking pace changes, and as well decreases the energy expenditure involved in ambulation.
- The ideal length of the bone stump is between 12 and 17 cm below the joint line of the knee, although shorter stumps up to the insertion of the patellar tendon may still present some benefit to the patient.
- It is the quality of the soft tissue envelope that will determine the length of the stump. Careful inspection and clinical evaluation, including tcP_{O_2} measurements, are required.
- Biomechanically, a longer stump provides a better lever arm and hence improved function. However, there is less soft tissue distally to adequately cover the bony stump, and this can lead to pressure sores, chronic ulceration, and challenging prosthetic fitting. In addition, some residual length is necessary to accommodate the pylon and the foot/ankle prosthetic unit.
- Approximately 90% of transtibial amputees successfully use a prosthesis, compared with a rate of less than 25% of geriatric dysvascular transfemoral amputation patients.
- The shortest useful transtibial amputation must include the tibial tubercle to preserve knee extension.
- In a very short transtibial amputation, the fibular head and neck should be removed and the common peroneal nerve transected high above the knee. Knee flexion during this maneuver may help achieve a higher transection of the nerve.
- Flap configuration is determined by the soft tissue envelope. Equal anterior-posterior, medial-lateral, or long posterior flaps may all be good options, as long as they allow myodesis to the tibia to prevent adherence of skin to bone and to provide good padding.
- Amputation with a long posterior flap, as popularized by Burgess (1971), is most desirable in patients with vascular disease. It leaves the patient with a scar on the anterior aspect of the residual limb, and due to the thick myofasciocutaneous flap there is very little risk of soft tissue problem at the end of the stump (Fig. 26–8).
- The anterior distal aspect of the tibia must be carefully beveled, removing a significant portion of bone. The fibula must be transected 1.5 cm proximal to the level of the tibial transection (Fig. 26–9).
- A knee contracture greater than 15° that does not respond to intensive physical therapy in a patient with limited ambulatory function is a contraindication to transtibial amputation. A higher level of amputation or knee disarticulation is necessary.
- Postoperative care should include a carefully molded cast extending proximally to the mid- or upper thigh in extension to avoid hamstring contractures. A good supracondylar mold to prevent cast slippage is helpful, or a waist band and suspension strap may be used. After 5-7 days, the cast may be changed to a prosthetic cast if wounds are healed. Serial prosthetic casts should be placed every 7-10 days, or whenever loose, until stump maturity (6-8 weeks), at which time the transition can be made to a preparatory or definitive prosthesis (requiring fitting).

Knee Disarticulation

- Knee disarticulation allows for end bearing (weight transmission) through the end of the stump (in a prosthesis).

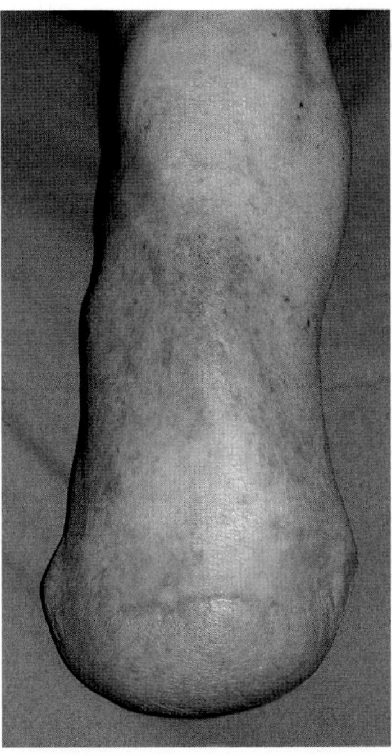

Figure 26–8: **Amputation with a long posterior flap, as popularized by Burgess, is most desirable in patients with vascular disease. It leaves the patient with a scar on the anterior aspect of the residual limb, and due to the thick myofasciocutaneous flap there is very little risk of soft tissue problem at the end of the stump.**

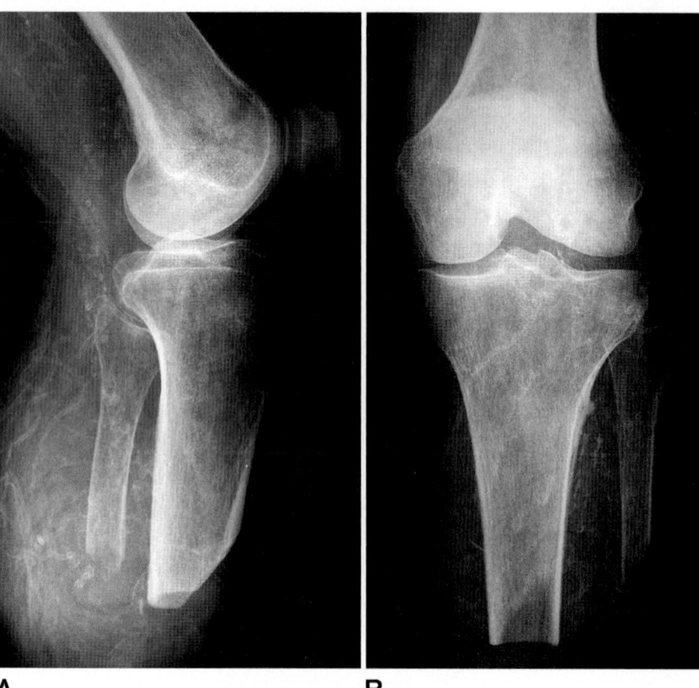

Figure 26–9: Radiographic views of transtibial amputation (anteroposterior and lateral). The anterior distal aspect of the tibia must be carefully beveled, removing a significant portion of bone. The fibula must be transected 1.5 cm proximal to the level of the tibial transection.

- Compared with a transfemoral amputation, it maintains a long active lever arm for control of the prosthesis, with excellent muscle attachments. The bulbous distal stump enhances suspension (of the prosthesis).
- The prosthesis is end bearing, which avoids the need for the ischial pressure and suspension belts that transfemoral amputation requires.
- In the non-ambulatory patient, it provides better balance for wheelchair activities and prevents hip flexion contractures, as compared with transfemoral amputation.
- The skin incisions are not much more proximal than those of a short transtibial amputation. Therefore, before deciding to perform a knee disarticulation one must be sure that a short transtibial amputation is not indicated.
- Prosthesis tolerance, compliance, and comfort are significantly higher than in those patients with a transfemoral amputation.
- In the past, there have been some concerns with regard to the difference in height of the knee joints between the sound limb and the disarticulated limb. However, with recent prosthetic technologies this is not an issue sufficient to deny its numerous advantages over a transfemoral amputation.
- The cruciate ligaments are detached from the tibia and retained for suturing to the patellar tendon without pulling the patella over the end of the femur.
- Bone excision is not required, nor is it necessary to remove articular cartilage.
- Medial and lateral sagittal flaps, with an incision extending from distal to posterior, allow the final suture line to stay posterior between the femoral condyles. This eliminates a surgical scar at the end of the stump in the weight-bearing area (Fig. 26–10).
- A method of closure of the disarticulation with use of the posterior calf skin and gastrocnemius muscle bellies as an integral flap has been described, with good results (Bowker et al. 2000).
- Postoperatively, a soft dressing or rigid cast should be applied depending on weight-bearing goals. Casts should be molded in a similar fashion to those in transtibial amputation in order to avoid slippage, and often require a suspension belt. Once wounds are fully healed, transition to a prostheses for weight bearing can begin, with serial fittings in 7- to 10-day increments until stump maturity.

Transfemoral Amputation

- Transfemoral amputation is associated with a high degree of disability.
- Prosthetic compliance is low in the geriatric population. Most elderly patients do not wear their prosthesis and will remain in a wheelchair.
- Energy expenditure is high and makes ambulation difficult in patients with associated comorbidities such as cardiopulmonary illnesses.
- Body image is negatively affected to the degree that some patients may become severely depressed.
- In particular, patients undergoing transfemoral amputation will greatly benefit from a multidisciplinary team approach aiming at improving their physical, psychologic, and social outcome.
- Healing is generally very good due to the large amount of soft tissue and rich vascular perfusion in the thigh, even in patients with vascular disease.

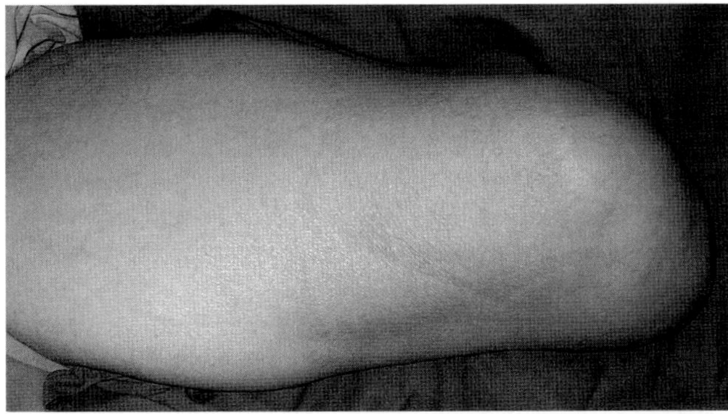

A

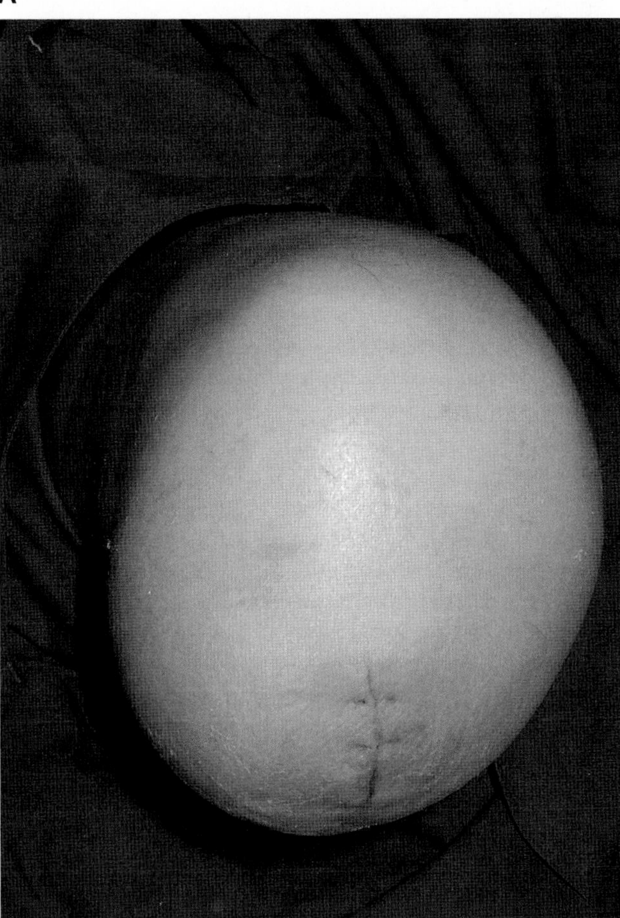

B

Figure 26–10: **Knee disarticulation with posterior suture line. Medial and lateral sagittal flaps, with an incision extending from distal to posterior, allow the final suture line to stay posterior between the femoral condyles. This eliminates a surgical scar at the end of the stump in the weight-bearing area.**

- Transfemoral amputation has been the most commonly used amputation level for vascular disease, because of its reliable healing rate. This should no longer be the case in developed countries, where patients may benefit from peripheral vascular surgery and objective assessment of skin perfusion through multilevel measurements.
- The technique of transfemoral amputation has evolved during the past decade, whereby muscle stabilization and biomechanical principles have gained new significance. Maintenance of the femoral shaft axis close to normal can be achieved by preservation of the adductor magnus and by myodesis of the muscle to the residual femur (Gottschalk 1999).
- The most common postoperative complication (after phantom limb pain) is a flexion and abduction contracture of the hip, which will interfere with ambulation and prosthetic fitting. Good surgical technique using myodesis of the adductors and myoplasty of hamstrings to quadriceps, as well as early postoperative physical therapy, will minimize this complication.
- Postoperative care for the transfemoral amputee is performed in a similar fashion to that of knee disarticulation.

References

Bosse MJ, MacKenzie EJ, Kellam JF et al. (2001) A prospective evaluation of the clinical utility of the lower-extremity injury-severity scores. J Bone Joint Surg Am 83: 3-14.

Prospectively evaluated 556 high-energy lower extremity injuries with use of five injury severity scoring systems for lower extremity trauma designed to assist in the decision-making process for the care of patients with such injuries. The analysis did not validate the clinical utility of any of the lower extremity injury severity scores. While low scores could be used to predict limb salvage potential, the converse was not true. The low sensitivity of the indices failed to support the validity of the scores as predictors of amputation. Scores at or above the amputation threshold should be cautiously used by a surgeon who must decide the fate of a lower extremity with a high-energy injury.

Bowker J, San Giovanni T. (2000) Amputations and disarticulations. In: Foot and Ankle Disorders (Myerson M, ed.). Philadelphia: Saunders. p. 486.

This book chapter is entitled *Amputations and Disarticulations*. Under the subheading of *Transmetatarsal Amputation*, the authors describe the indications for this level of amputation and the important surgical steps to be followed to provide a good outcome and maximum function.

Bowker JH, San Giovanni TP, Pinzur MS. (2000) North American experience with knee disarticulation with use of a posterior myofasciocutaneous flap. Healing rate and functional results in seventy-seven patients. J Bone Joint Surg Am 82: 1571-1574.

The authors describe the use of a posterior myocutaneous flap for closure of a knee disarticulation wound in 77 patients (31 with diabetes and PVD, 29 with PVD alone, 14 with a traumatic injury, and 3 with other diagnoses). This technique had been previously described, and the objective of this report was to determine the healing rate and functional results after use of such a flap for closure. The authors were pleased with the reliable healing, as well the comfortable end-bearing stump, which was thick and mobile.

Brakora MJ, Sheffield PJ. (1995) Hyperbaric oxygen therapy for diabetic wounds. Clin Podiatr Med Surg 12: 105-117.

Hyperbaric oxygen can be a useful adjuvant in the management of diabetic foot wounds when coordinated with medical-surgical treatment of the patient. Elevated tissue oxygen tensions improve leukocyte bacterial killing efficiency and enhance connective tissue regenerative systems for wound healing. In this article, the authors present an algorithm for the management of diabetic foot wounds.

Burgess EM, Romano RL, Zettl JH et al. (1971) Amputations of the leg for peripheral vascular insufficiency. J Bone Joint Surg Am 53: 874-890.

This article documents the lead authors' experience from 1964 to 1970 with 193 major lower extremity amputations (177 patients) for PVD. The article includes the selection of the level of amputation, surgical technique, and postsurgical management, with emphasis on rehabilitation. As far as surgical technique is concerned, the authors summarize their previously described technique and highlight its major features, including the now well-known modified long posterior myocutaneous flap and muscle stabilization.

Fitzpatrick MC. (1999) The psychologic assessment and psychosocial recovery of the patient with an amputation. Clin Orthop Relat Res 361: 98-107.

This article serves as an introduction to the importance of psychosocial issues in those patients undergoing amputation. A technically superb outcome is not the only end point following amputation. This paper reviews the necessity of a thorough preoperative assessment in those psychosocial areas most likely to impact how the patient perceives, reacts to, and ultimately accepts the recommendation for amputation.

Gottschalk F. (1999) Transfemoral amputation. Biomechanics and surgery. Clin Orthop Relat Res 361: 15-22.

In this review, the author discusses the significance of muscle stabilization and biomechanical principles as applied to transfemoral amputation. Maintenance of the femoral shaft axis close to normal can be achieved by preservation of the adductor magnus and by myodesis of the muscle to the residual femur. By following established biomechanical principles and satisfactory surgical techniques, patients undergoing transfemoral amputation are easier to fit with a prosthesis and more likely to remain able to ambulate. Reduction in stump problems can be achieved, and improvement in stump strength is seen.

Gregory RT, Gould RJ, Peclet M et al. (1985) The mangled extremity syndrome (M.E.S.): A severity grading system for multisystem injury of the extremity. J Trauma 25: 1147-1150.

Objective was to define the criteria for a mangled extremity and develop a retrospective graduated grading system. Evaluated 60 consecutive trauma patients with severely injured extremities using a graduated grading system directed at integument, nerve, artery, and bone. Developed a Mangled Extremity Severity Index, and their data suggest that a score of 20 is the dividing line below which functional limb salvage can be expected and above which limb salvage is improbable.

Helfet DL, Howey T, Sanders R et al. (1990) Limb salvage versus amputation. Preliminary results of the Mangled Extremity Severity Score. Clin Orthop Relat Res 256: 80-86.

Developed the MESS by reviewing 25 trauma victims with 26 severe lower extremity open fractures with vascular compromise. The four significant criteria (with increasing points for worsening prognosis) were skeletal/soft tissue injury, limb ischemia, shock, and patient age. This scoring system was then prospectively evaluated in 26 lower extremity open fractures with vascular injury over a 12-month period at two trauma centers. In both the prospective and retrospective studies, a MESS score of greater than or equal to 7 had a 100% predictable value for amputation. MESS was highly accurate in acutely discriminating between limbs that were salvageable and those that were unsalvageable and better managed by primary amputation.

Howe HR Jr., Poole GV Jr., Hansen KJ et al. (1987) Salvage of lower extremities following combined orthopedic and vascular trauma. A predictive salvage index. Am Surg 53: 205-208.

Retrospective review of 676 fractures of the tibia with 12 major vascular injuries (1.7%), and 985 fractures of the femur with 5 major vascular injuries (0.5%). Limb survival related to interval from injury to arrival in operating room, level of arterial injury, and the quantitative degree of muscle, bone, and skin injury. By combining these variables, a limb salvage index was established that identified lower extremity injuries likely to require amputation. The goal was to use this Predictive Salvage Index to avoid attempts to salvage a doomed or useless lower extremity, and thus permit early prosthetic rehabilitation to follow definitive primary amputation.

Johansen K, Daines M, Howey T et al. (1990) Objective criteria accurately predict amputation following lower extremity trauma. J Trauma 30: 568-572.

A prospective trial of the MESS in lower extremity injuries managed at two trauma centers demonstrated a significant difference between MESS values of 14 salvaged (mean 4.00 ± 0.28) and 12 doomed (mean 8.83 ± 0.53) limbs ($P < 0.01$).

Lind J, Kramhoft M, Bodtker S. (1991) The influence of smoking on complications after primary amputations of the lower extremity. Clin Orthop Relat Res 267: 211-217.

Review of 137 patients who underwent a total of 165 primary above-knee and below-knee amputations. Of the 77 patients who smoked, 44 smoked cigarettes, 30 cheroots, and 3 a pipe. There were 88 non-smokers. There was no discrepancy between smokers and non-smokers with regard to amputation level, the below-knee to above-knee ratio being 2:1. In cigarette smokers, the risk of infection and reamputation was 2.5 times higher than in cheroot smokers or non-smokers, which may be ascribed to the fact that only cigarette smokers tend to inhale. Inhalation of smoke leads to high concentrations of nicotine, which compromise the cutaneous blood flow velocity and increase the risk of the formation of microthrombi. Ideally, smoking should be discontinued 1 week before surgery, which is the requisite period for the process of coagulation and the fibrinogen level to normalize, and for free radicals to be eliminated.

MacKenzie EJ, Bosse MJ, Kellam JF et al. (2002) Factors influencing the decision to amputate or reconstruct after high-energy lower extremity trauma. J Trauma 52: 641-649.

Prospective review of 527 patients with type 3B and 3C open tibial fractures, dysvascular limbs resulting from trauma, type 3B ankle fractures, or severe open midfoot or hindfoot injuries. Data collected at enrollment relevant to the decision-making process included injury characteristics and its treatment, and the nature and severity of other injuries. The conclusion was that soft tissue injury severity has the greatest impact on decision making regarding limb salvage versus amputation. The data suggest that the injury factors that influence the decision to salvage limbs are muscle injury, absence of sensation, arterial injury, and vein injury.

McNamara MG, Heckman JD, Corley FG. (1994) Severe open fractures of the lower extremity: A retrospective evaluation of the Mangled Extremity Severity Score (MESS). J Orthop Trauma 8: 81-87.

The first part of the article was a retrospective evaluation of the MESS score in 24 patients with grade 3B and 3C open tibia fractures. A MESS value of ≥ 4 was most sensitive (100%), a MESS value of ≥ 7 was most specific, and a MESS value of ≥ 7 was found to have a positive predictive value of 100%. The authors subsequently addressed criticisms of the MESS by including nerve injury in the scoring system and by separating soft tissue and skeletal injury components of the MESS. They modified the MESS with a score called the Nerve, Ischemia, Soft Tissue, Skeletal, Shock, Age Index (NISSSA) and applied it retrospectively to their cases. After careful statistical comparison, they found both the MESS and the NISSSA to be highly accurate ($P < 0.005$) in predicting amputation. The NISSSA was found to be more sensitive (81.8 versus 63.6%) and more specific (92.3 versus 69.2%).

Pecoraro RE, Ahroni JH, Boyko EJ et al. (1991) Chronology and determinants of tissue repair in diabetic lower-extremity ulcers. Diabetes 40: 1305-1313.

Objective was to apply an objective method to quantify the rate of wound healing of full-thickness lower extremity ulcers in 46 diabetic outpatients who received local wound care under a standardized clinical protocol. Direct measures of local cutaneous perfusion, estimated by periwound measurements of transcutaneous O_2 tension (tcPO_2) and transcutaneous CO_2 tension (tcPCO_2), were significantly associated with the initial rate of tissue repair.

Pinzur M. (2003) Amputations in trauma. In: Skeletal Trauma (Browner B, Jupiter J, Levine A et al. eds), 3rd edn. Philadelphia: Saunders. pp. 2613-2614.

This chapter of the well-known textbook *Skeletal Trauma* takes a close look at amputation following traumatic injuries. The importance of early appropriate decision making is discussed, as well as the futile attempts at prolonged limb salvage from functional, psychosocial, and economic points of view.

Russell WL, Sailors DM, Whittle TB et al. (1991) Limb salvage versus traumatic amputation. A decision based on a seven-part predictive index. Ann Surg 213: 473-480.

Five-year review of 70 limbs with major lower extremity trauma and an associated arterial injury in 67 patients. Nineteen (27%) of the 70 limbs were amputated. Limb salvage was related to warm ischemia time and the quantitative degree of arterial, nerve, bone, muscle, skin, and venous injury. A Limb Salvage Index (LSI) was formulated based on the degree of injury to these systems. All 51 patients with an LSI score of less than 6 had successful limb salvage.

Waters R. (1992) The energy expenditure of amputee gait. In: Atlas of Limb Prosthetics. Surgical, Prosthetic and Rehabilitation Principles (Bowker J, Michael J, eds.), 2nd edn. St. Louis: Mosby. pp. 381-387.

This chapter looks at the energy involved in ambulation following amputation. The author points out that many studies do not specifically distinguish between the younger (usually traumatic) amputee and the older (usually vascular) amputee. In addition, the studies do not take into account the adequacy of prosthetic fit and prosthetic gait experience. This review describes the energy expenditure under different situations between different amputee populations.

Additional References

Adams PF et al. (1999) Current estimates from the National Health Interview Survey, 1996. Vital Health Stat 10: 200.

Czerniecki JM. (1996) Rehabilitation in limb deficiency. Gait and motion analysis. Arch Phys Med Rehabil 77(3 suppl): S3-S8.

Provides a good summary of energy expenditure following amputation.

Dillingham TR, Pezzin LE, Mackenzie EJ. (2002) Limb amputation and limb deficiency: Epidemiology and recent trends in the United States. South Med J 95(8): 875-883.

Good summary of the epidemiology of amputation.

CHAPTER 27

Ankle Arthroscopy

Richard J. de Asla* and Martin O'Malley§

*M.D., Instructor, Orthopaedic Surgery, Harvard Medical School, Massachusetts General Hospital, Boston, MA
§M.D., Attending Surgeon, Foot and Ankle Service, Hospital for Special Surgery, New York, NY

Indications

- Arthroscopy is now a well-established tool in the armamentarium of surgical care for foot and ankle diagnosis and treatment. With the advantage of shorter recovery times, and less pain and morbidity than with open techniques, ankle arthroscopy has become the modality of choice for treating a number of disorders.
- Arthroscopy allows for direct visualization and assessment of articular cartilage, synovium, and ligamentous structures. Arthroscopy can be useful in diagnosing certain conditions when history, physical examination, and imaging studies do not yield definitive results. Indications for diagnostic ankle arthroscopy include unexplained pain, swelling, locking, popping, stiffness, and hemarthrosis.
- Conditions well suited for arthroscopic treatment include removal of loose bodies, osteochondral lesions, synovectomy, biopsy, debridement of soft tissue impingement, excision of anterior osteophytes, and as an aid in fracture reduction.
- Arthroscopy is not recommended for more severe fractures, because the additional fluid could add to already present soft tissue injury.
- Relative contraindications to ankle arthroscopy include local soft tissue infection, severe edema, and severe peripheral vascular disease.

Equipment

Instruments

- Arthroscopes are available in a number of sizes, ranging from 1.9 to 4.0 mm. The authors prefer using a 2.7-mm scope. It allows for working in tight spaces, and the picture quality of the newer scopes is excellent. On occasion, we will use a 1.9-mm scope for tight joints or small ankles.
- Small joint scopes are shorter (67 mm) than scopes traditionally used in knee and shoulder arthroscopy, which makes working around the foot and ankle less cumbersome.
- Another variable to be aware of is the inclination of view. This is defined as the angle of projection at the objective end of the arthroscope relative to its axis. The 30° view is by far the most commonly used. Because the scope can be rotated, this allows the field of view to "sweep" over a greater area than would otherwise be permitted with a 0° scope.
- Arthroscopes are also available with a 70° view. It can be useful in seeing around corners such as in the medial and lateral gutters, or viewing the posterior aspect of the talar dome from an anterior portal. However, these scopes require practice and experience to use effectively.
- A variety of small joint instruments are available specifically for ankle arthroscopy (Box 27–1).

Box 27–1 Instruments for Ankle Arthroscopy

Instruments for ankle arthroscopy include probes, dissectors, graspers, basket forceps, ring and cup curettes, knives, osteotomes, rasps, suction baskets, and motorized instruments. Small joint motorized instruments are shorter and have smaller diameters than those used in large joint arthroscopy. A variety of disposable blades are available with different cutting surfaces and in different diameters. We most commonly use 2.9-mm tips. However, 2.0- and 3.5-mm tips are also available. Power burrs can be particularly useful in removing osteophytes, and are also available for small joints.

- Minidrill guides are available and can be quite useful for drilling osteochondral lesions of the talus (OLTs) while avoiding healthy cartilage (Fig. 27–1).
- Descriptions of arthroscopically assisted laser and radiofrequency use are becoming more common in the foot and ankle literature. These devices have been used for coagulation, synovectomy, trimming loose cartilage, ablating fibrous tissue and loose bodies, and treating instability with ligament shrinkage.

Inflow and Outflow

- A number of irrigation solutions can be used with ankle arthroscopy. Our preference is lactated Ringer's solution. Some surgeons prefer to add adrenaline (epinephrine) at 1:100 000 to help reduce bleeding.
- Inflow and outflow can be "toggled" through the same cannulae system. Generally, it is advisable to establish a third portal for outflow, as higher flow rates can be achieved.
- Gravity or an arthroscopic pump can be used for irrigation during the procedure. Caution must be taken if a pump is to be used. Fluid can extravasate into surrounding soft tissue, increasing compartment pressures.

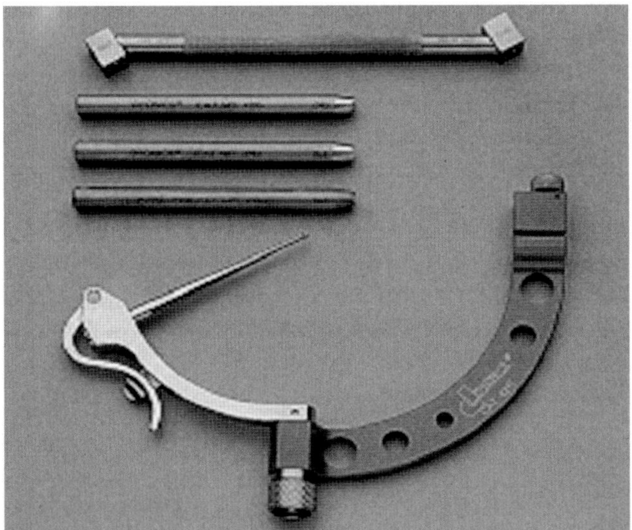

Figure 27–1: A small joint drill guide. (From Ferkel RD. (1996) Articular surface defects, loose bodies, and osteophytes. In: Arthroscopic Surgery: The Foot and Ankle. Philadelphia: Lippincott-Raven. p. 71).

Distraction

- In order to attain adequate visualization for an arthroscopic examination of the ankle, distraction of the joint is of major importance. An invasive external distraction device was popularized by Guhl but suffered from complications such as fracture and nerve injury. With the advent of commercially available non-invasive distraction systems, the indications for invasive distraction are very limited and may include certain fragile skin conditions or compromised circulation.
- A soft tissue distraction device, which consists of a heel and midfoot strap, is applied (Fig. 27–2). The distraction device is attached to a sterile bar that is fastened to a sterile clamp fixed to the side rail of the operating table over the drapes. An Ace wrap may be required to secure the thigh to the thigh rest to prevent the leg from sliding medially.

Arthroscopic Portals

Introduction

- Establishing proper portal placement is an essential first step in safe ankle arthroscopy.
- Perhaps the most common complication of ankle arthroscopy is nerve injury. Careful portal placement can minimize the risk.
- Plantar flexing the fourth toe can help visualize the intermediate branch of the superficial peroneal nerve (Fig. 27–3).
- Plantar flexing and dorsiflexing the joint helps identify the joint line.

Anterior Portals

- The anterolateral and anteromedial portals are the most commonly used portals.

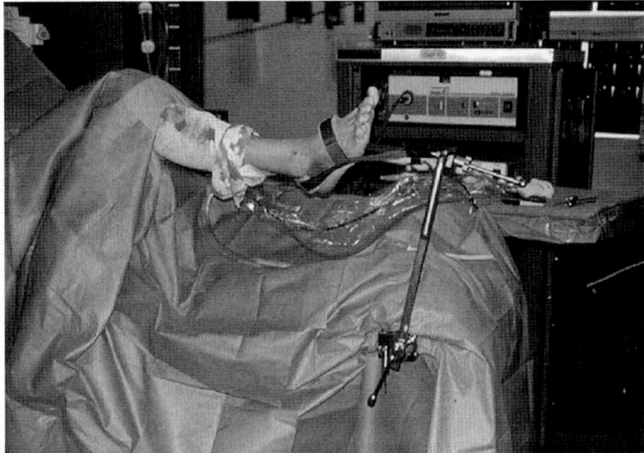

Figure 27–2: Non-invasive ankle distraction system. The sidebar is attached to the table over the drapes. The thigh holder is draped out of the field.

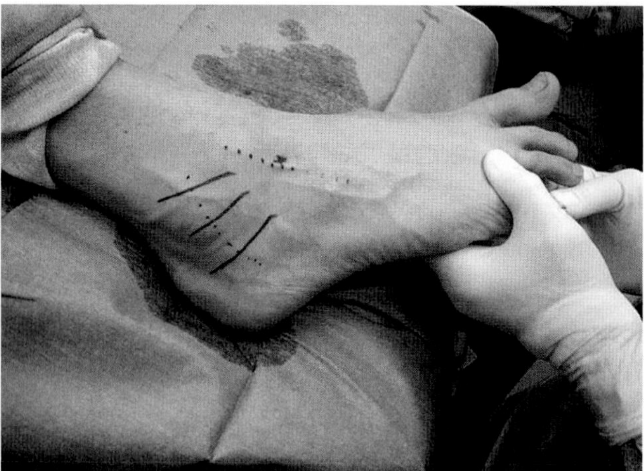

Figure 27–3: With the fourth toe plantar flexed, the intermediate branch of the superficial peroneal nerve can often be identified. Here, it is marked with a dotted line over the anterolateral aspect of the ankle joint.

- Prior to establishing the portals, the ankle joint is distended with approximately 15 cc of normal saline with adrenaline (epinephrine) using a 20-gauge needle just medial to the anterior tibial tendon. The injection site is helpful in determining the location of the anteromedial portal.
- An approximately 5-mm vertical incision is made through skin only at or near the fluid infiltration site. The remaining soft tissue layers are dissected bluntly with a straight mosquito clamp to the level of the joint capsule.
- This medial portal is established first because it is generally easy to do and safe, as the main anatomical landmark (i.e. the anterior tibial tendon) is readily identified (Fig. 27–4).
- Keeping the anteromedial portal close to the anterior tibial tendon will facilitate the passage of instruments posteriorly.

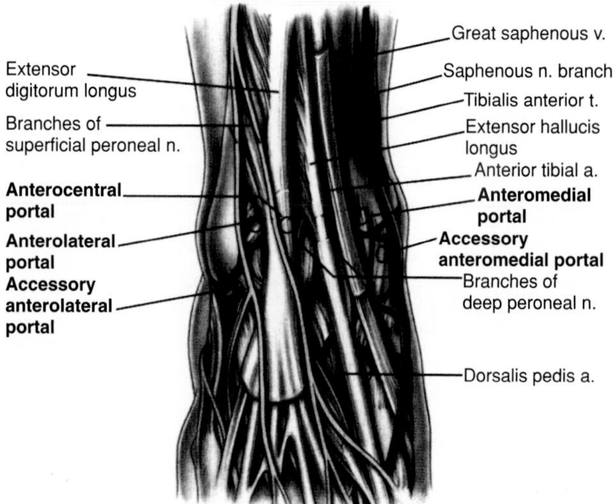

Figure 27–4: Anterior ankle joint portal placement sites and relevant anatomy. (From Ferkel RD. (1996) Articular surface defects, loose bodies, and osteophytes. In: Arthroscopic Surgery: The Foot and Ankle. Philadelphia: Lippincott-Raven. p. 104.)

- Classically, the anterolateral portal is established just lateral to the peroneus tertius tendon between the peroneus tertius and intermediate branch of the superficial peroneal nerve. However, the exact placement of this portal may vary, determined somewhat by the location of the pathology within the ankle joint as well as the location of the intermediate branch of the superficial peroneal nerve (see Fig. 27–4).
- It can be helpful to first place a 2-inch, 25-gauge needle under arthroscopic visualization to establish the most workable location. Transillumination of the anterolateral skin from within the joint can help avoid injury to the branches of the superficial peroneal nerve.
- An anterocentral portal has been described between the tendons of the extensor digitorum longus. This portal puts the dorsalis pedis artery and deep peroneal nerve at risk, because these structures pass between the extensor digitorum longus and extensor hallucis longus tendons.

Accessory Anterior Portals

- Accessory anteromedial and accessory anterolateral portals are used primarily for placing instruments in the medial and lateral ankle gutters while the scope remains in the ipsilateral standard portal.
- The accessory anteromedial portal is established about 0.5-1.0 cm inferior and 1.0 cm anterior to the anterior border of the medial malleolus.
- The accessory anterolateral portal is established 1.0 cm anterior to and at the level of the distal-most aspect of the lateral malleolus. This portal passes through the anterior talofibular ligament.

Posterior Portals

- The three posterior portals are the posterolateral portal, the posteromedial portal, and the trans-Achilles portal (Fig. 27–5).
- The posterolateral portal is the most commonly used of the posterior portals and is the safest. To establish the posterolateral portal, a 20-gauge spinal needle is inserted immediately lateral to the Achilles tendon approximately 1.0-1.5 cm proximal to the tip of the fibula. Placement can be visualized from the anteromedial portal with the scope directed posteriorly through an anatomical arch in the anteromedial plafond known as the "notch of Harty" (Fig. 27–6A).
- Initially, the posterolateral portal location can be used as the outflow portal site in systems that do not allow for both inflow and outflow from the cannulae. The needle is kept in place and allowed to drip into an underlying kidney basin. A formal portal can be established later if necessary (Fig. 27–6B).
- The posteromedial portal is created just medial to the Achilles tendon at the same level as the posterolateral portal.
- Multiple anatomical structures need to be protected establishing this portal, including the posterior tibial artery and nerve, the flexor hallucis tendon, and the

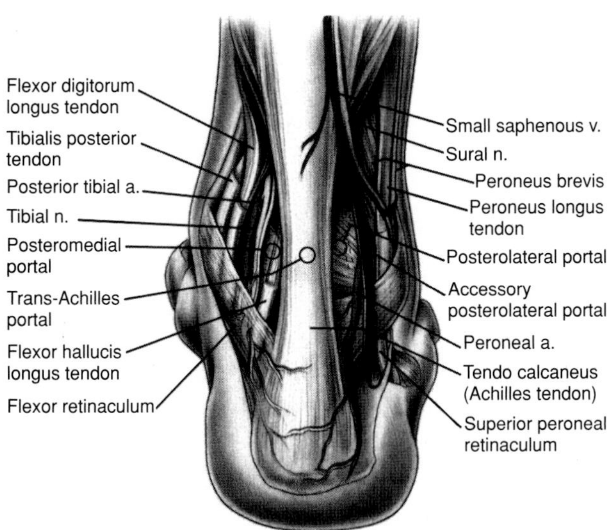

Figure 27–5: **Posterior ankle joint portal placement sites and relevant anatomy. (From Ferkel RD. (1996) Articular surface defects, loose bodies, and osteophytes. In: Arthroscopic Surgery: The Foot and Ankle. Philadelphia: Lippincott-Raven. p. 106.)**

flexor digitorum longus tendon. The calcaneal nerve and its branches may traverse the region between the medial border of the Achilles and posterior tibial nerve.

- Because of the potential for complication and better posterior portal options, we recommend against using this portal site routinely.
- The trans-Achilles portal site is established at the same level as the other portal sites but through the substance of the Achilles tendon. Theoretically, this allows for the establishment of two portals in the posterior aspect of the ankle, safe from injuring the neurovascular bundle.

Accessory Posterior Portal

- This portal is made 1.0-1.5 cm lateral to the standard posterolateral portal. This portal is useful when posterior ankle joint visualization is required along with posterior instrumentation. Extreme care must be used when creating this portal, as it is in the vicinity of the sural nerve and small saphenous vein.

Arthroscopic Examination

- Ferkel (1996) has described a 21-point arthroscopic evaluation (Box 27–2).

Osteochondral Lesions of the Talus (Osteochondritis Dissecans)

Introduction

- Osteochondritis dissecans (OCD) can be described as a local condition that results in the detachment of a segment of cartilage and its corresponding subchondral bone from an articular surface.

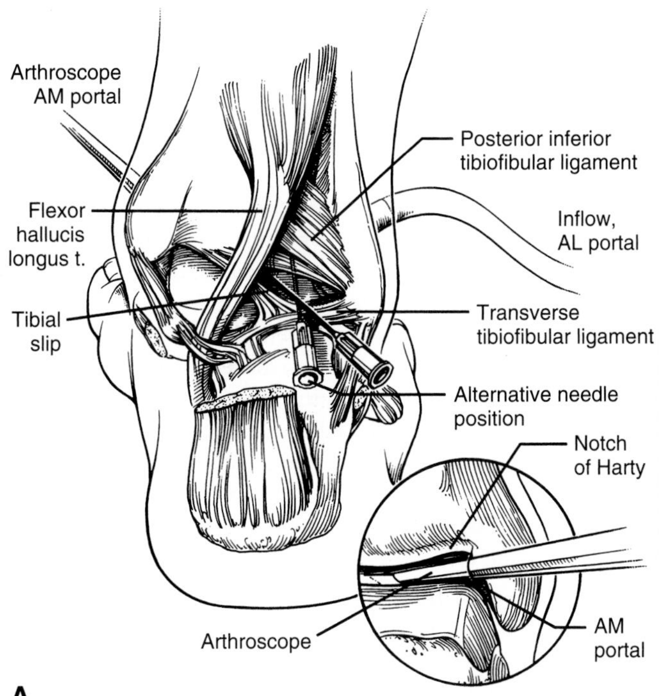

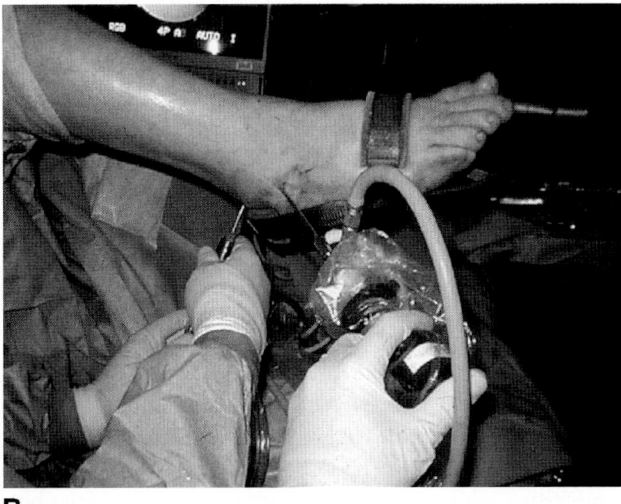

Figure 27–6: **A, Demonstrates the position of the arthroscope through the anteromedial (AM) portal across the "notch of Harty," visualizing the posterolateral ankle. B, A posterolateral portal is established. AL, anterolateral. (A, From Ferkel RD. (1996) Articular surface defects, loose bodies, and osteophytes. In: Arthroscopic Surgery: The Foot and Ankle. Philadelphia: Lippincott-Raven. p. 109.)**

Box 27–2 The 21-point Arthroscopic Examination

Anterior

- Deltoid ligament
- Medial gutter
- Medial talus
- Central talus and overhang
- Lateral talus
- Trifurcation of the talus, tibia, and fibula
- Lateral gutter
- Anterior gutter

Center

- Medial tibia and talus
- Central tibia and talus
- Lateral tibiofibular or talofibular articulation
- Posterior inferior tibiofibular ligament
- Transverse ligament
- Reflection of the flexor hallucis longus

Posterior

- Posteromedial gutter
- Posteromedial talus
- Posterocentral talus
- Posterolateral talus
- Posterior talofibular articulation
- Posterolateral gutter
- Posterior gutter

(From Stetson WB, Ferkel RD. (1996) Ankle arthroscopy. I. Technique and complications. II. Indications and results. J Am Acad Orthop Surg 4: 17.)

- The term *OCD* suggests an inflammatory process; however, investigators have not demonstrated the presence of inflammatory cells by histologic sections. To add further confusion to the nomenclature, many terms have been used to describe osteochondral lesions of the talar dome, such as *dome fractures*, *flake fractures*, *osteochondral fractures* and *avascular necrosis*.
- An acute fracture of a small piece of articular cartilage and bone is usually called a transchondral fracture or an acute OLT.
- OCD, when in reference to the ankle joint, has come to mean a chronic condition of osteochondral injury or non-union of an osteochondral fracture. The terms *acute OLT* and *chronic OLT* have gained favor in recent years.

Demographics

- The talar dome is the third most common location for OLT after the knee and elbow, representing 4% of cases.
- Although they can be present anywhere, OLTs are most commonly posteromedial (60%) or anterolateral (40%).
- Anterolateral lesions tend to be broad but superficial and waferlike, while posteromedial lesions tend to be deep but involve less articular surface area.
- Flick and Gould (1985) summarized findings in the English literature that addressed OLTs between 1947 and 1983 (534 patients). They noted a history of trauma in approximately 98% of lateral dome lesions, whereas trauma was noted in approximately 70% of medial lesions.
- Right- and left-sided lesions occur with relatively equal frequency, with a higher incidence in males.

Etiology

- Multiple etiologies have been proposed for OLTs, including direct trauma, repetitive microtrauma, ischemia, ossification defects, and genetic predisposition.
- Generally, the etiology of OLTs is known, as most authors agree that trauma is the principle predisposing factor, particularly for lateral lesions.
- Whether other etiologic factors are involved in certain medial OLTs is a matter of speculation. It is worthwhile to note that histologically both medial and lateral lesions appear the same.
- Ossification of the talar dome may be irregular during growth. Some adolescents will have what looks like an OLT but really is just normal ossification. Often, the contralateral ankle will have the same radiographic abnormality.
- In their classic paper, Berndt and Harty (1959) used 15 fresh cadaveric specimens to demonstrate the traumatic etiology of osteochondral lesions of the talar dome. Their four-stage classification of OLTs (Fig. 27–7) is the most widely recognized and is described as follows.
  - Stage 1: A small area of subchondral bone impaction.
  - Stage 2: Partial detachment of an osteochondral fragment.
  - Stage 3: Complete detachment of an osteochondral fragment not displaced from the articular surface.
  - Stage 4: Generation of an osteochondral loose body.
- They observed that anterolateral lesions were produced when a dorsiflexed ankle, allowing the wider anterior portion of the talus to fit snugly into the mortise, experienced an inverting force. The degree to which this force was imparted determined the stage of the lesion. Interestingly, they did not observe any damage to the malleoli.
- Berndt and Harty also proposed that posteromedial lesions resulted when a plantar-flexed ankle experienced an inversion force causing the posterior ridge of the tibia and medial ridge of the talus to impact.
- Loomer et al. (1993) proposed a "type 5" lesion whereby synovial fluid is forced into a defect in the articular cartilage. The hydraulic forces create a "blowout" in the talar dome under the subchondral bone.

History and Physical Examination

- There are no pathognomonic signs of OLT.
- In acute cases, the signs and symptoms are similar to those found in ankle sprains: ecchymosis, ligament pain, ankle swelling, and limited range of motion. The OLT typically occurs with an ankle sprain. Acute cases are

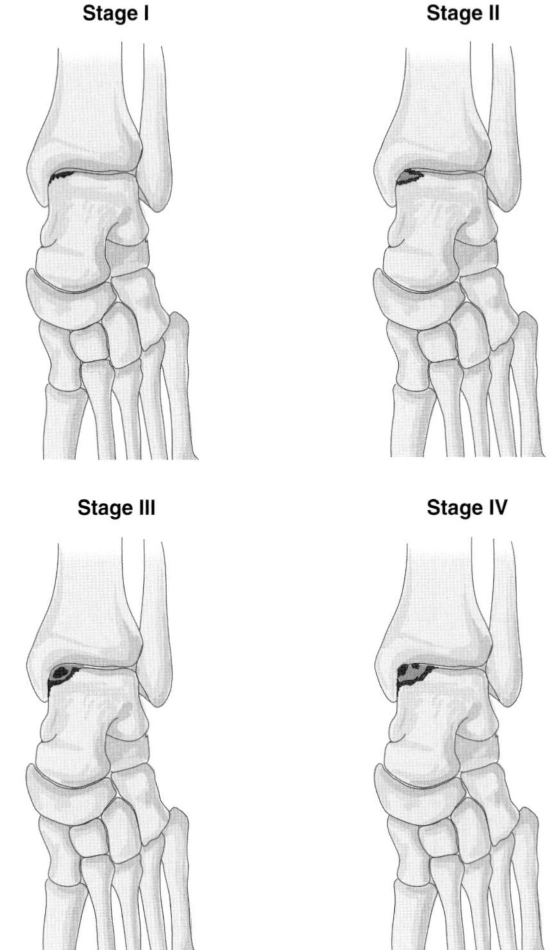

Figure 27–7: Berndt and Harty classification for osteochondral lesions of the talar dome.

often misdiagnosed or not detectable at the time of injury on plain radiographs.

- In chronic cases, activity-related pain and intermittent swelling are common complaints.
- Mechanical locking, although documented in the literature, is not a common complaint.
- Pain can sometimes be elicited in the interval between the talus and the tibiofibular ligament (i.e. over the anterolateral talar dome).
- Ankle joint stability should routinely be evaluated as part of the initial work-up.

Imaging

- A minimum work-up includes anteroposterior, lateral, and internal oblique (mortise view) radiographs of the ankle.
- The mortise view is most helpful and found to increase the sensitivity of plain radiographs, because the fibula does not overlap the lateral portion of the talus.
- An improved profile of the posteromedial lesion can be obtained with a mortise view of the ankle in plantar flexion, and anterolateral lesion profiles are aided by dorsiflexion.
- Accurate staging of the lesion by plain x-ray is often very difficult, if not impossible. Either magnetic resonance imaging (MRI) or computed tomography (CT) scan are indicated for further work-up.
- MRI is generally more helpful, although CT is useful to visualize the bone in cases of acute OLT (transchondral fracture).
- Ferkel and Sgaglione (1993-4) described a four-stage CT classification system (Fig. 27–8, Table 27–1). MRI has also been used to stage OLTs (Table 27–2) and found to correlate highly with arthroscopic findings of OLT stability.

Treatment

- The management of OLTs remains a challenging problem for the clinician, and controversy exists as to the best form of treatment.
- When surgery is deemed appropriate, arthroscopic treatment is currently the choice modality in most cases.
- When assessing an OLT, the following need to be considered: the age of the lesion (acute versus chronic), the size and stage of the lesion, the location of the lesion, and the age of the patient.

Non-operative Treatment

- Asymptomatic lesions, regardless of stage, require no specific treatment other than follow-up, as there is no evidence to suggest that such lesions progress to degenerative joint disease.
- Young patients with small, acute, low-grade lesions are the best candidates for non-operative therapy. Such treatment may consist of placement in a cast or walking boot for 3-6 weeks, followed by physical therapy.
- The duration of conservative treatment and the role of weight-bearing restriction are difficult to assess, because these variables have been poorly controlled for in the literature. It is probably prudent to observe the patient for at least several months prior to offering surgical intervention in acute cases.
- There is no good evidence that we are aware of to suggest that non-weight bearing has any advantages over weight bearing. Therefore the authors advocate weight bearing in these situations. Appropriate clinical and radiologic follow-up are important, as low-stage OLTs have the potential of progressing to higher stage lesions.
- Failure of conservative measures is a relative indication for surgical intervention.
- Treatment outcomes for lateral stage 3 lesions heavily favor surgical intervention.
- Some authors suggest approaching medial stage 3 lesions more conservatively, as these seem to have some potential to heal.

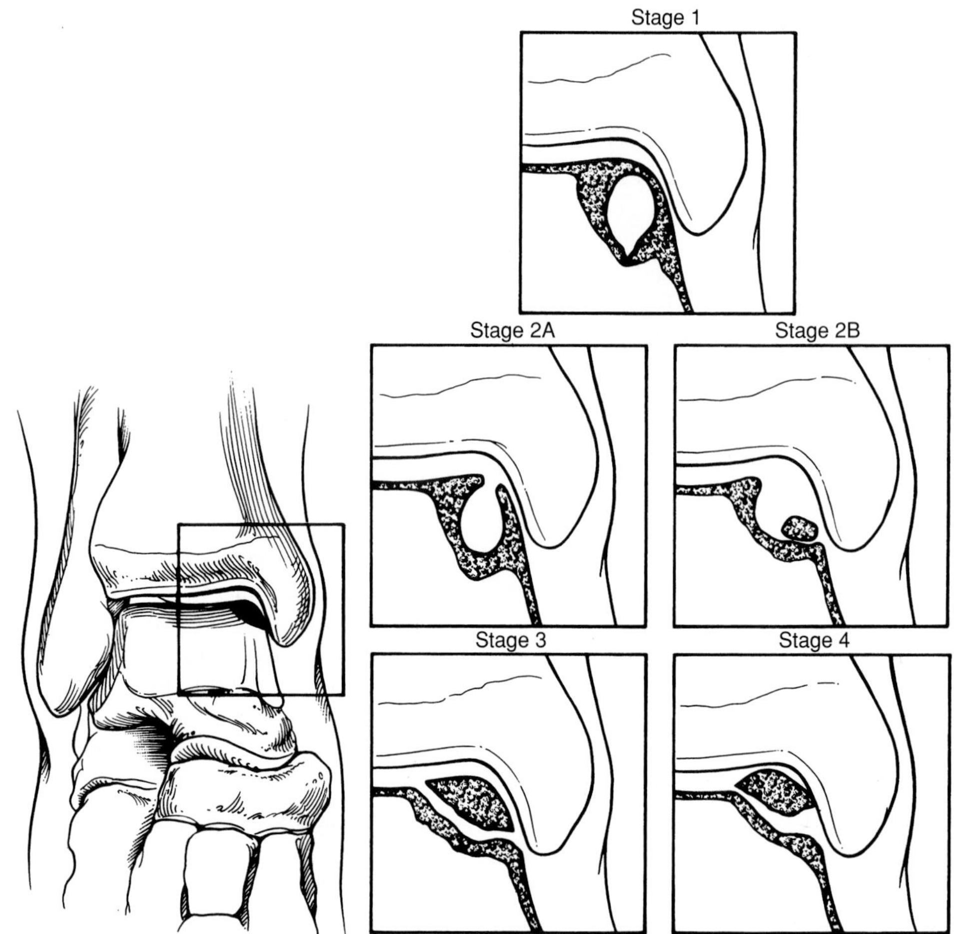

Figure 27–8: Computed tomography scan classification system. (From Ferkel RD. (1996) Articular surface defects, loose bodies, and osteophytes. In: Arthroscopic Surgery: The Foot and Ankle. Philadelphia: Lippincott-Raven. p. 151.)

Table 27–1: Computed Tomography Classification of Osteochondral Lesions of the Talus

STAGE	DESCRIPTION
1	Cystic lesion within dome of talus, intact roof on all views
2A	Cystic lesion with communication to talar dome surface
2B	Open articular surface lesion with overlying non-displaced fragment
3	Undisplaced lesion with lucency
4	Displaced fragment

(From Ferkel RD, Sgaglione NA. (1993-4) Arthroscopic treatment of osteochondral lesions of the talus: Long term results. Orthop Trans 17: 1011.)

Table 27–2: Magnetic Resonance Imaging Classification of Osteochondral Lesions of the Talus

STAGE	DESCRIPTION
1	Subchondral trabecular compression Negative plain radiographs Marrow edema on magnetic resonance imaging
2	Incomplete separation of the fragment
2A	Formation of a subchondral cyst
3	Unattached, undisplaced fragment with the presence of synovial fluid surrounding the fragment
4	Displaced fragment

(After Anderson IF, Crichton KJ, Grattan-Smith T et al. (1989) Osteochondral fractures of the dome of the talus. J Bone Joint Surg 71A(8): 1143-1152.)

- Surgery is indicated in all stage 4 lesions with acutely displaced fragments addressed urgently.

Surgical Treatment of Osteochondral Lesions of the Talus

- The decision to use either an open or an arthroscopic approach depends on the location and size of the lesion, the modality chosen to address the lesion, and the level of comfort the surgeon has with the various techniques.
- Compared with open techniques, arthroscopy offers advantages with regards to rehabilitation time and postoperative pain control. Results of arthroscopic treatment compare favorably with those of open treatment.

- With the advent of distraction and small joint arthroscopes, the arthroscopic approach to OLTs has become the preferred method of treatment. Still, despite experienced hands and improved technique, posteromedial lesions can create a significant challenge for the arthroscopist. Therefore one should be prepared for an open technique or malleolar osteotomy.
- The goals of surgical management of OLTs includes the debridement of the necrotic sequestrum, addressing cystic lesions, and the reestablishment of a joint surface by fibrocartilage ingrowth, hyaline cartilage replacement, or fixation of a loose fragment. Options to this end are dependent on its stage, and include:
  - drilling or abrading intact lesions
  - fixation of an intact or a displaced osteochondral fragment
  - bone grafting of cystic lesions
  - fragment excision followed by curettage of the defect and drilling subchondral bone
  - osteochondral autograft or allograft transfer.
- Direct visualization remains the most accurate way to determine the overall condition of the articular surface. An arthroscopic staging scheme has been described (Table 27–3).
- All loose bodies in the joint must be removed, the talar articular surface must be inspected, and stability of the osteochondral fragment needs to be established. It is critical to palpate the cartilage to determine the extent of the lesion and to judge the softness and intactness of the articular surface.
- Frankly loose cartilage flaps are excised and the defect debrided back to a rim of healthy well-attached cartilage. Soft or frayed areas adherent to the subchondral bone are left alone.

Acute Osteochondral Lesions of the Talus

- Acute OLTs can be classified as stable, unstable, or displaced. Retrograde drilling (from below) to avoid injury to the articular surface best treats stable lesions with intact overlying cartilage. If the overlying cartilage is not intact, it is debrided to a stable rim as mentioned above, and antegrade drilling of the lesion is carried out. It is recommended that a 0.062-inch smooth K wire be used to create holes approximately 1 cm deep in the subchondral bone every 3-5 mm. The tourniquet is let down, and the holes are observed for bleeding.
- The concept behind drilling is to allow for the egression of undifferentiated marrow mesenchymal stem cells into the defect, where they differentiate into cells capable of filling the defect with fibrocartilage. Fibrocartilage shares many of the characteristics of hyaline cartilage but lacks its biomechanical properties. Opportunistic second-look arthroscopy has confirmed fibrocartilage to be durable for many years.
- Unstable or displaced acute lesions can often be stabilized with internal fixation. The best candidates for internal fixation are young patients with acute traumatic lesions. Recommendations as to the size of the fragment that should be considered for fixation are not well established in the literature. Generally, this decision relies mainly on the fragment's viability and ability to accommodate fixation. Large fragments of unattached subchondral bone associated with healthy articular cartilage provide more secure fixation and increased likelihood of success. Acutely displaced OLTs should be urgently treated with internal fixation.
- Fixation options include countersunk Herbert screws, minifragment screws, K wires, and bioabsorbable pins and screws. Screw fixation provides good compression, but for medial lesions a medial malleolar osteotomy or a large transmalleolar tunnel must be created. Bioabsorbable fixation eliminates the need for hardware removal, which makes this option inviting (Fig. 27–9).

Table 27–3: Arthroscopic Staging System for Osteochondral Lesions of the Talus

GRADE	ARTHROSCOPIC APPEARANCE
A	Smooth and intact, but soft or ballottable
B	Rough surface
C	Fibrillations or fissures
D	Flap present or bone exposed
E	Loose, non-displaced fragment
F	Displaced fragment

(From Ferkel RD, Cheng MS, Applegate GR. (1995) A new method of radiologic and arthroscopic staging for osteochondral lesions of the talus. Presented at the 62nd Annual Meeting of the American Academy of Orthopaedic Surgeons, Orlando, FL, Feb 17, 1995.)

Chronic Osteochondral Lesions of the Talus

- The treatment options for chronic OLTs are determined by the grade of the lesion. In this section, we will use the MRI classification (see Table 27–2) when referring to the grade of an OLT.
- Chronic grade 1 and 2 lesions are treated with debridement and drilling using the technique described earlier. The direction from which drilling proceeds is determined by the condition of the overlying articular cartilage. Grade 2A (cystic) lesions require curettage. We find small, angled curettes useful for this purpose. Larger cysts may require bone grafting or osteochondral graft transfer. A thin, frail necrotic segment covers most cysts in the talus and will need to be removed. On rare occasions, the overlying surface is relatively healthy and worth preserving. In these cases, transtalar drilling and bone grafting can be done as described by Conti and Taranow (1996).
- Chronic grade 3 and 4 lesions with viable articular cartilage fixed to subchondral bone are candidates for

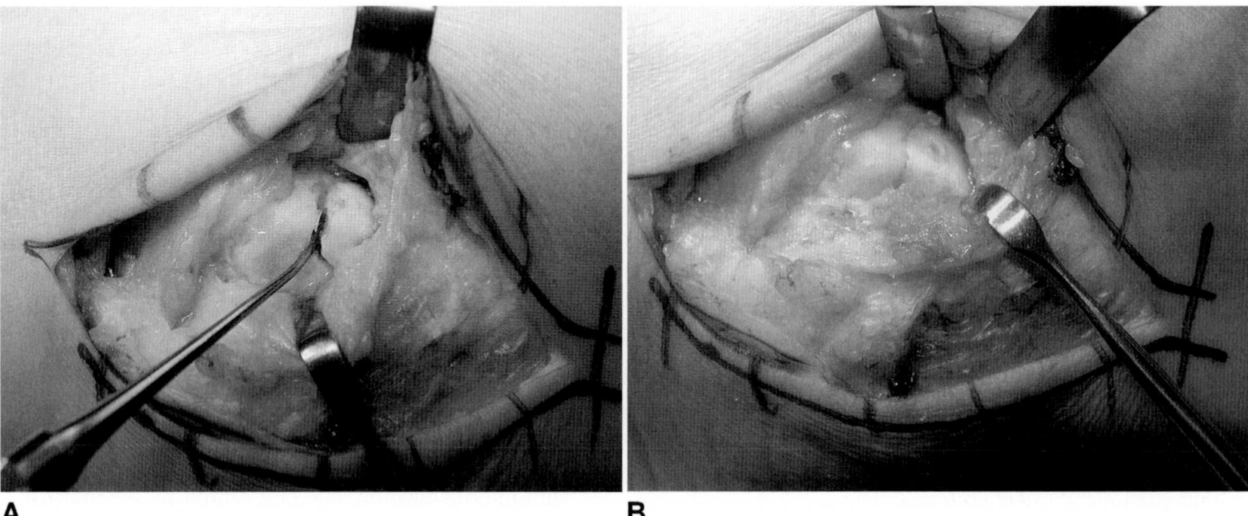

Figure 27–9: **A, A large undisplaced osteochondral fragment. B, The fragment is fixed in place with a bioabsorbable device.**

internal fixation. More often than not, the chronically loose fragment is not viable and is excised. After fragment excision, the underlying defect is debrided with drilling, curettage, or abrasion, and the crater filled with bone graft or osteochondral plugs. Before fixation of healthy fragments, the underlying bed is prepared in a similar manner, using bone graft when necessary.

- Large grade 5 lesions are addressed with aggressive debridement followed by autologous osteochondral grafting or allograft. Smaller grade 5 lesions may be amenable to drilling.
- Autologous osteochondral grafting (also known as mosaicplasty, osteochondral autograft transfer system, or CORE) for defects in the talar dome is a subject of much recent interest. The technique involves harvesting cylinder-shaped plugs of osteochondral tissue from a non-weight-bearing portion of an articular surface (usually the ipsilateral knee), and transferring it to a defect in the talar dome. The procedure can be done in an open or arthroscopically assisted fashion, depending on the location of the defect and the surgeon's preference.
- Osteochondral allografting is an option for patients who have failed other treatment modalities or to salvage particularly large lesions. Allografts are more commonly used for avascular necrosis but can be used in cases of failed autografting or large lesions. Early results are encouraging, but few studies are available. It is likely that with improved tissue storage technology this treatment modality will become more widespread.
- Autologous chondrocyte transplantation (ACT) is a process by which healthy chondrocytes are obtained, isolated after enzymatic digestion of the cartilage, and cultured in the laboratory for about 2 weeks. The cultured chondrocytes are then injected into the area of the defect under a periosteal cover. Using ACT in the knee demonstrates good results with more than 13 years' follow-up. With regards to the talus, reports of this technique in the literature are minimal.

Arthroscopic Approaches

Anterolateral Lesions

- Treatment should be preempted by a methodical evaluation of the ankle joint. Anterolateral lesions suitable for direct (antegrade) drilling or abrasion can usually be approached through the standard anteromedial and anterolateral portals.
- A transtalar approach is employed in lesions more appropriately addressed in a retrograde fashion. In this approach, a 0.062-inch K wire is placed percutaneously through the sinus tarsi and into the talus anterior to the insertion of the anterior talofibular ligament. The drilling proceeds from distal to proximal. Accuracy is improved by the use of commercially available drill guides and under the guidance of high-resolution fluoroscopy. The purpose of the technique is to avoid violating the overlying cartilage.
- Arthrotomy is required for osteochondral autograft transfer system and fixation of loose fragments. On rare occasions, a fibular osteotomy may be required.

Posteromedial Lesions

- Posteromedial lesions are more challenging to address arthroscopically. Lesions amenable to retrograde drilling can be addressed via the transtalar approach described above.
- For those lesions to be treated with antegrade drilling, a transmalleolar approach may be utilized. For this technique, the vector drill guide is inserted through the anteromedial portal and is positioned over the lesion as visualized from the anterolateral portal. A 0.062 K wire is used to drill across the medial malleolus and into the dome of the talus. The combination of multiple drill

tracks and varied ankle position in dorsiflexion and plantar flexion enables the entire lesion to be accessed.
- Extreme posterior lesions may sometimes need to be visualized through the posterolateral portal.
- Posteromedial lesions that require more extensive debridement, fixation, or grafting usually require a medial malleolar osteotomy.

Postoperative Care

- For drilling or abrasion chondroplasty: 4 weeks non- or partial weight bearing in a Cam Walker, followed by 4 weeks of full weight bearing in a Cam Walker with physical therapy-supervised range of motion exercises.
- For internal fixation: 6 weeks of no weight bearing in a short leg cast, followed by 4 weeks full weight bearing in a Cam Walker with physical therapy and range of motion.
- For osteochondral autograft transfers: 6 weeks of no weight bearing in a short leg cast, followed by 4 weeks in a weight-bearing cast. When the cast is removed, physical therapy and range of motion are begun.
- Some surgeons minimize the immobilization, and recommend early range of motion.

Loose Bodies

Introduction

- It is widely accepted that intraarticular loose bodies can damage articular surfaces, eventually leading to degenerative arthritis. Therefore loose bodies in the ankle joint are usually an indication for operative intervention. Large loose bodies may not produce symptoms or mechanical injury, because their size prohibits them from becoming lodged in between joint surfaces. Smaller loose bodies move more freely between articulating surfaces, where they are more likely to become symptomatic or do harm.
- Sometimes, the definitive origin of a loose body cannot be determined from history, radiographs, or findings at surgery.

Etiology

- Loose bodies can be generated in the ankle joint in a number of ways.
  - *OLTs*. Stage 4 OLTs are, by definition, loose bodies requiring surgical intervention in virtually all cases.
  - *Chronic ankle instability*. Until the advent of arthroscopy, there was little written about the intraarticular pathology affiliated with chronic ankle instability. The arthroscope has provided a method by which such evaluations may not only be diagnostic but also therapeutic in select cases with minimal morbidity. A number of intraarticular findings are now well described to be associated with chronic instability of the ankle, including synovitis, loose bodies, OLTs, chondromalacia, degenerative joint disease, meniscoid-type lesions, adhesions, and osteophytes (DiGiovanni et al. 2000, Komenda and Ferkel 1999).
  - *Synovial chondromatosis*. Synovial chondromatosis is a metaplastic process in which primitive mesenchymal cells in the subsynovial connective tissue differentiate into chondroblasts. The stimulus for this transformation is unknown. These cells then mature into chondrocytes that produce nodules of hyaline cartilage. As these bodies grow in size, they extrude through the synovial membrane into the joint space. While in the joint cavity, the surrounding synovial fluid nourishes them, allowing further peripheral growth. The demonstration of multiple cartilage foci within the synovial lining is the sine qua non of synovial chondromatosis. An accurate diagnosis is critical, in that synovectomy may be the choice procedure here, whereas in other causes of loose body formation, synovectomy may not be warranted.
  - *Degenerative joint disease of the ankle*. Chondral and osteochondral loose bodies are often associated with degenerative and posttraumatic osteoarthritis. Fragmentation of the joint surface, collapse of a subchondral cyst, or an area of avascular necrosis can generate loose bodies or nidi for loose bodies. Fractured osteophytes are also a source. Furthermore, production of de novo nodules in the synovium of the degenerated joint has been described, albeit uncommon. As in the knee, arthroscopic debridement of the degenerative ankle has not met with unvarying success. A review of the literature reveals that patients with advanced arthritis and joint space narrowing generally do not experience lasting relief with arthroscopic debridement. However, in patients with limited degenerative joint disease, symptomatic loose body removal is consistently successful.

History and Physical Examination

- Generalized pain, swelling, and decreased range of motion are common complaints for patients with loose bodies in the ankle. Passage of a loose body between joint surfaces may cause intermittent catching and locking, and serves as evidence of a mechanical issue.
- Physical examination usually does not contribute much to what was already learned in the history. It is uncommon to find local tenderness, and loose bodies generally cannot be palpated.

Imaging

- The diagnostic evaluation of an ankle suspected of containing loose bodies should start with orthogonal plain radiographs. These are generally helpful in revealing loose bodies containing bone or calcifications, but will not detect loose chondral bodies (Fig. 27–10).
- In 5-30% of cases of synovial chondromatosis, calcifications may not be seen.
- CT arthrography is helpful in detecting cartilaginous bodies or bodies whose calcifications are too faint to see

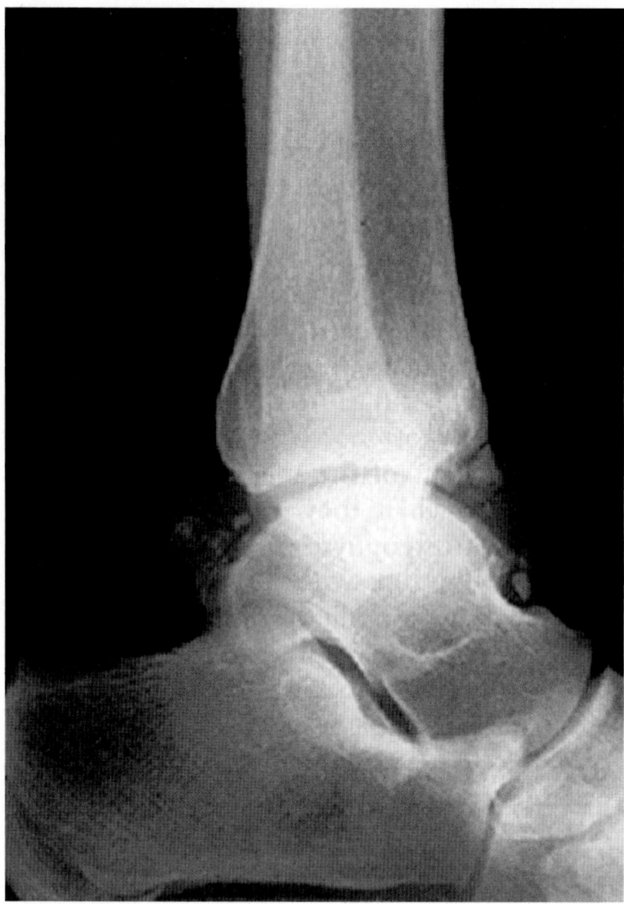

Figure 27–10: Lateral ankle x-ray demonstrating multiple loose bodies.

on plain radiographs. MRI is probably the preferred study for revealing chondral loose bodies. MRI with gadolinium may be helpful in detecting cartilage injuries, as well as differentiating simple joint effusion from chondral loose bodies.

Arthroscopic Approach to Loose Body Removal

- It is important to localize the loose body or bodies, if possible, prior to attempting removal. The number and location may predetermine the need to establish certain portals from the start.
- The use of distraction is extremely helpful. Most loose bodies, even ones located in the posterior compartment, can be reached utilizing distraction and the anterior portals. One technique is to coax the piece into the anterior compartment then release the distraction, effectively trapping it anteriorly.
- Large pieces can often be reduced in size by either a rongeur or a shaver for easier removal. Getting a grasp on an uncooperative loose body can be a frustrating task. A spinal needle can stabilize the piece while another instrument works on it through an accessory portal. Sometimes, a portal site needs to be enlarged to extract a large piece. The time saved and potential trauma averted wrestling a loose body trapped in the extracapsular soft tissue is worth enlarging the portal site another couple of millimeters.
- After all loose bodies are removed, a formal systematic examination of the ankle is warranted, with additional pathology treated accordingly.

References

Anderson IF, Crichton KJ, Grattan-Smith T et al. (1989) Osteochondral fractures of the dome of the talus. J Bone Joint Surg 71A(8): 1143-1152.
Correlates findings at arthroscopy with MRI.

Berndt AL, Harty M. (1959) Transcondylar fractures (osteochondritis dissecans) of the talus. J Bone Joint Surg 41-A: 988-1020.
The classic thesis whereby cadaver limbs are twisted until osteochondral fracture occurs. Although the authors were originally describing acute fractures in cadaver limbs, the staging has been extrapolated to all OLTs (which can sometimes be confusing).

Conti SF, Taranow WF. (1996) Transtalar retrograde drilling of medial osteochondral lesions of the talar dome. Oper Tech Orthop 6: 226-230.
Describes arthroscopic techniques for dealing with OLTs.

DiGiovanni BF, Fraga CJ, Cohen BE et al. (2000) Associated injuries found in chronic lateral ankle instability. Foot Ankle Int 21(10): 809-815.

Ferkel RD. (1996) Arthroscopic Surgery: The Foot and Ankle. Philadelphia: Lippincott-Raven.
This reviews general principles of ankle arthroscopy.

Ferkel RD, Sgaglione NA. (1993-4) Arthroscopic treatment of osteochondral lesions of the talus: Long term results. Orthop Trans 17: 1011.
Description of the MRI-based staging system.

Flick AB, Gould N. (1985) Osteochondritis dissecans of the talus: Review of the literature and new surgical approach for medial dome lesions. Foot Ankle 5: 165-185.
A thorough review of past experience with OLTs.

Guhl JF, Parisien JS, Boyton MD. (2004) Foot and Ankle Arthroscopy, 3rd edn. New York: Springer-Verlag.
This article reviews general principles of ankle arthroscopy.

Komenda GA, Ferkel RD. (1999) Arthroscopic findings associated with the unstable ankle. Foot Ankle Int 20(11): 708-713.

Loomer R, Fisher C, Lloyd-Smith R et al. (1993) Osteochondral lesions of the talus. Am J Sports Med 21(1): 13-19.
Introduction of the type 5 lesion.

CHAPTER 28

Nail Problems in the Foot

Mark Chong Lee* and Christopher W. DiGiovanni§

*M.D., Department of Orthopaedics, Brown Medical School, Providence, RI
§M.D., Associate Professor, Chief, Foot and Ankle Service, Department of Orthopaedic Surgery, Brown Medical School, Rhode Island Hospital, Providence, RI

- The primary functions of toenails are to protect the distal phalanx and to provide a mechanical support for the surrounding soft tissues.
- Secondary function is to enhance fine sensation by providing counterpressure for the fine touch organs in the pulp. This function is more evident in the hand.
- Toenail deformity and pathology results in both severe cosmetic and functional impairment.
- Toenail disorders can result from local mechanical problems, infection, and/or systemic disease.

Anatomy

- The toenail is divided into the nail plate (nail proper) and its soft tissue support.
- The nail plate is a translucent structure made up of three overlapping layers of keratinized germinal cells: a thin dorsal layer, a thick middle layer, and a deep layer.
- The nail plate's soft tissue support (Fig. 28–1A) consists of:
  - proximal and lateral nail folds
  - germinal matrix
  - nail bed (sterile matrix)
  - hyponychium.
- The nail folds are skin folds that border the nail plate in a "U" shape.
- The proximal nail fold is a complex structure that covers the base of the nail plate. Its dorsal surface is epithelial. As it folds over, its ventral surface, the *eponychium*, attaches to the dorsum of the forming nail plate.
- The *cuticle* is the translucent rim at the distal edge of the proximal nail fold.
- The germinal matrix is the main growth center for the toenail and lies plantar to the growing nail plate.
- The germinal matrix begins at the apex of the ventral surface of the proximal nail fold, usually 5-6 mm proximal to the cuticle. Its distal extent is visible through the nail plate as the opaque, crescent-shaped region called the *lunula*. It is continuous with the nail bed more distally.
- The width of the germinal matrix parallels the width of the nail plate.
- Proximally, the germinal matrix is closely related to the insertion of the extensor tendon on the distal phalanx and the distal interphalangeal joint (Fig. 28–1B).
- The nail bed is a grooved epithelial surface on which the nail plate rests, and to which the nail plate is tightly bonded.
- The hyponychium is the smooth border of skin at the distal end of the nail bed, and seals the area where the nail bed and nail plate separate.
- Nails are supplied by the dorsal branches of the proper plantar arteries and nerves. Venous drainage parallels arterial flow.

Physiology

- The normal adult toenail plate grows between 0.03 and 0.05 mm/day, and has a thickness of 0.5-1.0 mm. In contrast, the fingernails grow 2-4 times more quickly.

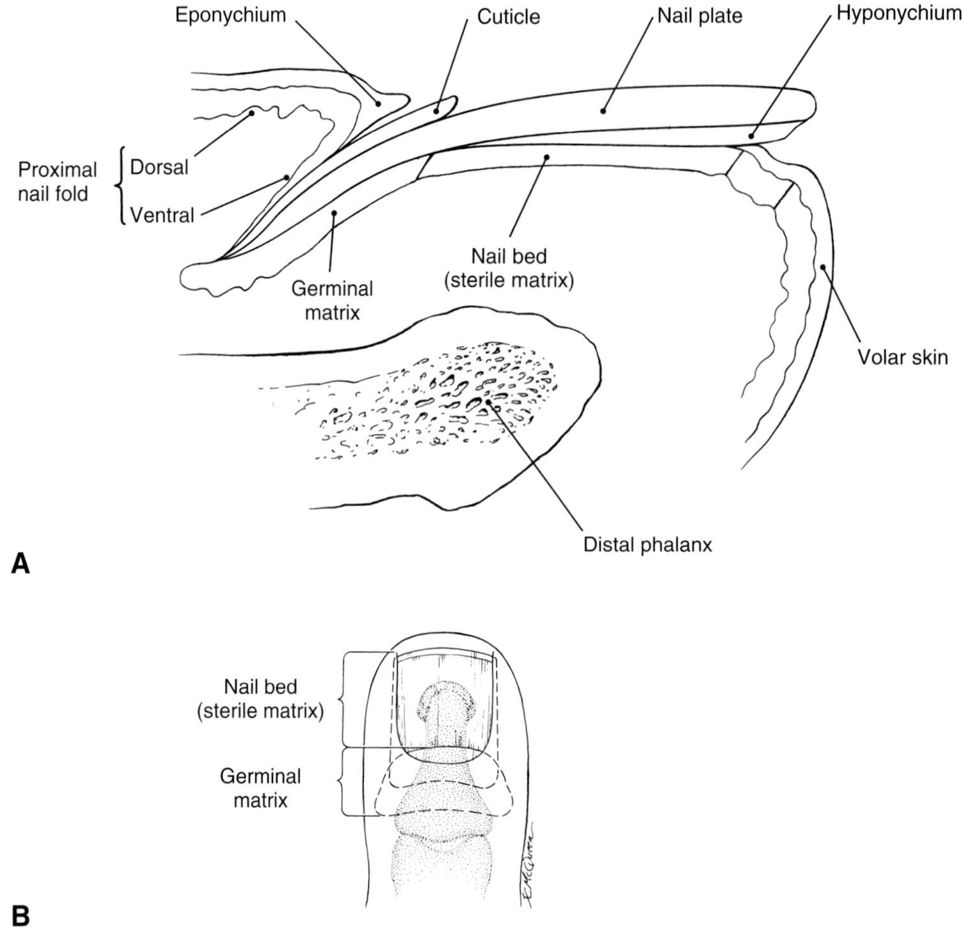

Figure 28–1: **A**, Anatomy of the toenail. **B**, Relationship of nail bed and matrix to distal interphalangeal joint. (A, From Richardson EG, Hendrix CL. (2003) Disorders of nails and skin. In: Campbell's Operative Orthopaedics, 10th edn. (Canale ST, ed.). Philadelphia: Mosby. p. 4172; B, From Tomczak R. (2000) Embryology of the nail unit. In: Foot and Ankle Disorders (Myerson M, ed.). Philadelphia: Saunders. p. 522.)

- Longitudinal growth of the nail plate is thought to result from the redirection of a vertically growing nail plate by the nail fold. As germinal matrix cells divide, they are flattened against the proximal nail fold by newly emerging cells beneath, and the net force vector of the growth is directed distally.
- The germinal matrix contributes 80% to the thickness of the nail plate, whereas the nail bed contributes the remaining 20% (Johnson and Shuster 1993). However, it is controversial whether the eponychium, nail bed, or lateral nail folds contribute to the longitudinal growth of the nail.
- More proximal sterile or germinal matrix components contribute to more superficial layers of the nail plate. The area of the germinal matrix proximal to the lunula produces the thin dorsal layer of the nail plate. The lunula produces the thicker and softer middle layer of the nail plate. The nail bed adds a layer to the ventral surface of the nail plate.
- The eponychium adds a thin layer to the nail dorsally to give it its shine.
- An intact nail bed or sterile matrix is required for the growth of a morphologically normal nail.
- Nail plate shape follows the shape of the bony contour of the distal phalanx and the soft tissue overlying the distal phalanx. Deformity can be caused by osseous malformation of the dorsum of the distal phalanx, or by hypertrophy and irregular thickening of the nail bed.
- The longitudinally growing nail plate gives structure to the soft tissue surrounding the nail. Removal of the nail can lead to upward deformation of the soft tissue around the nail bed.
- Traumatic disruption of the nail leads to slowed nail plate growth lasting approximately 3-4 months. Complete regrowth of a toenail can take 12-18 months.
- The hyponychium protects the nail bed and matrix from infection.

Nail Plate Disorders

Onychocryptosis (Ingrown Toenail)

- Occurs when the lateral border of the nail plate abuts the soft tissue of the lateral fold.
- Normally, the nail plate and lateral fold are separated by 1 mm.
- Nail plate shape irregularities from poor trimming, traumatic distortion, or progressive change from fungal infection can cause irritating contact with the lateral fold.
- Alternatively, primary lateral fold hypertrophy may lead to abnormal contact with the nail plate. Lateral fold hypertrophy may be due to abnormal pressures from shoe wear, direct trauma, tumor, or excessive pronation of the hallux.
- The condition probably results from a combination of nail plate and lateral fold pathology.
- The initial nail plate or lateral fold pathology or their combination will result in a cycle of chronic irritation that leads to further nail fold hypertrophy and contact of the lateral fold with the nail plate (Fig. 28–2A,B).
- Ultimately, the skin of the lateral fold is punctured by the nail, and secondary infection such as paronychia and eventually osteomyelitis may result (Fig. 28–2C,D).
- Most common in men of 20-30 years of age.
- In adults, the condition is typically acquired. In neonates, the condition is related to congenitally thick lateral nail folds.
- May be classified into three stages, with treatments specific for each stage (Table 28–1).
- General treatment involves instruction on proper nail trimming, shoe wear modification, and orthotics for excessive pronation of hallux.
- Late stage 2 and 3 lesions, as well as stage 1 lesions that have failed conservative treatment, require surgical management.
- Recurrence rates after total or partial nail plate removal without germinal matrix excision is frequent, and ranges from 32 to 73%.
- Partial nail plate and germinal matrix removal has a recurrence rate of 6% and is the most common surgical treatment (Pettine et al. 1988). A similar recurrence rate exists for either total nail plate and germinal matrix excision, or combined partial nail fold and germinal matrix removal.
- Phenol ablation of the germinal matrix has a slightly higher recurrence at 16% but is technically easier.

Onychomycosis

- A fungal infection of the toenails caused by dermatophytes, yeast, and molds.
- Accounts for approximately 50% of nail problems. Infects 20% of the population and increases to 75% in the subgroup over 60 years of age.
- Toenails are 4-10 times more frequently affected.
- Ninety percent are caused by dermatophytes, specifically *Trichophyton rubrum* (70%) and *T. mentagrophytes. Candida* infections are much less common.
- Four categories of onychomycosis: distal subungual, proximal subungual, white superficial, and candidal onychomycosis.
- Distal subungual onychomycosis is the most common type. Infection of the nail bed begins from the distal edge and proceeds proximally, causing yellowish, longitudinal streaks in the nail (Fig. 28–3A).
- Proximal subungual onychomycosis is the rarest type, with whitish discoloration extending from underneath the proximal nail fold distally. *T. rubrum* is the most frequent organism, and this form is found most commonly in immunocompromised patients.
- White superficial onychomycosis appears as white plaques on the surface of the nail plate that start at the cuticle and

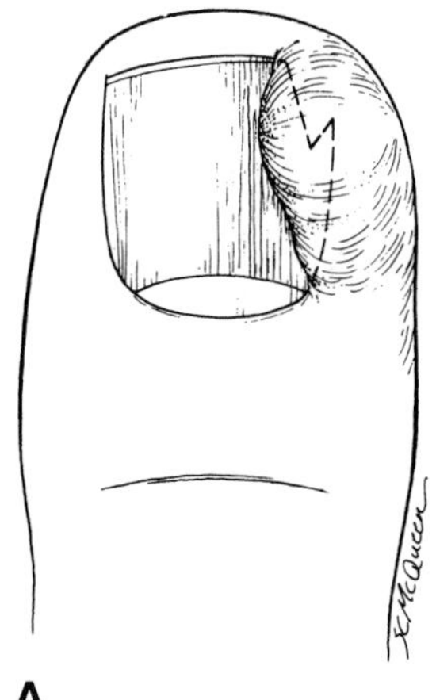
A

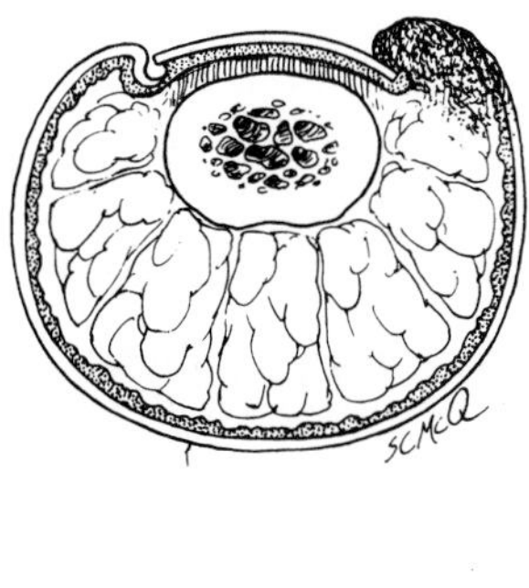
B

Figure 28–2: **A,** Anteroposterior view of lateral nail fold with hypertrophy from impinging nail plate with lateral "fish hook" irregularity. **B,** Cross-sectional view of toe with hypertrophy of lateral nail fold and obliteration of normal space between the nail plate and lateral fold.

Continued

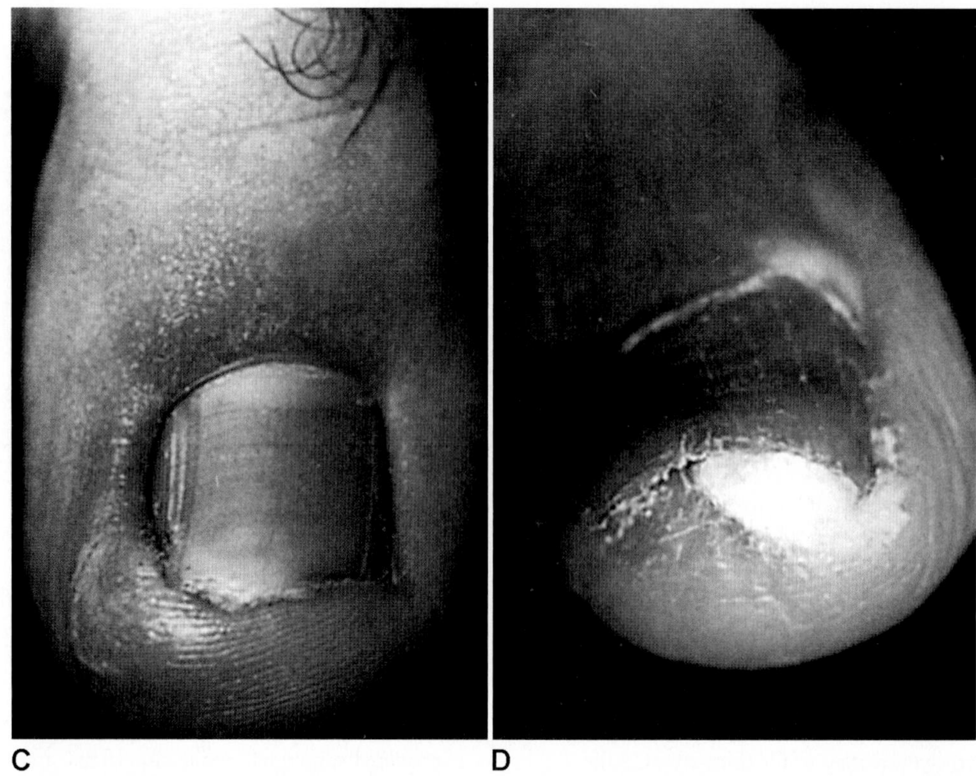

Figure 28–2: Cont'd **C,** Anteroposterior picture of ingrown toenail with surrounding erythema. **D,** Medial nail plate is lifted with cotton. (From Richardson EG, Hendrix CL. (2003) Disorders of nails and skin. In: Campbell's Operative Orthopaedics, 10th edn (Canale ST, ed.). Philadelphia: Mosby. p. 4172.)

then progress distally to erode the nail plate. The most common organism is *T. mentagrophytes*.

- Candidal onychomycosis is also a relatively rare form, with longitudinal white striations in the nail plate, nail bed thickening, and bulbous dilatation of the distal toe.
- Risk factors for onychomycosis include family history, increasing age, poor health, prior trauma, warm climate, participation in fitness activities, immunosuppression (e.g. HIV, drug-induced), communal bathing, and occlusive footwear.
- With chronic infection, the nail plate deforms, elevates, and sometimes becomes painful when compressed (Fig. 28–3B).
- Diagnosis may be made by nail scrapings in sodium hydroxide examined under light microscopy.
- Local therapy includes nail plate trimming with debridement of the subungual tissue. Most patients can be treated with good nail care.
- Systemic therapy with oral terbinafine, ketoconazole, and itraconazole has a variable efficacy, is of long duration, and has an extensive side effect and drug interaction profile, including liver toxicity and cardiovascular effects (Sigurgeirsson et al. 2002).
- Topical therapies with antibiotic creams have been historically ineffective. However, newer lacquer formulations may offer good alternatives as stand-alone or combination therapy.

Table 28–1: Classification and Treatment of Ingrown Toe Nails

STAGE	DESCRIPTION	TREATMENT
1 (inflammatory)	Erythema, swelling, and tenderness along lateral nail fold	Lift lateral edge of nail
2 (abscess)	Acute or active infection with drainage	Antibiotic therapy after culture and sensitivity Lift lateral edge of nail after drainage stops Surgical treatment
3 (granulation)	Granulation tissue develops in lateral nail fold from chronic infection	Surgical treatment

(After Heifetz CJ. (1945) Operative management of the ingrown toe nail. J Missouri Med Assoc 42: 213.)

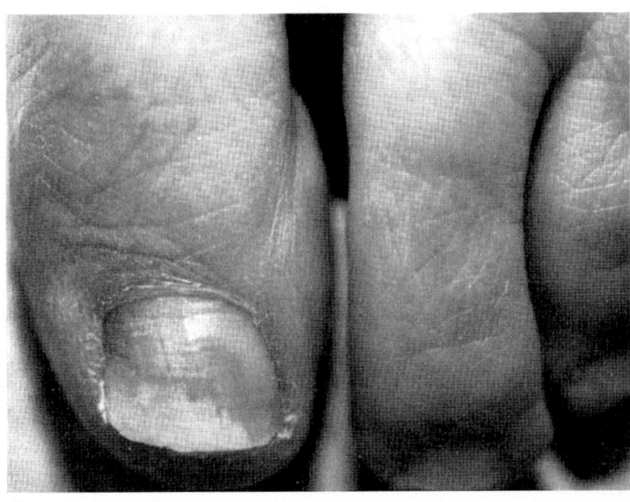

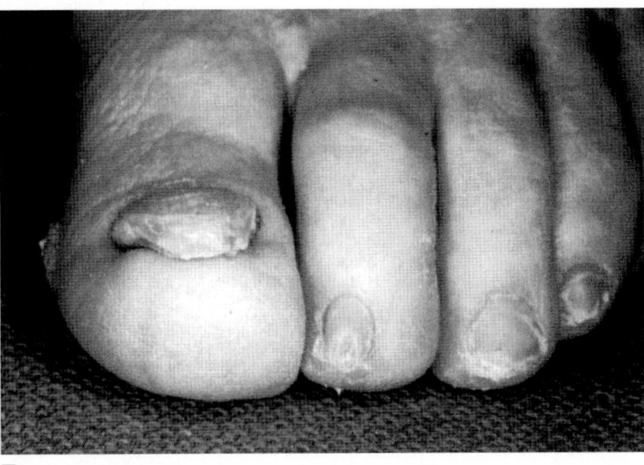

Figure 28–3: **A,** Advanced case of distal subungual onychomycosis with thickened and opaque nail. **B,** Late-stage chronic onychomycosis, with complete nail and nail bed deformity. (A, From Coughlin MJ. (1999) Toenail abnormalities. In: Surgery of the Foot and Ankle, 7th edn (Coughlin MJ, Mann RA, eds). Philadelphia: Mosby. p. 1054; **B,** From Tomczak R. (2000) Embryology of the nail unit. In: Foot and Ankle Disorders (Myerson M, ed.). Philadelphia: Saunders. p. 538.)

Onychauxis (Club Nail) and Onychogryphosis ("Hostler's Toe," "Ram Horn Nail")

- Onychauxis is hypertrophy of the nail plate and bed, without curving deformity. Yellow to black discoloration may also exist. The most frequent causes of onychauxis are tinea infection and local trauma.
- Onychogryphosis is longstanding hypertrophy of the nail plate with curving deformity of the nail, resembling a claw or horn (Fig. 28–4).
- Onychogryphosis is not related to tinea infections. Instead, it is the result of congenital or repeated trauma to the nail matrix along with poor hygiene.

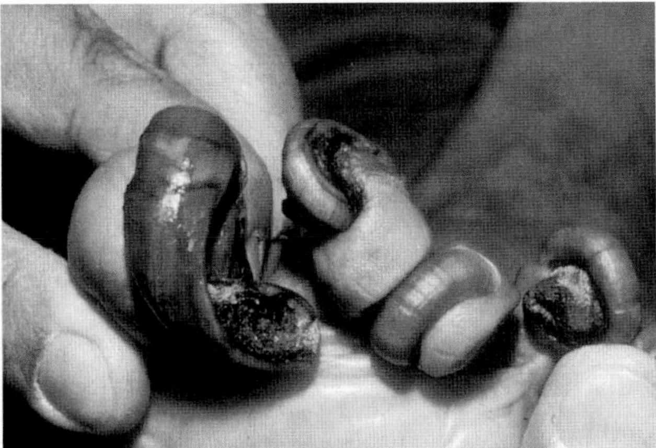

Figure 28–4: The curved, clawlike nails of onychogryphosis. All toes may be involved. (From Tomczak R. (2000) Embryology of the nail unit. In: Foot and Ankle Disorders (Myerson M, ed.). Philadelphia: Saunders. p. 538.)

- Nails with onychauxis and onychogryphosis may compromise the skin integrity of adjacent nails, or cause pain as pressure is applied to the nail bed through pressure on the nail plate.
- Treatment of onychauxis involves grinding the nail sequentially and topical antifungals. Severe deformity may require surgical ablation or a terminal Syme procedure.
- Treatment of onychogryphosis involves serial trimming of the nail to the hyponychia. Lambs' wool may be inserted between toes to prevent injury to adjacent toes.

Onycholysis and Onychomadesis

- Onycholysis refers to separation of the nail plate from the nail bed, usually beginning distally and advancing proximally.
- The reverse pattern is onychomadesis, with separation beginning proximally and extending distally. Onychomadesis can occur in psoriasis or scarlet fever.
- Nail discoloration may result from secondary infection of the exposed nail bed.
- Onycholysis occurs much more frequently in females than in males.
- May result from local trauma, contact dermatitis from nail products, chemotherapy, thyroid disorders, and primary infection.
- Diagnosis should include a thorough exposure history as well as nail scrapings to rule out infection.
- A chronic untreated onycholysis results in scarring of the nail bed with persistent nail plate deformity.
- Treatment consists of removing the precipitating cause.
- Trimming of the affected nail and topical antifungal medication for infection can then be used.
- Toenail ablation may be necessary in chronic cases.

Nail Bed Disorders

- In addition to the following disorders, benign soft tissue tumors such as fibromas, glomus tumors, and pyogenic granulomas can involve the nail bed and affect nail growth.

Subungual Hematoma

- Results when there is hemorrhage into the potential space between the nail bed and nail plate (Fig. 28–5).
- Typically occurs with trauma to the toenail.
- The hematoma is usually well demarcated and often involves the entire nail.
- Exquisite pain results from the pressure on the nail bed exerted by the mass effect of the hematoma.
- Fracture of the distal phalanx occurs in 25% of cases.
- In non-acute or non-traumatic presentations, one must exclude subungual melanoma through history and examination or, in difficult cases, nail biopsy.
- Acute decompression of the hematoma through a handheld cautery unit, a fine point no. 11 scalpel, or a needle will provide immediate relief.
- More aggressive surgical treatment for subungual hematomas with an intact nail plate is debatable, because evidence exists detailing no difference in the incidence of subsequent nail deformity (Seaberg et al. 1991).
- Some authors advocate nail plate removal and nail bed repair when > 50% of the nail bed is involved or a distal phalanx fracture is present (Simon and Wolgin 1987).
- Nail plate disruption with an underlying distal phalanx fracture should be treated as an open fracture with irrigation and debridement of the nail, with concomitant use of intravenous antibiotics (Kensinger et al. 2001).

Subungual Exostosis

- Benign bony growth occurring on the dorsomedial aspect of the distal phalanx of the hallux and, less commonly, on the lesser toes (Fig. 28–6A).
- Unilateral and slow growing.
- Histologically, is a fibrous proliferation that undergoes cartilage metaplasia and endochondral ossification with a characteristic fibrocartilaginous cap.
- Lesion may distort nail plate and lead to onychocryptosis with secondary infection.
- Most common between 20 and 40 years of age.
- Associated factors include trauma, as occurs in dance and gymnastics, and infection.
- Must be distinguished from chondrosarcoma and osteochondroma.
- Chondrosarcoma, unlike subungual exostosis, is a less well-demarcated, more cellular lesion with large and irregular nuclei.

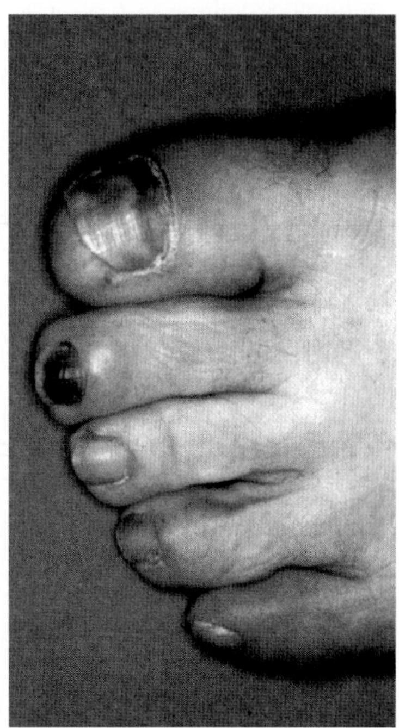

Figure 28–5: Subungual hematoma resulting from acute trauma. Note the partial involvement of the hallucial and second toenail beds. (From Tomczak R. (2000) Embryology of the nail unit. In: Foot and Ankle Disorders (Myerson M, ed.). Philadelphia: Saunders. p. 523.)

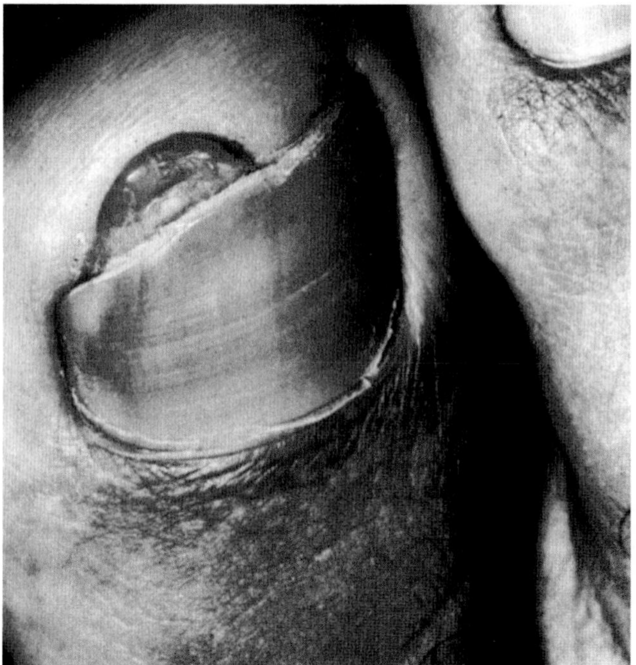

A

Figure 28–6: A, Subungual exostosis protruding from underneath the hallucial nail plate.

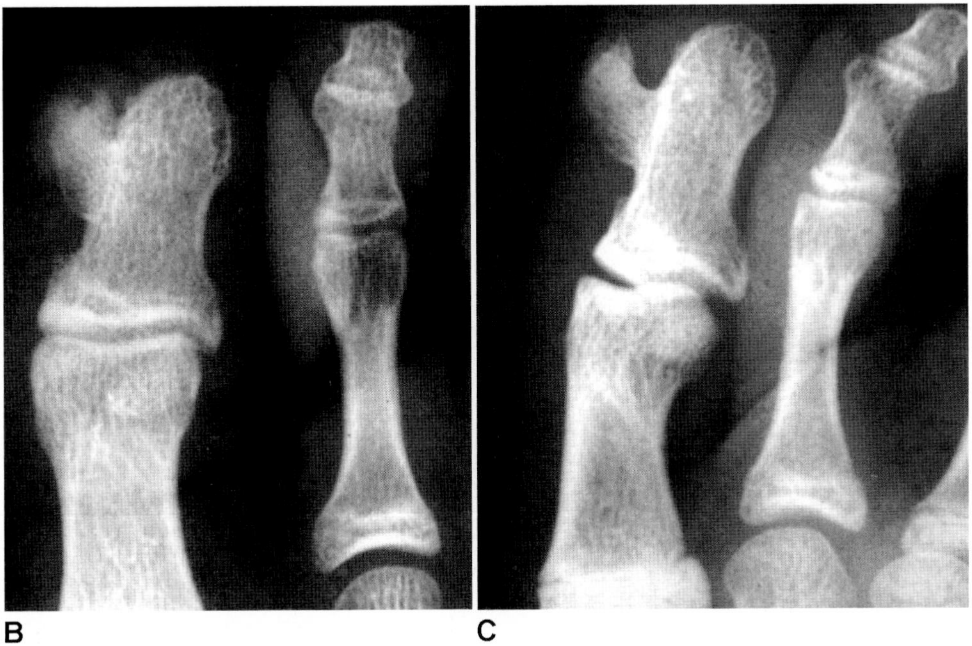

Figure 28–6: Cont'd **B,** Anteroposterior radiographic view of the subungual exostosis. **C,** Oblique radiographic view of the subungual exostosis. (From Jahss MJ. (1991) Disorders of the hallux and the first ray. In: Disorders of the Foot and Ankle: Medical and Surgical Management, 2nd edn (Jahss MJ, ed.). Philadelphia: Saunders. p. 1168.)

- Osteochondroma demonstrates a *hyaline cartilaginous cap* with enchondral ossification, similar to a growth plate.
- Diagnosis is made by radiographic demonstration of exostosis (Fig. 28–6B,C).
- Treatment is symptomatic resection including the overlying nail bed.
- Recurrence is common with subtotal surgical resection and has been reported to be 53% (Miller-Breslow and Dorfman 1988).

Nail Fold Disorders

Paronychia

- Paronychia is an infection of the nail fold and groove characterized by tenderness, erythema, and edema of the nail fold, often with a purulent collection underneath (Fig. 28–7).
- The most common isolates are polymicrobial aerobes, anaerobes, or both. *Candida albicans* is also frequently found.
- Usually affects the hallux but may also affect the other toes.
- Typically results from injury to the nail fold as caused by an ingrown toenail or trauma.
- Diabetics demonstrate a twofold higher incidence of infection. Also associated with antiretroviral therapy for HIV (Bouscarat et al. 1998).
- Secondary dystrophic changes to the nail plate may follow infection.
- Treatment begins with footwear modifications (such as a loose or open-toed shoe) to remove extrinsic pressure.
- Partial nail excision, with partial nail matrix ablation for ingrown toenail, and opening of the nail fold collection is used to treat the acute condition.
- Topical antibiotics or soaks may be continued until resolution of infection.

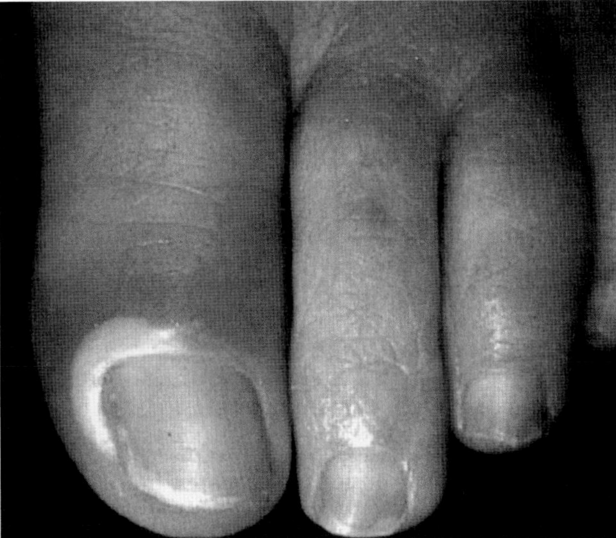

Figure 28–7: Acute paronychia of the hallux with involvement of the proximal and lateral nail fold. (From Coughlin MJ. (1999) Toenail abnormalities. In: Surgery of the Foot and Ankle, 7th edn (Coughlin MJ, Mann RA, eds). Philadelphia: Mosby. p. 1058.)

Pyogenic Granuloma

- A benign, painless, crusting, pedunculated or sessile vascular lesion with an appearance similar to that of a raspberry.
- Propensity for bleeding and ulceration results in a red, blue, or black coloration.
- Rapidly growing, with a size that varies from 2 mm to 1 cm.
- Common in children and young adults, but may develop at any age.
- Etiology is unknown, although trauma, chronic irritation, infection, and hormonal influences have been proposed.
- Frequently complicated by staphylococcal infection.
- Treatment involves surgical excision or cautery, accompanied by moist dressing and antibiotics as appropriate.

Herpetic Whitlow

- Relatively uncommon herpes simplex virus infection of the toe.
- Presents as painful vesicles on an erythematous base, mostly localized to the proximal nail fold (Fig. 28–8).
- Regional lymphangitis may be present.
- May elicit history of recurrent infection.
- Must be differentiated from a bacterial infection through Tzanck smear or antibody assay.
- Unlike bacterial infection, treatment is symptomatic, because antibiotics and surgical debridement have no effect on the course of infection.
- Antivirals such as acyclovir may be helpful in decreasing symptoms.

Periungual and Subungual Verruca (Warts)

- A verruca may be located along the nail folds (periungually) or under the nail plate (subungually).
- The appearance is typical, with a round, papular collection of brown or dark grey tissue with a cauliflower-like surface.
- Caused by human papillomavirus.
- Treatment involves ablation through chemical or thermal means or surgical excision.
- When removing warts from the periungual or subungual region, caution must be exercised to minimize damage to the nail matrix.

Nail Matrix Disorders

- Disorders of the nail matrix ultimately manifest as disorders in the nail plate.

Anonychia

- The absence of toenails, or anonychia, may be congenital or acquired.
- The congenital form may be an isolated anomaly or may be associated with ectrodactyly, the absence of phalangeal bones.
- Acquired anonychia may be a result of drug reactions, trauma, surgical ablation, frostbite, or vascular insufficiency.
- No treatment is needed for acquired or congenital anonychia.

Pterygium Unguis

- Describes an ingrowth of the cuticle and eponychium into the nail matrix, such that nail growth is obliterated at that site and a longitudinal splitting of the nail plate occurs distally.
- Most commonly occurs in the fourth and fifth digits.
- Can be congenital but most commonly found with leprosy and peripheral neuritis.

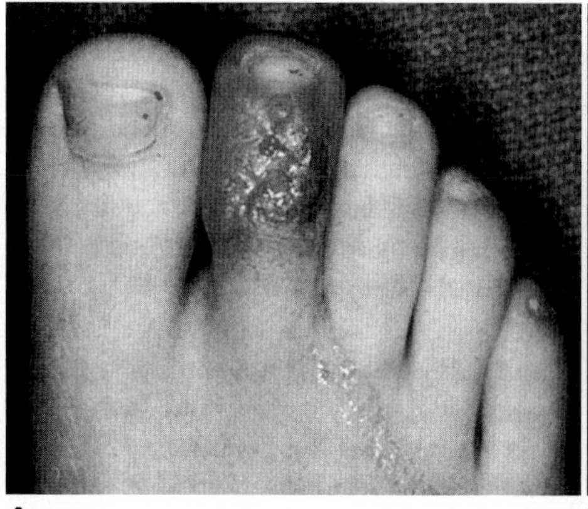
A

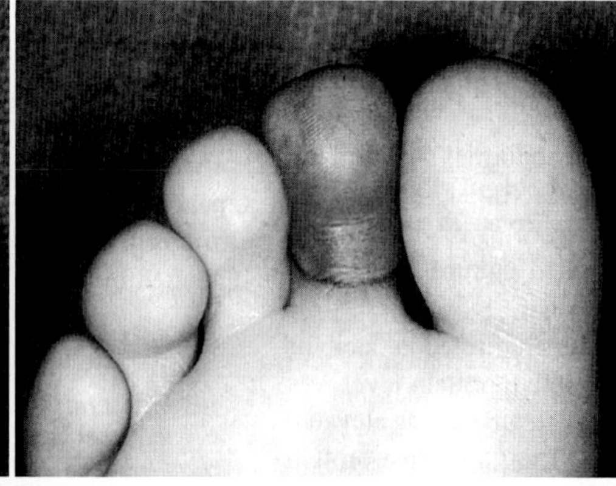
B

Figure 28–8: **A,** Herpetic whitlow of the second toe in a 28-year-old woman, with characteristic ruptured vesicles and erythema from the nail fold proximally. **B,** Erythema extends circumferentially to the plantar toe. (From Egan LJ, Bylander JM, Agerter DC et al. (1998) Herpetic whitlow of the toe: An unusual manifestation of infection with herpes simplex virus type 2. Clin Infect Dis 26(1): 196-197.)

Table 28–2: Genetic Disorders and Associated Nail Changes

DISEASE OR SYNDROME	INHERITANCE (DEFECTIVE GENE)[a]	PATHOLOGIC NAIL FINDINGS
Darier disease	AD (ATP2A2, intracellular Ca^{2+} channel pump)	Longitudinal red/white striations Atrophy/hypertrophy of nail plate Splinter hemorrhages Distal wedge-shaped keratoses
Pachyonychia congenita	AD (keratins 16 or 17 and isoforms)	Brown/yellow discoloration Massive nail plate hypertrophy
Nail-patella syndrome	AD (LMX1B homeodomain protein)	Nail atrophy Triangular-shaped lunula
Dyskeratosis congenita—X-linked type	X-linked (dyskerin, involved with cell cycle and nuclear function)	Atrophy of nail plate Ridging Fusion of proximal nail fold
DOOR syndrome[b]	AR (2-oxoglutarate decarboxylase)	Anonychia or atrophic nails

[a]AD, autosomal dominant; AR, autosomal recessive.
[b]Deafness, onychoosteodystrophy, mental retardation.
(After Coughlin MJ. (1999) Toenail abnormalities. In: Surgery of the Foot and Ankle, 7th edn (Coughlin MJ, Mann RA, eds). Philadelphia: Mosby. p. 1042.)

- Also results from trauma, vascular insufficiency, Raynaud phenomenon, scleroderma, and lichen planus.
- Surgical separation of the cuticle and eponychium from the nail matrix and interposition of a silicone sheet or sterile matrix graft have been shown to be effective.

Genetic Nail Disorders

- A variety of genetic disorders with collagen abnormalities can result in toenail changes.
- Many of the genetic disorders have been characterized at the level of molecular mechanisms (Table 28–2).
- The majority of familial nail disorders are autosomal dominant.
- Usually, no specific treatment is required for the nail disorder.

Tumors

- Primary nail tumors may be benign or malignant (Box 28–1).
- Secondary tumors may be metastatic or arise from underlying bone of the distal phalanx, as in subungual exostosis, osteochondroma, or enchondroma.
- Metastasis to the nail and digits is rare. However, it is most commonly from lung carcinoma, followed by kidney and breast carcinoma.
- Nail tumors may cause nail plate deformity through pressure effects on the nail bed and germinal matrix.
- Malignant tumors of greatest significance clinically are malignant melanoma and Bowen disease.

Box 28–1 Benign and Malignant Primary Nail Tumors

Benign

- Verruca (warts)
- Fibroma
- Fibrokeratoma
- Pyogenic granuloma
- Glomus tumor
- Pigmented nevus
- Keratocanthoma

Malignant

- Squamous cell carcinoma
- Malignant melanoma
- Basal cell carcinoma
- Metastatic carcinoma
- Bowen disease

Subungual Malignant Melanoma

- Malignant skin tumor derived from the pigment-producing cells called melanocytes.
- Subungual melanoma is a rare diagnosis and accounts for 2-3% of all cutaneous melanomas.
- In 2001, incidence for all cutaneous melanomas in men and women, respectively, was 21.9 and 13.8 per 100 000. Incidence has increased by 25-30% over the past decade and continues to rise.
- Subungual melanoma is more common in people of Asian and African descent, where it accounts for 20% of all cutaneous melanomas.
- More common in the fingers than in the toes.
- Median age of presentation is 50-60 years.
- History may be significant for longitudinal band along nail plate that has recently appeared or has changed appearance.
- The lesion is typically black, on a single toe, and may be accompanied by localized erythema, onycholysis, and/or ulceration.

- The Hutchinson sign is characteristic, and is described as a longitudinal band of pigmented tissue extending the length of the nail plate (Fig. 28–9).
- Unlike subungual hematoma, discoloration of the nail bed does not change as the nail grows distally and does not improve with time.
- Estimated 5-year survival rates vary between 26 and 80% (Moehrle et al. 2003).
- Poor prognostic factors include late clinical stage, deep level of invasion, ulceration, and histologic evidence of active cell division.
- Traditional treatment is early amputation through a metatarsophalangeal or transmetatarsal approach.
- Recent work has shown that limited resection with adequate margins and preservation of the distal phalanx in early disease did not change 5-year survival rate.
- It is extremely important to consider this lesion in the evaluation of nail disease so as to avoid a delay in diagnosis.

Squamous Cell Carcinoma

- Squamous cell carcinoma is very rare in the toenails.
- Typically presents as an ulcerative, friable, crusting lesion.
- Most common in men older than 50 years.
- Considered a low-grade lesion with relentless growth, at times invading bone and tendons.
- Although no standard treatment is available in light of the rarity of the lesion, recommended approach is with wide surgical excision and chemotherapy.
- *Bowen disease* is a squamous cell carcinoma variant that typically does not metastasize, termed in situ, and is associated with human papillomavirus.
- Treatment for Bowen disease is with surgical excision or curettage.

Nail Disorders from Systemic Disease

- The nail plate color, texture, shape, and rate of growth is often a signal to underlying systemic processes, and is manifested in numerous disease processes (Fig. 28–10 and Table 28–3).
- Although few of the nail changes in systemic disorders require treatment, it may alert the physician to a particular systemic disorder.
- Trauma should always be included in the differential for pathologic nail morphologies.

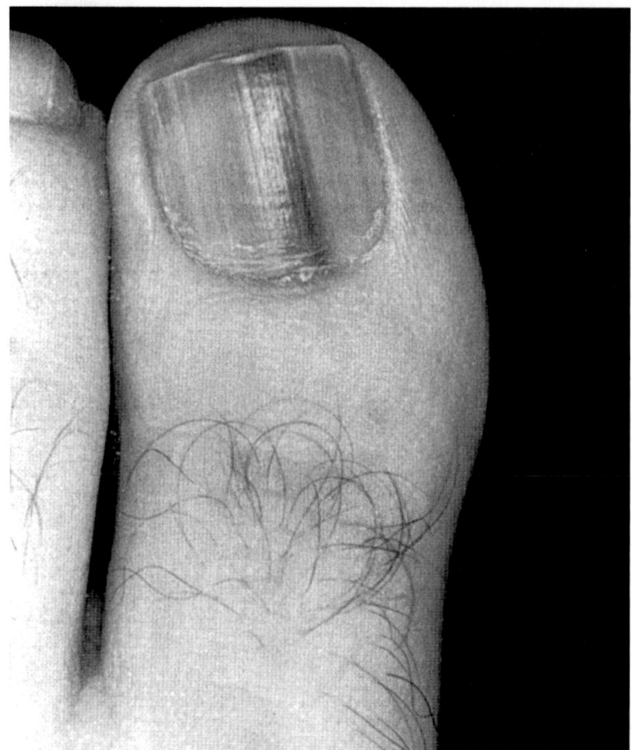

Figure 28–9: Hutchinson sign suggesting malignant melanoma. (From Tomczak R. (2000) Embryology of the nail unit. In: Foot and Ankle Disorders (Myerson M, ed.). Philadelphia: Saunders. p. 524.)

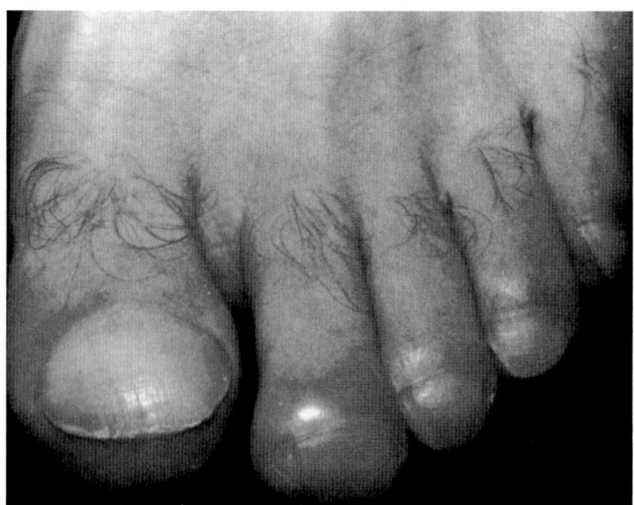

Figure 28–10: Clubbing of the toenails associated with systemic disease. (From Jahss MJ. (1991) Disorders of the hallux and the first ray. In: Disorders of the Foot and Ankle: Medical and Surgical Management, 2nd edn (Jahss MJ, ed.). Philadelphia: Saunders. p. 1158.)

Table 28–3: Toenail Changes as Manifestation of Systemic Disease

NAME	APPEARANCE	ASSOCIATED CONDITION
Pathologic lines		
Beau lines	Transverse depressions of up to 0.5 mm depth	Follow nail growth arrest Progress distally with continued nail growth Febrile illness, diabetes, trauma, Hodgkin disease
Mees lines	Transverse white bands of 1-3 mm width that involve more than one nail	Follow nail growth arrest Progress distally with continued nail growth Arsenic poisoning, Hodgkin disease, congestive heart failure, malaria, chemotherapy
Muehreke lines	Paired, transverse white lines that parallel the lunula and span the width of the nail	Do not progress distally with nail growth Hypoalbuminemia, nephritic syndrome, liver disease, malnutrition
Longitudinal striations	Ridges in the nail surface	Commonly seen in normal aging If involves all fingers and toes with absent luster, then lichen planus, alopecia areata, and psoriasis
Dark longitudinal lines	Pigmented band along direction of nail	Normal in 75% of adult black people Malignant melanoma, nevi, chemical staining
Pathologic shapes		
Koilonychia	Nail dorsum adapts a concavity such that nail resembles a spoon shape	Iron deficiency anemia, systemic lupus erythematosus, trauma, nail-patella syndrome, hemochromatosis
Clubbing	Thickening of the connective tissues under the nail bed and around the distal phalanx	May be autosomal dominant trait Cardiopulmonary insufficiency, metastatic tumor, lung carcinoma, cirrhosis, inflammatory bowel disease
Pitting	Punctate depressions in the surface of the nail plate	Psoriasis, autoimmune illness, sarcoidosis, alopecia areata
Onychoschizia	Fissuring or splitting of the nail plate with delamination of the layers of the nail plate	Hematologic disorders, infection, and hypovitaminosis
Pathologic colors		
Terry nail	Opacified nail plate with a 1- to 3-mm pinkish band located at the distal segment of the nail plate	Diabetes and liver disease
Blue nail, blue-gray nail	Bluish discoloration of the nail	Malignant melanoma and cyanotic diseases
Half and half nails	Distal portion of nail is colored brown, red, or pink, while the proximal portion has normal color	Renal failure or chronic liver disease
Splinter hemorrhages	Thin, short, longitudinal, dark red lines that lie in the nail bed	Classic for endocarditis, and thought to be more specific if occurs proximally in the nail Also systemic lupus erythematosus, rheumatoid arthritis, peptic ulcer disease, and psoriasis
Azure lunula	Blue discoloration of the lunula	Wilson disease and silver poisoning
Leukonychia	Whitish, spotty discoloration of nail plate	Most often normal, indicating minor nail bed trauma Typhoid fever, tuberculosis, trichinosis, nephritis, pneumonia
Yellow nail	Lunula is absent, nail plate thickens and yellows	Chronic bronchiectasis, pleural effusions, rheumatoid arthritis, immunodeficiency syndromes

Dermatologic Nail Disorders

Psoriasis

- Patients demonstrate pitting and crumbling of the nail plate, onycholysis, and subungual keratosis (Fig. 28–11).
- Eighty percent of patients with psoriatic arthritis have nail involvement.
- Nail problems cause pain in 52% of patients with psoriatic arthritis and interferes with activities of daily living in 58%, but is often left untreated by physicians (Williamson et al. 2004).
- The nail changes may be confused with infection, and scrapings of the nail should be sent for microscopy and cultures.
- Treatment involves symptomatic excision of loose nails or subungual keratosis.
- Topical steroids, vitamin D analogs, intralesional steroid injections, and topical cyclosporin A solutions have been shown to be effective therapies.

Eczema and Contact Dermatitis

- Chronic inflammation from eczema and contact dermatitis can lead to changes in the nail plate.

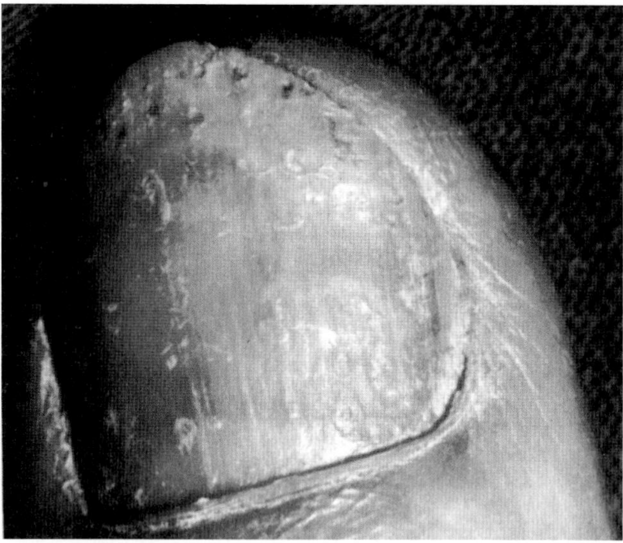

Figure 28–11: **Pitting of nail plate with onycholysis characteristic of psoriasis. (From Jahss MJ. (1991) Disorders of the hallux and the first ray. In: Disorders of the Foot and Ankle: Medical and Surgical Management, 2nd edn (Jahss MJ, ed.). Philadelphia: Saunders. p. 1158.)**

- Frequently involve the skin on the dorsum of toes and the lateral and proximal nail folds.
- With chronicity, transverse ridging, scaling, and discoloration of the nail plate may occur.
- Serous fluid may accumulate under the nail plate and lead to onycholysis.
- First step in treatment is to identify and remove inciting allergens such as nail polish, dyes, and detergents.
- Skin fissuring and dryness may then be treated with topical corticosteroids.

Cutaneous Bacterial Infections

- Can be associated with systemic disorders such as lymphoma, diabetes, or leukemia that compromise the immune system and predisposes to the infection.
- Divided into primary and secondary infections. Primary infections are established and maintained by the particular organism. Secondary infections are initiated and maintained by the dermal environment, typically the web space, as well as the organism.
- Culture and sensitivity should be obtained for most infections to establish appropriate antibiotic coverage.
- *Impetigo* is a primary superficial skin infection characterized by vesicles on an erythematous base. The lesion is caused by *Staphylococcus*, *Streptococcus*, or both and affects younger children, typically sparing the palms and soles. The infection readily responds to systemic antibiotics.
- *Ecthyma* is a primary skin infection characterized by ulcerating pustules or vesicles on an erythematous base secondary to group A β-hemolytic *Streptococcus*. It often occurs on the dorsum of the foot following minor trauma. As with impetigo, the infection readily responds to systemic antibiotics with concurrent topical antibiotics.
- *Infectious eczematoid dermatitis* is a secondary superficial skin infection that results from the spreading infected discharge of a primary cellulitis or pyoderma. Topical and systemic antibiotics are the mainstays of treatment.
- *Infected intertrigo* is a secondary infection that follows the maceration of the skin by moisture and heat in the web spaces. The infection is treated by promoting dryness in the web space and treating with an appropriate topical antibiotic.

References

Bouscarat F, Bouchard C, Bouhour D. (1998) Paronychia and pyogenic granuloma of the great toes in patients treated with indinavir. N Engl J Med 338(24): 1776-1777.

Retrospective case report of 42 HIV-1 patients presenting for treatment of paronychia of the great toe. All patients had been treated with indinavir for varying durations. In six patients with paronychia for 4-13 months, indinavir withdrawal was associated with partial to complete resolution of symptoms.

Fleckman P, Allan C. (2001) Surgical anatomy of the nail unit. Dermatol Surg 27(3): 257-260.

Clinical overview of the pertinent anatomy of the finger and toenail, as well as surgical precautions, with excellent diagrams of nail plate anatomy.

Johnson M, Shuster S. (1993) Continuous formation of nail along the bed. Br J Dermatol 128(3): 277-280.

Histologic study that examined 20 clinically normal big toenails avulsed from 14 men with a mean age of 25, and 6 women with a mean age of 56. Measurement of the nail thickness at multiple, specific anatomical points along the nail showed that rate of increasing thickness of the nail was greatest at the lunula, with 0.13 mm thickness/mm, and slowed along the nail bed, with 0.027 mm/mm. The total contribution to nail plate thickness was 80% for the germinal matrix and 20% for the nail bed.

Kensinger DR, Guille JT, Horn BD et al. (2001) The stubbed great toe: Importance of early recognition and treatment of open fractures of the distal phalanx. J Pediatr Orthop 21(1): 31-34.

Retrospective review of five cases of pediatric patients with open fractures of the distal phalanx of the great toe occurring over 1-year period. The two children whose injuries were recognized and treated early with antibiotics did not develop osteomyelitis. However, three children with delayed diagnoses and treatment developed osteomyelitis. At 10 months (range 9-11) after injury, all five fractures had healed, with no active signs of infection. However, variable growth arrest existed in four of the five children.

Miller-Breslow A, Dorfman HD. (1988) Dupuytren's (subungual) exostosis. Am J Surg Pathol 12(5): 368-378.

Retrospective case series examining 15 patients with subungual exostosis with a mean age of 24.6 years. Reported that 80% of cases occurred in the great toe, lesions typically occur over several months; 13-14% of patients had associated paronychia, and 53% of cases had recurrence after partial excision, whereas none had recurrence after total excision.

Moehrle M, Metzger S, Schippert W et al. (2003) "Functional" surgery in subungual melanoma. Dermatol Surg 29(4): 366-374.
Retrospective review of surgical treatment outcomes for 62 patients with American Joint Committee on Cancer stage 1 and stage 2 subungual melanoma. Thirty-one patients were treated with "functional surgery," in which the distal phalanx was preserved and a median margin of 10 mm was obtained, and 31 patients were treated with traditional surgery, with amputations through the interphalangeal or metatarsophalangeal/metacarpophalangeal joints and attainment of a median margin of 17.5 mm. There was no statistically significant difference in disease-free survival at 5 years for the "functional surgery" when compared with the amputation surgery, with values of 91.7% and 66.5%, respectively.

Nasca MR, Innocenzi D, Micali G. (2004) Subungual squamous cell carcinoma of the toe: Report on three cases. Dermatol Surg 30(2 part 2): 345-348.
Report of three cases of advanced squamous cell carcinoma of the toes. Discusses the presentation of squamous cell carcinoma of the toes, and notes that a standardized treatment protocol is absent.

Pettine KA, Cofield RH, Johnson KA et al. (1988) Ingrown toenail: Results of surgical treatment. Foot Ankle 9(3): 130-134.
One hundred patients with 142 ingrown toes were treated with five different surgical options and observed for a mean of 9.7 years. The study demonstrated that plastic nail reduction was effective for mild disease (stage 1 or early stage 2), with 0% recurrence; chemical ablation had a recurrence of 20%; marginal nail excision with nail matrix excision had a recurrence of 6%; nail ablation with matrix excision had a recurrence of 33%; and terminal amputation had a recurrence of 12%.

Richardson EG, Hendrix CL. (2003) Disorders of nails and skin. In: Campbell's Operative Orthopaedics, 10th edn (Canale ST, ed.). Philadelphia: Mosby. pp. 4171-4187.
Summary chapter on the various surgical and non-surgical options for the treatment of ingrown toenails. The chapter details each treatment and provides information on the recurrence rate of each approach.

Seaberg DC, Angelos WJ, Paris PM. (1991) Treatment of subungual hematomas with nail trephination: A prospective study. Am J Emerg Med 9(3): 209-210.
In a prospective study, 48 patients with subungual hematoma with an intact nail plate were treated with nail trephination. The subungual hematoma size was noted, and x-rays were obtained to detect distal phalanx fractures. During an average follow-up of 10.3 ± 4.3 months, no infections, osteomyelitis, or major nail deformities in any of the patients occurred. The authors argue that subungual hematomas with intact nail plates, regardless of size or distal phalanx fracture, should be treated only with nail trephination.

Sigurgeirsson B, Olafsson JH, Steinsson JB et al. (2002) Long-term effectiveness of treatment with terbinafine vs itraconazole in onychomycosis: A 5-year blinded prospective follow-up study. Arch Dermatol 138(3): 353-357.
In a prior randomized, placebo-controlled study, 496 patients were observed for 18 months after treatment with either terbinafine or itraconazole for onychomycosis. Between 75 and 80% of terbinafine recipients and 38-49% of itraconazole recipients in that study were mycologically cured, defined by negative microscopic and culture results. The Icelandic cohort of 151 patients from the prior study was followed for a further 5 years in this study. Only 46% of the terbinafine-treated patients and 13% of the itraconazole-treated patients remained disease-free at the end of the study, suggesting that relapses and reinfections were common despite one-time treatment.

Simon RR, Wolgin M. (1987) Subungual hematoma: Association with occult laceration requiring repair. Am J Emerg Med 5(4): 302-304.
X-rays and nail bed examinations were performed on 47 consecutive patients with subungual hematoma involving more than 25% of the nail bed. In those patients with an associated fracture, all had a laceration of the nail bed > 3 mm, defined as requiring repair by the authors. Patients with a subungual hematoma greater than 50% of the nail bed had a 60% incidence of a laceration requiring repair. The authors recommended that patients with a subungual hematoma involving greater than one-half of the nail surface and a fracture of the distal phalanx should have the nail lifted and the nail bed explored and repaired.

Williamson L, Dalbeth N, Dockerty JL et al. (2004) Extended report: Nail disease in psoriatic arthritis—clinically important, potentially treatable and often overlooked. Rheumatology (Oxford) 43(6): 790-794.
Sixty-nine patients with psoriatic arthritis were evaluated in a retrospective study through physical examination and questionnaires to assess a relationship between severity of nail disease and severity of psoriatic arthritis, as well as to distinguish patterns in clinical management of psoriatic nail disease. Results showed that 83% of patients had clinical evidence of psoriatic nail disease. Although 96% of patients had been treated for the skin disease, only 1% had received treatment for nail problems. Severity of nail disease was found to be directly correlated to severity of joint involvement and prevalence of anxiety and depression.

Zook EG. (2003) Anatomy and physiology of the perionychium. Clin Anat 16(1): 1-8.
Thorough review of the basic anatomy of each area of the nail, with discussion of the relevant physiology. Some clinical correlation offered.

CHAPTER 29

Enhancement of Bone Healing

Rahul Banerjee[*] and Christopher W. DiGiovanni[§]

[*]M.D., Clinical Instructor, Department of Orthopaedic Surgery, Texas Tech University Health Sciences Center, Interm Chief of Orthopaedic Trauma, William Beaumont Army Medical Center, El Paso, Texas, and Chief of Orthopaedics, 49th Medical Group, Holloman Air Force Base, New Mexico.
[§]M.D., Associate Professor, Chief, Foot and Ankle Service, Department of Orthopaedic Surgery, Brown Medical School, Rhode Island Hospital, Providence, RI

- At least 6 million fractures occur annually in the USA. Approximately 5-10% of these fractures will proceed to non-union or delayed union, resulting in severe consequences for patient and society. Non-union resulting from the failure of surgical arthrodesis is also a difficult situation.
- Many technologies exist to enhance bone healing, including internal fixation, bone grafts, bone graft substitutes, growth factors, and biophysical stimulation. Knowledge of methods to enhance bone healing is essential in order for the surgeon to succeed and minimize complications.

Factors Affecting Bone Healing and Fracture Repair

- A number of factors can disrupt bone healing and fracture repair. High-energy *trauma* with associated soft tissue damage results in injury to the vascular envelope surrounding the bone (Fig. 29–1). Such soft tissue injury can result in suboptimal fracture healing. In addition to careful soft tissue handling, rigid stabilization provides the best environment for soft tissue healing.
- Infection compromises the ability of bone to heal. Infection may be the result of severe trauma, as described above, or may be acquired by other routes. In order to improve bone healing in the setting of infection, the surgeon must follow two principles.
  - First, it is imperative that the underlying infection is treated with the appropriate antibiotics and complete debridement of all devitalized tissue.
  - Second, the affected region must be stabilized. Instability coupled with infection provides the worst environment for bone healing.
- Patients with *peripheral vascular disease* are also at risk for poor bone healing. Prior to surgery, vascular studies should be obtained, and if necessary revascularization procedures should precede orthopaedic surgical procedures.
- Optimizing the *nutrition* of a patient is one of the prerequisites to obtaining bone healing. Many patients suffer from poor nutrition, particularly the trauma patient, the elderly, and the chronically ill. Physical examination findings (Box 29–1) and laboratory indices (Table 29–1) can be used to monitor the nutritional status of the patient. Nutritional supplementation and involvement of hospital nutritional support services are important adjuncts to enhance bone healing.
- The diabetic patient poses a special problem in bone healing. The nature of *diabetes* and its multiple associated complications (e.g. peripheral vascular disease, neuropathy, increased risk of infection) all require specific management. The following measures should be adopted to optimize bone healing.
  - Following closed or surgical treatment of lower extremity fractures, diabetics should be kept non-weight bearing for approximately twice the amount of time as non-diabetic patients.

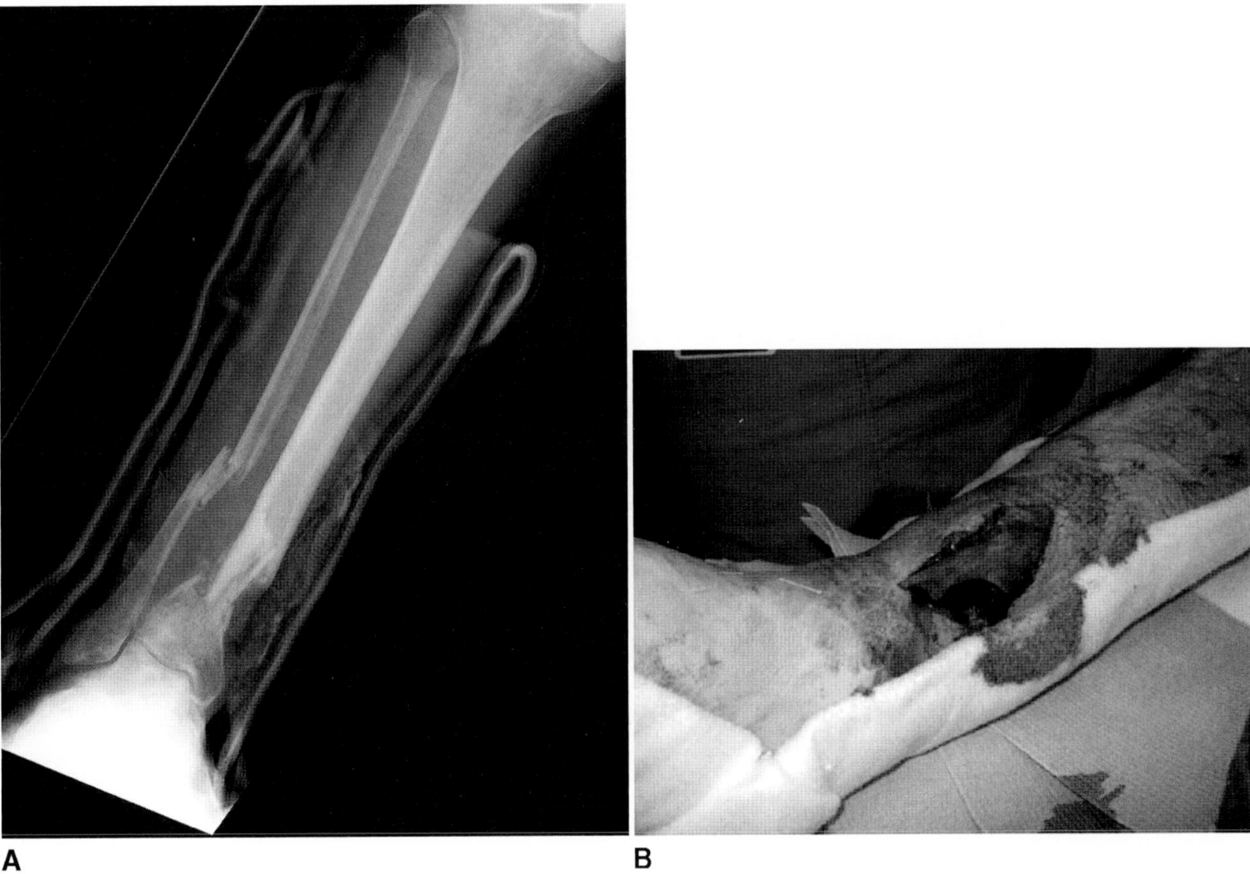

Figure 29–1: Severe soft tissue injury. This 50-year-old man fell off a roof and sustained this contaminated open distal tibia fracture. The high-energy nature of the injury and the severe damage and contamination of the soft tissues are evident from the clinical photograph.

Box 29–1 Physical Examination Findings Consistent With Nutritional Compromise

- General weakness
- Edema
- Pallor
- Ulcers
- Petechiae
- Ecchymoses
- Brittle hair
- Scaly, dry, or greasy skin
- Hyperpigmentation
- Poor skin turgor
- Fissured, beefy red tongue
- Fissured or inflamed lips
- Ulceration of lips or oral mucosa
- Nail abnormalities

Table 29–1: Laboratory Indexes to Monitor Nutrition

	NORMAL VALUE[a]	HALF-LIFE (DAYS)	MEASUREMENT
Albumin	3.5-5 mg/dL	18-21	Laboratory test
Prealbumin	15.7-29.6 mg/dL	2.5-3	Laboratory test
Transferrin	250-300 mg/dL	8-10	Laboratory test
Total lymphocyte count	> 2000	–	Percentage of lymphocytes/100 × white blood cells

[a]Normal values vary depending on which assay is used by the laboratory.

- Blood glucose should be optimized before, during, and after surgery.
- Diabetic patients should be trained in the routine examination of their feet and ankles, as neuropathy often prevents the early detection of sores.
    - Additional measures to ensure rigid fixation of fractures should be adopted (Fig. 29–2).
- *Smoking* diminishes the ability of bone to heal effectively. Patients should be counseled to stop all forms of nicotine use in order to enhance bone healing. Nicotine has been

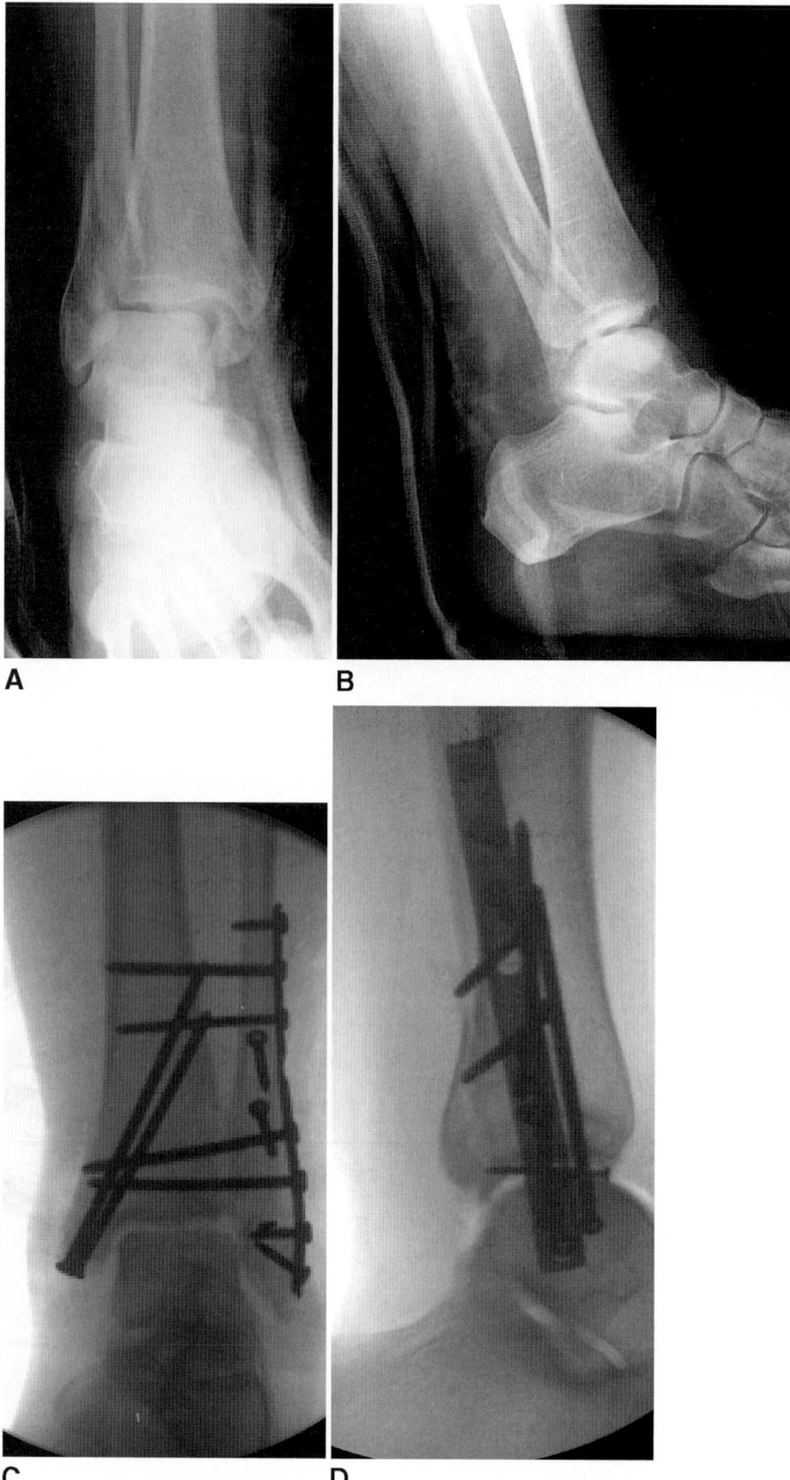

Figure 29–2: Management of lower extremity fractures in diabetics. **A** and **B**, This 56-year-old insulin-dependent diabetic patient sustained a closed ankle fracture. **C** and **D**, The patient was treated with open reduction and internal fixation. In this case, healing was augmented with extra fixation—specifically, fixation of the fibula to the tibia at multiple levels, and use of fully threaded bicortical screws for treatment of the medial malleolus fracture. Postoperatively, the patient remained non-weight bearing for 3 months.

demonstrated to interfere with vascularity and diminish fracture healing. Therefore nicotine substitutes (patches, chewing gum, etc.) should also be avoided. Antidepressants have been shown to be useful in patients who agree to cooperate with a program of smoking cessation.

- Finally, preservation of the vascular supply of bone requires careful attention from the operating surgeon. Use of surgical techniques that preserve periosteal blood supply and minimize bone stripping will help to enhance bone healing. The perils of iatrogenic insult to the vascular supply of bone are illustrated in Figure 29–3.

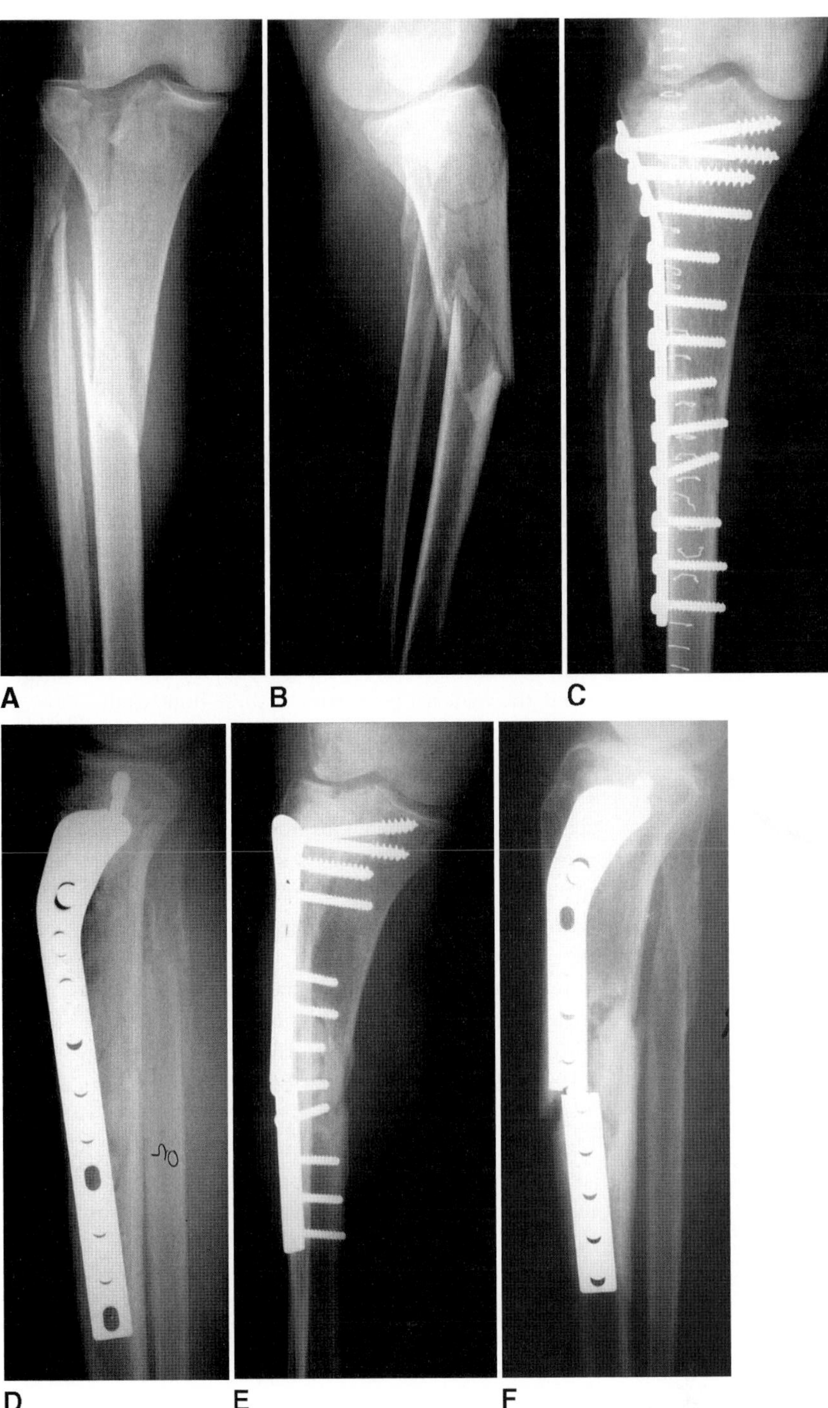
Figure 29–3: Peril of iatrogenic insult to the vascular supply of bone. The peril of iatrogenic injury to the blood supply at a fracture site is evident from this case. The injury films (**A** and **B**) demonstrate a midshaft tibia fracture, which was treated with open reduction and internal fixation (**C** and **D**) with direct exposure of the fracture site and extensive soft tissue stripping. The patient went on to develop a non-union (**E** and **F**), and eventually the plate failed.

Augmentation of Bone Healing and Fracture Repair

- The "gold standard" for enhancement of bone healing remains autogenous iliac crest bone graft.
- Bone grafts and bone graft substitutes can be broadly categorized by their properties.
  - *Osteoconductive* materials provide a temporary or permanent porous scaffold for bone ingrowth.
  - *Osteoinductive* materials influence the process by which primitive, pluripotential mesenchymal stem cells are

induced to mature into osteoprogenitor cells with bone-forming capacity.
- *Osteogenic* or *osteoproductive* materials contain osteoblasts or osteoblast precursors, which are able to form bone if placed in the appropriate environment.

Enhancing Bone Healing Through Osteoconductive Methods

- Osteoconductive materials must have structural and surface properties that favor the ingrowth of bone. The ideal osteoconductive material is adult human cancellous bone. The important structural properties that aid osteoconduction in human cancellous bone are:
  - porosity of 70-80%
  - mean trabecular width of 200 μm
  - an average intertrabecular pore size of 500 μm
  - ample pore interconnections.
- In order to maintain strength, most bone graft substitutes cannot reach porosity greater than 50%. An ideal material is inert, but the surface is osteophilic in order to attract the bone-forming osteoblasts.
- Materials that are osteoconductive include allogeneic bone grafts, ceramics, and bioactive glass.

Allogeneic Bone Grafts

- Allogeneic bone grafts are available in multiple forms, including cancellous grafts, cortical grafts, and osteochondral grafts. Allografts are helpful in avoiding the morbidity and complications associated with autogenous graft harvest. Furthermore, allograft bone can be used to supplement limited quantities of autogenous bone graft. Disadvantages include cost, lack of osteoinductive properties, and potential for disease transmission.
- Incorporation rate of allograft is slower than that of autograft. Incomplete remodeling and incorporation of corticocancellous allograft and osteochondral allograft has been seen as late as 7 years after implantation.
- Osteochondral (osteoarticular) allografts are available as whole bone or joint segments for reconstruction in situations of bone and/or cartilage loss, or limb salvage following tumor resection. Osteochondral allografts are osteoconductive and provide immediate structural support.
- Osteochondral allografts are available as fresh frozen grafts or fresh allografts without preservation. Fresh frozen allografts are prepared with a slow freezing process with a cryopreservative in order to maintain cartilage. This process yields 20-70% chondrocyte viability. Fresh allografts avoid the freezing process but can incite an extensive immune response. The advantages and disadvantages of the different allograft preparations are summarized in Table 29–2.
- Osteochondral allografts are associated with relatively high rates of non-union (10%), fracture (10%), and infection (15%).

Ceramics

- Ceramics and ceramic composites represent the majority of bone graft substitutes that are currently available. The material structure of ceramics is composed of individual crystals of highly oxidized substances that have been fused together.
- The first bone graft substitutes to be introduced to the market were crystalline hydroxyapatites. Obtained from coral, the material properties of these bone graft substitutes were very similar to those of human cancellous bone (pore diameter of 200-500 μm). Crystalline hydroxyapatite has a compressive strength similar to that of cancellous bone. The material is not resorbed by osteoclasts and is therefore not remodeled. As it remains in the bone as a permanent implant, there is a small risk that the grafted region may be subject to repeat fractures.
- Clinical studies have demonstrated that crystalline hydroxyapatites are equivalent to autologous bone graft for treatment of depressed tibial plateau fractures.
  - Both allow a small amount of settling of the articular surface during healing.
- Unlike hydroxyapatites, calcium sulfate grafts are highly soluble and are completely resorbed with bone remodeling. Although they may have some use in filling bone defects and cysts, limited information about their effectiveness and safety is available.
- Calcium phosphate ceramics are brittle and demonstrate poor tensile strength. These materials are useful in filling contained bone defects or in supporting the articular

Table 29–2: Characteristics of Allografts

TYPE	IMMUNOGENICITY	TORQUE STRENGTH	OSTEOCONDUCTIVE OR OSTEOINDUCTIVE?	CHONDROCYTE VIABILITY	RISK OF DISEASE TRANSMISSION
Fresh	High	High	Both	High	Intermediate (more than two cases of HIV transmission reported)
Fresh frozen	Minimal	High	Osteoconductive	20-70%	Low
Freeze-dried	Lowest	Intermediate	Osteoconductive	None	Low

surface fragments. Bony ingrowth is promoted by packing this material tightly into defects.

- Tricalcium phosphate is partially converted into hydroxyapatite once it is implanted. However, tricalcium phosphate is more porous than hydroxyapatite, and as a result it is resorbed faster after implantation. This results in a construct that is weaker in compression than hydroxyapatite alone. However, after conversion the hydroxyapatite remains in place for years and is remodeled slowly. Tricalcium phosphate is therefore incorporated quickly but remodeled slowly, and can provide support for longer periods of time.
- Injectable calcium phosphates are also available. For example, Skeletal Repair System (Norian, Cupertino, CA) is an injectable paste of inorganic calcium and phosphate. This material cures isothermically and hardens within minutes. This material provides some immediate structural support and is gradually resorbed and replaced by host bone.
  - There is some limited evidence to suggest these substances are better than autograft at providing subchondral support for tibial plateau fractures.
- Collagen can also function as an osteoconductive graft due to its three-dimensional structure. However, because collagen can bind circulating growth factors, it may also have osteoinductive properties. Collagen does not provide structural support, but it can be mixed with autogenous graft in order to expand graft volume.

Bioactive Glasses

- Bioactive glasses are another class of osteoconductive compounds that may help to enhance fracture healing.
- The components of these glass beads include silica and pyrophosphate, which allow the beads to bond to collagen, growth factors, and fibrin. The resulting matrix allows for the infiltration of osteogenic cells, and may provide some compressive strength.
- The ability of bioactive glass to bind to growth factors also makes it an attractive delivery system for growth factors.

Enhancing Bone Healing Through Osteoinductive Methods

- Osteoinduction is the process by which primitive, pluripotential mesenchymal stem cells are induced to mature into osteoprogenitor cells with bone-forming capacity.
- The process of osteoinduction is mediated by various growth factors and cytokines. A number of these growth factors may have potential in the enhancement of bone healing. The information regarding the growth factors and cytokines is summarized in Table 29–3.

Transforming Growth Factor-β

- TGF-β is a protein that is found in a number of tissues but is in higher concentrations in bone, platelets, and cartilage. TGF-β is a pleiotropic growth factor and affects a large number of processes, including growth, differentiation, and extracellular matrix synthesis.
- A number of animal studies have demonstrated the capacity of TGF-β to enhance fracture healing. These studies, however, are limited by the fact that different isoforms of TGF-β were used. Furthermore, the studies seem to indicate that frequent or high doses of the protein were needed to demonstrate efficacy. Finally, TGF-β enhances cellular proliferation among multiple cell types. These reasons may limit the usefulness of TGF-β in a clinical setting.

Fibroblast Growth Factors

- The FGFs are a family of nine related polypeptides that stimulate angiogenesis and mitogenesis. FGF-1 (α-FGF) and FGF-2 (β-FGF) are the two most abundant FGFs in normal adult tissue. Both of these forms promote growth and differentiation of a number of different cells. FGF-1 has been associated with chondrocyte proliferation. FGF-2 is more potent and is expressed by osteoblasts.
- Animal studies, including non-human primate studies, have demonstrated the ability of recombinant human FGF-2 to enhance fracture healing.
- FGF may have a future role in enhancement of fracture healing in the clinical setting.

Platelet-derived Growth Factor

- PDGF is secreted by platelets in the early phases of fracture healing. It has been identified at fracture sites in both mice and humans.
- PDGF has been shown to be mitogenic for osteoblasts in in vitro studies. PDGF has also been shown to be chemotactic, attracting inflammatory cells to fracture sites.
- Limited animal studies suggest that PDGF may play a role in the enhancement of fracture healing, but clinical studies have yet to be completed.

Growth Hormones and Insulin-like Growth Factors

- GHs and IGFs play a critical role in skeletal development and growth. GH is released by the anterior lobe of the pituitary gland in response to GH-releasing hormone. GH then travels to the liver and skeletal growth plates, where it stimulates its target cells to release IGF.
- Two IGFs have been identified. IGF-2 is the most abundant in bone. IGF-1 is more potent and has been localized to healing fractures in rats and humans.
- Animal studies have suggested that GH and IGF-1 may play a role in fracture healing, particularly in the enhancement of intramembranous ossification.

Parathyroid Hormone and Parathyroid Hormone-related Polypeptide

- PTH and PTHrP may play a role in fracture healing. Continuous exposure to PTH results in bone resorption,

Table 29–3: Growth Factors

GROWTH FACTOR	SOURCE	MECHANISM	ANIMAL STUDIES	CLINICAL TRIALS
Transforming growth factor-β	Platelets Bone ECM Cartilage ECM	Pleiotropic growth factor Induces ECM formation	Increases callus formation Enhances bone content of callus	No randomized clinical trials specifically studying bone healing
Fibroblast growth factor	Macrophages Mesenchymal cells Chondrocytes Osteoblasts	Angiogenic Mitogenic for mesenchymal cells, chondrocytes, osteoblasts	Enhances bone formation by intramembranous ossification Stimulates callus remodeling	No randomized clinical trials specifically studying bone healing
Platelet-derived growth factor	Platelets Osteoblasts	Mitogenic for osteoblasts Inflammatory cell chemotaxis	Increases callus formation and density	No randomized clinical trials specifically studying bone healing
Growth hormone/insulin-like growth factors	Pituitary gland	Induces bone cell proliferation Induces ECM proliferation	Enhances intramembranous ossification	Multiple studies showing positive but minimal effect of growth hormone on maintaining bone mineral density (?clinical significance) No randomized clinical trials specifically studying bone healing
Parathyroid hormone/-parathyroid hormone-related polypeptide	Parathyroid gland	Increases osteoblast number and activity Induces interleukin-6 production Stimulates chondrocyte differentiation	Increases concentration of insulin-like growth factor-1 and transforming growth hormone-β in bone Increases bone density in dose-dependent manner	Increases bone mass and decreases fracture rate No randomized clinical trials specifically studying bone healing
Prostaglandins	Released from traumatized bone and soft tissue	Stimulates type 1 collagen synthesis	Enhances bone formation Improves callus strength and size	No randomized clinical trials specifically studying bone healing
Bone morphogenetic protein	Osteoprogenitor cells Bone ECM	Promotes differentiation of mesenchymal cells into chondrocytes and osteoblasts	Used to heal bone defects in non-human primate models	Three randomized clinical trials: tibial non-unions (Friedlaender et al. 2001), spine fusion (Burkus et al. 2002), open tibial fractures (BMP-2 Evaluation in Surgery for Tibial Trauma Study Group 2002)

ECM, extracellular matrix.

yet administration at intermittent doses results in bone formation by increasing osteoblast number and activity. Clinical trials have demonstrated the anabolic action of PTH. Patients with osteoporosis who were treated with PTH demonstrated an increase in bone mass and a reduced fracture rate.

- In vitro, PTHrP induces interleukin-6 production by osteoblasts, and stimulates chondrocyte differentiation. Animal studies have demonstrated that PTH increases the concentration of IGF-1 and TGF-β in bone. In animal models of fracture healing, PTH increases the bone density in a dose-dependent manner, leading to faster repair and better fixation.

Prostaglandins

- Prostaglandins are released from traumatized bone and soft tissue, and stimulate the production of IGF.
- Animal studies suggest that prostaglandins stimulate the production of type 1 collagen.
- Prostaglandins may have a regulatory effect on fracture callus formation. Indomethacin has been reported to inhibit prostaglandins, resulting in fracture callus weakness.
- The role of prostaglandins in fracture healing needs further investigation.

Bone Morphogenetic Proteins

- BMP was initially described when Marshall R. Urist (1965) discovered that the extracellular matrix of bone contained a substance that could induce new bone formation when transplanted into extraskeletal sites. This substance was subsequently identified and named bone morphogenetic protein.
- Both BMP and TGF-β belong to a family of related proteins known as the TGF-β superfamily. At least 15 different forms of BMP have been identified. BMP-2, -4, and -7 are known to stimulate mesenchymal cells into the osteoblastic lineage.
- Critical-sized bone defects have been treated with BMP in animal models. Recombinant human BMP (rhBMP)-7 was used to effectively heal segmental ulnar and tibial defects in a non-human primate model. A number of

additional animal models support the role of rhBMP as a means of enhancing fracture healing.

- At time of writing, only three randomized clinical trials have supported the use of rhBMP.
  - A prospective randomized trial of 124 tibial non-unions was conducted with the use of rhBMP-7 (osteogenic protein [OP]-1). Patients treated with OP-1 showed equivalent radiographic and clinical healing to those treated with autogenous bone grafting (Friedlaender et al. 2001).
  - rhBMP-2 was used in a randomized, non-blinded, multicenter trial of single-level lumbar spine interbody fusion. Patients treated with rhBMP-2 demonstrated a higher fusion rate and also had decreased operative time and blood loss when compared with control subjects who did not receive rhBMP-2 (Burkus et al. 2002).
  - The BMP-2 Evaluation in Surgery for Tibial Trauma Study Group (2002) randomized 450 patients with open tibial shaft fractures to receive either standard treatment with debridement and intramedullary nailing, or debridement and nailing combined with high-dose or low-dose rhBMP-2. The results showed a 44% risk reduction for a secondary intervention in patients treated with rhBMP-2. Compared with the standard treatment group, patients who received high-dose BMP had faster healing, fewer infections, and fewer hardware failures.

Demineralized Bone Matrix

- DBM is based on Marshall Urist's original discovery that the extracellular matrix of bone could be used to stimulate new bone formation in extraskeletal tissue.
- When bone is demineralized in 0.5 N HCl, the result is DBM. The composition of DBM is 90% type 1 collagen and 10% non-collagen proteins, including growth factors and cytokines such as BMPs.
- DBM offers no structural support but is quickly revascularized when implanted. DBM is both osteoconductive and osteoinductive.
- The effects of DBM vary widely from donor to donor. Because of this variation, and due to safety reasons, the American Association of Tissue Banks and the US Food and Drug Administration require each batch of DBM to be obtained from a single human donor.
- The effects of DBM are further affected by the processing, storage, and sterilization procedures.
- DBM has been used successfully to treat contained skeletal defects such as bone cysts. Combined with stable fixation, DBM has also been used to treat long bone non-unions and acute defects in fractures. Autogenous bone marrow or even allograft combined with DBM may also have promise as a successful graft material. Finally, DBM can be used to augment the volume of autogenous bone graft when quantities are limited.
- To date, there are no randomized, controlled, prospective studies demonstrating the efficacy of DBM.

Synthetic Polymers

- Polylactic acid and polyglycolic acid have been used in absorbable suture material and in resorbable plates and screws. There may be future potential for use of these materials as carriers for growth factors.

Enhancing Bone Healing Through Osteogenic Methods

- Osteogenic materials include autogenous bone graft and autogenous bone marrow graft. Use of these materials combines the advantages of osteoinduction and osteoconduction. The structural properties of cancellous bone provide the ideal environment for osteoconduction. In addition, harvest of these materials may result in transfer of the bone matrix, which has osteoinductive properties.

Autogenous Bone Grafts

- Autogenous bone grafts have osteogenic properties in addition to varying degrees of osteoconductive and osteoinductive properties. The advantages of autogenous bone grafts include their well-described success rate, low risk of diseases transmission, and histocompatibility. Disadvantages include donor site morbidity and the limited quantity of autogenous graft.
- Four types of autogenous bone grafts are readily obtained for use: cancellous grafts, vascularized cortical grafts, non-vascularized cortical grafts, and autogenous bone marrow grafts. The different features of these grafts are summarized in Table 29–4.

Table 29–4: Properties of Autogenous Bone Grafts

GRAFT TYPE	OSTEOCONDUCTIVE	OSTEOINDUCTIVE	OSTEOGENIC	*IMMEDIATE*	*STRENGTH*[a] *6 MONTHS*	*1 YEAR*
Cancellous	++++	++	Yes	–	++	+++
Vascularized cortical	+	±	Yes	+++	+++	+++
Non-vascularized cortical	+	±	No	+++	+++	+++
Bone marrow	–	+++	Yes	n/a	n/a	n/a

[a]n/a, not applicable.
(After Finkemeier CG. (2002) Bone-grafting and bone-graft substitutes. J Bone Joint Surg Am 84: 454-464.)

- New bone formation from autogenous grafts occurs in two stages. During the first 4 weeks, cells from the graft are the main source of new bone formation. In the second phase, host cells contribute to the process.
- Autogenous cancellous graft is rapidly revascularized but does not provide structural support. It does, however, incorporate quickly and achieve strength comparably with that of cortical bone within 6-12 months. Incorporation of cancellous autograft occurs in three phases, as described in Table 29–5. Cancellous graft acts as primarily an *osteoconductive* substrate by supporting ingrowth of new blood vessels and the infiltration of osteoprogenitor cells. Although cancellous graft probably has *osteoinductive* properties, the activity of inductive growth factors in cancellous graft has never been demonstrated. Cancellous autograft can be obtained from a number of locations (Box 29–2).
- Autogenous cortical graft has different properties depending on whether it is harvested with its blood supply. Autogenous cortical grafts are primarily *osteoconductive*. However, particularly with vascularized grafts, the surviving autografts provide some osteogenic properties as well.
- Autogenous cortical grafts provide structural support at the recipient site. Vascularized cortical grafts maintain their structural support longer than non-vascularized grafts, which are generally resorbed and revascularized by 6 weeks after implantation. During the first 6 weeks after implantation, vascularized grafts provide stronger structural support. By 6-12 months, the strength of these grafts is equivalent.
- Autogenous cortical grafts can be used in cases of segmental bone defects. For typical defects, non-vascularized grafts may be used. Failure rates increase when the defects are greater than 12 cm. In these cases, vascularized grafts or bone transport may provide superior results.
- Autogenous iliac crest bone grafting continues to be the standard by which all other methods of bone grafting are judged. However, bone graft harvesting is associated with a major and minor complication rate of 8.6 and 20.6%. This complication rate, combined with the morbidity of bone graft harvesting procedures, has led many to consider bone graft substitutes.

Table 29–5: Three Phases of Incorporation of Cancellous Autograft

	PHASE	EVENT(S)	TIME PERIOD
1	Osteoconduction	0-3 weeks	
2	New bone formation and osteoclastic resorption	3-12 weeks	
3	Remodeling and reorientation of trabeculae	3-6 months	

Box 29–2 Potential Locations for Obtaining Cancellous Bone Graft

- Anterior iliac crest
- Posterior iliac crest
- Greater trochanter
- Distal lateral femoral metaphysis
- Gerdy's tubercle (proximal lateral tibial metaphysis)
- Medial distal tibial metaphysis
- Distal radius
- Distal tibia
- Calcaneus

Autogenous Bone Marrow Grafts

- Autogenous bone marrow grafts provide the surgeon with a source of osteogenic cells in addition to the *osteoinductive* properties of the cytokines and growth factors secreted by the transplanted bone marrow cells. Bone marrow can be aspirated from the iliac crest and transplanted to a fracture or arthrodesis site in order to stimulate healing.
- Marrow injection can be performed percutaneously with fluoroscopic guidance. Smaller defects (< 5 cm) and mechanical stability are prerequisites for success. Combination of bone marrow aspirate with carriers such as bone graft substitutes may provide an optimal method of delivery.
- Most recently, several case series have examined treatment of nonunions with injection of concentrated marrow aspirates. Results have been variable and may depend on the quality of progenitor cells aspirated.

Enhancement of Bone Healing Using Physical Forces

- In 1957, Fukada and Yasuda described the "piezoelectric potentials" that were generated by mechanical stress on the crystalline structure of bone. This has led to the theory that strain-generated electrical potentials may be a regulatory signal for cellular processes of bone formation.
- Two main modalities of physical force application are available for use: electromagnetic fields and ultrasound.
- Contraindications for use of physical forces to enhance fracture healing include unacceptable deformity that requires surgical correction, synovial pseudoarthrosis, and large gaps.

Electromagnetic Fields

- Electromagnetic fields can be applied through three different methods: direct electrical current (DC), capacitive coupling (CC), and inductive coupling (using a pulsed electromagnetic field, PEMF).
- DC is applied to bone through surgically implanted electrodes. Early research indicated that pO_2 is lowered and pH is raised near the cathode. A low-oxygen environment favors bone formation, and therefore for DC applications the cathode is placed into the site of bone healing. The anode is placed in nearby soft tissues. A constant current is applied to the bone for several months.
- DC decreases the O_2 concentration and stimulates collagen and proteoglycan synthesis.

- Clinical studies of tibial, humeral, and clavicular non-unions using DC all demonstrated favorable results for treatment of non-unions. Studies of DC techniques in enhancing spinal fusion have consistently shown 90-95% union rates, compared with 75-85% in the untreated control groups.
- DC eliminates the variable of patient compliance. However, the disadvantage of DC is that it requires surgical implantation of the cathode.
- DC is indicated in the treatment of established non-unions and for use in spinal fusion.
- CC is applied by placing skin electrodes on opposite sides of the bone that is to be stimulated. The induced field is the result of an oscillating electric current.
- CC has been demonstrated to increase bone cell proliferation, activate voltage-gated calcium channels, increase levels of prostaglandin E_2 and calcium, and increase the production of TGF-β mRNA.
- Clinical studies have shown effectiveness of CC in treatment of non-unions and enhancement of spinal fusion.
- CC may cause a mild skin reaction at the site of application of the electrodes. This method also requires patient compliance in order to work effectively.
- CC is indicated for non-unions of long bones and the scaphoid, and for enhancement of spinal fusion.
- Inductive coupling with a PEMF was developed in order to mirror the endogenous electrical fields produced by bone in response to strain. An external time-varying or PEMF is applied near the target bone. The external field induces a secondary electrical field in the bone.
- PEMF has been demonstrated to increase chondrogenesis, up-regulate the production of TGF-β, and increase mRNA for BMP-2 and BMP-4.
- At least 20 randomized trials have studied the effect of electrical and electromagnetic stimulation on bone repair. The majority of these trials used PEMF. Metaanalysis of these trials demonstrated a pooled difference of 0.26 in 765 combined cases, which supports the effectiveness of these techniques (Akai and Hayashi 2002). Inductive coupling techniques used in enhancement of spinal fusion have reported success rates of 75-92%.
- Gossling et al. (1992) reviewed the effectiveness of electric and electromagnetic stimulation of non-unions and delayed unions in a comprehensive review paper. Although a formal meta-analysis was not performed, the authors compared 28 studies of un-united tibia fractures with 14 studies of similar fractures treated with bone grafting with or without internal fixation. The combined results of these studies showed an 82% success rate for the surgical treatment of these tibial nonunions, compared with an 81% success rate for PEMF treatment.
- Modified PEMF was developed to reduce the energy requirements of standard PEMF. The devices used in modified PEMF are smaller. In vitro studies suggest that modified PEMF may work by stimulating neovascularization or "sprouting" of the blood vessels in endothelial tissue. Multicenter randomized trials of modified PEMF in the treatment of non-unions and spinal fusion have been favorable.
- The use of combined magnetic fields (CMFs) is based on the observation that combined dynamic and static magnetic fields affect ion transport across membranes and affect ion-dependent cell signaling. Combined alternate current and DC magnetic fields have been shown to have effects on calcium ion transport and cell proliferation. In vitro studies have also shown that CMFs can result in the increase of IGF-1 and IGF-2.
- Clinical studies have demonstrated a role for CMF in the treatment of nonunions and as an adjunctive device for spinal fusions.

Ultrasound

- In 1953, Corradi and Cozzolino used continuous wave ultrasound to stimulate fracture healing, resulting in an increase in callus formation (Corradi and Cozzolino 1953).
- Medical ultrasound has a variety of applications. Higher intensity ultrasound (5-300 W/cm^2) is used for diagnostic tools, surgical instruments, fragmentation of renal calculi, cataract ablation, and cement removal. Enhancement of bone healing utilizes low-intensity ultrasound (1-50 mW/cm^2).
- A variety of mechanisms have been suggested to explain how ultrasound enhances bone healing. In vitro studies have shown that ultrasound increases the influx and efflux of potassium, increases the level of calcium, stimulates adenylate cyclase activity, and increases the production of a number of cytokines and growth factors (TGF-β, prostaglandin E_2, and PDGF).
- Randomized, controlled clinical studies have shown that ultrasound can reduce the healing time in tibia and distal radius fractures. Additional studies have shown a role for ultrasound in decreasing the healing time in smokers, diabetic patients, patients with renal insufficiency, and patients on steroids.

Enhancement of Bone Healing in the Foot and Ankle

- Although iliac crest bone graft continues to be considered the gold standard for enhancement of fracture healing, the procedure is not without morbidity. During the initial postoperative period, at least 25% of patients undergoing foot and ankle surgery report that the pain at the iliac crest harvest site is more painful than the operative site. The ipsilateral proximal tibia, the distal tibia, or the calcaneus provides an alternative.
- There is anecdotal support for the use of bone graft substitutes in lower extremity reconstruction.
  - Scranton (2002) reported results of bone graft substitutes in the foot and ankle. Twenty-four of the 28 patients had a successful primary operation.
  - Weinraub and Cheung (2003) reported on 39 foot and ankle procedures in which they implanted

allograft tricortical iliac crest or DBM. Thirty-eight of 39 procedures were successful, with only 1 non-union.
  - Bibbo et al. (2005) showed a union rate of 94% with use of autologous platelet concentrate.
- Physical forces may also be useful in treating difficult foot and ankle problems.
  - CMF was used to treat patients in a prospective, randomized study of patients with acute, stage 1 Charcot neuropathy. The mean time to consolidation in the CMF group was 11.1 weeks, compared with 23.2 weeks in the control group (Hanft et al. 1998).
  - In another study, 13 patients with major risk factors for non-union were treated with an implantable electrical stimulator that was placed at the time of their hindfoot fusion. Successful fusion was achieved in 12 of 13 patients (Donley and Ward 2002).
- Many of these techniques can be applied in combination to address problems with bone healing in the lower extremity (Fig. 29–4).

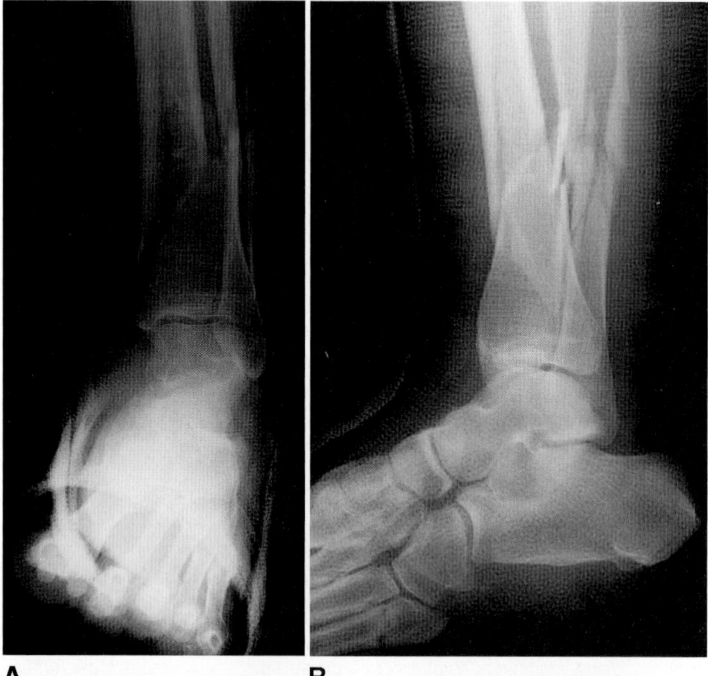

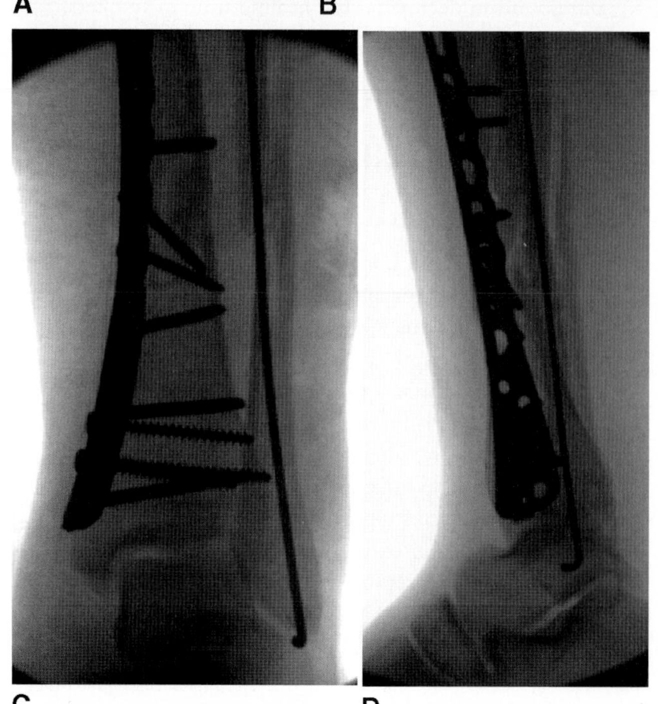

Figure 29–4: **Treatment of an infected non-union. Different methods of enhancement of bone healing can be used in combination, with successful results. This 52-year-old woman sustained a closed comminuted distal tibia and fibula fracture (A and B), and was treated with open reduction and internal fixation with a distal tibial locking plate and intramedullary fixation for her fibula (C and D).**

Continued

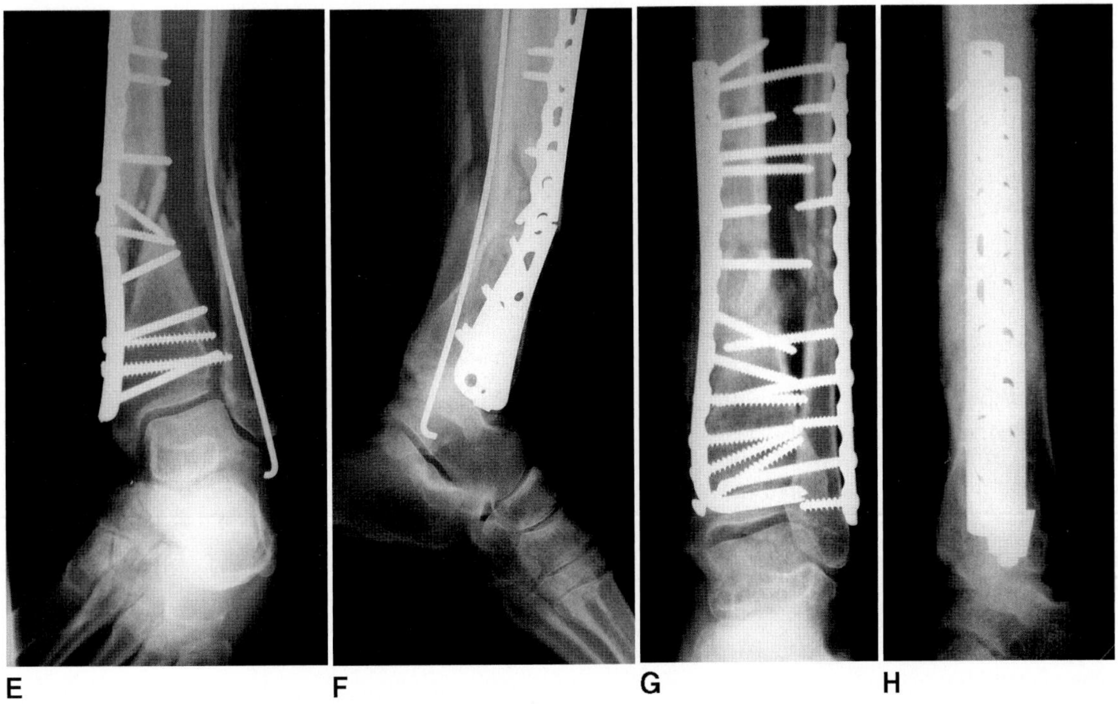

Figure 29–4: Cont'd **The patient went on to develop an infected non-union with failure of her hardware (E and F). After treatment of the infection, debridement, removal of hardware, and temporary external fixation, the patient was treated with revised internal fixation. The surgery was augmented with recombinant human bone morphogenetic protein-7 (osteogenic protein-1), autogenous bone graft from Gerdy's tubercle, and allograft. At 6 weeks, the fracture demonstrates extensive signs of healing (G and H).**

- Randomized controlled trials, or at least more clinical experience, is necessary to determine "how much is enough" and which agents are most effective. For most bone graft substitutes, there is little clinical evidence of efficacy.

References

Aaron RK, Ciombor DM, Simon BJ. (2004) Treatment of nonunions with electric and electromagnetic fields. Clin Orthop 419: 21-29.

Review of the different types of electric and electromagnetic fields and their effectiveness in the treatment of non-unions. Discusses the relevant basic science, in vitro studies, in vivo studies, and clinical research relating to the use of these technologies to enhance bone healing.

Akai M, Hayashi K. (2002) Effect of electrical stimulation as an adjunct to spinal fusion: A meta-analysis of controlled clinical trials. Bioelectromagnetics 23: 132-143.

A metaanalysis of 20 randomized controlled trials examining the role of electrical and electromagnetic stimulation in bone repair. Fifteen of the studied trials supported the effectiveness of electrical stimulation. Five trials (studying Perthes disease, bone grafts and chemotherapy, and fresh fractures) failed to show any significant effect.

Bibbo C, Bono CM, Lin SS. (2005) Union rates using autologous platelet concentrate alone and with bone graft in high-risk foot and ankle surgery patients. J Surg Orthop Adv 14: 17-22.

High-risk patients undergoing a number of different elective foot and ankle procedures were treated with autologous platelet concentrate. A total of 123 procedures were performed on 62 patients. The mean age of the patients was 51, and 39% of the patients were smokers. The union rate was 94% at a mean of 41 days. The results support a role for autologous platelet concentrate in high-risk foot and ankle surgery.

BMP-2 Evaluation in Surgery for Tibial Trauma (BESTT) Study Group. (2002) Recombinant human bone morphogenetic protein-2 for treatment of open tibial fractures: A prospective, controlled, randomized study of four hundred and fifty patients. J Bone Joint Surg Am 84-A: 2123-2134.

One of three randomized, controlled clinical trials demonstrating the effectiveness of BMP in improving bone healing. Patients with open tibia fractures receiving BMP had faster healing, fewer infections, and fewer hardware failures.

Burkus JK, Transfeldt EE, Kitchel SH et al. (2002) Clinical and radiographic outcomes of anterior lumbar interbody fusion using recombinant human bone morphogenetic protein-2. Spine 27: 2396-2408.

One of three randomized, controlled clinical trials demonstrating the effectiveness of BMP in improving bone healing. Randomized, non-blinded trial of BMP in single-level spinal fusion. Patients treated with rhBMP 2 had a higher fusion rate and decreased operative time.

Corradi C, Cozzolino A. (1953) Effect of ultrasonics on the development of osseous callus in fractures. Arch Orthop 66: 77-98.

One of the earliest reports of the effectiveness of ultrasound in stimulating fracture healing.

Day SM, Ostrum RF, Chao EYS et al. (2000) Bone injury, regeneration, and repair. In: Orthopaedic Basic Science, 2nd edn (Buckwalter JA, Einhorn TA, Simon SR, eds). Rosemont: American Academy of Orthopaedic Surgeons. pp. 371-399.

This chapter reviews the basic science behind the repair of injured bone, including brief discussions of growth factors, bone grafts, and physical forces used to enhance bone healing.

Donley BG, Ward DM. (2002) Implantable electrical stimulation in high-risk hindfoot fusions. Foot Ankle Int 23: 13-18.

Thirteen high-risk patients undergoing hindfoot fusions were treated with an implanted electrical stimulator. All patients had at least two major risk factors for non-union. Eleven of 13 patients were smokers. Twelve of 13 patients achieved a successful fusion. The results identify a use for direct electrical stimulation in high-risk foot and ankle surgery.

Einhorn TA. (2003) Clinical applications of recombinant human BMPs: Early experience and future development. J Bone Joint Surg Am 85: 82-88.

Review of the past, present, and future clinical research and applications of the BMPs.

Finkemeier CG. (2002) Bone-grafting and bone-graft substitutes. J Bone Joint Surg Am 84: 454-464.

Review of current methods and materials of bone grafts and bone graft substitutes.

Friedlaender GE, Perry CR, Cole JD et al. (2001) Osteogenic protein-1 (bone morphogenetic protein-7) in the treatment of tibial nonunions. J Bone Joint Surg Am 83-A(suppl 1): S151-S158.

One of three randomized, controlled clinical trials demonstrating the effectiveness of BMP in improving bone healing. One hundred twenty-four tibial non-unions were randomized to receive either autogenous bone grafting or treatment with BMP. Patients in both groups had equivalent radiographic and clinical healing.

Fukada E, Yasuda I. (1957) On the piezoelectric effect of bone. J Phys Soc Japan 12: 1158-1162.

The authors identified the presence of electrical fields in response to mechanical stimuli in bone.

Gossling HR, Bernstein RA, Abbott J. (1992) Treatment of ununited tibial fractures: A comparison of surgery and pulsed electromagnetic fields (PEMF). Orthopedics 15: 711-719.

Extensive review of published PEMF trials. Twenty-eight studies of ununited tibial fractures treated with PEMF were compared with 14 studies of patients treated with bone graft and internal fixation. Five hundred sixty-nine fractures treated with surgery achieved a union rate of 82%; 1718 fractures treated with PEMF achieved a union rate of 81%. Although no formal metaanalysis was performed, the results suggest that PEMF may be as effective as surgical treatment of tibial non-unions.

Hanft JR, Goggin JP, Landsman A et al. (1998) The role of combined magnetic field bone growth stimulation as an adjunct in the treatment of neuroarthropathy/Charcot joint: An expanded pilot study. J Foot Ankle Surg 37: 510-515.

Patient with acute, phase 1 Charcot neuroarthropathy treated with CMF showed a faster time to consolidation.

Lieberman JR, Daluiski A, Einhorn TA. (2002) The role of growth factors in the repair of bone: Biology and clinical applications. J Bone Joint Surg Am 84: 1032-1044.

Review of the basic science, research, and clinical applications of growth factors and cytokines as they relate to bone healing.

Nelson FRT, Brighton CT, Ryaby J et al. (2003) Use of physical forces in bone healing. J Am Acad Orthop Surg 11: 344-354.

Review of physical forces in bone healing, including electrical stimulation, electromagnetic fields, and ultrasound.

Schenk RK. (2003) Biology of fracture repair. In: Skeletal Trauma, 3rd edn (Browner BD, Jupiter JB, Levine AM et al., eds). Philadelphia: Saunders. pp. 29-73.

This chapter reviews the basic biology behind fracture repair and bone grafts.

Scranton PE Jr. (2002) Use of bone graft substitutes in lower extremity reconstructive surgery. Foot Ankle Int 23: 689-692.

Report of 28 patients undergoing lower extremity surgery who were treated with bone graft substitute. Twenty-four of the 28 patients had a successful primary procedure. Four patients required a second procedure.

Urist MR. (1965) Bone: Formation by autoinduction. Science 150: 893-899.

Urist's landmark paper in which he discovered that the extracellular matrix of bone could induce new bone formation when transplanted into extraskeletal sites.

Weinraub GM, Cheung C. (2003) Efficacy of allogenic bone implants in a series of consecutive elective foot procedures. J Foot Ankle Surg 42: 86-89.

Report of 26 patients who underwent 39 consecutive elective foot and ankle procedures utilizing allograft bone. Thirty-eight of 39 procedures were successful, leaving only one non-union.

Index

A
Accessory navicular 157–8
Achilles tendon 1, 2, 195, 200–8
  basic science 200–1
  contracture 38
  gastrocnemius contracture 204
  healing following acute injury 202
  magnetic resonance imaging 201
  overuse disorders 202–4
    Achilles tendinopathy 202
    insertional tendinosis 202–4
  partial gastrocnemius tears 207
  partial tears 204
  rupture 204–7
    chronic 207
    mini-incision repair 207
    non-operative treatment 205
    operative treatment 205–7
    treatment 205
  xanthomas 207–8
Acral metastases 330
Akin procedure 115
Alignment 13–15
Allogeneic bone grafts 380
Amputations 193, 339–51
  indications
    diabetic foot 88
    dysfunctional limb 341
    infection 341
    malignancies 341
    peripheral vascular disease 339–40
    trauma 340–1
  knee disarticulation 347–8
  level of 341–2
  metatarsal disarticulation (Lisfranc) 345–6
  midtarsal disarticulation (Chopart) 346
  physiology of 342–3
  ray resection of foot 344
  surgical technique 343–4
  Syme ankle disarticulation 346–7
  toe amputation or disarticulation 344
  transfemoral 348–9
  transmetatarsal 344–5
  transtibial 347
Aneurysmal bone cyst 325–6
Ankle 1, 3–4
  arthrodesis 185–9
  diabetic ulcers *see* diabetic foot
  examination 10–15
    anterior drawer test 12
    gastrocnemius contracture 11–12
    inspection 10–11
    motion 11
    palpation 11
    sensation 13
    stability 12
    strength 12–13
    vascular examination 10–15, 13
  fractures *see* malleolar fractures in gait 9
Ankle *(continued)*
  ligaments 4
    see also ankle sprains
  loss of motion 1
  overuse injuries 166–8
  rheumatoid arthritis 96–8
  total replacement 189–93
  valgus 52–6
  see also talus
Ankle arthritis 177–94
  biological aspects 177–8
  causes 178
  evaluation 178–9
  non-surgical treatment 179–80
  posttraumatic 177
  surgical treatment 180–93
    allograft 183–5
    amputation 193
    arthrodesis 185–9
    arthroplasty 189–93
    debridement 180
    distraction 181–3
    osteotomy 181
Ankle arthroscopy 352–62
  distraction 353
  examination 355, 356
  indications 352
  inflow and outflow 353
  instruments 352–3
  loose bodies 361–2
  osteochondritis dissecans 355–61
  portal placement 353–5
    accessory anterior portals 354
    accessory posterior portal 355
    posterior portals 354–5
Ankle instability
  orthotics 33
  see also ankle sprains
Ankle sprains 227–39
  acute lateral 227–30
    diagnostic evaluation 228–9
    history and physical examination 228
    treatment 229–30
  acute subtalar 234
  acute syndesmotic injuries 235–6
  anatomy and biomechanics 227
  chronic lateral instability 230–4
    anatomical repair 232
    diagnostic evaluation 230–1
    history and physical examination 230
    ligament reconstruction 233–4
    natural history 231
    postoperative care 234
    treatment 231–2
  chronic subtalar instability 234–5
  chronic syndesmotic pathology 236–7
  deltoid instability 237–8
  recurrent 59
Ankylosing spondylitis 100
Anonychia 370
Anterior drawer test 12
Anterior tarsal tunnel syndrome 173–4
Apes, foot structure 2
Arch 38
  collapse 48
  dynamic stabilizers 39
  height 7
  support 39
Arch pads 18
Arthritis 40
  ankle 177–94
  inflammatory 38
  psoriatic 100
  reactive 100
  rheumatoid *see* rheumatoid arthritis
  sesamoids 127
Arthrodesis 49–52
Arthrofibrosis 260, 262
Arthroplasty 189
Arthroscopy *see* ankle arthroscopy
Autogenous bone grafts 383–4
Autogenous bone marrow grafts 383–4
Autonomic neuropathy 79
Avascular necrosis 294

B
Balance, effects of orthoses 26
Beau lines 373
Bioactive glasses 381
Biomechanics 1–9
Body weight 10
Bone grafts
  allogeneic 380
  autogenous 383–4
Bone healing 376–88
  augmentation of 379–85
    osteoconduction 380–1
    osteogenesis 383–4
    osteoinduction 381–3
    physical forces 383–4
  enhancement of 385–7
  factors affecting 376–9
Bone lesions
  benign
    aneurysmal bone cyst 325–6
    chondroblastoma 329
    enchondroma 327–8
    giant cell reparative granuloma 330
    giant cell tumor 324–5
    intraosseous lipoma 327
    osteoblastoma 329
    osteochondroma 328
    osteoid osteoma 328–9
    subungual exostosis 328
    synovial chondromatosis 323–4
    unicameral bone cyst 326–7
  malignant
    acral metastases 330

Bone lesions *(continued)*
    chondrosarcoma 330
    Ewing sarcoma and peripheral primitive neuroectodermal tumors 330–1
    osteosarcoma 330
Bone morphogenetic protein 382–3
Bunion *see* hallux valgus
Bunionectomy 111
Bunionette deformity 139–42
  anatomy 140
  diagnostic tests 140
  history 140
  non-operative treatment 140
  operative treatment 140–2
  pathophysiology 140
  physical examination 140

C
Calcaneal apoplysitis 166–7
Calcaneal stress fracture 198
Calcaneofibular impingement 40
Calcaneus 5
Calcaneus fractures 267–82
  classification 270–5
  complications 280–1
    malunion 38
  extraarticular 277–8
  history 267
  initial evaluation and management 268–70
  intraarticular 278–80
  late reconstruction 281
  mechanism of injury 267–8
  operative versus non-operative treatment 275–7
  radiographic evaluation 270
  stress 198
Callusing 10–11
Cavovarus deformity 68
Cavus foot
  associated conditions 59
  claw toe deformity 65
  evaluation 59–61
  forefoot-driven 58
  hindfoot-driven 58
  imaging 61–3, 64
  neuromuscular 67–76
  non-neuromuscular 58–66
  pain 198
  pathomechanics 58
  treatment 63–5, 66
    orthotics 31–3, 64
Ceramics 380–1
Cerebral palsy 69
Charcot arthropathy 82–8
  classification 83, 84
  diagnosis 83
  examination 83
  natural history 84
  pathophysiology 83
  reconstruction 86–8
  treatment 83–6
    surgical 86
Charcot-Marie-Tooth disease 73–4
  diagnosis 73
  foot symptoms 73
  treatment 73–4
Cheilectomy 121
Children 147–70
  accessory navicular 157–8
  clubfoot 147–50
Children *(continued)*
    clinical presentation 147
    etiology 147
    non-operative treatment 148
    radiologic imaging 147–8
    surgical treatment 148–50
  congenital vertical talus 156–7
  curly toes and overlapping toes 160–1
  flatfoot 150–2
    etiology 150
    history 150
    physical examination 150–1
    radiographs 151
    treatment 151–2
  fractures 161–6
  metatarsus adductus 158–9
  overuse injuries of foot and ankle 166–8
  polydactyly and syndactyly 159–60
  tarsal coalitions 152–6
    clinical presentation 152–3
    treatment 153–6
Chimpanzee foot 2, 3
Chondroblastoma 329
Chondrosarcoma 330
Clawed hallux 75
Claw toes 65, 129–36
  anatomy 130–1
  definition 130
  diagnostic evaluation 133
  extrinsic muscles 131
  flexion/extension forces at joints 131–2
  history 133
  intrinsic muscles 131
  non-operative treatment 134
  operative treatment 134–6
  pathophysiology 132
  physical examination 133–4
Clear cell sarcoma 335
Clubfoot 147–50
  clinical presentation 147
  etiology 147
  non-operative treatment 148
  radiologic imaging 147–8
  surgical treatment 148–50
Coleman block test 14, 60
Comparative anatomy 2–3
Compartment syndrome 268
  untreated 71–3
    anterior compartment 71
    foot compartments 73
    four compartments 71–2
Complex regional pain syndrome 174–5
Congenital vertical talus 156–7
  history and physical examination 156
  radiographs 156–7
  treatment 157
Contact dermatitis 373–4
Crossover toe 130, 138
Crystalline arthropathy 178
Cuboid fractures 300–3
  evaluation 300–1
  malunion 38
  rehabilitation 301–3
  treatment 301–3
Cuneiform fractures 303–4
Curly toe 130
  children 160–1
Custom orthoses 19–22
  casting and models for 22–5

D
Dancer's fractures 316
Debridement 180
Demineralized bone matrix 383
Diabetic foot 77–89
  amputations 88
  Charcot arthropathy 82–8
    classification 83, 84
    diagnosis 83
    examination 83
    natural history 84
    pathophysiology 83
    reconstruction 86–8
    surgical treatment 86
    treatment 83–6
  diabetic neuropathy 78–9
    autonomic 79
    causes 78
    etiology 78
    motor 79
    neuropathic pain 79
    sensory 78–9
  diabetic vascular disease 77–8
    diagnostic tests 78
    evaluation 77–8
  foot and ankle ulcers 80–2
    classification 80–1
    infection 82
    pathophysiology 80
    risk factors 80
    treatment 81–2
  foot care and ulcer prevention 80
  forefoot deformity 88
  gastrocnemius contracture 79–80
  healing 79
  prescription footwear 80
Distal tibiofibular syndesmosis 4
Distraction arthroplasty 181–3
Double-limb heel rise test 14
Dynamic arch stabilizers 39

E
Eczema 373–4
Electromagnetic fields 384–5
Enchondroma 327–8
Enthesopathy 198
Ewing sarcoma 330–1
Extensor retinacula 218–19

F
Fat pad atrophy 198
Fibroblast growth factors 381
Fibromatosis 333
Fifth metatarsal apophysitis 167
First metatarsophalangeal joint
  arthrodesis 115
  disorders of 119–28
first ray
  hypermobility 105–6
  instability 7, 15
  mobility 12
    measurement of 106–7
Flatfoot 38–57
  arches of foot 38–9
  causes 38
  children 150–2
    etiology 150
    history 150
    physical examination 150–1

Flatfoot *(continued)*
radiographs 151
treatment 151–2
etiology 40, 42–3
imaging studies 44–6
pain from 40
physical examination 43–4
posterior tibial tendon dysfunction 41–2
tarsal coalition 43
three-dimensional deformity 39–40
treatment 46–56
advanced flatfoot 52
ankle valgus 52–6
arch collapse 48
combined medial and lateral procedures 52
compensatory forefoot supination 52
lateral column lengthening/arthrodesis 49–52
medial column stabilization 49
medial sliding calcaneal tuberosity osteotomy 48–9
non-operative 47
orthotics 33–6
selective fusions 52
stage 1 posterior tibial tendon dysfunction 47–8
surgical principles 47
Flexor hallucis longus 220–2
anatomy 220–1
clinical findings 221
epidemiology 221
function 220
treatment options 221–2
Flexor tendon lacerations 223–4
Foot
alignment 25
anatomy 3–7
bones of 1
cavovarus deformity 68
cavus *see* cavus foot
diabetic *see* diabetic foot
evolution of 2–3
examination 10–15
alignment 13–15
first ray mobility 12
gastrocnemius contracture 11–12
inspection 10–11
motion 11
palpation 11
sensation 13
stability 12
strength 12–13
vascular 13
in gait 9
joints of 4
neuromuscular deformity 67–76
overuse injuries 166–8
structural diversity 8–9
tripod model 7–8
Footwear
custom-made 110
and forefoot deformity 105
modifications 110
orthopedic 92
Forefoot 6
deformity in diabetic foot 88
disorders
orthotics 29–31
central metatarsalgia 30–1
first metatarsophalangeal pathologies 29–30
Forefoot *(continued)*
fractures *see* metatarsal/phalangeal fractures
rheumatoid arthritis 92
structure 310–11
Forefoot-driven hindfoot varus 8
Forefoot pads 17
Fractures
calcaneus 267–82
children 161–6
cuboid 300–3
cuneiform 303–4
malleolar 240–51
metatarsal/phalangeal 310–20
navicular 297–300
sesamoid 126–7
stress 167–8
calcaneal 198
calcaneus 198
malleolar 249–50
navicular 300
talus 283–96
tibial pilon 252–66
Freiberg infraction 142

G
Gait 9
Ganglion 333
Gastrocnemius
contracture 11–12, 38, 204
in diabetes 79–80
lengthening 115
partial tears 207
Giant cell reparative granuloma 330
Giant cell tumor 324–5
of tendon sheath 331–2
Gorilla foot 3
Gout 101
Great toe *see* hallux
Growth hormones 381
Gun barrel sign 133

H
Haglund deformity 195, 203
Hallux, in rheumatoid arthritis 93
Hallux elevatus primus 119–20
Hallux rigidus 119–24
etiology 119–20
history 120
physical examination 120
radiographs 120
treatment 120–4
Hallux valgus 104–18
adolescent 117
etiology 104–7
association with deformities and disease 105
gender 105
genetic 104
hypermobility of first ray 105–7
history 108
natural history 104
non-operative treatment 110
pain in 107–8
metatarsophalangeal joint 107
sesamoid-derived 108
transfer metatarsalgia and lesser toe pain 107–8
pathogenesis 107
physical examination 108–9
radiographic evaluation 109–10
Hallux valgus *(continued)*
surgery 110–15
Akin procedure 115
bunionectomy 111
complications 115
distal osteototomies 111–12
distal soft tissue realignment 111
first metatarsophalangeal joint arthrodesis 115
gastrocnemius lengthening 115
metatarsocuneiform arthrodesis 112–15
proximal osteotomies 112
resection arthroplasty 115
Hallux varus 116–17
diagnosis and treatment 116–17
pathogenesis 116
Hammertoes 129–36
anatomy 130–1
definition 130
diagnostic evaluation 133
extrinsic muscles 131
flexion/extension forces at joints 131–2
history 133
intrinsic muscles 131
non-operative treatment 134
operative treatment 134–6
pathophysiology 132
physical examination 133–4
Heel
peek-a-boo 13, 59
valgus 14
varus 14
see also calcaneal/calcaneus
Heel pads 17, 18
Heel pain 195–9
calcaneal stress fracture 198
cavus foot pain 198
in children 166
enthesopathy 198
fat pad atrophy 198
normal anatomy 195–6
orthoses 26, 31
plantar fasciitis 196–7
plantar nerve impingement 197
Heel rise test 14
Heel spur 196
Hemangioma 332–3
Hemochromatosis 178
Herpetic whitlow 370
Hindfoot
joints 1, 5–6
ligaments 6
loss of motion 1
rheumatoid arthritis 95–6
Hostler's toe 367

I
Imaging
Achilles tendon 201
calcaneus fractures 270
cavus foot 61–3, 64
clubfoot 147–8
congenital vertical talus 156–7
flatfoot 44–6
hallux rigidus 120
hallux valgus 109–10
metatarsal/phalangeal fractures 311
osteochondritis dissecans 357
Incisional/traumatic neuromas 174
Ingrown toenail 365

Insertional tendinosis 202–3
Insoles 19
Insulin-like growth factors 381
Interdigital corns 144–5
  diagnostic tests 145
  history 144
  non-operative treatment 145
  operative treatment 145
  physical examination 145
Interdigital (Morton) neuroma 171–2
Intraosseous lipoma 327
Iselin disease 167

J

Jones fractures 314, 316

K

Kaposi sarcoma 335
Keller procedure 115
Knee disarticulation 347–8
Koilonychia 373

L

Lapidus procedure 112–15
Lateral column lengthening 49–52
Lateral foot overload 59
Leg alignment, orthoses 25
Leukonychia 373
Ligaments
  ankle 4
    see also ankle sprains
  hindfoot 6
  Lisfranc 6
  syndesmotic 243–4, 247–8
    sprains 235–6
Lipoma 333
Lisfranc injuries 304–9
  evaluation 304–5
  rehabilitation 307, 309
  treatment 305–8
Lisfranc ligament 6
Longitudinal arch 3
Loose bodies 361–2

M

Malleolar fractures 240–51
  classification of injury 241
  complications 248–9
  general treatment 241
  mortise anatomy 240–1
  osteoporosis 249
  outcome 250
  posterior malleolus 247
  postoperative care 248
  pronation-abduction 245–7
  pronation-external rotation/Weber C 243–5
  soft tissue technique 248
  stress fractures 249–50
  supination-external rotation 242–3
  syndesmotic injuries 247–8
  Weber A/supination-adduction 242
Mallet toes 129–36
  anatomy 130–1
  definition 130
  diagnostic evaluation 133
  extrinsic muscles 131
  flexion/extension forces at joints 131–2
  history 133
  intrinsic muscles 131
Mallet toes *(continued)*
  non-operative treatment 134
  operative treatment 134–6
  pathophysiology 132
  physical examination 133–4
Mal perforans *see* diabetic foot, foot and ankle ulcers
Medial column stabilization 49
Medial sliding calcaneal tuberosity osteotomy 48–9
Mees lines 373
Melanoma 335, 336
  subungual 371–2
Metatarsal disarticulation (Lisfranc) 345–6
Metatarsalgia 59
Metatarsal/phalangeal fractures 310–20
  classification 311
  evaluation 311
  imaging 311
  lawn mower injuries 319
  metatarsals 311–17
    classification 311
    dancer's fractures 316
    fifth metatarsal 314
    first metatarsal 311–13
    Jones fracture 314–16
    mechanism 311
    multiple fractures 313
    second, third and fourth metatarsals 313
    stress fractures 316–17
    tuberosity avulsion fracture 314
  open fractures 319
  phalanges 317–19
    distal phalanx and nail bed 319
    first proximal phalanx 317
    lesser phalangeal fractures 317, 319
Metatarsocuneiform arthrodesis 112–15
Metatarsophalangeal joint
  dislocation 138
  pain 107
  see also individual joints
Metatarsophalangeals
  motion 1
  rheumatoid arthritis 93–5
Metatarsus adductus 158–9
Midfoot 1
  anatomy and function 297
  injuries 297–309
    cuboid fractures 300–3
    cuneiform fractures 303–4
    Lisfranc injuries 304–9
    navicular fractures 297–300
    navicular stress fractures 300
  joints 6
  rheumatoid arthritis 95
Midtarsal disarticulation (Chopart) 346
Motion 11
Motor neuropathy 79
Muehreke lines 373
Muscle imbalance 67

N

Nail bed disorders 319
  subungual exostosis 368–9
  subungual hematoma 368
Nail fold disorders
  herpetic whitlow 370
  paronychia 369
  periungual and subungual verruca 370
  pyogenic granuloma 370
Nail matrix disorders
  anonychia 370
  pterygium unguis 370–1
Nail plate disorders
  onychauxis (club nail) 367
  onychocryptosis (ingrown toenail) 365
  onychogryphosis (Hostler's toe; ram horn nail) 367
  onycholysis 367
  onychomadesis 367
  onychomycosis 365–7
Navicular
  accessory 157–8
  fractures 297–300
    evaluation 298
    rehabilitation 298
    stress 300
    treatment 298–300
Nerve disorders 171–6
  anterior tarsal tunnel syndrome 173–4
  complex regional pain syndrome 174–5
  incisional/traumatic neuromas 174
  interdigital (Morton) neuroma 171–2
  reflex sympathetic dystrophy 174–5
  tarsal tunnel syndrome 173
Nerve sheath and peripheral nerve tumours 333
Neuromuscular foot deformity 67–76
  causes 67–8
  Charcot-Marie-Tooth disease 73–4
  clawed hallux 75
  evaluation 69–70
  peroneal nerve palsy 70–1
  poliomyelitis 74–5
  symptoms 68–9
  treatment 70
    surgery 70, 75–6
  untreated compartment syndrome 71–3
Neuropathic arthropathy 178
Neuropathic pain 79

O

Onychauxis (club nail) 367
Onychocryptosis (ingrown toenail) 365
Onychogryphosis (Hostler's toe; ram horn nail) 367
Onycholysis 367
Onychomadesis 367
Onychomycosis 365–7
Onychoschizia 373
Orthopedic footwear 92
Orthotics 16–37
  cavus foot 31–3
  custom 19–22
    casting and models for 22–5
  flatfoot 33–6
  forefoot conditions 29–31
    central metatarsalgia 30–1
    first metatarsophalangeal pathologies 29–30
  hallux valgus 110
  heel pain syndrome 31
  indications 28–9
  lateral ankle instability 33
  materials
    rigid orthoses 28
    selection 27
    semirigid orthoses 28
    soft orthoses 27–8
  prefabricated 17–19
  treatment effects 25–6
    balance and postural control 26
    foot and leg alignment 25

Orthotics *(continued)*
heel pain syndrome 26
joint moments 26
patellofemoral pain syndrome 26
patient satisfaction 25
plantar pressures 25
types of 16–17
Os peroneum 212
pain 213
Osteoblastoma 329
Osteochondral allografting 183–4
Osteochondritis dissecans 295
arthroscopy 355–61
demographics 356
etiology 356
history and physical examination 356–7
imaging 357
non-operative treatment 357–8
surgical treatment 358–60
acute osteochondral lesions 359
arthroscopic approaches 360–1
chronic osteochondral lesions 359–60
postoperative care 361
Osteochondroma 328
Osteoid osteoma 328–9
Osteoporosis, post-fracture 249
Osteosarcoma 330
Osteotomy 181
Os trigonum 5, 222–3
anatomy 222
clinical conditions 222
diagnosis 222–3
epidemiology 222
treatment 223
Overlapping toes 160–1

P

Pain
cavus foot 198
flatfoot 40
hallux valgus 107–8
heel 195–9
metatarsophalangeal joint 107
neuropathic 79
os peroneum 213
Painful os peroneum syndrome 213
Palpation 11
Paratenonitis 209
Parathyroid hormone 381–2
Parathyroid hormone-related polypeptide 381–2
Paronychia 369
Patellofemoral pain syndrome 26
Peek-a-boo heel 13, 59
Peripheral primitive neuroectodermal tumors 330–1
Periungual and subungual verruca 370
Peroneal muscle spasm 38, 43
Peroneal nerve palsy 70–1
symptoms 71
treatment 71
Peroneal tendons 210–18, 270
anatomy 210–11
function 210
lacerations 224–5
longitudinal tears and rupture 213–15
painful os peroneum syndrome 213
paratenonitis 212–13
physical findings 211–13
subluxation and dislocation 215–18
tendonosis 212–13
Peroneus longus. and cavus foot 61
Pes planovalgus 99
Phalangeal fractures *see* metatarsal/phalangeal fractures
Pigmented villonodular synovitis 331–2
Plantar fascia 6
Plantar fasciitis 196–7
Plantar fat pad 6–7
Plantar keratosis, intractable 127, 142–4
diagnostic tests 143
history and physical examination 143
non-operative treatment 144
operative treatment 144
Plantar nerve impingement 197
Plantar pressures 25
Platelet-derived growth factor 381
Poliomyelitis 74–5
Polydactyly 159–60
Posterior tibial tendon
disease progression 41–2
dysfunction 38, 41
in gait cycle 39
treatment 47–8
Prefabricated orthoses 17–19
Prostaglandins 382
Psoriasis 373
Psoriatic arthritis 100
Pterygium unguis 370–1
Pump bump 195
Push-up test 134
Pyogenic granuloma 370

R

Ram horn nail 367
Ray resection of foot 344
Reactive arthritis 100
Reflex sympathetic dystrophy 174–5
Reiter syndrome 100
Retrocalcaneal bursitis 203
Rheumatoid arthritis 90–8
ankle 96–8
clinical evaluation 91
diagnosis 90–1
epidemiology 90
extraosseous manifestations 99
forefoot 92
hallux 93
hindfoot 95–6
lesser metatarsophalangeals/toes 93–5
midfoot 95
pathophysiology 90
treatment 91–2
Rheumatoid nodules 99
Rigid orthoses 28

S

Second metatarsophalangeal joint instability 136–9
additional procedures 139
anatomy and pathophysiology 136
diagnostic evaluation 136–7
history 137
non-operative treatment 137–8
physical examination 137
surgical treatment 138–9
Semirigid orthoses 28
Sensation 13
Sensory neuropathy 78–9
Seronegative inflammatory arthropathies 99–101
ankylosing spondylitis 100
Seronegative inflammatory arthropathies *(continued)*
gout 101
psoriatic arthritis 100
Reiter syndrome and reactive arthritis 100
Sesamoiditis 127
Sesamoids
complications of surgery 127
disorders of 126–7
arthritis 127
fracture 126–7
intractable plantar keratosis 127
sesamoiditis 127
pain 108
Sever disease 166–7
Silfverskiold test 137
Soft orthoses 30–1
Soft tissue lesions
benign
fibromatosis 333
ganglion 333
hemangioma 332–3
lipoma 333
nerve sheath and peripheral nerve tumours 333
pigmented villonodular synovitis/giant cell tumor of tendon sheath 331–2
malignant 333–6
clear cell sarcoma 335
Kaposi sarcoma 335
melanoma 335, 336
synovial sarcoma 334–5
Stability 12
Stieda's process 222–3
anatomy 222
clinical conditions 222
diagnosis 222–3
epidemiology 222
treatment 223
Strength 12–13
Stress fractures 167–8
calcaneus 198
malleolar 249–50
metatarsal 316–17
navicular 300
Subungual exostosis 328, 368–9
Subungual hematoma 368
Surgery
amputations 193, 339–51
ankle arthritis 180–93
Charcot arthropathy 86
clubfoot 148–50
flatfoot 47
hallux valgus 110–15
neuromuscular cavus foor 70, 75–6
neuromuscular foot deformity 70, 75–6
osteochondritis dissecans 358–60
second metatarsophalangeal joint instability 138–9
see also individual procedures
Syme ankle disarticulation 346–7
Syndactyly 159–60
Syndesmotic ligaments
injury 243–4, 247–8
sprains 235–6
Synovial chondromatosis 323–4
Synovial sarcoma 334–5
Synthetic polymers 383

T

Talocalcaneal impingement 40
Talonavicular coverage angle 45

Talus 4–5
congenital vertical 156–7
extraosseous arterial supply 284–5
skeletal anatomy 283–4
vascular anatomy 284
Talus fractures 283–96
complications
avascular necrosis 294
non-union and malunion 294–5
osteochondritis dissecans 295
lateral process 292
posteromedial talar body 287–8
talar body 285–7
talar neck 288–91
outcome 291–2
treatment 292–3
Tarsal coalitions 43
in children 152–6
Tarsal tunnel syndrome 173
Tendinitis 209
Tendinosis 209
Tendon disease 209–26
flexor hallucis longus 220–2
fluoroquinolones in 210
lacerations 223–5
flexors 223–4
peroneal tendons 224–5
tibialis anterior and toe extensors 224
os trigonum and Steida's process 222–3
peroneal tendons 210–18
rehabilitation 210
tibialis anterior 218–20
see also Achilles tendon
Tenosynovium 200
Tenovagium 200
Thompson test 205, 206
Tibialis anterior 218–20
anatomy 218
extensor retinacula 218–19
function 218
injury and diagnosis 219
lacerations 224
rupture 219–20
treatment 220
Tibial pilon fractures 252–66
classification 254
complications 260–3
arthrofibrosis 260, 262
osseous 262–3
wound problems and infection 260
context and mechanism 253–4
evaluation 255
external fixation 256–7
with limited internal fixation 256–7
non-spanning with/without limited internal fixation 257
fracture anatomy 252
historical discussion 255
non-operative treatment 255–6
normal anatomy 252
Tibial pilon fractures *(continued)*
open fractures 260
soft tissue anatomy 252–3
stage open reduction and internal fixation 257–60
fibula 258–9
postoperative 260
tibia 259–60
terminology 252
Toe extensors, lacerations 224
Toenails 363–75
anatomy 363, 364
clubbing 373
color 373
dermatologic disorders
cutaneous bacterial infections 374
eczema and contact dermatitis 373–4
psoriasis 373
disorders from systemic disease 372–3
genetic disorders 371
nail bed disorders
subungual exostosis 368–9
subungual hematoma 368
nail fold disorders
herpetic whitlow 370
paronychia 369
periungual and subungual verruca 370
pyogenic granuloma 370
nail matrix disorders
anonychia 370
pterygium unguis 370–1
nail plate disorders
onychauxis (club nail) 367
onychocryptosis (ingrown toenail) 365
onychogryphosis (Hostler's toe; ram horn nail) 367
onycholysis 367
onychomadesis 367
onychomycosis 365–7
physiology 363–4
pitting 373
tumors 371–2
squamous cell carcinoma 372
subungual malignant melanoma 371–2
Toes 1
amputation or disarticulation 344
great toe *see* hallux
lesser
disorders of 129–46
pain 107–8
rheumatoid arthritis 93–5
Too many toes sign 42, 43, 47, 59
Transfemoral amputation 348–9
Transfer metatarsalgia 106, 107–8
Transforming growth factor-β 381
Transmetatarsal amputation 344–5
Transtibial amputation 347
Tripod model 7–8
Tuberosity avulsion fracture 314
Tumors 321–38
benign bone lesions
Tumors *(continued)*
aneurysmal bone cyst 325–6
chondroblastoma 329
enchondroma 327–8
giant cell reparative granuloma 330
giant cell tumor 324–5
intraosseous lipoma 327
osteoblastoma 329
osteochondroma 328
osteoid osteoma 328–9
subungual exostosis 328
synovial chondromatosis 323–4
unicameral bone cyst 326–7
benign soft tissue lesions
fibromatosis 333
ganglion 333
hemangioma 332–3
lipoma 333
nerve sheath and peripheral nerve tumours 333
pigmented villonodular synovitis/giant cell tumor of tendon sheath 331–2
biopsy and surgical excision 322
clinical evaluation 321–2
malignant bone lesions
acral metastases 330
chondrosarcoma 330
Ewing sarcoma and peripheral primitive neuroectodermal tumors 330–1
osteosarcoma 330
malignant soft tissue lesions 333–6
clear cell sarcoma 335
Kaposi sarcoma 335
melanoma 335, 336
synovial sarcoma 334–5
nerve sheath 333
peripheral nerve 333
staging 322–3
toenails 371–2
squamous cell carcinoma 372
subungual malignant melanoma 371–2
Turf toe 124–6
etiology 125
grading 125–6
history and physical examination 125
treatment 126

U

Ultrasound 485
Unicameral bone cyst 326–7

V

Valgus
ankle 52–6
heel 14
Varus, heel 14
Vascular examination 13
Vasculitis 99

X

Xanthoma of Achilles tendon 207–8